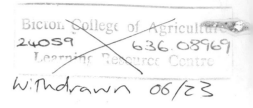

Veterinary Microbiology and Microbial Disease

P.J. Quinn   MVB, PhD, MRCVS
Professor of Veterinary Microbiology and Parasitology
Faculty of Veterinary Medicine
University College Dublin

B.K. Markey   MVB, PhD, MRCVS, Dip Stat
Senior Lecturer in Veterinary Microbiology
Department of Veterinary Microbiology and Parasitology

M.E. Carter   BVSc, MRCVS, Dip Bact, NDD
Former Senior Lecturer in Veterinary Microbiology
Department of Veterinary Microbiology and Parasitology

W.J.C. Donnelly   BVMS, MS, DVM, MRCVS, MIBiol
Former Senior Lecturer in Veterinary Pathology
Department of Veterinary Pathology

F.C. Leonard   MVB, PhD, MRCVS
Lecturer in Veterinary Microbiology
Department of Veterinary Microbiology and Parasitology

Computer graphics by
D. Maghire   AIMLS
Department of Veterinary Microbiology and Parasitology

Blackwell
Science

© 2002 by Blackwell Science Ltd,
a Blackwell Publishing Company
Editorial Offices:
Osney Mead, Oxford OX2 0EL, UK
  Tel: +44 (0)1865 206206
Blackwell Science, Inc., 350 Main Street,
Malden, MA 02148-5018, USA
  Tel: +1 781 388 8250
Iowa State Press, a Blackwell Publishing Company,
2121 State Avenue, Iowa 50014-8300, USA
  Tel: +1 515 292 0140
Blackwell Science Asia Pty, 54 University Street,
Carlton, Victoria, 3053, Australia
  Tel: +61 (0)3 9347 0300
Blackwell Wissenschafts Verlag, Kurfürstendamm 57,
10707 Berlin, Germany
  Tel: +49 (0)30 32 79 060

First published 2002 by Blackwell Science Ltd

Library of Congress
Cataloging-in-Publication Data is available

ISBN 0-632-05525-1

A catalogue record for this title is available from the
British Library

Printed and bound in Great Britain by
MPG Books Ltd, Bodmin, Cornwall

For further information on
Blackwell Publishing, visit our website:
www.blackwellpublishing.com

Contents

Section V
Viruses and Prions

Section VI
Microbial Agents and Disease Production

This book is dedicated to
the memory of
Margery E. Carter

Preface

Microbiology has undergone enormous change since the pioneering investigations of Pasteur and Koch elucidated the nature of infectious disease more than 120 years ago. This subject, which now occupies a central position in the veterinary curriculum, has developed into one of vast complexity ranging from cultural and biochemical characterization of pathogenic microorganisms to advanced molecular techniques used for identifying genes associated with virulence factors.

This book is intended primarily for undergraduate veterinary students. We hope that it will also be of value to veterinary colleagues engaged in teaching and diagnostic work and to those in allied professions who require information on microbial pathogens of animals. The contents reflect the many changes which may occurred in our understanding of infectious diseases in recent years.

The book is divided into sections dealing with bacteriology, mycology and virology. A final section, which is mainly concerned with the relationship between microbial agents and disease production, contains chapters on the principles of disinfection and immunity. The chapters relating to specific infectious agents are designed to facilitate easy access to information with emphasis on host-pathogen interactions and their clinical effects; appropriate chemotherapeutic and control measures are included. Major microbial pathogens of international or public health importance have been reviewed in detail. Tables, boxes and flow diagrams have been used extensively to summarize information relating to diseases and explain pathogenic mechanisms. Where relevant, a list of key points is included to emphasize those aspects of the topic central to the information presented in each chapter. Current international classification systems are used throughout. In addition to current references, recent review articles or textbooks are listed.

The authors would be pleased to receive notification of any errors or inaccuracies.

Margery E. Carter died in Hamilton, New Zealand on July 18, 2001 as this book was being completed. We acknowledge Margery's enormous contribution to the book and we mourn her passing.

Acknowledgements

We wish to acknowledge the constructive comments of the following colleagues who offered scientific, technical and editorial advise on individual chapters: Dr C. Budke, Dr M. Doherty, Ms K. Dunne, Dr J. Cassidy, Miss M. Gleeson, Mr S. Hogan, Dr H. Larkin, Ms H. McAllister, Mr M. Scanlon, Mr M. Nugent, Dr G. McCarthy, Dr T. Sweeney, Dr R. Vaughan and Ms R. Warner, Faculty of Veterinary Medicine, University College Dublin; Dr P. J. Hartigan, Trinity College Dublin; Professor O. Jarrett and Dr D. Addie, Faculty of Veterinary Medicine, University of Glasgow; Mr E. Weavers and Dr M. McElroy, Veterinary Research Laboratory, Abbotstown; Mr B. Meaney and Mr E. O'Callaghan, Research and Development Division, Teagasc, Moorepark, Co. Cork; Dr M. E. Di Menna, Hamilton, New Zealand; John, Michael, David and Joan Quinn.

We are deeply indebted to Mrs Lesley Doggett who cheerfully typed the entire text in a highly competent and efficient manner. We acknowledge with gratitude the many hours she devoted to revision and correction of the text.

Ms Antonia Seymour, and Mrs Sue Moore and their colleagues at Blackwell provided advice and encouragement throughout their constructive observations on both layout and presentation of text, tables and diagrams.

Dublin, August 2001

Author biographies

P.J. Quinn, MVB, PhD, MRCVS is Professor of Veterinary Microbiology and Parasitology and Head of the Department in the Faculty of Veterinary Medicine, University College, Dublin. After graduating from University College Dublin, in 1965, he spent some time in veterinary practice before enrolling as a postgraduate student in Ontario Veterinary College, University of Guelph, Canada. In 1970, he was awarded a PhD for research in veterinary immunology and he remained on the staff of Ontario Veterinary College until his return to the Faculty of Veterinary Medicine, University College Dublin in 1973.

His research interests have included allergic skin reactions in the horse to biting insects, the epidemiology of toxoplasmosis in sheep, immune mechanisms in the respiratory tract of calves, leptospirosis in dairy cattle, immuno-modulation, mechanisms of immunity in the respiratory tract of SPF and conventional cats, botulism in gulls around the Irish coastline, factors influencing the tuberculin test in cattle, airborne dispersal of bacteria during slurry spreading and evaluation of the efficacy of chemical disinfectants against *Brucella abortus* and *Mycobacterium bovis*.

In addition to many refereed publications in journals and chapters in books, he edited *Cell-mediated Immunity* (1984) and is senior co-author of *Animal Diseases Exotic to Ireland* (1992), *Clinical Veterinary Microbiology* (1994) and *Microbial and Parasitic Diseases of the Dog and Cat* (1997).

Bryan K. Markey, MVB, PhD, MRCVS, Dip. Stat, graduated from the Faculty of Veterinary Medicine, University College Dublin in 1985. Following a short period in general practice he was appointed house surgeon in the Faculty of Veterinary Medicine, University College Dublin. In 1986, he joined the academic staff as an assistant lecturer in the Department of Veterinary Microbiology and Parasitology. He spent one year on study leave at the Veterinary Sciences Division, Belfast and enrolled for a PhD degree at Queen's University. He was awarded a PhD from Queen's University, Belfast in 1991 and is currently a senior lecturer in veterinary microbiology.

His research interests include chlamydial infection of domestic animals, *Mycoplasma bovis* infection of cattle and the transmissible spongiform encephalopathies. He has contributed chapters to books on veterinary disinfection and is co-author of *Animal Diseases Exotic to Ireland* (1992), *Clinical Veterinary Microbiology* (1994) and *Microbial and Parasitic Diseases of the Dog and Cat* (1997).

Margery E. Carter, BVSc, MRCVS, Dip Bact, NDD, graduated from Sydney University, Australia in 1960. After graduation, she was in general practice in New Zealand for five years before engaging in postgraduate studies in Manchester University where she was awarded a Diploma in Bacteriology. She returned to work as a microbiologist at a veterinary investigation laboratory in Hamilton, New Zealand.

From 1980 until 1983 she was Associate Professor of Microbiology in Virginia-Maryland, College of Veterinary Medicine, Blacksburg, Virginia, U.S.A. She was appointed senior lecturer in microbiology, Faculty of Veterinary Medicine, University of Zimbabwe, Harare in 1984 and remained there until 1986. She held the position of Professor of Microbiology, Ross University, School of Veterinary Medicine, St. Kitts, West Indies from 1986 to 1987. She was appointed senior lecturer in the Department of Veterinary Microbiology and Parasitology, Faculty of Veterinary Medicine, University College Dublin in 1988, a position she held until 1997 when she relinquished her post. She remained in the Department of Veterinary Microbiology and Parasitology where she continued her scientific writing until her departure in 1999 for Hamilton, New Zealand.

Her publications include papers on mycoplasma mastitis, infectious bronchitis, mycotic pneumonia and placentitis in cattle, salmonellosis in foals, Newcastle disease, and leptospirosis. She has contributed chapters to a number of textbooks on veterinary microbiology. She is co-author of *Animal Diseases Exotic to Ireland* (1992), *Clinical Veterinary Microbiology* (1994) and *Microbial and Parasitic Diseases of the Dog and Cat* (1997).

William J.C. Donnelly, BVMS, MS, DVM, MRCVS, MIBiol, graduated from the University of Glasgow Veterinary School in 1954 and spent a number of years in general practice before joining the Irish Department of Agriculture in 1961 as a Veterinary Inspector. He was appointed Research Officer in the Department's Veterinary Research Laboratory in 1963.

He was the recipient of a Kellogg Foundation Fellowship in 1964 and enrolled as a postgraduate student in Michigan State University where he was awarded an MS degree in 1965. For published work on bovine GM1 gangliosidosis, he was awarded a DVM degree by the University of Glasgow in 1978. He retired as head of pathology at the Veterinary Research Laboratory in 1988 and joined the staff of the Department of Veterinary Pathology, University College Dublin as senior lecturer, a post he held until he retired in 1997.

His published work includes papers on salmonellosis in pigs, bovine mucormycosis, border disease and ruminant neuro-pathology. He was a contributor to *Animal Diseases Exotic to Ireland* (1992) and is co-author of *Microbial and Parasitic Diseases of the Dog and Cat* (1997). He is co-editor of *A Veterinary School to Flourish: The Veterinary College of Ireland 1900-2000* (2001).

Finola C. Leonard, MVB, PhD, MRCVS graduated from the Faculty of Veterinary Medicine, University College Dublin in 1983. She was house surgeon in the Department of Large Animal Medicine, Royal (Dick) School of Veterinary Studies, Edinburgh for one year and engaged in veterinary practice for three years. She commenced postgraduate studies in the Faculty of Veterinary Medicine, University College Dublin on leptospirosis in dairy cattle, while based at Teagasc, Moorepark, Co. Cork, and was awarded a PhD for research on this topic in 1991. She remained in Moorepark as a post-doctoral research worker until 1997. Her research was concerned with foot lameness in dairy cattle and the influence of housing on the behaviour and welfare of cattle and pigs.

She was appointed college lecturer in the Department of Veterinary Microbiology and Parasitology in the Faculty of Veterinary Medicine, University College Dublin in 1997. Her current research and publications relate mainly to food-borne pathogens especially *Salmonella* infections in pigs.

Section I

Introductory Bacteriology

Chapter 1

Microbial pathogens and infectious disease

Although the concept of infectious diseases is to be found in the works of classical Greek and Roman writers, their microbial aetiology was not clearly established until the mid-nineteenth century when it was confirmed by the scientific contributions of Louis Pasteur and Robert Koch. During the intervening centuries a number of investigators hypothesized about the nature of contagion and disease. Girolamo Fracastoro was one of the first to suggest, in his treatise *De contagione* published in 1546, that animate agents were responsible for disease. One hundred years later, Anthony van Leeuwenhoek demonstrated, in a sample of pus from his gums, microscopic 'animalcules', which were later identified as infectious agents.

For many centuries there had been philosophical and scientific discussion about the 'spontaneous generation' of small living entities. One of the most persuasive naked-eye observations which supported spontaneous generation, namely the occurrence of maggots on putrefying meat, had been put to rest by the experiments of Francesco Redi (1626-1697) an Italian physician and naturalist. He demonstrated that maggots developed in meat only when flies laid their eggs on it. However, van Leeuwenhoek's confirmation of the existence of microscopic 'animalcules' meant that the question of spontaneous generation remained unresolved. The concept was apparently supported by experiments conducted in the mid-eighteenth century by John Needham, an English naturalist. After boiling broth in containers which were then sealed, Needham detected microorganisms in the broth when the containers were opened after a few days. Subsequently, Needham's experimental technique was shown to be faulty. Boiling for a short time failed to eliminate all the microorganisms from the broth and the containers; an extended period of boiling was essential. When the broth was boiled for periods approaching three quarters of an hour and the flasks sealed immediately after boiling, microorganisms were not demonstrable even after prolonged storage. Despite these exacting experiments which were carried out by Lazzaro Spallanzani, protagonists of spontaneous generation continued to promote the concept up to the mid-1800s when Louis Pasteur became involved in biological investigations.

Pasteur's interest in spontaneous generation was prompted by experiments which he had conducted on spoilage during the fermentation of beet alcohol. He showed that a contaminating yeast, which produced lactic acid during fermentation and which differed morphologically from brewers' yeast, was responsible for the spoilage. He deduced that both alcoholic and lactic fermentation resulted from the metabolism and replication of the living yeast cells. The solution to the spoilage problem during fermentation of wine and beer products, lay in heating the raw materials to about 120°F, in order to kill contaminating microorganisms, prior to the addition of the appropriate yeast cells. This process, now known as pasteurization, is widely used to reduce microbial contamination in order to prolong the shelf-life of milk and some other foods.

Pasteur effectively ended the controversy about spontaneous generation through definitive confirmation of Spallanzani's experiments. Furthermore, he demonstrated that contamination of nutrient broth when exposed to air resulted from microorganisms in dust particles settling on the fluid.

An important technical advance, which stemmed from Pasteur's fermentation studies, was the development of a fluid medium suitable for culturing yeast cells. He then developed other liquid media containing specific ingredients which favoured the growth of particular pathogenic bacteria. It was this development which eventually allowed him to formulate the germ theory of disease. The germ theory formed the basis for Pasteur's experiments on vaccination against fowl cholera, anthrax and rabies. An additional practical application of the theory was the introduction of phenol as a disinfectant for surgical procedures by the British surgeon Joseph Lister.

Together with Pasteur, the German physician Robert Koch is considered to be a cofounder of modern microbiology. Having observed bacilli in the blood of animals which had died from anthrax, Koch demonstrated their pathogenicity by injecting mice with the blood. The injected mice died and the bacilli were present in preparations from their swollen spleens. He was also able to transfer the infection from mouse to mouse and to demonstrate the bacilli in each newly infected mouse. Initially, Koch used blood serum for growing the anthrax bacillus *in vitro*. Later, he developed solid media which allowed isolation of individual bacterial colonies. Using a solid medium, he was eventually able to isolate the tubercle bacillus from the tissues of an experimental animal in which he had demonstrated microscopically the presence of the organism. As a result of these observations, Koch formulated certain principles for proving that a specific microorganism caused a particular disease: the specific microorganism must be present in all affected animals and after isolation *in vitro*, must cause the disease when inoculated into susceptible animals. The identical microorganism must then be isolated from the inoculated animals.

Pasteur's germ theory of disease and Koch's postulates are the two corner-stones on which microbiology is based and without which, this branch of biology could not have advanced. During the past century, major developments have taken place in microbiological concepts, techniques and applications. Modern microbiology encompasses the study of bacteria, fungi, viruses and other microscopic and submicroscopic organisms (Box 1.1). In veterinary microbiology, emphasis is placed on those microorganisms associated with infectious diseases of animals. Immunology, the study of host responses to infectious agents, is a discipline closely related to microbiology and is sometimes considered as a distinct but cognate subject.

Living cells, the smallest units capable of independent existence, can be divided into two sharply differentiated groups, eukaryotes and prokaryotes. The main differentiating features of eukaryotic and prokaryotic cells are presented in Table 1.1. Eukaryotes possess true nuclei which contain chromosomes and individual cells replicate by mitosis. In addition, a typical eukaryotic cell contains organelles such as mitochondria, a Golgi apparatus, lysosomes and relatively large ribosomes. Organisms in the Archaebacteria and Eubacteria, which are less complex than eukaryotic organisms, are prokaryotes which lack true membrane-bound nuclei. Their genetic information is contained in a single circular chromosome. In some prokaryotic cells such as bacteria, extrachromosomal DNA, in the form of plasmids, encodes for certain characteristics of the organism. Although the origin of life is a much debated subject, it is probable that primitive microorganisms originated from ancestral life forms several billion years ago (Fig. 1.1). The degree of relatedness among microorganisms can be assessed by comparison of their ribosomal ribonucleic acid (rRNA). There is some evidence that all organisms developed from a group of primitive cells rather than from a single organism (Doolittle, 1999). Prokaryotes are considered as one branch of the phylogenetic tree and eukaryotes as the

Table 1.1 Comparative features of prokaryotic and eukaryotic cells.

Prokaryotic cell	Eukaryotic cell
Usually less than 5 μm in length	Usually more than 10 μm in diameter
Membrane-bound organelles absent	Membrane-bound organelles present
70S ribosomes	80S ribosomes in cytoplasm; 70S ribosomes in mitochondria and chloroplasts
Nucleic acid occurs as a single molecule, often circular	Nucleic acid is distributed in chromosomes
Nuclear membrane and nucleolus absent	Nuclear membrane and nucleolus present
Replicate by binary fission	Replicate by mitosis

second branch (Fig. 1.1). Lateral as well as horizontal transfer of genetic material probably occurred in the course of evolutionary development, with some eubacterial genes incorporated into members of the Archaebacteria and perhaps with some prokaryotic genes incorporated into eukaryotes. This lateral gene transfer may explain how complex eukaryotic cells acquired some of their genes and organelles. The endosymbiosis hypothesis proposes that, at some stage in their early development, eukaryotic cells became primitive phagocytes and acquired particular bacterial cell types which enhanced their respiratory activity (de Duve, 1996). It is proposed that the engulfed bacteria provided extra energy through this enhanced respiration to the host cell and eventually evolved into mitochondria. A similar phenomenon may account for the development of chloroplasts in plant cells. The cytoplasmic membrane is the site of respiratory or photosynthetic energy-generation in prokaryotes unlike eukaryotes, in which these activities occur in the membranes of mitochondria and chloroplasts.

Pathogenic microorganisms

Most microorganisms found in nature are not harmful to humans, animals or plants. Indeed, many bacteria and fungi make an important contribution to biological activities which take place in soil, in water and in the alimentary tract of animals. Those microorganisms which can cause disease in animals or humans are referred to as pathogenic microorganisms.

Bacteria
Microorganisms belonging to the Archaebacteria are not associated with diseases of domestic animals. Organisms (bacteria) belonging to the Eubacteria include many pathogens of veterinary importance.

Box 1.1 Subdivisions of microbiology.

- Bacteriology, the study of bacteria
- Mycology, the study of fungi
- Virology, the study of viruses
- The study of unconventional infectious agents including prions

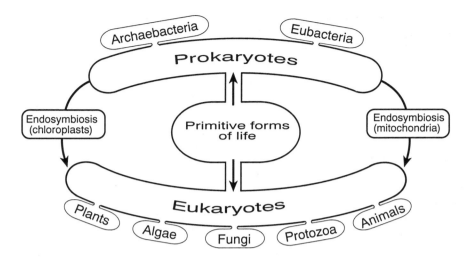

Figure 1.1 The evolutionary relationships of living organisms. Endosymbiosis is the postulated mechanism whereby eukaryotic cells acquired mitochondria or chloroplasts by incorporation of prokaryotic cells.

Bacteria are unicellular and are smaller and less complex than eukaryotic cells such as mammalian red blood cells (Table 1.2). They usually have rigid cell walls containing a peptidoglycan layer, multiply by binary fission and exhibit considerable morphological diversity. They occur as rods, cocci, helical forms and occasionally as branching filaments. Despite their morphological diversity, most bacteria are between 0.5 μm and 5 μm in length. Motile bacteria possess flagella by which they can move through liquid media. The majority of bacteria can grow on suitable inert media; some require special growth supplements and particular atmospheric conditions for growth. Two groups of small bacteria, rickettsiae and chlamydiae, which are unable to multiply on inert media, require living cells for *in vitro* growth. Cyanobacteria, formerly referred to as blue-green algae, utilize chlorophyll for some metabolic pathways. Unlike algae, which store chlorophyll in organelles referred to as chloroplasts, cyanobacteria have chlorophyll distributed inside their cell membranes.

Fungi

Yeasts, moulds and mushrooms belong to a large group of non-photosynthetic eukaryotes, termed fungi. Fungi may be either unicellular or multicellular. Multicellular fungi produce filamentous microscopic structures called moulds; yeasts which are unicellular, have a spherical or ovoid shape and multiply by budding. In moulds the cells are cylindrical and attached end-to-end, forming branched hyphae (Table 1.3). A notable feature of fungi is their ability to secrete potent enzymes which can digest organic matter. When moisture is present and other environmental conditions are favourable, fungi can degrade a wide variety of organic substrates. A small number of yeasts and moulds are pathogenic for humans and animals. Some fungi invade tissues whereas others produce toxic substances called mycotoxins which, if present on crops or in stored food such as grain or nuts, can cause disease in animals and humans.

Algae

A morphologically and physiologically diverse group of organisms, algae, are usually considered plant-like because they contain chlorophyll. Many algae are free-living in water; others grow on the surfaces of rocks and on other structures in the environment. Some algae produce pigments which impart distinct colouration to water

Table 1.2 A comparison of the morphology and size of bacterial cells relative to a mammalian red blood cell.

Cell	Morphology/size	Comments
Red blood cell	7 μm	Readily seen using conventional light microscopy
Bacillus	5 μm	Rod-shaped cells, usually stained by the Gram method. Using bright-field microscopy, a magnification of 1,000x is required to observe most bacterial cells.
Coccus	1 μm	Spherical-shaped cells, often occuring in chains or in grape-like clusters
Spirochaete	10 μm	Thin, helical bacteria. Dark-field microscopy (without staining) or special staining methods are required to demonstrate these unusual microorganisms.

Table 1.3 A comparison of the morphology and size of a bacterial cell and two fungal forms.

Structure	Morphology/size	Comments
Bacterial cell		
Coccus	☉ 1 µm	Often occur in chains or grape-like clusters
Fungal forms		
Yeast	⬭ 5 µm	Reproduce by budding
Mould	>30 µm	Branched structures (hyphae) composed of many cells

surfaces containing algal blooms. When water temperatures are high, algal growth may be marked, leading to the production of toxins which can accumulate in shellfish or in water containing algal blooms.

Viruses

Unlike bacteria and fungi, viruses are not cells. A virus particle or virion consists of nucleic acid, either DNA or RNA, enclosed in a protein coat called a capsid. In addition, some viruses are surrounded by an envelope. Viruses are much smaller than bacteria, and range in size from 20 nm to 300 nm in diameter (Table 1.4). Despite their simple structure, viruses occur in many shapes. Some are spherical, others are brick and bullet-shaped and a few have an elongated appearance. Because they lack the structures and enzymes necessary for metabolism and independent reproduction, viruses can multiply only within living cells. Both prokaryotic and eukaryotic cells are susceptible to infection by viruses. Those viruses which invade bacterial cells are called bacteriophages. Pathogenic viruses which infect humans and animals can cause serious disease by invading and destroying cells. A small number of viruses are aetiologically implicated in the development of malignant tumours in humans and animals.

Prions

Infectious particles which are smaller than viruses, have been implicated in the neurological diseases of animals and humans termed transmissible spongiform encephalopathies. These particles, called prions, are distinct from viruses and appear to be devoid of nucleic acid. Prions seem to be composed of an abnormally folded protein capable of inducing conformational changes in corresponding normal host cell protein. Following the induced changes, structurally altered abnormal protein accumulates in and damages long-lived cells such as neurons. Genetic factors seem to influence the susceptibility of humans and animals to prion diseases. Prions exhibit remarkable resistance to physical and chemical inactivation procedures.

Biological classification and nomenclature

Microscopic living organisms were formerly classified on the basis of phenotypic expression including morphology and distinct attributes reflecting unique metabolic properties. Increasingly, classification methods for microorganisms have come to rely heavily on genotypic analysis. In recent years, this has led to changes in the classification and nomenclature of microorganisms.

Species are groups of organisms with similar genetic and metabolic characteristics. Closely related species are initially grouped into genera and thereafter into families, orders, classes, phyla and kingdoms (Box 1.2). Organisms are usually referred to by their generic and specific names, for example, the bacterium which causes anthrax in humans and animals is termed *Bacillus anthracis*, *Bacillus* being the generic name and *anthracis* the specific name. This binomial system of nomenclature was devised in the eighteenth century by the Swedish naturalist, Linnaeus. Viruses are not classified according to the Linnaean system because they are not cells and cannot reproduce independently. They are generally grouped in families based on virion morphology and nucleic acid type. Further subdivision of pathogenic animal viruses relates to the species of host affected and to the clinical disease which is produced.

Table 1.4 A comparison of a bacterial cell and a large and a small virus[a].

Structure	Morphology/size	Comments
Bacterial cell		
Coccus	1 µm	Readily seen at magnification of 1,000x.
Viruses		
Poxvirus	300 nm	Viruses cannot be seen using conventional bright-field microscopy. Electron microscopy at a magnification of up to 100,000x is used to demonstrate viruses in clinical specimens or in laboratory preparations.
Parvovirus	⊛ 20 nm	

a   not drawn to scale

Box 1.2 Categories used for the taxonomic classification of microorganisms.

Kingdom (includes all microorganisms)
—Phylum (group of related classes in kingdom)
  —Class (group of related orders in phylum)
    —Order (group of related families in class)
      —Family (group of related genera in order)
        —Genus (group of related species in family)
          —Species (organisms with similar features)

Microscopical techniques

A number of different microscopic methods are employed for examining microorganisms. These include bright-field, dark-field, phase contrast and electron microscopy. Table 1.5 summarizes common staining methods used in microscopy and the particular types of microorganisms for which the techniques are appropriate. Units of measurement employed in microscopy are indicated in Table 1.6.

The maximum magnification obtainable by bright-field microscopy, using oil-immersion objectives, is approximately 1000x. With bright-field microscopy, suitably stained bacteria as small as 0.2 μm in size can be visualized. With dark-field microscopy, the scattering of light by fine microorganisms such as spirochaetes suspended in liquid allows them to be observed against a dark background. In common with dark-field techniques, phase-contrast microscopy can be used to examine

Table 1.5 Microscopical techniques used in microbiology.

Technique	Comments
Bright-field microscopy	Used for demonstrating the morphology and size of stained bacteria and fungi; staining affinity may allow preliminary classification of bacteria and the morphology of fungal structures permits identification of the genus
Phase-contrast microscopy	Used for examining unstained cells in suspension
Dark-field microscopy	Used for examining unstained bacteria such as spirochaetes in suspension
Fluorescent microscopy	Used for identifying microorganisms with specific antibodies conjugated with fluorochromes
Transmission electron microscopy	Used for demonstrating viruses in biological material and for identifying ultrastructural details of bacterial, fungal and mammalian cells
Scanning electron microscopy	Used for demonstrating the three-dimensional structure of microorganisms

Table 1.6 Units of measurement used in microbiology.

Unit	Abbreviation	Comments
Millimetre	mm	One thousandth of a metre (10^{-3} m). Bacterial and fungal colony sizes are usually measured in mm. When growing on a suitable medium, bacterial colonies range in size from 0.5 mm to 5 mm
Micrometre (micron)	μm	One thousandth of a millimetre (10^{-6} m). Used for the size of bacterial and fungal cells. Most bacteria range in size from 0.5 μm to 5 μm. A small number of bacteria may exceed 20 μm in length
Nanometre	nm	One thousandth of a micrometre (10^{-9} m). Used for expressing the size of viruses. Most viruses of veterinary importance range in size from 20 nm to 300 nm

unstained specimens. This procedure is more appropriate for research purposes than for routine diagnostic microbiology.

In transmission electron microscopy, beams of electrons are used in place of visible light to visualize small structures such as viruses. Specimens, placed on grids, are negatively stained with electron-dense compounds such as potassium phosphotungstate and viewed as magnified images on a fluorescent screen. Magnifications greater than 100,000x are possible with modern instruments. Scanning electron microscopy is used to obtain three-dimensional views of microorganisms when coated with a thin film of heavy metal. With this technique, a wide range of magnifications up to 100,000x is feasible.

References

de Duve, C. (1996). The birth of complex cells. *Scientific American*, **274**, 38–45.

Doolittle, W.F. (1999). Phylogenetic classification and the universal tree. *Science*, **284**, 2124–2128.

Further reading

Debré, P. (1998). *Louis Pasteur*. Johns Hopkins University Press Ltd., London.

Lechevalier, H.A. and Solotorovsky, M. (1965). *Three Centuries of Microbiology*. McGraw-Hill Book Company, New York.

Madigan, M.T., Martinko, J.M. and Parker, J. (1997). *Brock Biology of Microorganisms*. Eighth Edition. Prentice Hall International, London.

Schlegel, H.G. (1993). *General Microbiology*. Seventh Edition. Cambridge University Press, Cambridge.

Chapter 2

The structure of bacterial cells

A typical bacterial cell is composed of a capsule, cell wall, cell membrane, cytoplasm containing nuclear material and appendages such as flagella and pili (fimbriae). Certain species of bacteria can produce forms termed spores or endospores, which are resistant to environmental influences. Some of the structural features of pathogenic bacteria which are important in the production of disease or may be useful for the laboratory diagnosis of infection are reviewed in Chapters 5 and 7. The principal structural components of bacterial cells are presented in Table 2.1.

Capsule

Bacteria can synthesize extracellular polymeric material which is usually described as glycocalyx. In some bacterial species this polymeric material forms a capsule, a well-defined structure closely adherent to the cell wall. A slime layer is formed when the polymeric material is present as a loose meshwork of fibrils around the cell. Most capsules are composed of polysaccharides; *Bacillus* species such as *B. anthracis* produce polypeptide capsules. Defined capsules can be visualized by light microscopy using negative staining techniques. Bacteria with well-defined capsular material produce mucoid colonies on agar media. However, the capsules of most species of bacteria can be demonstrated only by electron microscopy or by immunological methods using antisera specific for the capsular (K) antigens. The main function of capsular material appears to be protection of the bacterium from adverse environmental conditions such as desiccation. In the body, capsules of pathogenic bacteria may facilitate adherence to surfaces and interfere with phagocytosis.

Cell wall

The tough, rigid cell walls of bacteria protect them from mechanical damage and osmotic lysis. As cell walls are non-selectively permeable, they exclude only very large molecules. Differences in the structure and chemical composition of the cell walls of bacterial species account for variation in their pathogenicity and influence other characteristics including staining properties. Peptidoglycan, a polymer unique to prokaryotic cells, imparts rigidity to the cell wall. This polymer is composed of chains of alternating subunits of N-acetylglucosamine

Table 2.1 Structural components of bacterial cells.

Structure	Chemical composition	Comments
Capsule	Usually poly-saccharide; polypeptide in *Bacillus anthracis*	Often associated with virulence; interferes with phagocytosis; may prolong survival in the environment
Cell wall	Peptidoglycan and teichoic acid in Gram-positive bacteria. Lipopolysacch-aride (LPS), protein, phospho-lipid and peptido-glycan in Gram-negative bacteria	Peptidoglycan is responsible for the shape of the organism. LPS is responsible for endotoxic effects. Porins, protein structures, regulate the passage of small molecules through the phospholipid layer.
Cytoplasmic membrane	Phospholipid bilayer	Selectively permeable membrane involved in active transport of nutrients, respiration, excretion and chemoreception.
Flagellum (plural, flagella)	Protein called flagellin	Filamentous structure which confers motility
Pilus (plural, pili)	Protein called pilin	Also known as fimbria (plural, fimbriae). Thin, straight, thread-like structures present on many Gram-negative bacteria. Two types exist, attachment pili and conjugation pili.
Chromosome	DNA	Single circular structure with no nuclear membrane
Ribosome	RNA and protein	Involved in protein synthesis
Storage granules or inclusions	Chemical composition variable	Present in some bacterial cells; may be composed of polyphosphate (volutin or metachromatic granules), poly-beta-hydroxybutyrate (reserve energy source), glycogen

and N-acetylmuramic acid cross-linked by short tetrapeptide side chains and peptide cross-bridges.

Bacteria can be divided into two major groups, Gram-positive and Gram-negative, on the basis of colour when stained by the Gram method. This colour reaction is determined by the composition of the cell wall. Gram-positive bacteria which stain blue have a relatively thick uniform cell wall which is composed mainly of peptidoglycan and teichoic acids. In contrast, Gram-negative bacteria, which stain red, have cell walls with a more complex structure, consisting of an outer membrane and a periplasmic space containing a comparatively small amount of peptidoglycan (Fig. 2.1). The outer membrane is a protein-containing asymmetrical lipid bilayer. The structure of the inner surface of the membrane resembles that of the cytoplasmic membrane, whereas that of the outer surface is composed of lipopolysaccharide (LPS) molecules. Low molecular weight substances such as sugars and amino acids enter through specialized protein channels, known as porins, in the outer membrane. The outer membrane LPS, the endotoxin of Gram-negative bacteria, is released only after cell lysis. The major components of LPS molecules are core polysaccharides bound to lipid A and long external polysaccharide side chains. The polysaccharide side chains of the LPS molecules stimulate antibody production and correspond to the somatic (O) antigens used for serotyping of Gram-negative cells. Lipid A is the molecular component in which endotoxic activity resides. On account of its composition, the outer membrane excludes hydrophobic molecules and renders Gram-negative bacteria resistant to some detergents which are lethal to most Gram-positive bacteria.

The mycoplasmas comprise an important group of bacteria without cell walls. Conventional bacteria, exposed to the action of antibiotics such as penicillin, or other substances which interfere with the synthesis of peptidoglycan, cannot produce cell walls and are termed L forms.

Cytoplasmic membrane

The cytoplasmic membranes of bacterial cells are flexible structures composed of phospholipids and proteins. They can be observed only by electron microscopy and are structurally similar to the plasma membranes of eukaryotic cells. However, bacterial cytoplasmic membranes, with the exception of those present in mycoplasmas, do not contain sterols. The inner and outer faces of cytoplasmic membranes are hydrophilic while the interior is hydrophobic, forming a barrier to most hydrophilic molecules. Only a limited range of small molecules such as water, oxygen, carbon dioxide and some lipid-soluble compounds can enter bacterial cells by passive diffusion. Two major functions of the cytoplasmic membrane, the active transport of nutrients into the cell and the elimination of waste metabolites, require the expenditure of energy. The energy required by permeases and other carrier molecules for active transport of nutrients derives from adenosine triphosphate. The cytoplasmic membrane is also the site of electron transport for bacterial respiration, of phosphorylation systems and of enzymes and carrier molecules that function in the biosynthesis of DNA, cell wall polymers and membrane lipids.

Cytoplasm

The cytoplasm, which is enclosed by the cytoplasmic membrane, is essentially an aqueous fluid containing the nuclear material, ribosomes, nutrients and the enzymes and other molecules involved in synthesis, cell maintenance

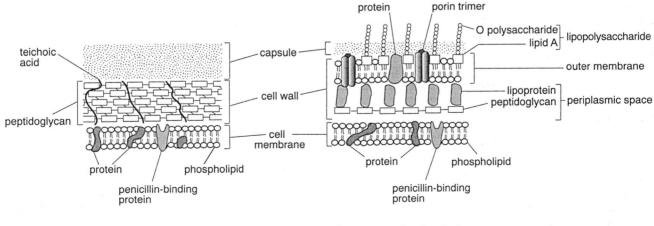

Gram-positive bacterium   **Gram-negative bacterium**

Figure 2.1 Comparison of the capsule, cell wall and cell membrane of a Gram-positive bacterium and a Gram-negative bacterium. Structures of importance in staining, virulence and toxicity, antigenicity, and susceptibility to antibiotics are illustrated.

and metabolism. Storage granules may be present under certain environmental conditions, usually those unfavourable for bacterial growth. These granules, which may be composed of starch, glycogen, polyphosphate or other compounds, can often be identified using particular dyes.

Ribosomes

All protein synthesis takes place on ribosomes. These structures are composed of ribonucleoproteins and are up to 25 nm in size. They consist of two subunits, a larger 50S subunit and a smaller 30S subunit. The Svedberg (S) unit is a measure of sedimentation rate, which is dependent on both the size and shape of a particle. Ribosomal ribonucleic acid (rRNA) is complexed with many different proteins and accounts for about 80% of the RNA of the cell. Smaller amounts of transfer RNA (tRNA) and messenger RNA (mRNA) account for the remaining cellular RNA. Ribosomes may be present either in the cytoplasm or associated with the inner surface of the cytoplasmic membrane. During active bacterial growth and rapid protein synthesis, individual ribosomes are joined by mRNA into long chains known as polysomes.

Nuclear material

The bacterial genome is composed of a single haploid circular chromosome containing double-stranded DNA. Small amounts of protein and RNA are also associated with nuclear material. The genes in the bacterial chromosome code for all the vital functions of the cell. Bacterial genomes vary in size depending on the species. Because of its length, the bacterial chromosome is extensively folded to form a dense body which can be seen by electron microscopy. The nuclear material can also be demonstrated by light microscopy when stained by the Feulgen method which is specific for DNA. During replication, the DNA helix unwinds and both daughter cells, produced by binary fission, receive a copy of the original genome.

Plasmids, small circular pieces of DNA which are separate from the genome, are capable of autonomous replication. Several different plasmids may be present in individual bacterial cells. Copies of plasmids can be transferred from cell to cell during binary fission or through conjugation (*see* Chapter 4). Plasmid DNA may code for characteristics such as antibiotic resistance and exotoxin production.

Flagella

Bacteria which possess flagella are motile. Many species of Gram-negative bacteria have flagella. Although they are rarely present in cocci, some species of enterococci and the zoospores of *Dermatophilus congolensis* possess flagella. Flagella are usually several times longer than the bacterial cell and are composed of a protein called flagellin. They consist of a filament, hook and basal body. The hook functions as a universal joint between the filament and the basal body. The basal body is anchored to the cell wall and to the cytoplasmic membrane. The positions at which flagella are inserted into the bacterial cell vary and may be characteristic of a genus or family (Fig. 2.2). Motile bacteria can move into suitable micro-environments in response to physical or chemical stimuli.

Flagella can be demonstrated by electron microscopy, by light microscopy using special methods and by serology using antibodies specific for flagellar antigens. Motility can be confirmed in young broth cultures using the hanging drop technique or in a semisolid motility medium containing tetrazolium salts.

Pili

Fine, straight, hair-like appendages called pili or fimbriae, composed of the protein pilin, are attached to the cell wall of many bacteria. The number of pili on each bacterial cell varies widely. They are most common on Gram-negative bacteria and they may have different functions. In pathogenic bacteria, pili function as adhesins for receptors on mammalian cells (*see* Chapter 7). A unique type of pilus, the F (sex or conjugation) pilus, functions in male or donor cells of Gram-negative bacteria as a conduit for the transfer of DNA to female or recipient cells. Conjugation will be discussed further in Chapter 4.

Endospores

Dormant highly resistant bodies, termed endospores, are formed by some bacteria to ensure survival during adverse environmental conditions. The only genera of pathogenic bacteria which contain endospore-forming species, are *Bacillus* and *Clostridium*. Endospores, which are produced inside the bacterial cell, show species variation

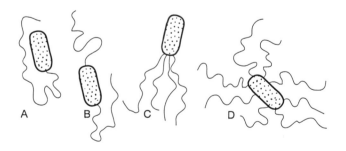

Figure 2.2 Bacterial flagella.
A. Monotrichous (polar) flagellum
B. Amphitrichous flagella
C. Lophotrichous flagella
D. Peritrichous flagella

in shape, size and position within the mother cell. Because of the resistance and impermeability of the spore coat, special staining procedures which employ heat are required to demonstrate endospores. The resistance of endospores is attributed to their layered structure, their dehydrated state, their negligible metabolic activity and their high content of dipicolinic acid (Fig. 2.3). Dipicolinic acid, which is not found in vegetative cells, occurs in the spore wall in combination with large amounts of calcium. The high calcium content may explain the extended survival times of endospores in calcium-rich soils. In areas of low soil calcium or in acidic soils, calcium may be leached from spores, shortening their survival times. Because spores are thermostable, they can be destroyed with certainty only by moist heat at 121°C for 15 minutes.

When an endospore is reactivated, germination occurs in three stages namely activation, initiation and outgrowth. Activation may occur in response to factors such as brief exposure to heat, abrasion of the spore coat or environmental acidity. If other environmental conditions including the presence of adequate nutrients are favourable, initiation of germination will occur. The spore cortex and coat are degraded, water is absorbed, calcium dipicolinate is released and outgrowth develops. Outgrowth is a period of active biosynthesis and terminates with division of the new vegetative cell.

The spores produced by some of the filamentous actinomycetes are different from endospores in that their function is mainly concerned with reproduction rather than survival.

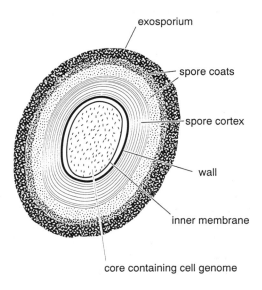

exosporium

spore coats

spore cortex

wall

inner membrane

core containing cell genome

Figure 2.3 Structural features of a mature bacterial endospore.

Further reading

Balows, A. and Duerden, B.I. (1998). *Topley and Wilson's Microbiology and Microbial Infections*. Volume 2, *Systematic Bacteriology*. Ninth Edition. Arnold, London.

Brooks, G.F., Butel, J.S. and Morse, S.A. (1998). *Jawetz, Melnick and Adelberg's Medical Microbiology*. Twenty-first Edition. Appleton and Lange, Stamford, Connecticut.

Singleton, P. (1997). *Bacteriology in Biology, Biotechnology and Medicine*. Fourth Edition. Wiley, Chichester.

Volk, W.A. (1992). *Basic Microbiology*. Seventh Edition. HarperCollins, New York.

Chapter 3

Cultivation, preservation and inactivation of bacteria

Appropriate conditions of moisture, pH, temperature, osmotic pressure, atmosphere and nutrients are required for bacterial growth. Bacteria increase in number by binary fission (Fig. 3.1). The generation time, that is the length of time required for a single bacterial cell to yield two daughter cells, is influenced by both genetic and nutritional factors. *Escherichia coli*, a common enteric organism, has a generation time of approximately 20 minutes. Bacterial pathogens have generation times ranging from 30 minutes to 20 hours. Long-term preservation of microorganisms usually involves freezing procedures. Heat treatment or chemicals can be used to inactivate bacteria.

Bacterial growth

Following inoculation of bacterial cells into fresh broth medium, the growth curve of the culture exhibits lag, exponential and stationary phases, and a final decline phase (Fig. 3.2). The lag phase is characterized by active metabolism of the cells as they acquire various essential constituents prior to division. Binary fission of the young cells results in an exponential increase in numbers. A straight line relationship is obtained when the logarithmic number of viable cells is plotted against incubation time. Exponential growth in a broth culture is limited and eventually ceases because essential nutrients are depleted and toxic metabolic products accumulate in the medium. During this stationary phase, no increase in bacterial

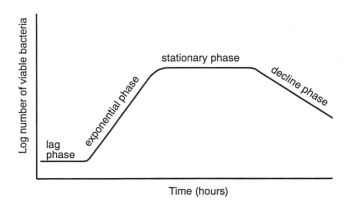

Figure 3.2 The pattern of growth and decline of viable bacterial cell numbers in liquid medium.

numbers occurs; slow growth and division of a few bacteria is balanced by death of others. As the bacterial population enters the decline phase, old cells die rapidly followed eventually by the younger cells. The resulting rate of cell death is exponential. Abnormally shaped cells, known as involution forms, may be seen in stained smears from cultures in the decline phase. When maintenance of bacteria in the exponential growth phase is required, a chemostat consisting of a growth chamber connected to a reservoir of fresh medium is used. As fresh medium enters the growth chamber, bacteria are harvested and exhausted medium and waste products are removed.

The size of bacterial populations is usually expressed either as the number or the density of the cells present. Cell numbers can be determined either as a total cell count or as a viable cell count. The standard methods for counting bacterial cell numbers are presented in Table 3.1. Bacteria may be counted by direct microscopy, by colony counting, by membrane filtration and by electronic methods. Accurate cell counts may be required for specific purposes such as vaccine preparation and for bacterial testing of water.

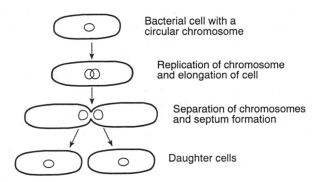

Bacterial cell with a circular chromosome

Replication of chromosome and elongation of cell

Separation of chromosomes and septum formation

Daughter cells

Figure 3.1 Bacterial replication by binary fission. The time required to produce two daughter cells in rapidly growing bacteria is referred to as the generation time.

Bacterial nutrition

Bacteria acquire nutrients from their immediate environment. Most are chemoheterotrophs, using organic chemicals as sources of energy and carbon. Small

Table 3.1 Methods for counting bacteria.

Method	Technique	Comments
Microscopic counting		
Direct smear (Breed's method)	Counts carried out on a fixed and stained smear prepared from a defined volume of fluid; 50 microscopic fields counted	Traditional method for counting bacteria in milk. Slow and unreliable. Cannot differentiate viable from non-viable bacteria
Counting chamber	Counts carried out on a fixed volume of bacterial suspension using a calibrated slide	Does not differentiate viable from non-viable bacteria
Colony counting		
Spread plate	Following serial ten-fold dilution of a bacterial suspension, a fixed volume of each dilution is spread on the surface of agar plates and incubated for 24 to 48 hours	Colony counts are carried out on plates with 30 to 300 colonies after incubation. The number of viable organisms in the suspension is calculated and expressed as colony-forming units (CFU)/ml of suspension
Pour plate	Following serial ten-fold dilution as in the spread plate technique, 0.1 ml of each dilution is placed in Petri dishes and approximately 20 ml of molten agar at 45°C to 48°C is added, and thoroughly mixed	Colony counting is carried out as in the spread plate technique and results are expressed as CFU/ml of suspension
Miles-Misra	Following serial ten-fold dilution, 0.02ml of each dilution is placed on a sector of an agar plate, five dilutions per plate	Colony counting is carried out as in the spread plate technique and the average colony count from the five drops is used for calculating the number of viable bacterial cells expressed as CFU/ml of fluid
Membrane filtration	Following filtration of a known volume of fluid through a filter of 0.22 μm pore size, the filter, placed on the surface of an agar plate, is incubated for 24 to 48 hours	The number of viable bacteria is expressed as CFU/ml of fluid
Other counting methods		
Opacity tubes	The bacterial suspension is matched visually with McFarland's opacity standard tubes	Tables indicating the total bacterial cell numbers/ml equivalent to matching opacities are supplied with the standard tubes
Electronic counting	Electronic counting instruments, such as the Coulter counter, when carefully calibrated, give accurate rapid results	Reliability of results is dependent on rigorous quality control. Provides total cell count only

molecules may be metabolized rapidly or utilized to synthesize macromolecules. Nutrient media for the isolation of pathogenic bacteria are formulated to supply particular growth factors for specific groups of organisms.

Most bacteria require carbon and nitrogen in relatively large amounts. In culture media, peptones are usually the main source of nitrogen. Peptones, which are mixtures of peptides and amino acids obtained by the digestion of meat and other sources of protein, frequently supply other essential nutrients such as phosphate, sulphate, potassium, magnesium, calcium and iron. Phosphates are essential for the production of nucleic acids and molecules containing energy-rich bonds. Sulphates are required for the synthesis of sulphur-containing amino acids, and magnesium, potassium, calcium and iron are important co-factors for certain enzymes. Trace elements and certain growth factors such as vitamins are also essential for bacterial growth.

Physical and chemical factors which influence growth

In addition to nutritional factors, growth of bacteria is influenced by genetic factors and by chemical, physical and other environmental factors. Awareness of those factors which limit growth is essential for the successful culture and long-term preservation of microorganisms. Growth of bacteria in culture is influenced by temperature, hydrogen ion concentration, availability of moisture, atmospheric composition and osmotic pressure. Most pathogenic bacteria can be grown aerobically on a nutrient medium at 37°C, close to normal body temperature. Although the optimal temperature for growth of these bacteria, termed mesophiles, is 37°C, they can grow at temperatures between 20°C and 45°C. In contrast, many environmental bacteria grow at temperatures outside this range. Those with an optimal incubation temperature of 15°C are termed psychrophiles and those with an optimal incubation temperature close to 60°C are termed thermophiles (Fig. 3.3).

As most bacteria grow optimally at neutral pH, it is standard practice to buffer culture media close to pH 7. Bacteria require water for growth and species vary widely in their susceptibility to desiccation. The ability to tolerate desiccation is determined by the cell wall composition and the surrounding microenvironment. Moreover, the cell wall composition accounts for the ability of bacteria to withstand changing osmotic pressures. Change in the cell wall composition, induced by the action of lysozyme or of antibiotics such as penicillin, results in protoplast formation. These spherical structures lack rigidity and are susceptible to osmotic change. In the animal body, pathogenic bacteria without cell walls (L forms) can replicate, causing chronic or persistent infections. Bacterial cells in the environment are usually present in hypotonic solutions and, provided that the cell wall is intact, they remain in a state of turgor and do not lyse. In hypertonic solutions, bacterial cells undergo shrinkage. Some bacteria, however, have adapted to hypertonic environments and can grow in solutions with high salt concentrations. *Staphylococcus aureus*, an important pathogen of humans and animals, can grow in media containing up to 7.5% sodium chloride.

Based on their preference for particular levels of oxygen, bacteria can be assigned to four main groups, namely aerobes, anaerobes, facultative anaerobes and microaerophiles (Fig. 3.4). Capnophiles, a fifth group, are aerobic bacteria with a requirement for carbon dioxide. Because they utilize metabolic pathways in which oxygen is the final electron acceptor, aerobic bacteria require oxygen for growth and they are incubated in air. In

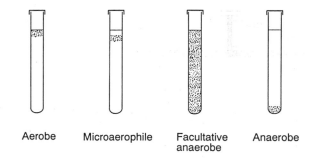

Aerobe Microaerophile Facultative anaerobe Anaerobe

Figure 3.4 The pattern of growth at different depths in semi-solid agar, reflecting the preference of various bacterial species for aerobic, microaerophilic and anaerobic conditions.

contrast, anaerobic bacteria are unable to grow in an atmosphere containing oxygen. These organisms use fermentative pathways in which organic compounds serve as final electron acceptors. As they lack enzymes such as superoxide dismutase and catalase, obligate anaerobes survive only briefly in the presence of oxygen. Facultative anaerobes are bacteria which have the ability to grow well under both aerobic and anaerobic conditions. Microaerophilic bacteria require a reduced oxygen concentration for growth.

The cultivation of bacteria other than aerobes requires special laboratory techniques. Strict anaerobes are cultured in tightly sealed jars in an atmosphere from which free oxygen has been removed. One commercially available system employs a gas-producing envelope. On the addition of water to the envelope, hydrogen and carbon dioxide are released into the jar. A palladium catalyst, either in the jar or attached to the envelope, accelerates the reaction of the hydrogen with free oxygen in the jar to form water. In addition, the release of carbon dioxide enhances the growth of anaerobes. A more convenient alternative system, in which oxygen is removed by reacting with ascorbic acid contained in a porous envelope, has been developed (Fig 3.5). This system, which eliminates the need to generate hydrogen, releases carbon dioxide into the jar (Brazier and Hall, 1994). Moreover, this method is suitable for culturing strict anaerobes. Other methods for the cultivation of anaerobic bacteria include the use of specially designed anaerobic chambers and media, such as thioglycollate broth and cooked meat broth, with low redox potentials.

For the cultivation of microaerophiles reduced oxygen levels are required. A gas-producing envelope, which delivers up to 10% carbon dioxide into a sealed jar, is available commercially. This system is also suitable for the cultivation of capnophilic bacteria.

Preservation of microorganisms

In order to produce modified-live vaccines and to maintain stock cultures of the bacteria and fungi used in teaching

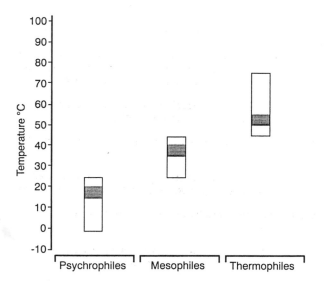

Figure 3.3 Categories of bacteria based on temperature ranges at which they can grow. Shaded areas indicate temperature ranges for optimal growth.

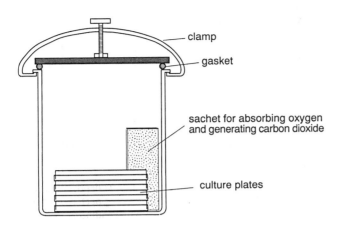

Figure 3.5 Jar for culturing anaerobic bacteria. When the porous sachet containing ascorbic acid is placed in the jar, which is then tightly sealed, oxygen is absorbed and carbon dioxide is generated. Anaerobic growth is enhanced by the released carbon dioxide.

and research, microorganisms must be preserved. Preservation should ensure viability, freedom from contamination and genetic stability. Subculturing can be used for the short-term preservation of bacteria. Limitations of this procedure include death of some cells and a risk of contamination and mutation. Long-term methods of preservation include freeze-drying (lyophilization), ultra-freezing in liquid nitrogen at −190°C and freezing at −70°C. If properly used, these preservation methods can maintain organisms in a hypobiotic state for more than 30 years and they ensure that the organisms remain unchanged and uncontaminated. However, because

freezing can harm microorganisms, chemicals must be employed to minimize the damage and ensure that the majority of organisms remain viable. Cryoprotective agents such as dimethyl sulphoxide or glycerol can minimize the negative effects of freezing on the viability of cells. Young actively-growing cultures are less affected by freezing than older cultures. As bacteria are easily damaged if desiccation takes place, freeze-drying must be carried out under vacuum. The microorganisms are subsequently stored in the dark in sealed evacuated ampoules.

Physical methods for inactivating microorganisms

Physical and chemical methods can be used for microbial inactivation or inhibition. Chemical agents include antimicrobial drugs (*see* Chapter 6), disinfectants (*see* Chapter 83) and food preservatives. Techniques which either inactivate bacteria or interfere with their metabolism include elevated temperature, low pH values, desiccation and high osmotic pressures. Some of the methods for preventing spoilage or limiting microbial growth in food are presented in Table 3.2. Sterilization is the method employed for the destruction of microorganisms on equipment used in microbiological and surgical procedures. Physical methods for sterilizing equipment or fluids are presented in Table 3.3. Sterilization procedures are effective for the destruction of bacterial, fungal and viral agents. However, unconventional infectious agents such as prions require more rigorous sterilization procedures. When dealing with bacterial endospores, such as those of *Clostridium* species, heating at a temperature of 121°C for 15 minutes is required for inactivation. Factors which may

Table 3.2 Methods for preventing spoilage and limiting microbial growth in food.

Method	Application	Comments
Refrigeration at 4°C	Prevention of growth of spoilage organisms and pathogenic bacteria	Pathogens such as *Listeria monocytogenes, Yersinia* species and many fungal species can grow at 4°C
Freezing at -20°C	Long-term storage of food. Microbial multiplication prevented	Surviving microorganisms can multiply rapidly when thawed food is left at ambient temperatures
Boiling at 100°C	Inactivation of vegetative bacteria and fungi in food	Many endospores can withstand prolonged boiling
Pasteurization at 72°C for 15 seconds	Inactivation of most vegetative bacteria	Heat treatment should be followed by rapid cooling. If present in high numbers, some bacteria may survive
Acidification	Adjustment of pH to a low level inhibits bacterial growth	Applicable to a limited range of foods such as vegetables
Increasing osmotic pressure	Inhibition of microbial multiplication; used for preservation of food	Addition of salts or sugars increases osmotic pressure; applicable to a limited range of foods
Vacuum packing	Packaging of meat and other perishable foods	Removal of oxygen prevents the growth of aerobes
Irradiation	Inactivation of spoilage organisms and pathogenic bacteria	Not permitted in some countries

Table 3.3 Physical methods for sterilizing equipment or fluids and for disposing of contaminated material.

Method	Comments
Moist heat (autoclaving) employing steam under pressure to generate 121°C for 15 minutes or 115°C for 45 minutes	Used for sterilizing culture media, laboratory items and surgical equipment. Inappropriate for heat sensitive plastics or fluids. Prions are not inactivated by this treatment
Dry heat in a hot-air oven at 160°C for 1 to 2 hours	Used for sterilizing metal, glass and other solid materials. Unsuitable for rubber and plastics
Incineration at 1,000°C	Used for destruction of infected carcasses and other contaminated material; environmental pollution a possible outcome
Flaming	Used for sterilizing inoculating loops in the naked flame of a Bunsen burner
Gamma irradiation	Ionizing rays used for sterilizing disposable plastic laboratory and surgical equipment. Unsuitable for glass and metal equipment
UV light	Non-ionizing rays with poor penetration. Used in biosafety cabinets
Membrane filtration	Used for filtering out bacteria from heat-sensitive fluids such as serum and tissue culture media. Pore size of filter should be 0.22 μm or less

influence the effectiveness of sterilization by heat are listed in Box 3.1.

When a population of microorganisms is exposed to high temperatures, there is an exponential decline in the numbers of viable organisms. Susceptibility to moist heat, used in autoclaving, can be expressed in terms of the thermal death time, which is the time required to kill all bacteria in suspension at a given temperature. The thermal death time is dependent on the initial size of the microbial population. The decimal reduction time (D value) is the time in minutes, at a particular temperature, required to reduce the viable cell population by 90%. The D value is inversely related to temperature and is independent of the size of the initial population.

Biosafety cabinets

Personnel handling hazardous materials require suitable protection. Biological safety cabinets protect operators from aerosols containing microbial pathogens. Different levels of protection can be provided depending on the type of cabinet used. At higher levels of protection, all contact between the operator and infective material is prevented through the use of closed cabinets fitted with rubber gloves. Air extracted from biosafety cabinets is filtered through high efficiency particulate air (HEPA) filters designed to trap particulate matter such as micro-organisms.

Box 3.1 Factors which influence the outcome of sterilization by heat.

- Temperature and holding time
- Degree of contamination
- Presence of endospores or prions
- Nature of the material being heat-treated
- Quantity of material being heat-treated

Reference

Brazier, J.S. and Hall, V. (1994). A simple evaluation of the AnaeroGen™ system for the growth of clinically significant anaerobic bacteria. *Letters in Applied Microbiology*, **18**, 56–58.

Further reading

Brooks, G.F., Butel, J.S. and Morse, S.A. (1998). *Jawetz, Melnick and Adelberg's Medical Microbiology*. Twenty-first Edition. Appleton and Lange, Stamford, Connecticut.

Pelczar, M.J., Chan, E.C.S. and Krieg, N.R. (1993). *Microbiology Concepts and Applications*. McGraw-Hill, New York.

Quinn, P.J., Carter, M.E., Markey, B.K. and Carter, G.R. (1994). Bacterial pathogens: microscopy, culture and identification. In *Clinical Veterinary Microbiology*. Mosby-Year Book, London. pp. 21–66.

Singleton, P. (1997). *Bacteriology in Biology, Biotechnology and Medicine*. Fourth Edition. Wiley, Chichester.

Chapter 4

Bacterial genetics and mechanisms of genetic variation

Bacteria are haploid with one circular chromosome consisting of double-stranded DNA. The chromosome, which is free in the cytoplasm in a coiled configuration, is much longer than the parent cell and contains a large number of genes. Each gene is a segment of chromosomal DNA with nucleotide sequences encoding a specific protein required for essential cellular structures or metabolic processes. Plasmids, bacteriophages and transposable elements may contribute additional genetic information, some of which may influence phenotypic expression (Fig. 4.1).

Replication of bacterial DNA

As bacteria replicate by binary fission, daughter cells are usually identical genetically. During replication, the sequence of purine and pyrimidine nucleotides in the DNA is copied into two double stranded daughter molecules. Each of these molecules is composed of a strand from the parent molecule and a newly synthesized complementary strand, a process termed semiconservative replication. As the two parent strands of the helical DNA unwind under the influence of DNA gyrase, each acts as a template for the synthesis of a complementary strand. In this manner, two identical helical DNA molecules are formed through the action of DNA polymerase. The ends of the new, fully formed strands are joined by DNA ligase to form circular chromosomes.

Transcription and translation

During transcription, one strand of DNA, the positive strand, is transcribed to messenger RNA (mRNA). The enzyme DNA-dependent RNA polymerase binds to the promoter region, a special sequence of DNA nucleotides on the positive strand. The two strands of DNA separate and a complementary strand of mRNA is synthesized. Transcription to mRNA stops when the enzyme reaches the termination sequence of the gene. The information encoded in the mRNA is translated into protein on a ribosome through the involvement of transfer RNA (tRNA). Each tRNA molecule has a particular triplet of three bases, the anticodon, which is complementary to a codon on the mRNA. Each triplet of tRNA transfers a specific amino acid to the mRNA on the ribosome where the amino acids are linked together to form a polypeptide chain. Following the linking of two amino acids, the tRNA of the first amino acid is released from the ribosome. Synthesis of the protein chain stops when a nonsense codon on the mRNA is encountered by the ribosome.

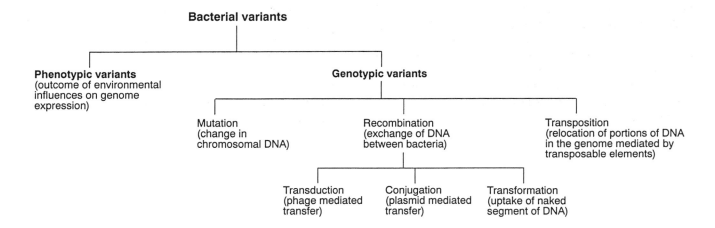

Figure 4.1 The basis of bacterial variation. A bacterium which has acquired DNA from another bacterial cell by recombination is termed a recombinant.

Plasmids

Many bacteria contain small genetic elements, termed plasmids, which are located in the cytoplasm and can replicate independently. The majority of plasmids are circular and composed of double-stranded DNA. They vary in size but are usually less than one tenth of the size of a bacterial genome and they may contain genes which can be utilized by the cell. In some pathogenic bacteria, plasmids encode virulence factors and antibiotic resistance.

Plasmids may use host cell enzymes for replication. Some plasmids, such as the F plasmid, can be integrated into the bacterial genome and are transferred during replication to daughter cells. However, replication of most plasmids is not directly related to multiplication of the host bacterium. Moreover, the distribution of plasmids between daughter cells is random. Plasmids in the bacterial cytoplasm may be transferred not only during replication but also by conjugation and by transformation. Transfer of genetic material by transformation rarely occurs in nature but can be accomplished by genetic manipulation of organisms under laboratory conditions.

Bacteriophages

Viruses which infect bacteria are termed bacteriophages (phages). There is considerable morphological diversity among bacteriophages. Some are filamentous with helical symmetry and others have icosahedral or pentagonal heads with tails of different lengths (Fig. 4.2). Structural features of a DNA phage are illustrated in Fig. 4.3. Phages may be either virulent or temperate depending on their method of replication. Virulent phages undergo a lytic cycle in bacteria, culminating in the production of phage progeny with lysis of host cells. Temperate phages, prophages, are usually integrated into the bacterial genome but they may also be present as circular DNA in the cytoplasm like plasmids. Temperate phages can also undergo a lytic cycle, either as a rare natural event or when exposed experimentally to UV light or to other mutagens (Fig. 4.4). A

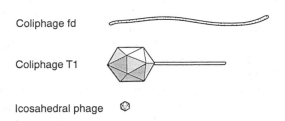

Figure 4.2 Types of bacteriophages indicating their shapes and relative sizes. The majority contain double-stranded DNA, but some contain single-stranded DNA, double-stranded RNA or single-stranded RNA.

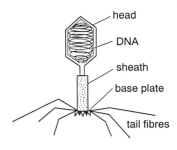

Figure 4.3 Schematic representation of a DNA phage.

prophage in a bacterial cell may be responsible for changes in phenotypic characteristics, a phenomenon referred to as lysogenic conversion. The production of neurotoxins by certain types of *Clostridium botulinum* is associated with lysogenic conversion of host cells (Table 4.1).

The phage genome may be composed of DNA or RNA, either single-stranded or double-stranded. Replication of phages is similar in many respects to that of animal viruses (Fig. 4.5). However, the capsid usually remains outside the bacterial cell after introduction of phage nucleic acid into the cytoplasm. The host specificity of phages relates to chemical affinity between attachment structures on the phages and specific receptor sites on the bacterium. A repressor protein, synthesized following entry of the DNA of temperate phage, inhibits production of virion proteins. The DNA of temperate phages is incorporated into host genomes, usually at specific integration sites, and is transmitted to progeny bacteria during binary fission.

Mechanisms contributing to genetic variation

Genetic variation may occur following mutation, in which a change occurs in the nucleotide sequence of a gene, or by recombination, in which new groups of genes are introduced into the genome or into the cytoplasm (Fig. 4.1). The genotype of a cell determines its inheritable potential. However, only a small proportion of the genetic information is expressed under defined environmental conditions. The phenotype represents those recognizable characteristics expressed by the cellular nucleic acid. *Bacillus anthracis*, the cause of anthrax, has a capsule which is expressed only *in vivo* and not when it is growing in laboratory media. Thus, both the genotype of an organism and its environment can influence phenotypic expression.

Mutation

A stable inheritable alteration in a bacterial genome is termed a mutation. Because a gene with altered base pairs may code incorrectly for an amino acid in a protein, mutation may result in phenotypic change. Mutational changes may be beneficial or damaging for the organism.

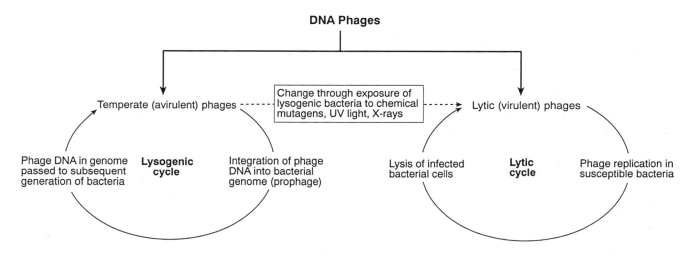

Figure 4.4 Lysogenic and lytic cycles of bacteriophages illustrating sporadic conversion of phages in the lysogenic cycle to lytic phages.

Under defined environmental conditions, selective mutations may provide growth advantage for the mutant over the parent or wild type bacterium. Mutations can be either spontaneous or experimentally induced by physical, chemical or biological mutagens. Spontaneous mutations can arise during replication because of errors in pairing of nucleotide bases. Such mutations occur at a frequency of 10^{-7} to 10^{-11} per base pair and are maintained at a low level because of the regulatory activity of repair enzymes. The types of mutation which may occur in bacteria are listed in Box 4.1. Point mutations involving one base pair or a limited number of base pairs may not result in phenotyp-

ic changes. In contrast, mutations in which many base pairs are deleted or inserted result in the formation of non-functional proteins. Extensive changes which affect protein synthesis influence bacterial viability.

Genetic recombination

Recombination occurs when sequences of DNA from two separate sources are integrated. In bacteria, recombination induces an unexpected inheritable change due to the introduction of new genetic material from a different cell. This new genetic material may be introduced by conjugation, transduction or transformation.

Conjugation

The transfer of genetic material during conjugation is a complex process which has been extensively studied in the enteric bacterium *Escherichia coli*. These studies have shown that two strains of *E. coli*, F$^+$ and F$^-$, participate in the process. The F$^+$ strains are the source of donor cells, which contain a fertility (F) plasmid whereas organisms in F$^-$ strains, having no F plasmid, are recipient cells. During conjugation, F$^+$ bacteria synthesize a modified pilus, the F or sex pilus. This pilus, through which genetic material can be transferred, can attach to F$^-$ bacteria. One strand of F plasmid DNA is passed to the recipient F$^-$ bacterium in which a complementary strand is then synthesized. After a new F plasmid is formed, the recipient is converted into an F$^+$ bacterium.

Individual bacteria may contain several different types of plasmids. Plasmid incompatibility-group genes control the types of plasmids within the cell and the ability of these plasmids to replicate. Plasmids belonging to the same incompatibility group cannot exist together in the same cell but can do so with plasmids of other incompatibility groups. Plasmids which govern their own transfer between cells are designated conjugative plasmids.

Table 4.1 Virulence factors of pathogenic bacteria mediated by defined genetic elements.

Pathogen	Virulence factors / Genetic elements
Bacillus anthracis	Toxins, capsule / plasmid
Clostridium botulinum, types C, D and E	Neurotoxins / bacteriophages
Escherichia coli	Shiga-like toxin / bacteriophage Adherence factors, enterotoxins / plasmids Heat-stable toxin, siderophore production / transposons
Salmonella Dublin	Serum resistance factor / plasmid
Staphylococcus aureus	Enterotoxins (A,D,E), toxic shock syndrome factor-1 / bacteriophages Coagulase, exfoliating toxins, enterotoxins / plasmids
Yersinia pestis	Fibrinolysin, coagulase / plasmid

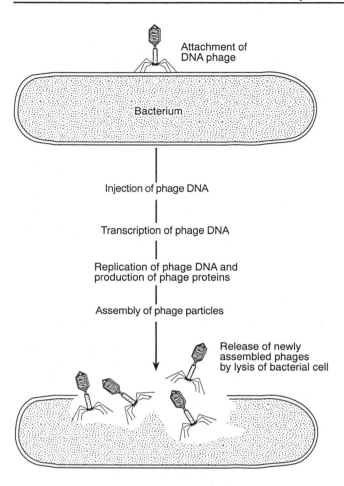

Attachment of
DNA phage

Bacterium

Injection of phage DNA

Transcription of phage DNA

Replication of phage DNA and
production of phage proteins

Assembly of phage particles

Release of newly
assembled phages
by lysis of bacterial cell

Figure 4.5 Replication of a double-stranded DNA phage. Attachment of phage to a specific receptor is followed by injection of phage DNA. Mature phages are released after lysis of the host cell.

Because of the complexity of conjugation, conjugative plasmids are relatively large, with genes occupying 30 kilobase pairs or more. During conjugation, plasmid DNA is the genetic material usually transferred. However, chromosomal DNA can sometimes be transferred especially when the F plasmid is integrated into the bacterial genome, forming a high frequency recombination (Hfr) strain. The F plasmid can integrate at specific sites in the bacterial chromosome. These sites represent regions of homology between the DNA of the bacterium and that of the plasmid. During conjugation of Hfr strains, the genes closest to the transferring end of the F plasmid are transferred first. The potential exists for transfer of the entire chromosome. However, this is an unlikely occurrence because transfer, which can take up to 100 minutes, is usually interrupted before completion.

Although conjugation is most frequently associated with Gram-negative bacteria, it can also occur in Gram-positive organisms. A sex pilus is not formed in Gram-positive bacteria; plasmid DNA can be transferred when the bacteria are in close contact.

Transduction

In transduction, DNA from a donor bacterium incorporated into the nucleic acid of a phage may be transferred by progeny of the phage to susceptible recipient cells. During a lytic cycle, DNA derived from any part of the host genome may be incorporated into the phage genome. In temperate phages, transduction affects only those bacterial genes adjacent to the prophage when a lytic cycle is induced. Transduction which occurs during a lytic cycle is termed generalized transduction. It occurs at a low frequency of one cell in 10^6 to 10^8 transduced for a particular bacterial characteristic or genetic marker. Specialized transduction may occur when a prophage is induced to undergo a lytic cycle by exposure to mutagens (Fig. 4.4). This type of transduction can result in the transfer of bacterial genes to many other cells because the bacterial genes are copied to all phage progeny. A small number of bacterial genes are excised with the prophage and some phage genes remain integrated in the bacterial chromosome when lysis occurs. Thus, the phage progeny are defective because some phage genes are missing.

Transformation

This process involves the transfer of genes in a free segment of chromosomal DNA from a lysed donor bacterium to a competent recipient. Natural transformation is uncommon and occurs in few bacterial genera. Transformation is limited to particular bacterial cells and such cells are termed 'competent'. The competent cells can bind naked DNA which is transported into the cell. A specific protein binds to the DNA and protects it from intracellular nucleases; the DNA subsequently integrates into the bacterial genome.

Box 4.1 Mutations which occur in bacteria.

- Base-pair substitution producing:
  — silent mutations
  — nonsense mutations
  — mis-sense mutations
- Microinsertions or microdeletions of base pairs
  — frame shift mutations
- Reversions
  — back mutations reversing point mutations
    (base-pair substitution)
- Deletions of multiple base pairs
- Insertions during recombination resulting in errors
- Translocation of DNA segments within the genome
- Inversions
  — inverted orientation of a segment of DNA within
    the chromosome

Transposons

These genetic elements, sometimes called 'jumping genes' can move from one location to another in the genome. They can also become integrated into plasmid DNA. Simple transposons, termed insertion sequences, have only those genes required for incorporation into new locations. Complex transposons have additional genes such as those encoding antibiotic resistance which can ensure survival in the face of antimicrobial therapy. Insertion of a transposon into a gene essential for bacterial survival results in cell death. Transposons cannot replicate independently. Replication occurs only during the replicative process of a bacterial chromosome or plasmid into which they are inserted.

Integrons and gene cassettes

In addition to transposons, another system for providing bacteria with genetic diversity involves integrons. These genetic units contain information for the recognition of the specific recombination site of a gene cassette, a 'mobile' genetic element usually coding for antibiotic resistance. Gene cassettes encoding for other biochemical reactions and for virulence factors have been described (Ploy *et al.*, 2000). Excision and insertion of gene cassettes is facilitated by an integrase present in integrons. In addition, integrons provide promoters for the expression of the genes carried by the gene cassette. The ability to acquire and express new genes allows integrons to contribute to genetic variability in chromosomal and non-chromosomal DNA. Moreover, they appear to play a major role in the transmission, through conjugation, of antibiotic resistance among Gram-negative bacteria.

Functions of bacterial genetic elements

The bacterial chromosome codes for all essential metabolic functions of the cell. Other elements such as plasmids and transposons code for additional functions that may be advantageous for cell survival. Genes which encode functions such as toxin production and antibiotic resistance may be carried on these genetic elements. The attributes of some pathogenic bacteria mediated by particular genetic elements are presented in Table 4.1. Antibiotic resistance, a property encoded by plasmids, is significant in both human and veterinary medicine. When the genes for antibiotic resistance are located on conjugative plasmids, the resistance can be transmitted between bacterial species and sometimes between different bacterial genera. Options for effective chemotherapy may be severely limited by transfer of antibiotic resistance between pathogenic bacteria and by transfer from pathogens to bacteria in the normal flora of humans and animals.

Phage typing

Techniques employing lytic phages can be used for the identification of human and veterinary pathogens. These techniques are based on observations that particular phages infect and lyse specific bacterial strains. The pattern of susceptibility of a bacterial isolate, tested against a panel of typing phages, establishes its phage type. Some phages, which lyse all members of a bacterial species, can be used to identify organisms to species level. More often, phages infect only some strains of a bacterial species and they can be used to characterize organisms at subspecies level. Phage typing is frequently used on isolates of *Staphylococcus aureus*, *Salmonella* Typhimurium and *Salmonella* Enteritidis to identify sources of infection in outbreaks of food-poisoning.

Molecular typing

In addition to phage typing, bacteria can be characterized according to the composition of their chromosomal and extrachromosomal DNA (*see* Chapter 5). Characterization of organisms based on the genetic composition of their plasmids or transposable elements may be used for typing purposes. Definitive identification of a pathogen, based on possession of the genes for virulence factors such as those listed in Table 4.1, can be carried out using gene probes regardless of gene location.

Genetic manipulation of bacteria

Genetic variation, which occurs naturally in bacteria, can be utilized in the laboratory for genetic engineering. Genes can be inserted into plasmids to form recombinant plasmids. These can be introduced into bacterial cells and propagated. The genes, which are required for insertion into the plasmid, can be produced by cleaving donor DNA containing the genes using restriction enzymes. These enzymes, which cleave the nucleic acid asymetrically, produce DNA fragments with cohesive 'sticky' ends. If recipient plasmid DNA is cut using the same restriction endonuclease as that used for donor DNA, the cohesive ends of donor and plasmid DNA are complementary. The donor fragment can be incorporated using DNA ligase into the cleaved plasmid which is restored to its circular form. The plasmid can then be acquired by bacteria through the process of transformation. Although transformation through plasmids rarely occurs naturally, uptake of plasmids by host cells in the laboratory can be facilitated by manipulating environmental conditions. Exposure to electrical stimuli can also facilitate uptake of plasmid DNA. Propagation of the host cell produces a population of identical cells, a clone in which each cell contains a copy of the new genetic material. The plasmid used to introduce the new genes is termed the cloning vector. Plasmids are used as cloning vectors because they replicate independently without integration into the bacterial chromosome. Bacteriophages can also be used as cloning vectors.

Genetic engineering is currently used for the production of vaccines, hormones and other pharmaceutical products. Vaccines produced in this manner are potentially safer than conventional vaccines. The genes which code for the vaccine antigens can be cloned separately from genes encoding replication of the parent organism. Genetically engineered vaccines, therefore, may stimulate an effective immune response without the risk of introducing a pathogen capable of replicating in vaccinated animals.

Reference

Ploy, M.C., Lambert, T., Couty, J-P. and Denis, F. (2000). Integrons: An antibiotic resistance gene-capture expression system. *Clinical Chemistry and Laboratory Medicine*, **38**, 483–487.

Further reading

Berg, D.E. and Howe, M.M. (1989). *Mobile DNA*. American Society for Microbiology, Washington, DC.

Holloway, B.W. (1993). Genetics for all bacteria. *Annual Reviews of Microbiology*, **47**, 659–671.

Madigan, M.T., Martinko, J.M. and Parker, J. (1997). Microbial genetics. In *Brock, Biology of Microorganisms*. Eighth Edition. Prentice Hall International, London. pp. 304-356.

Pelczar, M.J., Chan, E.C.S. and Krieg, N.R. (1993). Inheritance and variability. In *Microbiology: Concepts and Applications*. McGraw-Hill, New York. pp. 350–379.

Riley, M. and Drlica, K. (1990). *The Bacterial Chromosome*. American Society for Microbiology, Washington, DC.

Schlegel, H.G. (1993). Constancy, change, recombination and transfer of genetic information. In *General Microbiology*. Seventh Edition. Cambridge University Press, Cambridge. pp. 484–537.

Singleton, P. (1997). Bacteriophages. In *Bacteriology, Biotechnology and Medicine*. Fourth Edition Wiley, Chichester. pp. 204–214.

Chapter 5

Laboratory diagnosis of bacterial disease

Laboratory investigation of bacterial disease is necessary for identifying the aetiological agent and, sometimes, for determining the antimicrobial susceptibility of pathogens. A full clinical history including the age, sex, species and number of animals affected and treatment administered should accompany the specimens, together with a tentative clinical diagnosis. In the absence of adequate clinical information, procedures for the detection of relevant pathogens may not be carried out.

Selection, collection and transportation of specimens

The accuracy and validity of the results of laboratory examinations are largely influenced by the care taken in the selection, collection and submission of samples to the laboratory. Particular points should be considered when dealing with clinical specimens.

- Ideally, specimens should be obtained from live animals before administration of antimicrobial therapy. Samples from dead animals should be collected, if possible, before autolytic or putrefactive changes occur.
- Specimens, from a site most likely to yield a pathogen, should be collected using procedures which minimize contamination.
- In warm weather, refrigeration of samples may be required.
- Samples must be submitted in separate leak-proof containers. Each container should be labelled with the identity of the animal, the type of specimen and the date of collection.
- In some circumstances, specimens may be required for particular diagnostic procedures.

Identification of pathogenic bacteria

The presence of pathogenic bacteria can be confirmed by examination of stained smears, cultural and biochemical characteristics and detection by immunological and molecular methods.

Examination of stained smears

Staining methods routinely used in diagnostic bacteriology are presented in Table 5.1. Gram-stained smears from tissues or exudates are useful rapid procedures for demonstrating bacteria present in large numbers. The contrast between Gram-positive bacteria and tissue debris is marked rendering them easier to detect in smears than Gram-negative organisms. The Ziehl-Neelsen stain is used to detect pathogenic mycobacteria. *Coxiella burnetii*, *Brucella* species, *Nocardia* species and chlamydiae can be demonstrated in smears using the modified Ziehl-Neelsen stain. The fluorescent antibody staining method gives rapid, specific identification of bacterial pathogens in smears and cryostat tissue sections. Although this technique is suitable for identifying many bacterial species, it is particularly useful for pathogens, such as *Clostridium chauvoei*, spirochaetes, *Campylobacter fetus* and *Lawsonia intracellularis*, which are difficult to culture.

Table 5.1 Routine staining methods for bacteria.

Method	Comments
Gram stain	Widely used for the routine staining of bacteria in smears. The crystal violet, which is retained in cell walls despite decolourization, stains Gram-positive bacteria blue. In contrast, Gram-negative bacteria which do not retain the crystal violet are counterstained red
Giemsa	Useful for demonstrating *Dermatophilus congolensis*, rickettsiae and *Borrelia* species which stain blue
Dilute carbol fuchsin	Especially useful for recognizing *Campylobacter* species, *Brachyspira* species and *Fusobacterium* species which stain red
Polychrome methylene blue	Used for the identification of *Bacillus anthracis* in blood smears. The organisms stain blue with distinctive pink capsules
Ziehl-Neelsen stain	Hot concentrated carbol fuchsin which penetrates mycobacterial cell walls is retained after acid-alcohol decolourization. The red-staining bacteria are described as acid-fast or Ziehl-Neelsen positive
Modified Ziehl-Neelsen stain	Unlike the Ziehl-Neelsen stain, this method employs dilute carbol fuchsin with decolourization by acetic acid

Cultural and biochemical characteristics

The selection of culture medium, atmospheric conditions and other features essential for isolation are determined by the pathogenic bacterium suspected. Routine isolation of many pathogens involves inoculation of blood agar and MacConkey agar plates followed by incubation for 24 to 48 hours.

Media used in diagnostic bacteriology are indicated in Table 5.2. Nutrient agar is a basic medium which supplies essential nutrients for the growth of non-fastidious bacteria. However, nutrient agar is unsuitable for the primary isolation of fastidious pathogenic bacteria. The growth characteristics and reactions on blood agar and MacConkey agar form the basis for the preliminary identification of many bacterial pathogens. Blood agar, which supports the growth of most pathogens, is

Table 5.2 Laboratory media used for the isolation and presumptive identification of bacterial pathogens.

Medium	Comments
Nutrient agar	A basic medium on which non-fastidious bacteria can grow. Suitable for demonstrating colonial morphology and pigment production; also used for viable counting methods
Blood agar	An enriched medium which supports the growth of most pathogenic bacteria and is used for their primary isolation. Allows the recognition of bacterial haemolysin production
MacConkey agar	A selective medium containing bile which is especially useful for isolation of enterobacteria and some other Gram-negative bacteria. Allows differentiation of lactose fermenters and non-lactose fermenters. Colonies of lactose fermenters and the surrounding medium are pink
Selenite broth, Rappaport-Vassiliadis broth	Selective enrichment media used for the isolation of salmonellae from samples containing other Gram-negative enteric organisms
Edwards medium	A blood agar-based selective medium used for the isolation and recognition of streptococci
Chocolate agar	Heat-treated blood agar which supplies special growth requirements (X and V factors) for the isolation of *Haemophilus* species and for the culture of *Taylorella equigenitalis*
Brilliant green agar	An indicator medium for the presumptive identification of *Salmonella* species. Salmonella colonies and surrounding medium have a pink colour
Buffered peptone water	A non-selective enrichment medium often used for isolation of pathogens when present in low numbers in samples collected from foods and environmental sources

appropriate for routine primary isolation. Selective media may be used for particular organisms. Some media are designed to give a presumptive identification of bacterial colonies on the basis of biochemical reactions. MacConkey agar, which contains bile salts, is selective for many Gram-negative bacteria. This medium contains lactose with neutral red as a pH indicator. If an organism growing on this medium ferments lactose, the acidic byproducts turn the medium red. Non-lactose fermenting bacteria metabolize the peptones in the medium, generating alkaline byproducts which impart a yellowish colouration to the medium and the colonies.

Plates should be inoculated using a streaking technique which facilitates growth of isolated colonies (Fig. 5.1). This is an essential step for the identification of pathogens in clinical specimens which may contain microbial contaminants. Such contaminants may derive from the normal flora or from environmental sources. Definitive identification of a potential pathogen involves subculture of an isolated colony to obtain a pure growth which can then be subjected to biochemical or other tests.

Morphological characteristics and biochemical tests allow presumptive identification of a bacterial pathogen (Box 5.1). Additional features, which may aid identification, include pigment and odour production on both blood agar and MacConkey agar and the production of haemolysis on blood agar. Definitive identification of bacteria is usually based on biochemical tests and serology. Additional tests can be used to aid identification of particular organisms (Table 5.3).

Biochemical techniques

Catalase, an enzyme produced by many aerobes and facultative anaerobes, causes the breakdown of hydrogen peroxide to oxygen and water. A positive oxidase test indicates the presence of cytochrome oxidase C in the bacterial cell. Reactions in oxidation-fermentation medium can be used to identify the atmospheric requirements of certain pathogens (Fig. 5.2).

Biochemical tests relate to the catabolic activities of bacteria and an indicator system is usually employed to demonstrate the utilization of a particular substrate (Table 5.4). Because the range of sugars utilized by individual bacterial species is usually limited, catabolism of different

---

Box 5.1 Criteria for the presumptive identification of bacterial pathogens.

- Colonial morphology and colour
- Presence or absence of haemolysis on blood agar
- Appearance when stained by the Gram method
- Motility
- Ability to grow on MacConkey agar
- Reaction in the oxidation-fermentation test
- Reactions in catalase and oxidase tests

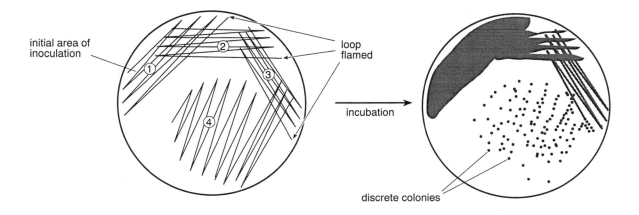

Figure 5.1 Plate culture technique for obtaining isolated colonies on an agar medium. With a sterile inoculating loop, a sample of the specimen (the inoculum) is spread over a small area at the edge of the plate, the 'well' (1). The inoculum is spread from the well sequentially over three contiguous areas of the plate (2, 3, 4). The loop is sterilized by flaming before inoculation of each area. When carried out carefully, the procedure results in a reduction in bacterial numbers at each step. In area 4, discrete bacterial colonies can be recognised after incubation.

sugars is frequently used for identification. Several commercial companies produce miniaturized versions of biochemical tests for the identification of bacteria. These usually consist of a strip of plastic cupules containing the requisite reagents for each test to which a suspension of the bacterium for identification is added. The identity of the organism can be deduced from the pattern of the reactions in the cupules. Strips are available for different

Table 5.3 Tests used in the identification of particular bacterial pathogens.

Test	Pathogens	Comments
CAMP reaction	*Streptococcus agalactiae* *Rhodococcus equi* *Actinobacillus pleuropneumoniae* *Listeria monocytogenes*	Haemolysis caused by *Staphylococcus aureus* is enhanced by pathogenic bacteria growing close to staphylococcal colonies
Pitting of Loeffler's serum slope	*Arcanobacterium pyogenes*	Proteolytic digestion of the medium around colonies
Haem-agglutination	*Bordetella bronchiseptica*	Agglutination of suspended ovine red blood cells by the bacteria
Nagler test	*Clostridium perfringens*	Breakdown of lecithin in egg yolk agar by alpha toxin (lecithinase) produced by the organism. Surface application of antitoxin inhibits the alpha toxin activity

categories of bacteria including the enterobacteria, non-enteric Gram-negative organisms, anaerobes and strepto-cocci.

Immunological techniques

Serotyping is based on the immunological identification of surface antigens on pathogens such as *Escherichia coli* and other members of the *Enterobacteriaceae, Listeria monocytogenes, Pasteurella multocida* and *Actinobacillus pleuropneumoniae.*

Immunological techniques such as fluorescent antibody staining can be used for identifying bacterial pathogens. Antigen capture and direct enzyme-linked immunosorbent assays have been developed for some bacterial pathogens and require the immobilization of specific antibody on a solid phase. The bacterial agent, if present in the diagnostic specimen, is bound by the specific antibody and can be demonstrated by an enzyme-labelled antibody. Techniques using immune reactions may be combined with other methods for improving detection of pathogens. Immunomagnetic separation, in which magnetic particles coated with antibodies to the particular pathogen bind the organism, combines physical and immunological methods. Immunomagnetic separation is usually followed by either cultural identification or molecular characterization of the organism.

Phage typing

The fact that a particular phage is specific for a limited number of susceptible strains of bacteria allows differentiation by phage typing. Using this method, bacterial species can be subdivided into subtypes which are defined by their susceptibility to particular phages. Phage typing is commonly used to differentiate isolates of

Aerobic bacteria

Colour change (acid production) indicating utilization of glucose by aerobic bacteria confined to top layer of medium, exposed to air

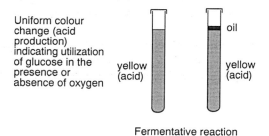

yellow (acid)

green

oil

green

Oxidative reaction   No reaction

Facultative anaerobic bacteria

Uniform colour change (acid production) indicating utilization of glucose in the presence or absence of oxygen

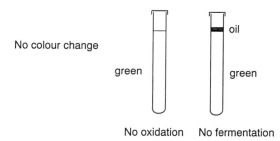

yellow (acid)

oil

yellow (acid)

Fermentative reaction

Bacteria unable to grow or, alternatively, to utilize glucose

No colour change

green

oil

green

No oxidation   No fermentation

Figure 5.2 The possible reactions produced by bacteria in oxidation-fermentation medium which has a green colour before inoculation (Indicator: bromothymol blue).

Staphylococcus aureus and *Salmonella enterica* subspecies *enterica* serotypes Typhi, Typhimurium and Enteritidis. Detailed typing may be employed in epidemiological investigations when tracing the origin of a pathogen.

Molecular techniques
Selected molecular techniques can be used for the detection and enumeration of pathogenic bacteria. These techniques, along with phage typing and serotyping, may also be of use in epidemiological investigations. In addition, molecular techniques assist in determining the virulence of an isolate by identifying genes associated with pathogenic properties.

The main molecular biological techniques for pathogen

detection are nucleic acid hybridization and the polymerase chain reaction (PCR). In nucleic acid hybridization, synthetic nucleic acid probes, specific for a particular pathogen, are applied either to prepared clinical specimens or to genetic material extracted from the pathogen. Probes can be designed to detect DNA or RNA. However, the usefulness of RNA probes is limited by the lability of the RNA molecule. Nevertheless, diagnostic tests based on the detection of RNA can be particularly useful in specific areas such as food microbiology because they allow discrimination of viable from dead microorganisms. Probes can be designed to detect all members of a particular genus or to detect strains of organisms within a species. For example, a probe for the detection of the gene which encodes 16S ribosomal RNA can often detect all members of a genus because it is highly conserved in the species within a genus. In contrast, intergenic regions display more variability and are useful for designing probes to discriminate between different strains within a species.

Assays based on the direct detection of DNA or RNA are relatively insensitive because they usually require large numbers of bacteria (10^4 to 10^5) in the specimen. For specimens containing small numbers of bacteria, amplification of the nucleic acid of the target organisms by PCR can be used. After amplification of a specific fragment of DNA, using either a DNA or RNA template, the PCR product can then be identified by its electrophoretic

Table 5.4 Biochemical tests used for the presumptive identification of bacterial pathogens.

Test	Indicator	Comments
Sugars in peptone water	Andrade's	Used for differentiating *Streptococcus* species
Triple sugar iron	Phenol red	Used for presumptive identification of *Salmonella* species
Hydrogen sulphide production	Iron or lead compounds	Employed in tests for *Salmonella* and *Brucella* species
Decarboxylase	Bromocresol purple	Used for presumptive identification of enterobacteria
Urease	Phenol red	Used for the presumptive identification of *Proteus* species and *Corynebacterium renale*
Indole test Methyl red test Voges-Proskauer test Citrate utilization	Kovac's reagent Methyl red Oxidation of acetoin Bromothymol blue	Used for identification of enterobacteria; collectively known as IMViC tests

pattern using appropriate size-marker molecules.

Restriction endonuclease analysis and gene probes are two methods employed for epidemiological investigations. The selected technique must be convenient to use and must discriminate between closely related strains by detecting genetic differences of epidemiological significance. Restriction endonucleases can be used to cleave chromosomal or plasmid DNA to generate fragments which can then be separated by gel electrophoresis. Analysis of the resulting electrophoretic patterns allows comparison of isolates. Restriction enzymes which cleave DNA in only a few places produce large fragments which can be separated using pulsed-field gel electrophoresis, a method frequently used in epidemiological studies.

Serology

Many potentially pathogenic bacteria are present as part of the normal flora of a host or are common in the environment. As animals are frequently exposed to these bacteria, they may produce antibodies to the organisms. Antibodies demonstrable in a serum sample are, therefore, evidence of exposure to an infectious agent but they do not necessarily confirm an aetiological role for that agent. Despite these limitations, serological tests are used extensively for confirming infection with particular pathogens in susceptible animals.

Further reading

Murray, P.R., Baron, E.J., Pfaller, M.A., Tenover, F.C. and Yolken, R.H. (1999). *Manual of Clinical Microbiology*. Seventh Edition. American Society for Microbiology, Washington, DC.

Quinn, P.J., Carter, M.E., Markey, B.K. and Carter, G.R. (1994). *Clinical Veterinary Microbiology*, Mosby-Year Book Europe, London.

Smith, T.J., O'Connor, L., Glennon, M. and Maher, M. (2000). Molecular diagnostics in food safety: rapid detection of food-borne pathogens. *Irish Journal of Agricultural and Food Research*, **39**, 309–319.

Chapter 6

Antimicrobial agents

Antibiotics are low molecular weight microbial metabolites which can kill or inhibit the growth of susceptible bacteria. The term 'antibiotic' is also often loosely used to describe synthetic antimicrobial agents which may or may not be derived from microbial metabolites.

Antibiotic activity was first recorded in 1929 by Alexander Fleming when he observed the lytic effect of a colony of the mould *Penicillium notatum* on neighbouring staphylococcal colonies on a culture plate. The active principle of the mould was called penicillin. Early attempts to purify penicillin from fluid cultures of the mould were unsuccessful. Moreover, the sulphonamides, synthetic antibacterial agents, were developed in the 1930s by Domagk. As a result, the therapeutic potential of penicillin remained unrealized. The successful purification of penicillin in 1940 by Florey and Chain allowed clinical testing of the antibiotic to proceed. After a relatively short time, with the participation of the pharmaceutical industry, large scale production of penicillin commenced and the antibiotic became freely available. The discovery and development of many other antibacterial agents followed (Table 6.1). It was widely accepted that antibiotic therapy could signal the end of bacterial infections as a significant cause of mortality in human and animal populations. However, this premature optimism has been dispelled by the emergence of antibiotic resistance, an intractable problem, in many bacterial pathogens.

The therapeutic use of antibiotics depends on their selective toxicity; these drugs kill or inhibit bacterial pathogens without direct toxicity for animals receiving treatment. The basis of the selective toxicity of many antibiotics is poorly understood. However, biochemical differences in structures or metabolic pathways between mammalian and bacterial cells frequently account for selective antibacterial toxicity. Penicillin, for example, inhibits cell wall synthesis by acting on peptidoglycan, a component unique to bacterial cell walls. Only a small percentage of the large number of known antibiotics exhibit sufficient selective toxicity to be therapeutically useful. Individual antibacterial agents are not effective against all pathogenic bacteria. Some are active against a narrow range of bacterial species while broad spectrum antibiotics such as the tetracyclines and chloramphenicol are active against many species.

Mode and site of action

In order to interfere with bacterial cell growth, antibacterial agents must interact with a vital structure or block a metabolic pathway. The modes and sites of action of antibacterial drugs are indicated in Fig. 6.1. At therapeutic levels, antibacterial agents are usually either bacteriostatic or bactericidal. Bacteriostatic agents inhibit

Table 6.1 Antimicrobial agents derived from microorganisms.

Microorganism	Antimicrobial agent
Bacillus colistinus	Colistin (polymyxin E)
B. polymyxa	Polymyxin B
B. subtilis	Bacitracin
Cephalosporium species (F)[a]	Cephalosporins
Chromobacterium violaceum	Monobactams
Micromonospora purpurea	Gentamicin
Penicillium notatum (F) and other species	Penicillin G
P. griseofulvin (F)	Griseofulvin (anti-fungal activity only)
Streptomyces species	Spectinomycin Tetracyclines
S. cattleya	Carbapenems
S. erythreus	Erythromycin
S. fradiae	Neomycin
S. griseus	Streptomycin
S. kanomyceticus	Kanamycin
S. lincolnensis	Lincomycin
S. mediterranei	Rifamycin
S. nodosus	Amphotericin B (anti-fungal activity only)
S. orientalis	Vancomycin
S. venezuelae	Chloramphenicol

a   (F), fungus

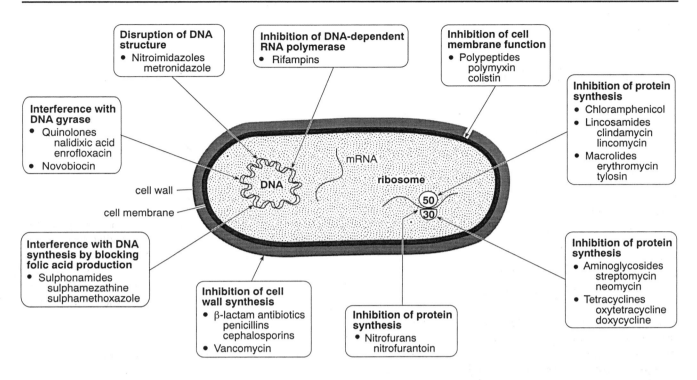

Figure 6.1 Modes and sites of action of antibacterial drugs.

the growth of bacteria, allowing host immune defenses to eliminate the infection. If this type of therapeutic agent is not maintained at effective concentrations in the tissues, dissociation of the drug-cell structure complex can occur, permitting bacterial survival. In contrast, bactericidal agents cause irreparable damage and bacterial cell death by binding irreversibly to target structures. At high concentrations some bacteriostatic agents can be bactericidal. Antibacterial agents may inhibit the synthesis of cell walls, proteins or nucleic acids. In addition, they may disrupt cell membrane function. The major classes of antibacterial drugs and their modes of action are listed in Table 6.2.

Inhibition of cell wall synthesis

Because peptidoglycan is a unique component of bacterial cell walls, antibacterial agents which prevent cross-linking of peptidoglycan chains inhibit cell wall synthesis and are selectively toxic for bacteria. The penicillins and cephalosporins comprise the largest and most important class of antibacterial drugs which inhibit cell wall synthesis. Their bactericidal activity relates to this effect in actively growing cells. The basic structure of β-lactam antibiotics is illustrated in Figure 6.2. Semi-synthetic penicillins and cephalosporins can be produced by incorporating various chemical side chains into the basic molecules. Differences in side chains of the particular antibiotic influence their spectrum of activity, stability and resistance to β-lactamases. The mode of action of β-lactam antibiotics involves binding to cell receptors

known as penicillin binding proteins (PBPs). In addition to interfering with transpeptidation, many of these drugs promote autolysin activity causing cell lysis.

Bacteria which produce β-lactamases are resistant to β-lactam antibiotics. β-lactamases cleave the β-lactam ring rendering the antibiotic ineffective. These enzymes may be plasmid-mediated as in staphylococci, or they may be chromosomally encoded as in many Gram-negative bacteria. Tolerance to β-lactam antibiotics exhibited by some bacteria may relate to an inability of the antibiotic to induce autolysin activity. In these circumstances, although the cell wall is damaged and growth is inhibited, the bacteria survive. Differences in the structure and composition of the cell walls of Gram-positive and Gram-negative determines their susceptibility to β-lactam antibiotics. Because some antibacterial agents cannot penetrate the outer membrane of Gram-negative cells, their antimicrobial spectrum is confined to Gram-positive bacteria.

Inhibition of cell membrane function

If the functional integrity of the cell membrane is disrupted, macromolecules and ions escape from the cell, leading to cell damage and death. Comparatively few antibacterial agents act on the cell membrane; those which target it are usually bactericidal. Because antibacterial agents with this activity are more toxic for animal cells than other classes of antibiotics, their use is generally limited to topical application.

Table 6.2 Major classes of antimicrobial drugs and their modes of action.

Antimicrobial drug	Mode of action	Effect	Comments

β-Lactam antibiotics
  Penicillins
  Cephalosporins
	Inhibition of cell wall synthesis	Bactericidal	Low toxicity. Many are inactivated by β-lactamases

Vancomycin	Inhibition of cell wall synthesis	Bactericidal	Used against methicillin-resistant *Staphylococcus aureus*

Polypeptides
  Polymyxin
  Colistin
	Inhibition of cell membrane function	Bactericidal	Resistance slow to develop. Potentially nephrotoxic and neurotoxic

Nitrofurans Nitrofurantoin	Inhibition of protein synthesis	Bacteriostatic	Synthetic agents with broad-spectrum activity. Relatively toxic

Aminoglycosides
  Streptomycin
  Neomycin
	Inhibition of protein synthesis. Block 30S ribosomal activity	Bactericidal	Active mainly against Gram-negative bacteria. Ototoxic and nephrotoxic

Tetracyclines
  Oxytetracycline
  Doxycycline
	Inhibition of protein synthesis. Block 30S ribosomal activity	Bacteriostatic	Formerly used in feed for prophylactic medication. Development of resistance common

Chloramphenicol Florfenicol	Inhibition of protein synthesis. Block 50S ribosomal activity	Bacteriostatic	Use prohibited in food-producing animals in some countries. Potentially toxic

Lincosamides
  Clindamycin
  Lincomycin
	Inhibition of protein synthesis. Block 50S ribosomal activity	Bactericidal or bacteriostatic	May be toxic in many species. Contraindicated in horses and neonatal animals. Oral administration is hazardous in ruminants

Macrolides
  Erythromycin
  Tylosin
	Inhibition of protein synthesis. Block 50S ribosomal activity	Bacteriostatic	Active against Gram-positive bacteria. Some macrolides active against mycoplasmal pathogens

Quinolones
  Nalidixic acid
  Enrofloxacin
	Inhibition of nucleic acid synthesis by blocking DNA gyrase	Bactericidal	Synthetic agents used for treating enteric infections and for intracellular pathogens

Novobiocin	Inhibition of nucleic acid synthesis by blocking DNA gyrase	Bactericidal or bacteriostatic	Often used along with other compatible drugs for treatment of mastitis
Rifampins	Inhibition of nucleic acid synthesis by blocking DNA-directed RNA polymerase	Bacteriostatic	Antimycobacterial activity; used with erythromycin for treating *Rhodococcus equi* infections

Sulphonamides
  Sulphamezathine
  Sulphamethoxazole
	Inhibition of nucleic acid synthesis by competitive blocking of para-aminobenzoic acid (PABA) incorporation into folic acid	Bacteriostatic	Synthetic structural analogues of PABA active against rapidly growing bacteria

Trimethoprim	Inhibition of nucleic acid synthesis by combining with the enzyme dihydrofolate reductase	Bacteriostatic	Usually administered with sulphamethoxazole. This combination, referred to as a potentiated sulphonamide, is bactericidal
Nitroimidazoles Metronidazole	Disruption of DNA structure and inhibition of DNA repair	Bactericidal	Particularly active against anaerobic bacteria; also active against some protozoa

Inhibition of protein synthesis

A number of classes of antibacterial agents inhibit protein synthesis. The selective toxicity of some antibiotics relates to the difference in structure between prokaryotic (70S) and eukaryotic (80S) ribosomes. Such antibiotics bind to receptors on the 30S or 50S subunits of bacterial ribosomes. Aminoglycosides bind to 30S ribosomal subunits and affect a number of different steps in protein synthesis. This results in the formation of non-functional proteins. Resistance to aminoglycosides may be intrinsic due to lack of a specific receptor on the subunit. Extrinsic resistance is conferred by plasmids, which may encode a number of enzymes capable of degrading antimicrobial drugs. In some bacteria, particularly anaerobes, the active

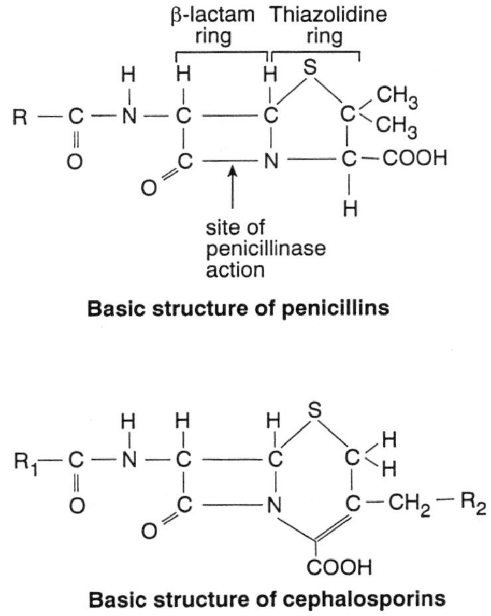

Basic structure of penicillins

Basic structure of cephalosporins

Figure 6.2 Basic structure of penicillin and cephalosporin molecules. Biological activities of different penicillins and cephalosporins are influenced by their side chain structures (R).

transport system essential for the intake of aminoglycosides may be lacking.

Tetracyclines also enter cells by an active uptake process and bind to receptors on the 30S subunit. They block attachment of tRNA molecules to acceptor sites preventing the addition of amino acids to the polypeptide chain. Chloramphenicol, an antibiotic which binds to the 50S subunit, also prevents the linking of amino acids to growing polypeptide chains. The antibacterial activity of both of these classes of drugs is diminished if effective concentrations are not maintained for the required period.

Macrolide antibiotics also inhibit protein synthesis by blocking 50S subunit activity. Although these antibiotics are bacteriostatic, at high concentrations they can be bactericidal. Resistance to macrolide antibiotics is plasmid-mediated and involves alteration of the binding site on the 50S ribosomal subunit.

Inhibition of nucleic acid synthesis

Many antibacterial agents including quinolones, novobiocin, rifampin, nitroimidazoles and sulphonamides inhibit nucleic acid synthesis (Table 6.2). The quinolones and novobiocin act on DNA gyrase, the enzyme which separates the strands of DNA during bacterial replication. Although novobiocin is active against staphylococci and streptococci, its use is limited to local intramammary therapy because of its toxicity. Rifampin, by interfering with the activity of DNA-dependent RNA polymerase, prevents RNA synthesis. This antibiotic is active against Gram-positive bacteria including mycobacteria. It is usually used in combination with other antibacterial agents

because of the rapid development of resistant organisms. Metronidazole, the most commonly used drug of the nitroimidazole class, causes breaks in DNA strands and is particularly effective against obligate anaerobic bacteria.

Sulphonamides interfere with the formation of folic acid, an essential precursor for nucleic acid synthesis. Their action relates to their structural similarity to para-aminobenzoic acid (PABA). When present at sufficient concentrations, sulphonamides are utilized by the enzyme dihydropteroate synthetase instead of PABA (Fig. 6.3), forming non-functional analogues of folic acid. The synthetic pyrimidine derivative, trimethoprim, inhibits the activity of dihydrofolate reductase, a later step in the synthesis of folic acid by bacteria. When used in combination, the action of each drug is potentiated resulting in enhanced activity against bacteria. Potentiated sulphonamides are selectively toxic for bacteria because animals can absorb preformed folic acid from their feed.

Combined antibacterial therapy

When antibacterial drugs are combined for the treatment of disease, the outcome is influenced by the particular combinations in use. An additive effect is produced when the combined action of the drugs is equivalent to the sum of the actions of each drug when administered separately. A synergistic effect results when the combined action of two drugs is significantly greater than the sum of effects of each drug used separately. Indifference is defined as lack of an enhancement effect when two drugs are administered in combination. Antagonism describes the reduced effectiveness of combined antibacterial therapy when compared to the effectiveness of each drug alone.

These effects, which can be demonstrated *in vivo* and *in vitro*, must be considered when selecting drugs for combined treatment of infected animals. If a bacteriostatic drug is combined with a bactericidal drug, antagonism may occur. Bactericidal drugs, particularly the β-lactam

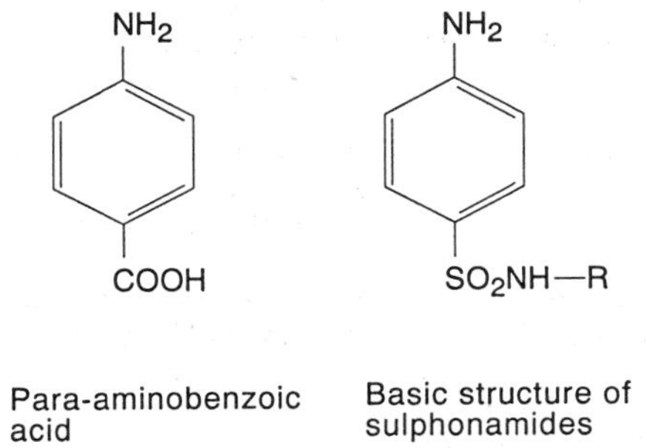

Para-aminobenzoic acid

Basic structure of sulphonamides

Figure 6.3 Sulphonamides, analogues of para-aminobenzoic acid, competitively inhibit the enzyme dihydropteroate synthetase preventing folate production, an essential step in the production of bacterial DNA. This type of activity is known as competitive inhibition.

antibiotics, are effective against actively dividing cells. If they are combined with a bacteriostatic drug, which inhibits bacterial growth, their bactericidal activity may be abolished. Drugs which act synergistically include sulphonamides and trimethoprim, which act at two different sites in the folic acid pathway, and clavulanic acid and penicillin combinations, in which clavulanic acid inhibits β-lactamase activity preventing inactivation of penicillin.

Factors influencing antibacterial activity

The activity of antibacterial agents is influenced *in vivo* by the site and rate of absorption, the site of excretion and the tissue distribution and metabolism of a particular agent. In addition, antibacterial activity can be affected by interactions between pathogen and drug and between host and pathogen.

Drug-pathogen interactions

The response of a bacterial pathogen to exposure to a drug *in vivo* may differ considerably from that *in vitro*. The environment *in vitro* tends to be constant whereas pathogens may encounter different environments in various organs and tissues of a host. Following therapeutic administration, the distribution and concentration of a drug can vary widely. For example, some drugs can cross the blood-brain barrier while others are concentrated in the urine during excretion. If pathogens are quiescent in the presence of bactericidal drugs such as penicillin, they may survive and multiply later producing clinical disease. Because of their location, intracellular bacteria tend to be resistant to chemotherapeutic agents. A drug, bound to proteins and other tissue components, may have reduced effectiveness. Moreover, products of inflammatory reactions such as pus and necrotic debris may adsorb antibacterial agents. The acidic environment in necrotic tissue can also inhibit the activity of some antibacterial drugs.

Host-pathogen interaction

Antimicrobial drug administration can alter the host's immune response and may change the normal flora, particularly on the skin and in the intestinal tract. Disturbance of the normal intestinal flora, following therapy for salmonellosis, may allow the development of a prolonged carrier state. In addition, major disturbance of the normal flora may permit overgrowth of resistant organisms leading to disease. In horses treated orally with antibiotics, *Clostridium difficile* overgrowth can cause acute colitis. Many inflammatory responses may be modified by drug administration. Acute responses can become chronic if drug therapy suppresses the growth of a pathogen while permitting its survival.

Antibacterial drug resistance

Resistance to antibacterial drugs is an increasingly important problem in both humans and animals. The widespread, sometimes indiscriminate, use of these drugs results in the selection of bacteria which are inherently resistant. Not only may these resistant bacteria become the predominant species in a population but they may also transfer genetic material to susceptible bacteria which then acquire resistance. Antibacterial drug resistance can be encoded either in the bacterial chromosome or in plasmids. Resistance genes can be transferred between bacteria through transduction, conjugation, transposable elements or transformation (Table 6.3). Resistance to an antibacterial agent often results in cross-resistance to other agents in the same class. This form of resistance is encountered with the sulphonamides, tetracyclines, aminoglycosides and macrolides. Plasmids and transposable elements often mediate multiple resistance, in which organisms become resistant to a number of drugs from different classes. This type of resistance can be transferred rapidly between different bacterial species and genera. It is particularly common in members of the *Enterobacteriaceae*, *Pseudomonas* species and anaerobes of the intestinal tract. Multiple drug resistance is of particular concern in *Salmonella* Typhimurium, which is one of the most common causes of human food poisoning in the developed world (Glynn *et al.*, 1998). Resistant strains of non-pathogenic *E. coli* were found in healthy children in cities in the USA, Venezuela and China (Lester *et al.*, 1990). The realization that non-pathogens can acquire resistance to antibacterial compounds is a cause for concern. The resistance patterns of the strains in the study correlated with the types and amount of antibiotics used in the general population. The findings suggest that there can be high levels of resistance in the endogenous bacterial flora of healthy human populations and there is, therefore, a risk of this resistance extending to pathogenic organisms also.

Resistance mechanisms

Mechanisms producing resistance to antibacterial drugs include production of enzymes by bacteria which destroy or inactivate the drug and reduction of bacterial cell permeability. Bacteria may also develop alternative metabolic pathways to those inhibited by the drug. The antibiotic may be eliminated from the cell or the target site of the drug may be structurally altered. Alteration of the target site and enzymatic destruction of the agent are probably the most common mechanisms whereby resistance can occur. Examples of resistance mechanisms in particular bacteria are presented in Table 6.3.

Strategies for limiting antibacterial resistance

Antibacterial resistance is widespread and control measures in a country may be ineffectual as a result of

Table 6.3 Antibacterial drug resistance.

Drug	Target	Examples of resistant bacteria / Genetic basis	Comments
Erythromycin	Ribosomal protein	*Staphylococcus aureus* / Chromosomal-based	Ribosomes unaffected by drug action due to structural change
Streptomycin	Ribosomal protein	*Enterobacteriaceae* / Chromosomal-based	Mutation results in altered ribosome
Tetracycline	Ribosomal protein	*Enterobacteriaceae* / Plasmid-mediated	Ribosome protection proteins produced
	Transport mechanisms	*Enterobacteriaceae* / Plasmid-mediated	Decreased absorption or development of energy-dependent efflux mechanism
Rifampin	DNA-dependent RNA polymerase	*Enterobacteriaceae* / Chromosomal-based	Mutation results in alteration of enzyme
Fluoroquinolones	DNA gyrase	*Enterobacteriaceae* / Chromosomal-based	Mutation results in structurally altered enzyme
	Cell membrane	*Enterobacteriaceae* / Chromosomal-based	Decreased permeability
β-lactam antibiotics	Penicillin-binding proteins (PBP)	*Staphylococcus aureus* / Chromosomal-based	Decreased affinity of PBP for drug
	Penicillin-binding proteins	*Enterobacteriaceae* / Chromosomal-based	Outer membrane of most Gram-negative bacteria inherently impermeable to drug
	Penicillin-binding proteins	*Staphylococcus aureus, Enterobacteriaceae* / Plasmid- or chromosomal-based	Enzymatic degradation of drug by β-lactamases.
Chloramphenicol	Peptidyltransferase	*Staphylococcus* species, *Streptococcus* species / Plasmid- or chromosomal-based	Inactivation of drug by a specific acetyltransferase
Sulphonamides	Dihydropteroate synthetase	*Enterobacteriaceae* / Plasmid- or chromosomal-based	New folic acid synthetic pathway employing sulphonamide-resistant enzyme

importing resistant bacteria in food or in the normal flora of animals or humans from countries in which controls are less stringent. Health professionals and the general public should be aware of the risks associated with resistance so that realistic control measures can be implemented. It is probable that measures to restrict antibiotic usage, combined with the control of bacterial contamination, may reduce the occurrence and dissemination of resistant organisms.

Recommendations for dealing with resistance to antibacterial drugs are contained in 'The Copenhagen Recommendations' (Rosdahl and Pedersen, 1998). Similar recommendations have been issued by expert committees in the UK (Anon., 1998, 1999) and the USA (Cohen, 1998). Effective surveillance systems to collect data on resistant organisms should be established at local, national and international levels. The supply and use of antibacterial drugs should be closely monitored to allow evaluation of the risks and benefits of therapy. Prescription of antimicrobial drugs should be based on sound medical and veterinary therapeutic principles. Ideally, antibiotic therapy should be dictated by the results of laboratory examinations and drugs should be administered at the recommended therapeutic dose and for

the prescribed period of time. There should be strict adherence to drug withdrawal periods following treatment of food-producing animals. Antimicrobial agents should not be used for growth promotion and greater reliance should be placed on improved hygiene measures, disinfection and vaccination for the prevention and control of infectious disease.

Antibacterial susceptibility testing

Tests to determine the most suitable antibiotic for the effective treatment in a given disease can be conducted on isolates from clinical cases. However, these tests which are carried out *in vitro* cannot allow for the various factors which may affect antibacterial activity *in vivo*. The results obtained following treatment may not reflect the susceptibility pattern of an isolate as determined in the laboratory. A number of antibacterial susceptibility tests are available including broth dilution, disc diffusion, agar gradient and some automated methods (Jorgensen *et al.*, 1999). The Kirby-Bauer disc diffusion method is a flexible and relatively inexpensive technique which is commonly used in diagnostic laboratories. This standard procedure (National Committee for Clinical Laboratory Standards, 1997) is

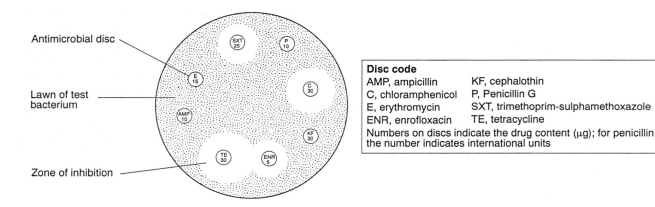

Figure 6.4 An antibiogram of *Escherichia coli* using a lawn of bacteria on Mueller-Hinton-based medium. Following the application of antimicrobial discs, the inoculated plate is incubated at 37°C for 18 hours. The diameters of the zones of inhibition are measured (mm) and compared to internationally-accepted measurements to determine the susceptibility or resistance of the isolate (Quinn *et al.*, 1994).

used mainly for testing rapidly-growing aerobic bacteria. Filter paper discs containing specified amounts of antibacterial agents are placed on agar uniformly seeded with the test bacterium. The procedure and the method of interpretation are indicated in Fig. 6.4. The diameter of each zone of inhibition is measured in millimetres and the results compared with standards for interpretation of the zone size (Quinn *et al.*, 1994). Susceptibility to an antibacterial drug indicates that the infection caused by the bacterium may respond to treatment if the drug reaches therapeutic levels in the affected tissues.

Determination of the minimum inhibitory concentration

Laboratory procedures for determining minimum inhibitory concentration (MIC) are illustrated in Fig. 6.5. The MIC of an antibacterial agent for a specific bacterium can be determined *in vitro*. The MIC is the highest dilution of an antibacterial agent which inhibits growth of an isolate. The minimum bactericidal concentration is the highest dilution of a drug which can kill a particular bacterium (Fig. 6.5).

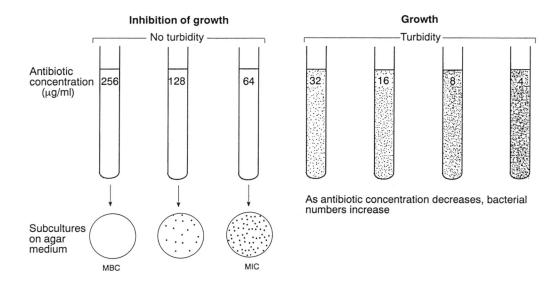

Figure 6.5 Dilution method for determining the minimal inhibitory concentration (MIC) and minimal bactericidal concentration (MBC) of an antibiotic for a test bacterium. Doubling dilutions of antibiotic are made in broth, a standard amount of bacterial inoculum is added to each tube and the test is incubated at 37°C for 24 hours. The MIC is the highest dilution of an antibiotic which inhibits the growth of the test bacterium, indicated by the absence of turbidity in the tube (64 μg/ml in the example given). The MBC is the highest dilution of an antibiotic which kills all the bacterial cells (256 μg/ml in the example given) demonstrated by subculturing the broth on agar. Below the MBC growth occurs in the subcultures of broth from tubes without turbidity.

References

Anon, (1998). Standing Medical Advisory Committee, Sub-Group on Antimicrobial Resistance. Main Report: *The Path of Least Resistance*. Department of Health, U.K.

Anon, (1999). Advisory Committee on the Microbiological Safety of Food. *Report on microbial antibiotic resistance in relation to food safety*. Department of Health, U.K.

Cohen, M.L. (1998). Antibiotic use. In *Antimicrobial Resistance: Issues and Options*. Workshop Report. National Academy Press, Washington, DC.

Glynn, M.K., Bopp, C., Dewitt, W., Dabney, P., Mokhtar, M. and Angulo, F.J. (1998). Emergence of multidrug-resistant *Salmonella enterica* serotype Typhimurium DT104 infections in the United States. *New England Journal of Medicine*, **338**, 1333–1338.

Jorgensen, J.H., Turnidge, J.D. and Washington, J.A. (1999). Antibacterial susceptibility tests: dilution and disk diffusion methods. In *Manual of Clinical Microbiology*. Seventh Edition. Eds. P.R. Murray, E.J. Barron, M.A. Pfaller, F.C. Tenover and R.H. Yolken. ASM Press, Washington, D.C. pp. 1526–1543.

Lester, S.C., del-Pilar-Pla, M., Wang, F., Perez-Schael, I., Jiang-H and O'Brien, T.F. (1990). The carriage of *Escherichia coli* resistant to antimicrobial agents by healthy children in Boston, in Caracas, Venezuela and in Qin Pu, China. *New England Journal of Medicine*, **323**, 285–289.

National Committee for Clinical Laboratory Standards (1997). *Performance standards for antimicrobial disk susceptibility tests*. Approved standard M2-A6 National Committee for Clinical Laboratory Standards, Wayne, Pa.

Quinn, P. J., Carter, M.E., Markey, B., Carter, G.R. (1994). *Clinical Veterinary Microbiology*, Mosby-Year Book Europe, London.

Rosdahl, V.T. and Pedersen, K.B. (1998). *The Copenhagen Recommendations: Report from the Invitational EU Conference on the Microbial Threat*. Copenhagen, Denmark. 9–10 September, 1998. Ministry of Health, Ministry of Food, Agriculture and Fisheries, Denmark.

Further reading

Bennett, P.M. (1995). The spread of drug resistance. In *Population Genetics of Bacteria*. Eds. S. Baumberg, J.P.W. Young, E.M.H. Wellington and J.R. Saunders. Cambridge University Press, Cambridge. pp. 317–344.

Gold, H.S. and Moellering, R.C. (1996). Antimicrobial-drug resistance. *New England Journal of Medicine*, **335**, 1445–1453.

Levy, S.B. (1998). The challenge of antibiotic resistance. *Scientific American*, **278**, 32–39.

Nicolaou, K.C. and Boddy, C.N.C. (2001). Behind enemy lines. *Scientific American*, **284**, 46–53.

Prescott, J.F. and Baggot, J.D. (1993). *Antimicrobial Therapy in Veterinary Medicine*. Second Edition. Iowa State University Press, Ames, Iowa.

Chapter 7

Bacterial colonization, tissue invasion and clinical disease

Although most bacteria are saprophytes which grow on organic matter in the environment, a small number, referred to as bacterial pathogens, produce infection and disease in animals and humans. Infections with some bacteria, such as anthrax caused by *Bacillus anthracis*, are invariably fatal. The development and severity of infections with other pathogenic bacteria are influenced by host-related determinants such as physiological status and immune competence. The skin is an important defence barrier consisting of several layers including an outer keratinized layer. Most bacteria cannot penetrate the skin unless it is damaged by trauma. Bacterial disease can also result from opportunistic infection by the commensals which normally colonize epithelial surfaces without deleterious effects. Opportunistic infections may also be caused by environmental saprophytes, such as *Nocardia asteroides* and *Pseudomonas* species, when these organisms enter the body through wounds or by inhalation.

In the 1870s, Robert Koch proposed a number of criteria which had to be fulfilled for a particular microorganism to be confirmed as the cause of a specific disease. For Koch's postulates to be fulfilled, the organism must be demonstrated by isolation in pure culture from the tissues of all animals with the disease. Moreover, when introduced into a susceptible healthy animal, it should cause the disease. It should also be possible to isolate the organism from the experimentally infected animal and the isolate should be identical to the original organism. Although many infectious diseases of animals can be shown to fulfil Koch's postulates, it is clear that some do not. Koch's postulates do not apply to diseases caused by opportunistic pathogens. In addition, they are not fulfilled by diseases associated with multiple infectious agents or by those precipitated by immunosuppression or stressful environmental factors.

Infection of susceptible animals

Animals may be exposed to infection from exogenous or endogenous sources. Exogenous infections occur after direct or indirect transmission from an infected animal or from the environment. Endogenous infections can be caused by commensal bacteria when an animal is subjected to stress factors.

The sequence of events following infection of a susceptible animal with a bacterial pathogen is outlined in Fig. 7.1.

Infection can be acquired by a number of routes which may be important in determining the outcome. In exogenous infections, pathogens may enter a host through the skin, the conjunctiva or the mucous membranes of the respiratory, gastrointestinal or urogenital tracts. Other possible routes of entry include the teat canal and the umbilicus. In addition, enterotoxigenic strains of *Escherichia coli* can cause enteritis in newborn farm animals without invasion by adhering to the mucosal lining and producing toxins.

The virulence of a bacterium relates to its ability to invade and produce disease in a normal animal. Highly virulent organisms produce serious disease or death in many affected animals whereas bacteria of low virulence rarely produce serious illness. Factors which influence the outcome of interaction between host and pathogen are illustrated in Fig. 7.2. Bacteria can attach to epithelial surfaces. Some commensals have an affinity for mucus; in contrast, pathogens frequently possess specific surface molecules which allow adherence to receptors on host cells. Adhesins on the tips of the fimbriae of Gram-negative bacteria usually bind to the carbohydrate components of glycoproteins and glycolipids in host cell membranes. Strains of a given bacterial species may possess different types of fimbriae, each with specificity for a particular receptor. This may account for the various enteric disease syndromes associated with different strains of the same enteropathogen. Some adhesins are present on the surface of Gram-negative bacteria and not on fimbriae. Invasin, an adhesin present on the surface of *Yersinia enterocolitica*, recognizes receptors called integrins on host cells. Although integrins are primarily involved in inflammatory processes such as adherence of white blood cells to endothelial surfaces, pathogenic bacteria can utilize these structures for attaching to cells. Enteropathogenic *E. coli* possess an adhesin, an outer membrane protein called intimin. Unlike other adhesins, intimin binds to a receptor protein, Tir (translocated intimin receptor), which is produced by the bacterium and incorporated into the host cell membrane. However, there is evidence that intimin can bind to cells in the absence of Tir (Hartland *et al.*, 1999).

Gram-positive bacteria can bind to extracellular matrix

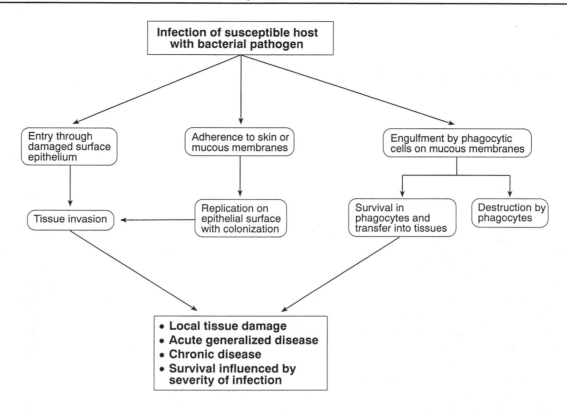

Figure 7.1 Possible sequelae following infection of a susceptible animal with a bacterial pathogen.

proteins such as fibrinogen, fibronectin, laminin and collagen. A fibronectin-binding protein, protein F, is necessary for adherence of streptococci to respiratory epithelial cells. The coagulase associated with pathogenic staphylococci promotes adherence to fibrinogen-coated surfaces. The interaction of *Klebsiella pneumoniae* with human intestinal cells is enhanced by possession of capsule-like material (Favre-Bonte *et al.*, 1995). In contrast, the capsules of some bacteria such as those of *Pasteurella multocida* (Jacques *et al.*, 1993), *Actinobacillus pleuropneumoniae* (Rioux *et al.*, 2000) and group B streptococci (Kallman *et al.*, 1993) may hinder adherence to host cells. It is postulated, therefore, that expression of capsules by some bacterial species may be down-regulated early in infection to avoid interference with adhesion and up-regulated in the later stages of infection (St. Geme *et al.*, 1996).

Colonization and growth

Pathogens bound to host cell receptors must replicate to avoid total elimination in desquamated cells. This surface replication is referred to as colonization. In order to replicate, pathogens must compete successfully for nutrients with the normal flora, tolerate host micro-environmental conditions and evade host defence mechanisms.

   Availability of iron is a limiting factor for the growth of bacteria. Iron, as a component of the cytochromes and the iron-sulphur proteins involved in electron transport, plays a major role in bacterial respiration. Most iron in the animal body is unavailable to bacteria because it is bound by iron-binding proteins such as lactoferrin and transferrin. However, many pathogenic bacteria have evolved mechanisms for obtaining iron from their hosts. These include the production of iron-chelating compounds (siderophores) which can remove iron from transferrin and lactoferrin. Some bacteria can extract iron from these molecules in the absence of siderophores; others can lyze erythrocytes to obtain iron from haemaglobin.

Dissemination in the host

Avoidance of defence mechanisms is essential for successful invasion of the host by pathogens. Some of the mechanisms which assist bacterial survival in hosts are presented in Table 7.1. Certain bacteria remain at the site of primary infection with local extension only. This localized invasion may be facilitated through breakdown of host tissues by collagenases, lipases, hyaluronidases and fibrinolysin produced by the bacteria. Bacteria can be disseminated throughout the body in the bloodstream either free in the plasma or in phagocytes. In bacteraemia, bacteria are present transiently in the blood stream without replicating. In septicaemia, pathogenic organisms multiply and persist in the blood stream producing systemic disease. The mechanisms used by bacteria for crossing epithelial barriers are poorly understood. In neonatal animals,

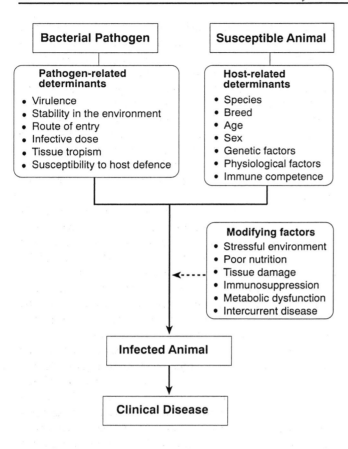

Figure 7.2 Determinants and modifying factors which can influence the outcome of bacterial infections in susceptible animals.

incomplete junctions between enterocytes may permit entry of enteropathogens. The passage of bacteria through the interior of enterocytes or M cells, transcytosis, is the common route of entry of enteropathogens. The M cells, specialized epithelial cells overlying Peyer's patches, periodically engulf intestinal bacteria and present them to the underlying cells of the immune system. *Yersinia* species and *Campylobacter jejuni* enter the host in this manner. Salmonellae can invade either through enterocytes or through M cells by a unique mechanism which involves inducing membrane ruffling followed by internalization by the host cell. Dissemination of *Mycobacterium bovis* throughout the body can occur following phagocytosis by macrophages. Following ingestion, *Listeria monocytogenes* can spread from the oral cavity to the CNS in cranial nerves.

Damage to host tissues and associated clinical signs

Bacteria can damage host tissues directly through the effects of exotoxins and endotoxins. Moreover, tissue damage can result indirectly from the activity of enzymes secreted by the bacteria from the inflammatory reactions and immune responses of the host. Bacterial exotoxins and endotoxins differ in their structures and modes of

action (Table 7.2). Exotoxins are produced by Gram-positive and Gram-negative bacteria. Endotoxins, which are lipopolysaccharides present in the outer membrane of Gram-negative bacteria, are released when the cells are lyzed.

Exotoxins are often produced within the body and exert their effects either locally or systemically. Occasionally, exotoxins, such as the potent toxin of *Clostridium botulinum* are ingested in contaminated food and produce systemic effects. The effects of exotoxins are summarized in Box 7.1. Some exotoxins cause cell death either by digesting lipids in cytoplasmic membranes or by insertion into the membranes, forming protein pores. Lecithinase

Table 7.1 Mechanisms which assist bacterial survival in the host.

Mechanism	Comments
O antigen polysaccharide chain	Length of polysaccharide chain hinders binding of the membrane attack complex of complement to the outer membrane of many Gram-negative bacteria
Capsular antigen	Incorporation of sialic acid by some Gram-negative bacteria has an inhibitory effect on complement activity
Capsule production	Antiphagocytic role in many bacteria
M protein production	Antiphagocytic activity in *Streptococcus equi*
Production of Fc-binding proteins	Staphylococci and streptococci produce protein which bind to the Fc region of IgG and prevent interaction with the Fc receptor on membranes of phagocytes
Production of leukotoxins	Cytolysis of phagocytes by toxins produced by *Mannheimia haemolytica*, *Actinobacillus* species and other pathogenic bacteria
Interference with phagosome-lysosome fusion	Allows the survival of pathogenic mycobacteria within phagocytes
Escape from phagosomes	Survival mechanism used by *Listeria monocytogenes* and rickettsiae
Resistance to oxidative damage	Allows survival of salmonellae and brucellae within phagocytes
Antigenic mimicry of host antigens	Adaptation of surface antigens by *Mycoplasma* species to avoid recognition by the immune system
Antigenic variation of surface antigens	Permit survival of *Mycoplasma* species and borrelliae despite the host's immune response to these pathogens
Coagulase production	Conversion of fibrinogen to fibrin by *Staphylococcus aureus* can isolate site of infection from effective immune responses

Table 7.2 Comparison of exotoxins and endotoxins.

Exotoxins	Endotoxins
Produced by live bacteria, both Gram-positive and Gram-negative	Component of the cell wall of Gram-negative bacteria released following cell death
Proteins, usually of high molecular weight	Lipopolysaccharide complex containing lipid A, the toxic component
Heat labile	Heat stable
Potent toxins, usually with specific activity; not pyrogenic. Highly antigenic; readily converted into toxoids which induce neutralizing antibodies	Toxins with moderate, non-specific generalized activity; potent pyrogens, weakly antigenic; not amenable to toxoid production. Neutralizing antibodies not associated with natural exposure
Synthesis determined extrachromosomally	Encoded in chromosome

and phospholipase degrade phospholipids in cytoplasmic membranes. The α toxin of *Staphylococcus aureus* and streptolysin O produced by some streptococci form pores in the cytoplasmic membranes of target cells. Certain exotoxins disrupt intracellular processes. The structure of these toxins is similar in that they consist of two moieties; one moiety binds to the cell membrane and the other, the toxic moiety which has enzymatic activity, disrupts cell function. In tetanus and botulism, the toxic moiety acts on synaptobrevins, the proteins responsible for release of neurotransmitters and inhibitory mediators.

Endotoxins of Gram-negative bacteria contain a hydrophobic glycolipid (lipid A) and a hydrophilic polysaccharide composed of a core oligosaccharide and an O-polysaccharide (O antigen). The toxicity of this complex lipopolysaccharide molecule resides in the lipid A portion. The effects of endotoxin are summarized in Box 7.2. Cells with which endotoxin interacts include mononuclear phagocytes, neutrophils, platelets and B lymphocytes. Effects of endotoxin depend on the amount present in the circulation and may be influenced by previous exposure to the toxin. In low concentrations, endotoxin elicits fever through the release of endogenous

---

Box 7.1 Effects of exotoxins.

- Cell membrane damage
  — Enzymatic digestion
  — Formation of pores
- Interference with protein synthesis
- Elevation of cAMP levels
- Disruption of functions relating to nervous tissue
- Digestion of components of interstitial tissue: collagen, elastin, hyaluronic acid

---

pyrogens such as interleukin-1 and tumour necrosis factor from leukocytes and through the promotion of inflammatory responses involving activation of complement and macrophages. High doses of endotoxin induce disseminated intravascular coagulation associated with hypotension and shock. Endotoxin stimulates coagulation by activating clotting factor XII, by causing platelet degranulation and by stimulating neutrophils to release proteins which stabilize fibrin clots. Pyrexic and inflammatory reactions, elicited by cell wall components, are also features of infections with many Gram-positive bacteria.

Local and systemic inflammatory responses, while essential for counteracting infection, can induce damage to host tissues. The host immune response may also cause tissue damage. This is a feature of the pathogenesis of the chronic inflammatory reactions associated with myco-bacterial infections which are related to the immune response of the host. Moreover, in infections caused by *Borrelia burgdorferi*, immune complex formation may contribute to the pathogenesis of Lyme disease.

Bacteria such as *Staphylococcus aureus* can subvert the immune response by producing superantigens. These superantigens are proteins which can bind non-specifically to T lymphocyte receptors as well as to the major histocompatibility complex class II molecule on antigen-presenting cells. This non-specific interaction results in activation of large numbers of T lymphocytes with the copious production of cytokines and generalized toxic effects.

Box 7.2 Effects of endotoxins.

- Interaction with polymorphonuclear and mononuclear phagocytes, platelets and B lymphocytes
- Release of interleukin-1, leading to fever
- Activation of complement, promoting inflammatory changes

Types of bacterial infections

Disease is not an inevitable consequence of infection. When susceptible animals become infected with bacterial pathogens the clinical outcome is determined by the virulence of the pathogen and the response of the host. This response may range from mild disease to sudden death. The host-pathogen relationship can also influence the nature of the tissue reaction and the transmission of the infectious agent to other animals. Some individual pathogens tend to produce a predictable clinical picture following infection of a susceptible host. Anthrax in ruminants is invariably peracute and fatal. In contrast, infections with bacteria such as *Salmonella* Dublin in cattle may produce many different forms of disease.

Bacterial infections can be conveniently categorized as

acute, subacute, chronic or persistent. Acute infections usually have a short severe clinical course, often a matter of days, and the invading bacteria are usually cleared from the body by the host's immune response. The host may shed the agent in large numbers for a short period. Subacute infections produce clinical effects of less intensity.

Chronic infections tend to occur when the host fails to eliminate the pathogen. Frequently, the infectious agent replicates initially to a high level and is subsequently cleared from most sites in the body by the host's immune response. Persistence occurs in certain sites such as the uriniferous tubules and the CNS in which the effects of cell-mediated and humoral immunity are minimal. Persistent shedding may occur from some of these sites as in bovine leptospirosis, in which leptospires may be shed in urine for more than a year. Some other chronic infections may be characterized by persistence with or without shedding of the aetiological agent. Cattle which have mounted an effective cell-mediated immune response to *Mycobacterium bovis* infection may remain chronically infected, with the organism persisting in localized foci without shedding. Intermittent shedding may occur in chronic bovine mastitis caused by *Staphylococcus aureus*. Latent bacterial infections are characterized by persistence of the pathogen in the host without shedding, although it can occur occasionally. *Salmonella* Dublin can establish latent infection in the bovine gall bladder with intermittent faecal shedding precipitated by stress.

References

Favre-Bonte, S., Darfeuille-Michaud, A. and Forestier, C. (1995). Aggregative adherence of *Klebsiella pneumoniae* to intestine-407 cells. *Infection and Immunity*, **63**, 1318–1328.

Hartland, E.L., Batchelor, M., Delahay, R.M., Hale, C., Matthews, S. Dougan G, Knutton, S., Connerton, I. and Frankel, G. (1999). Binding of intimin from enteropathogenic *Escherichia coli* to Tir and to host cells. *Molecular Microbiology*, **32**, 151-158.

Jacques, M., Kobisch, M., Belanger, M. and Dugal, F. (1993). Virulence of capsulated and noncapsulated isolates of *Pasteurella multocida* and their adherence to porcine respiratory tract cells and mucus. *Infection and Immunity*, **61**, 4785–4792.

Kallman, J., Schollin, J., Hakansson, S., Andersson, A. and Kihlstrom, E. (1993). Adherence of group B streptococci to human endothelial cells *in vitro*. *Acta Pathologica Microbiologica et Immunologica Scandanavica*, **101**, 403–408.

Rioux, S., Galarneau, C., Harel, J., Kobisch, M., Frey, J., Gottschalk, M. and Jacques, M. (2000). Isolation and characterization of a capsule-deficient mutant of *Actinobacillus pleuropneumoniae* serotype I. *Microbial Pathogenesis*, **28**, 279–289.

St. Geme, J.W. III and Cutter, D. (1996). Influence of pili, fibrils and capsule on in vitro adherence by *Haemophilus influenzae* type G. *Molecular Microbiology*, **21**, 21–31.

Further reading

Brooks, G.F., Butel, J.S. and Morse, S.A. (1998). Pathogenesis of bacterial infection. In *Jawetz, Melnick and Adelberg's Medical Microbiology*. Twenty-first Edition. Appleton and Lange, Stamford, Connecticut. pp 134–144.

Gyles, C.L. and Thoen, C.O. (1993). *Pathogenesis of Bacterial Infections in Animals*. Second Edition. Iowa State University Press, Ames, Iowa.

Madigan, M.T., Martinko, J.M. and Parker, J. (1997). Host-parasite relationships. In *Brock, Biology of Microorganisms*. Eighth Edition. Prentice Hall International, London. pp. 785–812.

Section II

Pathogenic Bacteria

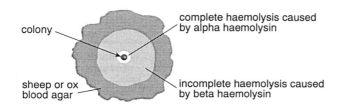

Figure 8.2 The characteristic double haemolysis of *S. aureus* and *S. intermedius* on sheep or ox blood agar.

Diagnostic procedures

- Exudative epidermitis in piglets and tick pyaemia of lambs are the only clinical conditions of domestic animals specifically attributable to pathogenic staphylococci. In suppurative conditions, the likelihood of staphylococcal infection must be considered and appropriate specimens such as exudates and mastitic milk collected for laboratory procedures.
- Gram-stained smears of pus or other suitable specimens may reveal typical staphylococcal clusters.
- Specimens are cultured on blood agar, selective blood agar and MacConkey agar and incubated aerobically at 37°C for 24 to 48 hours. Selective blood agar, which contains nalidixic acid and colistin, is used to inhibit *Proteus* species and other Gram-negative contaminants.
- Identification criteria for isolates:
  — Colonial characteristics
  — Presence or absence of haemolysis
  — Absence of growth on MacConkey agar
  — Catalase production
  — Coagulase production
  — Biochemical profile
- Phage typing is applicable in epidemiological investigations such as those relating to outbreaks of staphylococcal food poisoning in man.

Clinical infections

Because staphylococci occur both as commensals on skin and mucous membranes and as environmental contaminants, infections can be either endogenous or exogenous in origin. Many infections are opportunistic and associated with trauma, immunosuppression, intercurrent parasitic or fungal infections, allergic conditions or endocrine and metabolic disturbances. Coagulase-positive staphylococci are responsible for the majority of infections (Table 8.1). Some strains of low virulence which are coagulase negative are also capable of causing disease in animals (Table 8.2). Currently available vaccines are ineffective for preventing staphylococcal infections. Antibiotic susceptibility testing should precede treatment.

Staphylococcal diseases of importance in domestic animals include mastitis, tick pyaemia, exudative epidermitis, botryomycosis and pyoderma.

Bovine staphylococcal mastitis

Staphylococcal mastitis, usually caused by *S. aureus*, is a common form of bovine mastitis worldwide. It may be subclinical, acute or chronic. The majority of infections are subclinical. Peracute and gangrenous forms are associated with severe systemic reactions and can be life-threatening. In gangrenous mastitis the affected quarter, which becomes cold and blue-black, eventually sloughs. Tissue necrosis is attributed to the alpha-toxin which causes contraction and necrosis of smooth muscle in blood vessel walls, impeding blood flow in the affected quarter. In addition, this toxin causes release of lysosomal enzymes from leukocytes. Bovine staphylococcal mastitis is discussed in Chapter 81.

Tick Pyaemia

Tick pyaemia, an infection of lambs with *S. aureus*, is confined to hill-grazing regions of Britain and Ireland, where there are suitable habitats for the tick *Ixodes ricinus*.

Table 8.5 Virulence factors, including toxins, of *Staphylococcus aureus* and their pathogenic effects.

Virulence factor	Pathogenic effects
Coagulase	Conversion of fibrinogen to fibrin. Fibrin deposition may shield staphylococci from phagocytic cells
Lipase, esterases, elastase, staphylo-kinase, deoxyribonu-clease, hyaluronidase, phospholipase	Enzymes which contribute to virulence
Protein A	Surface component which binds Fc portion of IgG and inhibits opsonization
Leukocidin	Cytolytic destruction of phagocytes of some animal species
Alpha-toxin (alpha-haemolysin)	The major toxin in gangrenous mastitis. It causes spasm of smooth muscle and is necrotizing and potentially lethal
Beta-toxin (beta-haemolysin)	A sphingomyelinase which damages cell membranes
Exfoliative toxins	Responsible for desquamation in staphylococcal scalded skin syndrome in man
Enterotoxins	Heat-stable toxins associated with staphylococcal food poisoning in man
Toxic shock syndrome toxins (TSST)	Induce excessive lymphokine production, resulting in tissue damage. Bovine and human strains of *S. aureus* produce TSST-1. Sheep and goat strains produce a variant of this toxin. The significance of these toxins in animals is unclear

Lambs can carry *S. aureus* on their skin and nasal mucosa and infection occurs through minor skin trauma including tick bites. *Ixodes ricinus* is a vector for the rickettsial agent of tick-borne fever, *Ehrlichia phagocytophila*, which can cause immunosuppression in lambs and may predispose to staphylococcal infection.

Tick pyaemia is characterized either by septicaemia and rapid death or by localized abscess formation in many organs. Clinical manifestations include arthritis, posterior paresis and ill-thrift. The condition can be of considerable economic importance on some farms where up to 30% of lambs between 2 and 10 weeks of age can be affected in spring and early summer.

Diagnosis

- In young lambs, grazing rough pasture in Britain or Ireland, clinical signs may be indicative of the disease.
- Microscopic demonstration of the bacteria in pus, followed by isolation and identification of *S. aureus* from lesions, is confirmatory.

Treatment and control

Treatment is of limited value in severely affected lambs. Efforts should be directed at control within the flock.

- Prophylactic treatment of lambs with antibiotics, such as long-acting tetracycline, can be initiated at one week of age. Tetracyclines also protect lambs against *E. phagocytophila*.
- Tick-control measures such as dipping should be introduced.

Exudative epidermitis (greasy-pig disease)

This disease, caused by *S. hyicus*, occurs worldwide in sucklers and weaned pigs up to 3 months of age. It is highly contagious and characterized by widespread excessive sebaceous secretion, exfoliation and exudation on the skin surface. Affected pigs, which are anorexic, depressed and febrile, have an extensive, non-pruritic dermatitis with a greasy exudate. Piglets under 3 weeks of age may die within 24 to 48 hours. Morbidity rates range from 20 to 100%, and mortality rates can reach 90% in severely affected litters. *Staphylococcus hyicus* can be isolated from the vaginal mucosa and skin of healthy sows. The organisms probably enter the skin of young pigs through minor abrasions such as bite wounds.

Predisposing stress factors include agalactia in the sow, intercurrent infections and weaning. Injection of a toxin of *S. hyicus* into the skin of young pigs can produce exfoliation (Amtsberg, 1979).

Diagnosis

- A high mortality rate in young pigs with exudative, non-pruritic skin lesions is typical of the disease.

- Isolation and identification of *S. hyicus* from the dermal lesions is confirmatory.

Treatment and control

- Early systemic antibiotic therapy, combined with topical treatment with antiseptic or antibiotic suspensions may be effective.
- Strict isolation of affected pigs is essential.
- Cleaning and disinfection of contaminated buildings should be carried out.
- Sows should be washed with a suitable antiseptic soap before farrowing.
- Prior colonization of the skin with an avirulent strain of *S. hyicus* prevented experimental infection with virulent *S. hyicus* (Allaker *et al.*, 1988).

Botryomycosis

Botryomycosis is a chronic, suppurative granulomatous condition, often caused by *S. aureus*. It can occur within a few weeks of castration in the horse due to infection of the stump of the spermatic cord (scirrhous cord). Botryomycosis can also occur in mammary tissues of sows. The lesion is composed of a mass of fibrous tissue containing foci of pus and sinus tracts.

Staphylococcal infections in dogs and cats

Staphylococcus intermedius is commonly isolated from pyoderma, otitis externa and other suppurative conditions including mastitis, endometritis, cystitis, osteomyelitis and wound infections. Occasionally, similar suppurative conditions are caused by *S. aureus*.

References

Allaker, R.P., Lloyd, D.H. and Smith, I.M. (1988). Prevention of exudative epidermitis in gnotobiotic pigs by bacterial interference. *Veterinary Record*, **123**, 597–598.

Amtsberg, G. (1979). Demonstration of exfoliation-producing substances in cultures of *Staphylococcus hyicus* of pigs and *Staphylococcus epidermidis* biotype 2 of cattle. *Zentralblatt für Veterinärmedizin (B)* **26**, 257–272.

Davis, G.H.G. and Hoyling, B. (1973). Use of a rapid acetoin test in the identification of staphylococci and micrococci. *International Journal of Systematic Bacteriology*, **23**, 281–282.

Igimi, S., Kawamura, S., Takahashi, E. and Mitsuoka, T. (1989). *Staphlococcus felis*, a new species from clinical specimens from cats. *International Journal of Systematic Bacteriology*, **39**, 373–377.

Igimi, S., Takahashi, E. and Mitsuoka, T. (1990). *Staphylococcus schleiferi* subsp. *coagulans* subsp. nov., isolated from external auditory meatus of dogs with external ear otitis. *International Journal of Systematic Bacteriology*, **40**, 409–411.

Quinn, P.J., Carter, M.E., Markey, B. and Carter, G.R. (1994). *Staphylococcus* species. In *Clinical Veterinary Microbiology*. Mosby-Year Book Europe, London. pp. 118–126

Thomson-Carter, F.M., Carter, P.E. and Pennington, T.H. (1989). Differentiation of staphylococcal species and strains by ribosomal RNA gene restriction patterns. *Journal of General Microbiology*, **135**, 2093–2097.

Further reading

Brodie, T.A., Holmes, P.H. and Urquhart, G.M. (1986). Some aspects of tick-borne diseases of British sheep. *Veterinary Record*, **118**, 415–418.

Cox, H.U., Newman, S.S., Roy, A.F. and Hoskins, J.D. (1984). Species of *Staphylococcus* isolated from animal infections. *Cornell Veterinarian*, **74**, 124–135.

Lloyd, D. (1996). Dealing with cutaneous staphylococcal infections in dogs. *In Practice*, **18**, 223–231.

Mason, I.S., Mason, K.V. and Lloyd, D.H. (1996). A review of the biology of canine skin with respect to the commensals *Staphylococcus intermedius*, *Demodex canis* and *Malassezia pachydermatis*. *Veterinary Dermatology*, **7**, 119–132.

Chapter 9

Streptococci

The streptococci are a group of bacteria that can infect many animal species, causing suppurative conditions such as mastitis, metritis, polyarthritis and meningitis. The group contains the genera *Streptococcus*, *Enterococcus* and *Peptostreptococcus*. Most pathogenic species are in the genus *Streptococcus*. These organisms are Gram-positive cocci, approximately 1.0 μm in diameter, which form chains of different lengths (Fig. 9.1).

Streptococcus species are catalase-negative, facultative anaerobes, which are non-motile. They are fastidious bacteria and require the addition of blood or serum to culture media. *Streptococcus pneumoniae* (pneumococcus) occurs as slightly pear-shaped cocci in pairs. Pathogenic strains have thick capsules and produce mucoid colonies. These bacteria cause pneumonia in humans, guinea-pigs and rats.

Enterococcus species are enteric streptococci which are found in the intestinal tract of animals and man. They are opportunistic pathogens and differ from the *Streptococcus* species in two important respects:

— They tolerate bile salts and grow on MacConkey agar as red, pin-point colonies.
— Some isolates are motile.

Peptostreptococcus indolicus is an anaerobic streptococcus, which is aetiologically implicated in bovine 'summer mastitis' in association with *Arcanobacterium pyogenes*.

Usual habitat

The streptococci are distributed worldwide. Most species

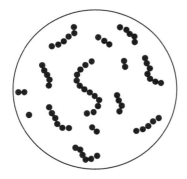

Figure 9.1 Streptococcal chains.

Key points

- Gram-positive cocci in chains
- Fastidious, requiring enriched media
- Small, usually haemolytic, translucent colonies
- Catalase-negative
- Facultative anaerobes, usually non-motile
- Commensals on mucous membranes
- Susceptible to desiccation
- Cause pyogenic infections

live as commensals on the mucosae of the upper respiratory tract and lower urogenital tract. These fragile bacteria are susceptible to desiccation and survive only for short periods off the host. The enterococci are opportunistic pathogens.

Differentiation of the streptococci

Three laboratory procedures are used for differentiating streptococci, namely type of haemolysis, Lancefield grouping and biochemical testing.

- Type of haemolysis on sheep or ox blood agar:
  - Beta-haemolysis is complete haemolysis indicated by clear zones around colonies.
  - Alpha-haemolysis is partial or incomplete haemolysis indicated by greenish or hazy zones around colonies.
  - Gamma-haemolysis denotes no observable changes in the blood agar around colonies.
- Lancefield grouping is a serological method of classification based on the group-specific C-substance (polysaccharide) in the cell wall. Test methods include:
  - Ring precipitation test. The C-substance is extracted by acid or heat from the *Streptococcus* species under test. This antigen extract is layered over antisera of different specificities, in narrow tubes placed in plasticine on a slide. A positive reaction is indicated by the formation of a white ring of precipitate close to the interface of the two fluids within 30 minutes (Fig. 9.2).

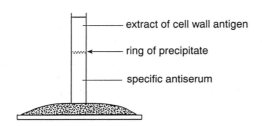

Figure 9.2 Ring precipitation test for streptococci.

—Latex agglutination test. Specific C-substance antisera for groups A to G (with the exception of group E) are commercially available. Suspensions of latex particles are coated with each of the group-specific antibodies. The group antigen is extracted enzymatically from the streptococcus under test. A drop of antigen is mixed on a plate with a drop of each latex-antibody suspension and rocked gently. A positive reaction, which usually occurs within one minute, is indicated by agglutination (Fig. 9.3).

• Biochemical testing:
  —A number of commercial test systems are available for rapid biochemical identification of streptococci.
  —A short range of biochemical tests are used for differentiating equine group C streptococci.

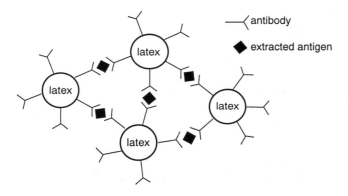

Figure 9.3 Diagrammatic representation of the latex agglutination test for streptococcal identification.

Pathogenesis and pathogenicity

Pyogenic streptococci are associated with abscess formation, other suppurative conditions and septicaemias. Beta-haemolytic streptococci are generally more pathogenic than those producing alpha-haemolysis. Virulence factors include enzymes and exotoxins such as streptolysins (haemolysins), hyaluronidase, DNase, NADase, streptokinase and proteases. The specific action and significance of some of these factors are poorly understood. Polysaccharide capsules, which are major virulence factors of *S. pyogenes*, *S. pneumoniae* and some strains of

S. equi, are antiphagocytic. The cell wall M proteins of *S. pyogenes*, *S. equi* and *S. porcinus* are also antiphagocytic. In the absence of antiphagocytic factors, these bacteria are rapidly killed by phagocytes.

Diagnostic procedures

History, clinical signs and pathology may be indicative of certain streptococcal infections such as strangles.

• Streptococci are highly susceptible to desiccation and specimens should be cultured promptly. Pus or exudate collected on swabs should be placed in transport medium if specimens cannot be processed immediately.
• A sensitive technique using the polymerase chain reaction has been developed for detecting both viable and non-viable *S. equi* in nasal swabs (Timoney and Artiushin, 1997).
• Chains of Gram-positive cocci may be demonstrable in smears from specimens.
• Specimens should be cultured on blood agar, selective blood agar and MacConkey agar. Plates are incubated aerobically at 37°C for 24 to 48 hours.
• Identification criteria for isolates:
  —Small, translucent colonies, some of which may be mucoid
  —Type of haemolysis on blood agar
  —Chains of Gram-positive cocci
  —No growth on MacConkey agar with the exception of *E. faecali*s
  —Negative catalase test
  —Lancefield grouping
  —Biochemical test profile

Clinical infections

Streptococci are often commensals on mucous membranes and, consequently, many streptococcal infections are opportunistic. Infections may be primary as in strangles or secondary as in streptococcal pneumonia following a viral infection. Lymph nodes, genital tract or mammary glands may become infected. Neonatal septicaemias are often related to maternal genital tract infection. *Streptococcus pyogenes*, a human pathogen, occasionally causes bovine mastitis, tonsillitis in dogs and lymphangitis in foals.

Streptococci of animal origin are of limited public health significance with the exception of *S. suis*, which can cause severe infections in individuals working with pigs. The group B streptococci, which cause disease in human infants, appear to be distinct from animal strains in this group.

Streptococcus canis, a significant pathogen of dogs, is associated with neonatal septicaemia, many suppurative conditions and recently with toxic shock syndrome (Miller *et al.*, 1996). Strangles, porcine streptococcal meningitis and bovine streptococcal mastitis are important specific

Table 9.1 Pathogenic streptococci, their habitats, hosts and consequences of infection.

Species	Lancefield group	Haemolysis on blood agar[a]	Hosts	Consequences of infection	Usual habitat
S. pyogenes	A	β	Man	Scarlet fever, septic sore throat, rheumatic fever	Mainly upper respiratory tract
S. agalactiae	B	β (α, γ)	Cattle, sheep, goats	Chronic mastitis	Milk ducts
			Man, dogs	Neonatal septicaemia	Vagina
S. dysgalactiae	C	α (β, γ)	Cattle	Acute mastitis	Buccal cavity, vagina, environment
			Lambs	Polyarthritis	
S. equisimilis (*S. dysgalactiae* subsp. *equisimilis*)	C	β	Horses	Abscesses, endometritis, mastitis	Skin, vagina
			Pigs, cattle, dogs, birds	Suppurative conditions	
S. equi (*S. equi* subsp. *equi*)	C	β	Horses	Strangles, suppurative conditions, purpura haemorrhagica	Upper respiratory tract, guttural pouch
S. zooepidemicus (*S. equi* subsp. *zooepidemicus*)	C	β	Horses	Mastitis, pneumonia, navel infections	Mucous membranes
			Cattle, lambs, pigs, poultry	Suppurative conditions, septicaemia	Skin, mucous membranes
Enterococcus faecalis	D	α (β, γ)	Many species	Suppurative conditions following opportunistic invasion	Intestinal tract
S. suis	D	α (β)	Pigs	Septicaemia, meningitis, arthritis, bronchopneumonia	Tonsils, nasal cavity
			Cattle, sheep, horses, cats	Suppurative conditions	
			Man	Septicaemia, meningitis	
S. porcinus	E	β	Pigs	Submandibular lymphadenitis	Mucous membranes
S. canis	G	β	Carnivores	Neonatal septicaemia, suppurative conditions, toxic shock syndrome	Vagina, anal mucosa
S. uberis	Not assigned	α (γ)	Cattle	Mastitis	Skin, vagina, tonsils
S. pneumoniae	Not assigned	α	Man, primates	Septicaemia, pneumonia, meningitis	Upper respiratory tract
			Guinea-pigs, rats	Pneumonia	

a   types of haemolysis occurring less frequently are shown in brackets infections. Vaccines for the control of streptococcal infections are usually ineffective. The clinical consequences of streptococcal infections are listed in Table 9.1.

Strangles

Strangles is a highly contagious disease of horses caused by *Streptococcus equi* (*S. equi* subsp. *equi*). It is a febrile disease involving the upper respiratory tract with abscessation of regional lymph nodes.

Epidemiology
Although non-immune *Equidae* of all ages are susceptible, outbreaks of the disease occur most commonly in young horses. Assembling horses at sales, shows and race courses increases the risk of acquiring infection. Transmission is via purulent exudates from the upper respiratory tract or from discharging abscesses. A chronic, convalescent carrier state can develop with bacteria present in the guttural pouch. An atypical mild form, in which *S. equi* is present in small purulent foci has been described. Infected animals may shed *S. equi* for at least 4 weeks after development of clinical signs.

Clinical signs
The incubation period is 3 to 6 days and the course of the uncomplicated disease is 5 to 10 days. There is a high fever, depression and anorexia followed by an oculonasal discharge that becomes purulent. The lymph nodes of the head and neck are swollen and painful. Characteristically the submandibular nodes are affected and they eventually rupture discharging purulent, highly infectious material. Guttural pouch empyema is a common finding. The morbidity may be up to 100% and mortality rate is usually less than 5%. Reinfection may occur in some recovered horses.

    Death may result from complications such as pneumonia, neurological involvement, asphyxia due to pressure on the pharynx from enlarged lymph nodes, or purpura haemorrhagica. Purpura haemorrhagica, considered to be an immune-mediated disease, may occur in some affected horses 1 to 3 weeks after initial illness.

    Streptococcus zooepidemicus and *S. equisimilis,* which produce mild upper respiratory tract infections, must be differentiated from *S. equi*.

Table 9.2 Differentiation of equine group C streptococci by sugar fermentation.

	Trehalose	Sorbitol	Lactose	Maltose
S. equi	–	–	–	+
S. zooepidemicus	–	+	+	+(–)
S. equisimilis	+	–	v	+

v variable reactions   (–) a few strains are negative

Bastard strangles, in which abscessation develops in many organs, is a serious complication in about 1% of affected animals.

Diagnosis
- Clinical signs and a history of recent exposure to suspect animals may allow a presumptive diagnosis of strangles.
- Colonies are usually mucoid, up to 4 mm in diameter, and surrounded by a wide zone of beta-haemolysis.
- *Streptococcus equi* must be distinguished from other Lancefield group C streptococci, particularly *S. equisimilis* and *S. zooepidemicus*, by sugar fermentation in peptone water containing serum (Table 9.2) and by other confirmatory biochemical tests.
- Asymptomatic carriers can be detected using the polymerase chain reaction test.

Treatment and control
- Administration of penicillin to in-contact and infected horses is recommended. Antibiotic therapy may be of limited benefit if abscesses have formed.
- Clinically suspect animals should be isolated.
- Horses should be isolated for 10 days when first introduced or returning to a property.
- An inactivated vaccine (bacterin) which is available in some countries is of questionable efficacy. Research on vaccines is now targeting the development of subunit or vectored strangles vaccines.
- Predisposing factors such as over-crowding and mixing of different age groups should be avoided.
- Following outbreaks of the disease, buildings and equipment should be cleaned and disinfected.

Streptococcus suis infections

Streptococcus suis is recognized worldwide as a cause of significant losses in the pig industry. It is associated with meningitis, arthritis, septicaemia and bronchopneumonia in pigs of all ages, and with sporadic cases of endocarditis, neonatal deaths and abortion.

Serological and biochemical characteristics of isolates
Streptococcus suis properly belongs to Lancefield group D, although strains were previously assigned to groups R, S, (RS) and T. Serological testing is based on antigenic differences in capsular material, largely carbohydrate in nature. At least 34 serotypes of varying virulence have been recognized. About 70% of *S. suis* isolates belong to serotypes 1 to 9 and to serotype 1/2, which has both type 1 and type 2 antigens. Of these, serotype 2 is the most prevalent serotype with carrier rates up to 90%. This serotype is associated with meningitis in both pigs and man. Two biotypes, *S. suis* I and *S. suis* II, are identifiable using commercial test systems.

Table 9.3 Differentiation of streptococci which cause bovine mastitis.

	Haemolysis on blood agar	CAMP test	Aesculin hydrolysis (Edwards medium)	Growth on MacConkey agar	Lancefield group
Streptococcus agalactiae	β (α, γ)	+	–	–	B
S. dysgalactiae	α	–	–	–	C
S. uberis	α	–	+	–	not assigned
Enterococcus faecalis	α	–	+	+	D

Clinical signs and epidemiology

Asymptomatic carrier pigs harbour *S. suis* in tonsillar tissue. Disease outbreaks are most common in intensively-reared pigs when they are subjected to overcrowding, poor ventilation and other stress factors. Sows carrying the organisms can infect their litters, leading either to neonatal deaths or to carrier animals in which characteristic signs develop later in life. Meningitis, which is often fatal, is characterized by fever, tremors, incoordination, opisthotonos and convulsions.

In North America, *S. suis* is often isolated from cases of respiratory disease in conjunction with *Mycoplasma* and *Pasteurella* species. Serious infections occur periodically in humans directly involved in pig husbandry or processing. Infections with *S. suis* have also been recorded in cattle, small ruminants, horses and cats.

Control

These bacteria tend to become endemic in a herd and eradication is not feasible. Improved husbandry may decrease the prevalence of clinical disease.

Most strains of *S. suis* are susceptible to penicillin or ampicillin. Prophylactic long-acting penicillin, given by injection to sows one week prior to farrowing and to piglets during the first 2 weeks of life, has proved worthwhile in herds experiencing neonatal deaths or meningitis at weaning.

Bovine streptococcal mastitis

Streptococcus agalactiae, *S. dysgalactiae* and *S. uberis* are the principal pathogens involved in streptococcal mastitis. *Enterococcus faecalis*, *S. pyogenes* and *S. zooepidemicus* are less commonly isolated from cases of mastitis.

- *Streptococcus agalactiae* colonizes the milk ducts and produces persistent infection with intermittent bouts of acute mastitis.
- *Streptococcus dysgalactiae*, which is found in the buccal cavity and genitalia and on the skin of the mammary gland, causes acute mastitis.
- *Streptococcus uberis,* a normal inhabitant of skin, tonsils and vaginal mucosa, is a major cause of clinical mastitis, usually without systemic signs.

Diagnosis

- Clinical signs include inflammation of mammary tissue and clots in the milk.
- Milk samples should be collected carefully to avoid contamination.
- Samples should be cultured on blood agar, Edwards medium and MacConkey agar and incubated aerobically at 37°C for 24 to 48 hours.
- Differentiation of the mastitis-producing streptococci is outlined in Table 9.3. A positive CAMP test (Christie, Atkins and Munch-Petersen) is illustrated in Fig. 9.4.
- Sugar fermentation tests.

Treatment and control

A detailed description of bovine mastitis including streptococcal mastitis is presented in Chapter 81.

References

Miller, C.W., Prescott, J.F., Mathews, K.A., Betschel, S.D., Yager, J.A., Guru, V. *et al.* (1996). Streptococcal toxic shock syndrome in dogs. *Journal of the American Veterinary Medical Association*, **209**, 1421–1426.

Timoney, J.F. and Artiushin, S.C. (1997). Detection of

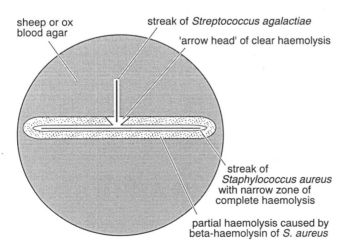

sheep or ox blood agar

streak of *Streptococcus agalactiae*

'arrow head' of clear haemolysis

streak of *Staphylococcus aureus* with narrow zone of complete haemolysis

partial haemolysis caused by beta-haemolysin of *S. aureus*

Figure 9.4 CAMP test. *Streptococcus agalactiae* elaborates a factor which completely lyses the red cells already damaged by the beta-haemolysin of *Staphylococcus aureus*, producing a characteristic clear 'arrow head' pattern of complete haemolysis.

Streptococcus equi in equine nasal swabs and washes by DNA amplification. *Veterinary Record*, **141**, 446–447.

Further reading

Fox, L.K. and Gay, J.M. (1993). Contagious mastitis. *Veterinary Clinics of North America: Food Animal Practice*, **9**, 475–487.

Hillerton, J.E. (1988). Summer mastitis – the current position. *In Practice*, **10**, 131–137.

MacLennan, M., Foster, G., Dick, K. *et al.* (1996). *Streptococcus suis* serotypes 7, 8 and 14 from diseased pigs in Scotland. *Veterinary Record*, **139**, 423–424.

Newton, J.R., Verheyen, K., Talbot, N.C. *et al.* (2000). Control of strangles outbreaks by isolation of guttural pouch carriers identified using PCR and culture of *Streptococcus equi*. *Equine Veterinary Journal*, **32**, 515–526.

Reams, R.Y., Glickman, L.T., Harrington, D.D. *et al.* (1994). *Streptococcus suis* infection in swine: a retrospective study of 256 cases. Part II. Clinical signs, gross and microscopic lesions and coexisting microorganisms. *Journal of Veterinary Diagnostic Investigation*, **6**, 326–334.

Sweeney, C.R., Benson, C.E., Whitlock, R.H. *et al.* (1987). *Streptococcus equi* infection in horses. Parts I and II. *Compendium on Continuing Education for the Practicing Veterinarian*, **9**, 689–695 and 845–852.

Welsh, R.D. (1984). The significance of *Streptococcus zooepidemicus* in the horse. *Equine Practice*, **6**, 6–16.

Chapter 10

Corynebacterium species

Corynebacterium species are small, pleomorphic Gram-positive bacteria which occur in coccoid, club and rod forms (coryneform morphology). In stained smears, they occur singly, in pallisades of parallel cells and in angular clusters resembling Chinese letters (Fig. 10.1). The type species is *Corynebacterium diphtheriae*, the cause of diphtheria in children.

The genus *Corynebacterium* formerly contained a miscellaneous collection of bacteria. Recently, DNA and 16S rRNA studies have assigned several former members of the corynebacteria to other genera.

Most corynebacteria are catalase-positive, oxidase-negative, non-spore-forming facultative anaerobes which require enriched media for growth. Pathogenic corynebacteria are non-motile. Tissue trauma usually precedes the establishment of pathogenic corynebacteria and the resulting lesions are characterized by suppuration.

Usual habitat

Many *Corynebacterium* species are commensals on mucous membranes (Table 10.1). *Corynebacterium pseudotuberculosis* (formerly *C. ovis*) can survive for months in the environment.

Differentiation of the corynebacteria

Most pathogenic corynebacteria are relatively host specific and produce identifiable clinical syndromes. The host species and the nature of the disease may suggest the

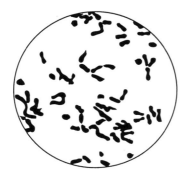

Figure 10.1 Characteristic pleomorphism of corynebacteria showing their typical arrangement in stained smears.

> **Key points**
> - Gram-positive, pleomorphic bacteria
> - Fastidious, requiring enriched media
> - Majority are commensals on mucous membranes
> - Cause pyogenic infections
> - *Corynebacterium* species:
>   —non-motile facultative anaerobes
>   —catalase-positive, oxidase-negative

causal agent. Identification criteria include bacterial cell morphology, colonial appearance and biochemical reactions. An enhancement of haemolysis test is used for the identification of *C. pseudotuberculosis*.

- Colonial characteristics:
  - *Corynebacterium bovis* is a lipophilic bacterium which produces small, white, dry, non-haemolytic colonies in the well of plates inoculated with a bovine milk sample.
  - *Corynebacterium kutscheri* produces whitish colonies. Occasional isolates are haemolytic.
  - *Corynebacterium pseudotuberculosis* has small, whitish colonies surrounded by a narrow zone of complete haemolysis, which may not be evident for up to 72 hours. After several days, the colonies become dry, crumbly and cream-coloured.
  - Members of the *C. renale* group produce small non-haemolytic colonies after incubation for 24 hours. Pigment production after incubation for 48 hours is one of the differentiating features of the three species in the group (Table 10.2).
- Biochemical reactions:
  - Conventional or commercially-available biochemical tests can be used to differentiate the corynebacteria.
  - Two biotypes of *C. pseudotuberculosis* are recognised. The ovine/caprine strains lack nitrate-reducing capacity, while the equine/bovine strains usually reduce nitrate. Cross-infection by biotypes is thought to be minimal.
  - The biochemical reactions used to distinguish

Table 10.1 The pathogenic corynebacteria, their hosts, usual habitats and the disease conditions which they produce.

Pathogen	Host	Disease condition	Usual habitat
Corynebacterium bovis	Cattle	Subclinical mastitis	Teat cistern
C. kutscheri	Laboratory rodents	Superficial abscesses, caseopurulent foci in liver, lungs and lymph nodes	Mucous membranes, environment
C. pseudotuberculosis			
Non-nitrate-reducing biotype	Sheep, goats	Caseous lymphadenitis	Skin, mucous membranes, environment
Nitrate-reducing biotype	Horses, cattle	Ulcerative lymphangitis, abscesses	Environment
C. renale group			
C. renale (type I)	Cattle	Cystitis, pyelonephritis	Lower urogenital tracts of cows and bulls
	Sheep and goats	Ulcerative (enzootic) balanoposthitis	Prepuce
C. pilosum (type II)	Cattle	Cystitis, pyelonephritis	Bovine urogenital tract
C. cystitidis (type III)	Cattle	Severe cystitis, rarely pyelonephritis	Bovine urogenital tract
C. ulcerans	Cattle	Mastitis	Human pharyngeal mucosa

members of the *C. renale* group are indicated in Table 10.2.

—Urease is produced by all pathogenic corynebacteria with the exception of *C. bovis*.

• Enhancement of haemolysis test:
The haemolysis produced by *C. pseudotuberculosis* is enhanced when the organisms are inoculated across a streak of *Rhodococcus equi* (Fig. 10.2).

Pathogenesis and pathogenicity

Many corynebacteria are opportunistic pathogens. Corynebacteria, with the exception of *C. bovis*, are pyogenic organisms which cause a variety of suppurative conditions in domestic animals. *Corynebacterium bovis*, which is found in the teat canal of up to 20% of apparently healthy dairy cows, provokes a mild neutrophil response. It has been suggested that this response may protect the mammary gland against invasion by more virulent pathogens (Pociecha, 1989).

Corynebacterium pseudotuberculosis is a facultative intracellular pathogen, capable of surviving and replicating in phagocytes. The virulence of this pathogen is linked to its cell wall lipid and to the production of an exotoxin, phospholipase D (PLD). This enzyme hydrolyzes sphingomyelin in mammalian cell membranes, releasing choline. In the early stages of infection, PLD may enhance survival and multiplication of *C. pseudotuberculosis* in the host. Both *C. ulcerans* and *C. pseudotuberculosis* can produce diphtheria toxin when lysogenized by corynephage beta which possesses the *tox* gene. Although

the effect of this toxin in animals is unclear, its presence in raw milk from cows infected with *C. ulcerans* may have public health implications.

Bacteria in the *C. renale* group are urinary tract pathogens which cause cystitis and pyelonephritis in cattle. These organisms produce urease, and hydrolyse urea. Members of the *C. renale* group possess fimbriae which allow attachment to the urogenital mucosa.

Minor trauma to the skin may allow entry of *C. kutscheri* and *C. pseudotuberculosis*, whereas the urinary tract pathogens avail of diminished immunological defences or local tissue damage following parturition.

Table 10.2 Differentiation of bacteria in the *Corynebacterium renale* group.

Feature	*C. renale* (type I)	*C. pilosum* (type II)	*C. cystitidis* (type III)
Colour of colony	Pale yellow	Yellow	White
Growth in broth at pH 5.4	+	−	−
Nitrate reduction	−	+	−
Acid from xylose	−	−	+
Acid from starch	−	+	+
Casein digestion	+	−	−
Hydrolysis of Tween 80	−	−	+

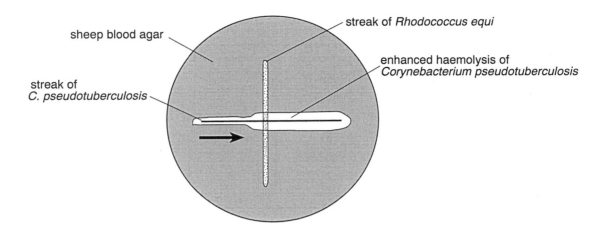

Figure 10.2   Enhancement of haemolysis test for *Corynebacterium pseudotuberculosis*. When a streak of *C. pseudotuberculosis* is drawn at right angles (arrow) across a streak of *Rhodococcus equi*, enhancement of haemolysis occurs.

Diagnostic procedures

- The species of animal affected and the clinical signs may suggest a specific diagnosis.
- Suitable specimens for laboratory examination include pus, exudate, samples of affected tissue and mid-stream urine.
- Direct microscopic examination of Gram-stained smears from specimens may reveal coryneform organisms (Fig. 10.1).
- Culture media for routine use include blood agar, selective blood agar and MacConkey agar. Inoculated plates are incubated aerobically at 37°C for 24 to 48 hours.
- Identification criteria for isolates:
  — Colonial characteristics
  — Presence or absence of haemolysis
  — Aerobic or anaerobic incubation requirements
  — Absence of growth on MacConkey agar
  — Typical coryneform pleomorphism in a Gram-stained smear from culture (Fig. 10.1)
  — Results of conventional or commercially available biochemical tests
  — Specific tests for distinguishing members of the *C. renale* group (Table 10.2)
  — Enhancement of haemolysis test for *C. pseudotuberculosis*

Clinical infections

The main diseases caused by infections with *Corynebacterium* species are summarized in Table 10.1. *Corynebacterium pseudotuberculosis* causes occasional human infections; some acquired from infected animals and others from environmental sources.

Caseous lymphadenitis

Caseous lymphadenitis, caused by the non-nitrate-reducing biotype of *C. pseudotuberculosis,* is a chronic suppurative condition of sheep, goats and rarely cattle. Infection results in abscessation and enlargement of superficial or internal lymph nodes. The incubation period is about 3 months. The disease is prevalent in Australia, New Zealand, the Middle East, Asia, Africa and parts of North and South America. Caseous lymphadenitis is being reported more frequently in Britain and other European countries. Ill-thrift may be evident in affected animals, and the disease invariably results in condemnation of carcases and devaluation of hides. Infection is spread by pus from ruptured abscesses and from nasal and oral secretions. The organism can survive in the environment for several months. *Corynebacterium pseudotuberculosis* has been isolated from the milk of affected goats.

Sheep become infected through contamination of shearing wounds, by arthropod bites or from contaminated dips. Affected lymph nodes are enlarged and exhibit characteristic encapsulated abscesses which have an 'onion ring' appearance in cross-section. The abscess material is caseous, initially greenish and later putty-coloured. Haematogenous spread can lead to abscessation of internal lymph nodes without obvious superficial lesions. Ill-thrift and pneumonia may be present. The visceral form of the disease may not be detectable antemortem. Goats usually develop the superficial form of the disease with subcutaneous abscesses in the head and neck regions.

Diagnosis
- The disease may be suspected on clinical grounds or at postmortem examination.
- Smears from lesions may reveal Gram-positive coryneform bacteria.

- Isolation and identification of *C. pseudotuberculosis* from abscess material is confirmatory.
- A sandwich ELISA, which detects circulating antibodies directed against the exotoxin (PLD), has been developed for identifying infected sheep (Schreuder *et al.*, 1994).

Treatment

Because of the chronic nature of lesions and the ability of the organisms to survive intracellularly, therapy is usually ineffective.

Control

Appropriate control measures for individual countries are determined by the prevalence of the disease.

- Exclusion of caseous lymphadenitis from countries free of the disease:
  — Sheep and goats should be imported only from countries which are either free of the disease or have a low incidence of infection. Animals must be selected from flocks or herds officially certified to be free of infection for 3 years.
  — Animals should be subjected to pre-importation ELISA testing.
  — Imported animals should be quarantined for several months and infected animals should be slaughtered.
- Eradication of caseous lymphadenitis from countries with a low prevalence of the disease:
  — Animals with obvious lesions should be segregated and culled.
  — Regular testing of flocks or herds using ELISA should be followed by culling of animals with positive or doubtful results.
  — Lambs can be removed from seropositive dams at birth and reared artificially.
  — Contaminated buildings and equipment should be thoroughly disinfected.
- Control measures in countries with a high prevalence of caseous lymphadenitis:
  — Strict hygienic measures should be applied in buildings such as shearing sheds. Shearing and docking equipment should be regularly and thoroughly disinfected.
  — Inactivated vaccines, available for use in some countries, may have a place in control programmes.

Ulcerative lymphangitis

The nitrate-reducing biotype of *C. pseudotuberculosis* causes sporadic cases of ulcerative lymphangitis in horses and cattle. Ulcerative lymphangitis occurs in Africa, the Americas, the Middle East and India. In the USA, the disease is prevalent in autumn and early winter and is more common in horses than in cattle. Infection occurs through skin wounds, arthropod bites or by contact with contaminated harness. The condition presents either as lymphangitis of the lower limbs or abscessation in the pectoral region. The onset of lymphangitis is slow and the condition usually becomes chronic. Affected lymphatic vessels are swollen and firm and nodules form along their length. Oedema develops in affected limbs, and ulcerated nodules exude a thick, odourless, greenish, blood-tinged pus. Infection in cattle manifests as lymphadenitis and lymphangitis with abscess formation and ulceration. Lesions of the coronary band with resulting lameness in affected dairy cattle have been reported (Steinman *et al.*, 1999).

Diagnosis is based on isolation and identification of *C. pseudotuberculosis* from lesions, since lymphangitis can also result from infection with other pyogenic bacteria. Systemic antibiotic therapy may be combined with topical treatment using an iodophor shampoo. Affected animals must be isolated and contaminated areas should be disinfected.

Bovine pyelonephritis

Organisms belonging to the *C. renale* group can be isolated from the vulva, vagina and prepuce of apparently normal cattle. The stress of parturition and the shortness of the urethra in the cow predispose to infection of the urinary tract. Although infection by any member of the group can cause cystitis, the most severe form is associated with *C. cystitidis*. Ascending infection from the bladder through the ureters can result in pyelonephritis. Clinical signs of pyelonephritis include fever, anorexia and decreased milk production. Restlessness and kicking at the abdomen may indicate renal pain. Dysuria, an arched back and blood-tinged urine are invariably present. Long-standing infections lead to extensive renal damage.

Diagnosis

- Clinical signs may suggest urinary tract disease.
- Thickened ureters and enlarged kidneys may be detected by rectal palpation. The condition is often unilateral.
- Red blood cells and protein are present in the urine.
- Culture of *C. renale* from urinary deposits, in association with characteristic clinical signs, is confirmatory.

Treatment

Antibiotic therapy, based on susceptibility testing, must be instituted early in the disease and should be continued for at least 3 weeks. Because penicillin is excreted in the urine, treatment with this antibiotic is particularly effective for susceptible isolates.

Ulcerative balanoposthitis

Ulcerative (enzootic) balanoposthitis (pizzle rot), particularly common in Merino sheep and Angora goats, is caused by *C. renale* and characterized by ulceration around the preputial orifice, with a brownish crust developing over the lesion. Similar lesions sometimes occur on the vulva in ewes. *Corynebacterium renale* can hydrolyse urea to ammonia which may cause mucosal irritation and ulceration. A high urinary urea level, a consequence of high protein intake, may predispose to the development of disease. Animals grazing pastures containing high oestrogen levels are also prone to the condition. Castrated sheep are affected more frequently than rams. A heavy wool or mohair cover around the prepuce predisposes to infection. Untreated cases may progress to total occlusion of the preputial orifice.

References

Pociecha, J.Z. (1989). Influence of *Corynebacterium bovis* on constituents of milk and dynamics of mastitis. *Veterinary Record*, **125**, 628.

Schreuder, B.E.C., terLaak, E.A. and Derck, D.P. (1994). Eradication of caseous lymphadenitis in sheep with the help of a newly developed ELISA technique. *Veterinary Record*, **135**, 174–176.

Steinman, A., Elad, D. and Spigel, N.Y. (1999). Ulcerative lymphangitis and coronet lesions in an Israeli dairy herd infected with *Corynebacterium pseudotuberculosis*. *Veterinary Record*, **145**, 604–606.

Further reading

Brown, C.C. and Ollander, H.J. (1987). Caseous lymphadenitis of goats and sheep. A review. *Veterinary Bulletin*, **57**, 1–11.

Carr, J., Walton, J. and Done, S. (1995). Cystitis and ascending pyelonephritis in the sow. *In Practice*, **17**, 71–79.

Lloyd, S. (1994). Caseous lymphadenitis in sheep and goats. *In Practice*, **16**, 24–29.

Rebhun, W.C., Dill, S.G., Perdrizet, J.A. and Hatfield, C.E. (1989). Pyelonephritis in cows: 15 cases (1982–1986). *Journal of the American Veterinary Medical Association*, **194**, 953–955.

Chapter 11

Rhodococcus equi

Rhodococcus equi, formerly called *Corynebacterium equi*, is a Gram-positive, aerobic soil saprophyte which occurs worldwide. It is an opportunistic pathogen of foals under 6 months of age. *Rhodococcus equi* grows on non-enriched media such as nutrient agar and produces characteristic mucoid salmon-pink colonies, features reflecting capsule formation and pigment production. Some strains of *R. equi* appear as cocci and others as rods up to 5 μm in length (Fig. 11.1). The organism is non-motile, catalase-positive, oxidase-negative and weakly acid-fast.

Usual habitat

Rhodococcus equi is an inhabitant of both soil and the intestinal tracts of animals. It can replicate at warm temperatures in soils enriched with faeces of herbivores.

Clinical infections

Suppurative bronchopneumonia of foals is the major disease caused by this pyogenic organism. Superficial abscesses due to *R. equi* have been recorded in horses over 6 months of age. Pigs, cats and cattle can occasionally be infected (Table 11.1). Pneumonia, caused by *R. equi* acquired from environmental sources, has been reported in patients with human immunodeficiency virus infection.

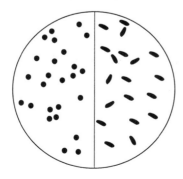

Figure 11.1 Cocci and rods, the two distinct morphological forms of *Rhodococcus equi*.

> **Key points**
> - Gram-positive rods or cocci
> - Growth on non-enriched media
> - Salmon-pink mucoid colonies with no haemolysis
> - Aerobic, non-motile
> - CAMP test-positive
> - Soil saprophyte
> - Respiratory pathogen of foals

Suppurative bronchopneumonia of foals

This important disease of foals 1 to 4 months of age is characterized by bronchopneumonia and lung abscessation. It is generally acquired by inhalation of dust contaminated with *R. equi*. The organism is often present in large numbers in the faeces of healthy foals under 3 months of age, and can also be isolated from the faeces of older horses and many other mammals and birds. A buildup of *R. equi* can occur on pastures heavily stocked with horses, leading to outbreaks of disease. Granulomatous ulcerative enterocolitis and mesenteric lymphadenitis sometimes occur when affected foals swallow sputum containing large numbers of *R. equi*. Ingestion of low numbers of organisms does not result in disease. Foals over 6 months of age appear to be refractory to pulmonary infection.

Pathogenesis and pathogenicity
The virulence of *R. equi*, an intracellular pathogen, is principally associated with specific surface antigens encoded in the DNA of a large plasmid. Production of these antigens is temperature dependent and they are expressed at 34 to 41°C (Takai *et al.*, 1992). Only virulent strains of *R. equi* are isolated from lesions of naturally infected foals and thus these virulence-associated antigens and plasmids can be used as epidemiological markers. Other factors enhancing virulence include capsular poly-saccharides and mycolic acids in the cell wall, which retard phagocytosis, and also various exoenzymes. The particular susceptibility of foals under four months of age

Table 11.1 Clinical conditions associated with *Rhodococcus equi*.

Host	Clinical condition
Foals of 1 to 4 months of age	Suppurative bronchopneumonia and pulmonary abscessation
Horses	Superficial abscessation
Pigs, cattle	Mild cervical lymphadenopathy
Cats	Subcutaneous abscesses, mediastinal granulomas

to bronchopneumonia caused by this pathogen is attributed to impaired cellular immunity in the lungs (Songer and Prescott, 1993).

Clinical signs

Clinical signs vary with the age at which the foal becomes infected. Acute disease often occurs in one month-old foals, with sudden onset of fever, anorexia and signs of bronchopneumonia. The disease tends to be insidious in 2 to 4 month-old foals and lesions can be well advanced before the animal exhibits coughing, dyspnoea, weight loss, exercise intolerance and characteristic loud, moist rales on auscultation of the lungs. Affected foals may occasionally have diarrhoea.

Diagnosis

- A history of the disease on the farm, the age of the affected foal and clinical signs may suggest infection with *R. equi*.
- Auscultation and radiography of the thorax provide confirmatory evidence of pulmonary involvement.
- Specimens for laboratory examination include tracheal aspirates and pus from lesions.
- Blood and MacConkey agar plates inoculated with suspect material are incubated aerobically at 37°C for 24 to 48 hours.
- Identification criteria for isolates:
  — Colonies on blood agar are non-haemolytic, salmon-pink and mucoid.
  — Absence of growth on MacConkey agar.
  — CAMP-test positive (Fig. 11.2).
  — Unreactive in the oxidation-fermentation test and in sugar fermentation tests.
  — Biochemical profile using commercially available kits.
- Quantitative faecal culture on a selective medium demonstrating over 10^6 *R. equi*/g of faeces may be of diagnostic value (Woolcock *et al.*, 1979).

Treatment

- A combination of oral rifampin and erythromycin for 4 to 10 weeks, although expensive, is the preferred treatment. However, severely affected foals may fail to respond. The response to therapy can be evaluated radiographically.
- Supportive therapy includes rehydration and the use of bronchodilatory agents or expectorants.

Control

- No commercial vaccines are available.
- On farms where the disease has occurred, foals should be kept under observation and examined clinically twice weekly until they are 4 months of age.
- Prevention of a buildup of *R. equi* in the environment of young foals is desirable:
  — Foal manure should be removed from pastures at frequent intervals.
  — Foals and their dams should be moved regularly to

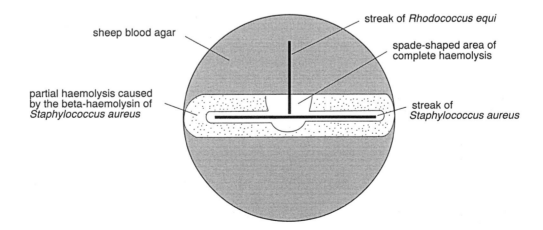

Figure 11.2 CAMP test. *Rhodococcus equi* produces a factor which completely lyses the red cells previously damaged by the beta-haemolysin of *Staphylococcus aureus*, producing a spade-shaped pattern of complete haemolysis which extends across the streak of *S. aureus*.

fresh pasture.
— Dusty conditions in paddocks and holding yards should be minimized.

• Hyperimmune serum from the dam, administered to the foal in the first month of life, is claimed to reduce the prevalence of disease on some farms.

References

Songer, J.G. and Prescott, J.F. (1993). *Rhodococcus equi.* In *Pathogenesis of Bacterial Infections in Animals*, Second Edition. Eds. C.L. Gyles, and C.O. Thoen. Iowa State University Press, Ames, Iowa. pp. 64–65.

Takai, S., Iie, M., Watanabe, Y., Tsubaki, S. and Sekizaki, S. (1992). Virulence-associated 15 to 17 kilodalton antigens in *Rhodococcus equi*: Temperature-dependent expression and localization of the antigens. *Infection and Immunity*, **60**, 2995–2997.

Woolcock, J.B., Farmer, A.M.T. and Mutimer, M.D. (1979). Selective medium for *Corynebacterium equi* isolation. *Journal of Clinical Microbiology*, **9**, 640–642.

Further reading

Giguere, S. and Prescott, J.F. (1997). Clinical manifestations, diagnosis, treatment and prevention of *Rhodococcus equi* infections in foals. *Veterinary Microbiology*, **56**, 313–334.

Knottenbelt, D.C. (1993). *Rhodococcus equi* infection in foals: a report of an outbreak on a thoroughbred stud in Zimbabwe. *Veterinary Record*, **132**, 79–85.

Takai, S. (1997). Epidemiology of *Rhodococcus equi* infections: a review. *Veterinary Microbiology*, **56**, 167–176.

Chapter 12

Actinomycetes

The actinomycetes are a phylogenetically diverse group of Gram-positive bacteria, which tend to grow slowly and produce branching filaments. Because of filament formation and granulomatous responses to tissue invasion, these organisms were originally regarded as fungi. However, filaments of the prokaryotic actinomycetes rarely exceed 1 μm in width, whereas hyphae of the eukaryotic fungi are usually more than 5 μm wide. The actinomycetes which cause disease in domestic animals belong to the genera *Actinomyces*, *Arcanobacterium*, *Actinobaculum*, *Nocardia* and *Dermatophilus* (Fig. 12.1). The comparative features of these genera, which are not closely related genetically, are summarized in Table 12.1.

Some thermophilic actinomycetes, such as *Micropolyspora faeni* found in poor-quality overheated hay, produce spores which can induce allergic pulmonary disease in cattle, horses and man. *Streptomyces* species are saprophytic soil actinomycetes and are common contaminants on laboratory media. They elaborate a variety of antimicrobial substances, many with therapeutic activity.

Actinomyces, Arcanobacterium and *Actinobaculum* species

The species in these genera are non-motile, non-spore-forming, Gram-positive bacteria which require enriched media for growth. *Arcanobacterium pyogenes* has undergone two name changes in recent years; it was formerly called *Actinomyces pyogenes* and before that *Corynebacterium pyogenes*. *Actinobaculum suis* has also undergone a number of recent name changes and is closely related to the genus *Arcanobacterium* (Lawson *et al.*, 1997). Both of these organisms have a coryneform morphology whereas the *Actinomyces* species are usually long and filamentous although short V, Y and T configurations also occur (Fig. 12.2). The species of veterinary importance in the group are *Arcanobacterium pyogenes*, *Actinobaculum suis*, *Actinomyces bovis*, *Actinomyces viscosus* and *Actinomyces hordeovulneris*. The main diseases are summarized in Table 12.2.

Key points

- Gram-positive bacteria, many species with branching filaments
- Relatively slow growth on laboratory media
- Opportunistic pathogens producing diverse inflammatory responses
- *Actinomyces, Arcanobacterium* and *Actinobaculum* species
  —anaerobic or facultatively anaerobic
  —morphologically heterogeneous
  —non-spore-forming, non-motile
  —MZN-negative
  —colonize mucous membranes
- *Nocardia* species
  —aerobic, non-motile
  —spores from aerial filaments
  —growth on Sabouraud dextrose agar
  —MZN-positive
  —soil saprophytes
- *Dermatophilus congolensis*
  —aerobic and capnophilic
  —motile zoospores
  —no growth on Sabouraud dextrose agar
  —found in scabs and in foci on skin of carrier animals

Usual habitat

With the exception of *A. hordeovulneris*, pathogenic members of these genera colonize the mucous membranes of mammals. *Actinomyces bovis* is found in the oropharynx of cattle and other domestic animals, and *Actinomyces viscosus* is a commensal in the oral cavity of dogs and humans. *Arcanobacterium pyogenes* is commonly present on the nasopharyngeal mucosa of cattle, sheep and pigs. The usual habitat of *Actinobaculum suis* is the preputial mucosa of boars. Although the habitat of *Actinomyces hordeovulneris* is uncertain, the organism appears to be closely associated with awns in the seed

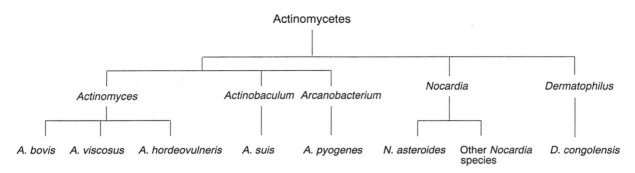

Actinomycetes

Actinomyces — Actinobaculum Arcanobacterium — Nocardia — Dermatophilus

A. bovis   *A. viscosus*   *A. hordeovulneris*   *A. suis*   *A. pyogenes*   *N. asteroides*   Other *Nocardia* species   *D. congolensis*

Figure 12.1   Pathogenic actinomycetes of veterinary importance.

heads of grasses of the genus *Hordeum*. The seed heads of these grasses are often referred to as foxtails in North America.

Differentiation of the genera

Differentiating features of the genera are presented in Table 12.3.

* Morphology of individual species in stained smears aids differentiation. *Arcanobacterium pyogenes* and *Actinobaculum suis* have coryneform morphology.
* Each species has a defined atmospheric growth requirement.
* Colonial morphology and haemolytic activity:
  —*Arcanobacterium pyogenes* produces a characteristic hazy haemolysis along streak lines after aerobic incubation for 24 hours. Pin-point colonies become visible after 48 hours.
  —*Actinomyces bovis* and *A. hordeovulneris* colonies typically adhere to agar media and are usually non-haemolytic.

—*Actinomyces viscosus* can produce two colony types, one large and smooth and the other small and rough. The large colony is composed of V, Y and T cell configurations and the smaller colonies are formed of short branching filaments.
—*Actinobaculum suis* produces colonies which are up

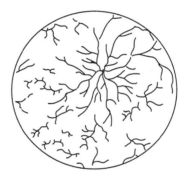

Figure 12.2   Long branching filaments and shorter V, Y and T forms, typical of many *Actinomyces* species as they appear in smears from lesions.

Table 12.1   Comparative features of actinomycetes of veterinary importance.

Feature	*Actinomyces* species	*Arcanobacterium pyogenes*	*Actinobaculum suis*	*Nocardia* species	*Dermatophilus congolensis*
Atmospheric growth requirements	Anaerobic or facultatively anaerobic and capnophilic	Facultatively anaerobic and capnophilic	Anaerobic	Aerobic	Aerobic and capnophilic
Aerial filament production	−	−	−	+	−
Modified Ziehl-Neelsen staining	−	−	−	+	−
Growth on Sabouraud dextrose agar	−	−	−	+	−
Usual habitat	Nasopharyngeal and oral mucosae	Nasopharyngeal mucosa of cattle, sheep and pigs	Prepuce and preputial diverticulum of boars	Soil	Skin of carrier animals, scabs from lesions
Site of lesions	Many tissues including bone	Soft tissues	Urinary tract of sows	Thoracic cavity, skin and other tissues	Skin

Table 12.2 Disease conditions produced by *Actinomyces, Arcanobacterium* and *Actinobaculum* species in domestic animals.

Species	Hosts	Disease conditions
Arcanobacterium pyogenes	Cattle, sheep, pigs	Abscessation, mastitis, suppurative pneumonia, endometritis, pyometra, arthritis, umbilical infections
Actinomyces hordeovulneris	Dogs	Cutaneous and visceral abscessation, pleuritis, peritonitis, arthritis
Actinomyces bovis	Cattle	Bovine actinomycosis (lumpy jaw)
A. viscosus	Dogs	Canine actinomycosis: — cutaneous pyogranulomas — pyothorax and proliferative pyogranulomatous pleural lesions — disseminated lesions (rare)
	Horses	Cutaneous pustules
	Cattle	Abortion
Actinomyces species (unclassified)	Pigs	Pyogranulomatous mastitis
	Horses	Poll evil and fistulous withers
Actinobaculum suis	Pigs	Cystitis, pyelonephritis

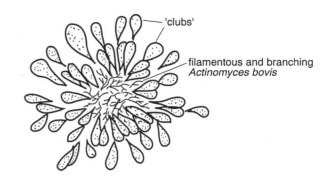

Figure 12.3 A club colony with a core of branching filaments of *Actinomyces bovis* surrounded by club-shaped structures. These structures are part of the host response to this chronic infection.

laboratories, are required for definitive identification of most of these fastidious, slow-growing organisms. In routine diagnosis, a presumptive identification of *A. pyogenes* is based on colonial morphology and pitting of a Loeffler's serum slope within 24 hours, which indicates proteolytic activity. It also hydrolyses gelatin.

• Granules in pus
  Granules can be detected when pus is diluted with distilled water in a Petri dish. In infections caused by *A. bovis*, pinhead-sized, yellowish 'sulphur granules' are found. Whitish, soft, grey granules are demonstrable in pus from animals infected with *A. viscosus*. Granules in lesions caused by *A. bovis* contain characteristic clubs (Fig. 12.3). Club colony formation is a feature of other chronic infections such as bovine actinobacillosis caused by *Actinobacillus lignieresii* and botryomycosis usually associated with *Staphylococcus aureus*.

to 3 mm in diameter, with a shiny raised centre and a dull edge. Poorly defined haemolysis is observed on ruminant blood agar.

• Biochemical reactions
  Specialized techniques, usually conducted in reference

• Urease is produced by *A. suis*.

Table 12.3 Differentiation of *Actinomyces, Arcanobacterium* and *Actinobaculum* species of veterinary importance.

Characteristic	*Actinomyces bovis*	*Actinomyces viscosus*	*Actinomyces hordeovulneris*	*Arcanobacterium pyogenes*	*Actinobaculum suis*
Morphology	Filamentous branching, some short forms	Filamentous branching, short forms	Filamentous branching, short forms	Coryneform	Coryneform
Atmospheric requirements	Anaerobic + CO_2	10% CO_2	10% CO_2	Aerobic	Anaerobic
Haemolysis on sheep blood agar	±	−	±	+	±
Catalase production	−	+	+	−	−
Pitting of Loeffler's serum slope	−	−	−	+	−
Granules in pus	'Sulphur granules'	White granules	No granules	No granules	No granules

Pathogenesis and pathogenicity

Arcanobacterium pyogenes produces a haemolytic exotoxin which has dermonecrotizing activity and is lethal for laboratory animals. This bacterium also produces a protease and a neuraminidase, neither of which has a defined role in virulence. Toxin production by the other *Actinomyces* species has not been established. Purulent reactions are typical of infections with *A. pyogenes* whereas *A. bovis* and *A. viscosus* provoke pyogranulomatous reactions.

Diagnostic procedures

- Clinical presentation, species affected and type and location of lesions may suggest the species involved.
- Specimens suitable for laboratory procedures include exudates, aspirates and tissue samples for culture and histopathology.
- Gram-stained smears may reveal morphological forms typical of the aetiological agent (Fig. 12.2). Unlike *Nocardia* species, these bacteria are modified Ziehl-Neelsen (MZN) negative.
- Histopathological examination of specimens from lesions caused by *A. bovis* reveals aggregates of filamentous organisms surrounded by eosinophilic club-shaped structures (Fig. 12.3).
- Blood and MacConkey agars are inoculated with the specimen and incubated at 37°C for up to 5 days. The atmospheric requirements for different species are indicated in Table 12.3. Species identification is difficult except in the case of *A. pyogenes*.
- Identification criteria for isolates:
  — Colonial characteristics
  — Morphology in stained smears
  — Presence or absence of haemolysis on blood agar
  — Absence of growth on MacConkey agar
  — Absence or presence of growth when subcultured onto Sabouraud dextrose agar
  — Pitting of a Loeffler's serum slope (*A. pyogenes*)
  — Urease production (*A. suis*)

Clinical infections

The disease conditions produced by the pathogenic *Actinomyces*, *Arcanobacterium* and *Actinobaculum* species are presented in Table 12.2. In some conditions the identity of the actinomycete has not been clearly defined. An unclassified *Actinomyces* species, resembling *A. bovis*, has been isolated from pyogranulomatous mastitis in sows. Abortion in sows has been ascribed to *A. naeslundii*, an organism usually associated with human dental caries (Palmer *et al.*, 1979). An *Actinomyces* species, probably *A. bovis*, has been identified in the suppurative discharges from poll evil and fistulous withers in horses.

Infections with *Arcanobacterium pyogenes*

Arcanobacterium pyogenes is a common cause of suppurative lesions in many domestic species worldwide, especially cattle, pigs and sheep. Any organ system may be affected. Cases of lymphadenitis, osteomyelitis, peritonitis and neural abscessation are commonly encountered. The organism has also been associated with pyometra, metritis and acute mastitis in cows. In the acute bovine mastitis, referred to as 'summer mastitis' in Britain and Ireland, the anaerobic bacterium *Peptostreptococcus indolicus* is usually associated with *A. pyogenes*. *Arcanobacterium pyogenes* also occurs in association with anaerobes in other mixed infections such as foot abscesses in cattle and sheep (*see* Chapter 32). Diagnosis is based on the typical pleomorphic cell morphology in Gram-stained smears from specimens, colonial characteristics and the ability of *A. pyogenes* to pit a Loeffler's serum slope. The organism is usually susceptible to penicillin but broad-spectrum antibiotics may be necessary as *A. pyogenes* often occurs in mixed infections.

Canine actinomycosis

Actinomyces viscosus is the aetiological agent of canine actinomycosis. Infection can result in subcutaneous pyogranulomatous lesions and extensive fibrovascular proliferation on the peritoneal or pleural surfaces with sanguinopurulent exudate in the affected cavity. The thoracic lesions closely resemble those of canine nocardiosis. The main clinical finding is respiratory distress. *Actinomyces viscosus* has also been isolated from cutaneous lesions in a horse (Specht *et al.*, 1991) and from an aborted heifer (Okewole *et al.*, 1989). The lesions associated with *A. hordeovulneris* infection in the dog include cutaneous and visceral pyogranulomas, pleuritis, peritonitis and arthritis. In uncomplicated infections, *A. viscosus* is usually responsive to treatment with penicillin. Recently a new species, *Actinomyces canis*, has been described which was isolated from a number of differing clinical conditions in dogs (Hoyles *et al.*, 2000).

Bovine actinomycosis (lumpy jaw)

Invasion of the mandible and, less commonly, the maxilla of cattle by *A. bovis* causes a chronic rarefying osteomyelitis. The organism is presumed to invade the tissues following trauma to the mucosa from rough feed or through dental alveoli during tooth eruption. A painless swelling of the affected bone enlarges over a period of several weeks. The swelling becomes painful and fistulous tracts, discharging purulent exudate, develop. Spread to contiguous soft tissues may occur but there is minimal involvement of regional lymph nodes.

Diagnosis

- Clinical signs are often distinctive in advanced cases.
- Radiography can be used to determine the degree of bone destruction.
- Other appropriate diagnostic techniques (*see* Diagnostic procedures).
- Lumpy jaw should be distinguished from other conditions which result in swelling of the bones of the jaw and from actinobacillosis which may involve the soft tissues of the head.

Treatment

- When lesions are small and circumscribed, surgery is the therapy of choice. In advanced cases, surgical treatment is frequently unrewarding.
- Prolonged therapy with penicillin, given parenterally to animals early in the disease, may be of value. Isoniazid *per os* for 30 days has also been recommended.

Porcine cystitis and pyelonephritis

This specific disease, which affects the urinary tract of pregnant sows, is transmitted at coitus and is potentially fatal. The pathogen, *Actinobaculum suis*, can be isolated from the prepuce and preputial diverticulum of healthy boars but not from the urogenital tract of healthy sows. Boars are rarely affected clinically and sows usually develop evidence of disease 3 to 4 weeks after mating. Anorexia, arching of the back, dysuria and haematuria are prominent signs. If both kidneys are extensively damaged death may result. The diagnostic procedures and therapeutic measures appropriate for this disease are similar to those for bovine pyelonephritis (*see* Chapter 10).

Nocardia asteroides and other *Nocardia* species

Members of the *Nocardia* species are Gram-positive, aerobic, saprophytic actinomycetes. In smears of exudate from infected tissue, they appear as long, slender branching filaments with a tendency to fragment into rods and cocci (Fig. 12.4). When cultured, these organisms produce aerial filaments which may form spores. Components of the cell wall, especially mycolic acid, render *Nocardia* species partially acid-fast (MZN-positive). In this genus, *Nocardia asteroides* is the pathogen of greatest significance in domestic animals (Table 12.4).

Usual habitat

Nocardia species are saprophytes found in soil and decaying vegetation.

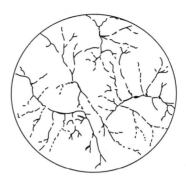

Figure 12.4 Branching filaments of *Nocardia asteroides* as they appear in smears from lesions. The filaments have a tendency to fragment.

Differentiation of *Nocardia* species

At least 12 *Nocardia* species are recognized, including *N. asteroides*, *N. farcinica* and *N. nova*, which is a human pathogen. These three species are closely related (Wallace *et al.*, 1991). Identification of individual species is usually carried out in reference laboratories and is based on specialized biochemical tests, analyses of mycolic acid composition and DNA probes.

Pathogenesis and pathogenicity

Infection, which is opportunistic, is usually associated with immunosuppression or, alternatively, may follow a heavy challenge. The usual mode of infection is by inhalation but it may also occur through skin wounds or via the teat canal. An intestinal form of nocardiosis may result from ingestion of the organisms.

Table 12.4 Disease conditions produced by *Nocardia* species in domestic animals.

Species	Hosts	Disease conditions
Nocardia asteroides	Dogs	Canine nocardiosis: — cutaneous pyogranulomas — pyogranulomatous pleural lesions and pyothorax — disseminated lesions
	Cattle	Chronic mastitis, abortion
	Pigs	Abortion
	Sheep, goats, horses	Wound infections, mastitis, pneumonia, other pyogranulomatous conditions
Nocardia farcinica	Cattle	Bovine farcy[a]

a some mycobacteria have also been implicated in bovine farcy

Virulent strains of *N. asteroides* survive intracellularly. The production of superoxide dismutase and catalase and the presence of a thick peptidoglycan layer in the cell wall confer resistance to microbiocidal activity of phagocytes. Cell-mediated immunity is essential for protection against infection by this facultative, intracellular bacterium (Deem *et al.*, 1982).

Diagnostic procedures

A presumptive diagnosis of infection with *N. asteroides* is based on clinical findings and laboratory procedures.

* Specimens suitable for laboratory examination include exudates, aspirates, mastitic milk, tissue from granulomas and fixed tissue for histopathology.
* Smears of exudate should be stained by the Gram and MZN methods. *Nocardia asteroides* is MZN-positive, unlike *Actinomyces* species which are MZN-negative.
* Histopathological examination of tissue specimens may reveal clusters of nocardial filaments.
* The organism can be cultured on blood agar or on selective growth-enhancing media such as charcoal-yeast extract medium. Plates are incubated aerobically at 37°C for up to 10 days.
* Identification criteria for isolates:
  — Colonies on blood agar are usually visible after incubation for about 5 days. They are white, powdery and firmly adherent to the agar. Colonies are variably haemolytic and odourless.
  — Subculture onto Sabouraud dextrose agar yields dry, wrinkled, orange-coloured colonies after incubation for up to 5 days.
  — Gram-stained smears from colonies show some filamentous forms with a preponderance of rod and coccal forms.
* *Nocardia asteroides* requires differentiation from *Streptomyces* species which may contaminate laboratory media. Features of *Streptomyces* species which distinguish them from *Nocardia asteroides* include a strong, earthy odour, MZN-negative filaments and colonies on Sabouraud dextose agar which are powdery-white in appearance.

Clinical infections

Nocardia asteroides accounts for most nocardial infections in domestic animals (Table 12.4). The most commonly encountered conditions are cutaneous and systemic infections in dogs and mastitis in cattle. Nocardial infection has been reported occasionally in horses, immunosuppression being an important predisposing factor (Biberstein *et al.*, 1985). *Nocardia asteroides* has also been associated with abortion in sows (Koehne, 1981). *Nocardia farcinica* is implicated in bovine farcy. *Nocardia brasiliensis* and *N. otitidiscaviarum* (*N. caviae*)

Table 12.5 Differentiation of *Nocardia asteroides* and *Actinomyces viscosus*.

Characteristic	Nocardia asteroides	Actinomyces viscosus
MZN-staining of filaments	+	−
Atmospheric requirement	Aerobic	10% CO$_2$
Growth on Sabouraud dextrose agar	+	−
Susceptibility to Penicillin G	−	+

MZN modified Ziehl-Neelsen stain

are pathogenic for man and rarely cause disease in domestic animals.

Canine nocardiosis

Infections in dogs, usually due to *N. asteroides*, are acquired by inhalation, through skin wounds or by ingestion. Thoracic, cutaneous and disseminated forms of the disease are recognised. The thoracic form is characterised by fever, anorexia and respiratory distress. There is a fibrovascular proliferative reaction on the pleura and sanguinopurulent fluid accumulates in the thoracic cavity. The cutaneous form presents either as an indolent ulcer or as a granulomatous swelling with discharging fistulous tracts. In the disseminated form, which occurs typically in dogs less than 12 months of age, clinical signs are non-specific and are referable to the organ system mainly affected.

Diagnosis
Although canine nocardiosis is clinically similar to canine actinomycosis, antibiotic therapy for nocardiosis is less effective. Consequently, it is essential to distinguish the two main aetiological agents, *N. asteroides* and *A. viscosus*. The main differentiating features of these two organisms are listed in Table 12.5.

Treatment
Nocardia asteroides strains show a marked variation in their susceptibility to antibiotics. Effective antibiotics, which include amikacin, imipenem-cilastatin and co-trimoxazole, should be administered systemically for at least 6 weeks.

Bovine nocardial mastitis

A chronic form of bovine mastitis results from infection with *N. asteroides*. Fibrosis, either diffuse or multifocal, develops and white clots are evident intermittently in the milk. Multifocal fibrosis can be detected clinically as discrete hard masses, up to 5 cm in diameter, palpable in the affected gland after milking. Infection during early lactation may occasionally induce a systemic reaction with fever, depression and anorexia. Nocardial mastitis is usually sporadic, affecting only one or two cows in a herd and is usually refractory to chemotherapy.

Bovine farcy

This disease, also known as bovine nocardiosis, is limited to the tropics. It is a chronic infection of superficial lymphatic vessels and lymph nodes. Early lesions consist of small cutaneous nodules, often on the medial aspect of the legs and on the neck. These nodules enlarge slowly and coalesce to form swellings, up to 10 cm in diameter, which rarely ulcerate. The lymphatic vessels may become thickened and cord-like. Internal organs may be affected occasionally and the condition is important because lesions resemble those of tuberculosis. Because *Nocardia farcinica*, *Mycobacterium farcinogenes* and *M. senegalense* have been isolated from such lesions, the aetiology of bovine farcy requires clarification.

Dermatophilus congolensis

Dermatophilus congolensis is a Gram-positive, filamentous, branching actinomycete with distinctive morphology (Fig. 12.5). This actinomycete is unusual because it produces motile coccal zoospores about 1.5 μm in diameter. Mature zoospores produce germ tubes which develop into filaments 0.5 to 1.5 μm in width. Within these filaments, transverse and longitudinal divisions form segments which ultimately develop into zoospores. Mature filaments may be more than 5 μm in width and contain columns of zoospores which impart a 'tram-track' appearance to the filaments. Although skin infections caused by *D. congolensis* occur worldwide, dermatophilosis is most prevalent in tropical and subtropical regions.

Usual habitat

The organism seems to persist in foci in the skin of many clinically normal animals, particularly in endemic areas. Dormant zoospores may become activated when microenvironmental moisture and temperature levels are favourable. Duration of zoospore survival in the environment is usually limited but may be up to three years in dry scabs.

Pathogenesis and pathogenicity

Dermatophilus congolensis does not usually invade healthy skin. Trauma and persistent wetting predispose to

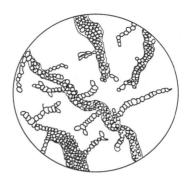

Figure 12.5 *Dermatophilus congolensis* in a smear from scab material. Wide filaments contain coccal zoospores. Side branches divide into segments prior to the formation of zoospores.

skin invasion. Microenvironmental conditions which interfere with normal surface protective mechanisms, such as sebaceous secretions, also lead to activation of dormant zoospores. When activated, zoospores produce germ tubes and these develop into filaments which invade the epidermis. The ability of individual strains to invade the epidermis is related to their virulence. Keratinolytic activity may be a virulence factor.

Invasion leads to an acute inflammatory response characterized by large numbers of neutrophils which ultimately form microabscesses in the epidermis. A cyclical pattern of invasion by the pathogen of regenerating epithelial cells, together with serous exudation and microabscess formation, leads to the development of raised scab-like crusts containing numerous branching filaments. Factors which depress specific immune responses, including intercurrent diseases and pregnancy, may increase host susceptibility to dermatophilosis.

Diagnostic procedures

- The clinical picture is usually indicative of the infection, particularly in endemic areas.
- Specimens suitable for laboratory examination include scab material and samples of skin fixed in formalin.
- Smears from the undersurface of scabs or from softened scab material, stained by the Giemsa method, reveal the characteristic branching filaments containing zoospores (Fig 12.5). When there is difficulty demonstrating the organism in smears, histopathological or immunofluorescent techniques may be employed.
- Scab material softened with water can be cultured on blood agar at 37°C in an atmosphere of 2.5–10% CO_2 for up to 5 days.
- Zoospores, which exhibit chemotaxis for CO_2, can be recovered from heavily contaminated specimens by placing infected scab material in distilled water at room temperature for 3.5 hours, followed by exposure to an atmosphere of CO_2 for 15 minutes. A sample from the surface of the water contains motile zoospores which

can be cultured.

- Identification criteria:
  - After incubation for 48 hours, colonies are up to 1 mm in diameter, yellow and haemolytic. When incubated for 3 to 4 days, they become rough, golden-yellow and embedded in the agar. Older colonies may have a mucoid appearance.
  - Giemsa-stained smears from colonies reveal solidly-staining filaments.
  - No growth occurs on Sabouraud dextrose agar.
  - Biochemical tests are rarely required for identification. The organism liquefies Loeffler's serum medium, hydrolyzes gelatin and casein, and produces acid from glucose and fructose.

Clinical infections

Infections with *D. congolensis* are usually confined to the epidermis. However, invasion of subcutaneous tissue has been described in a cat (Jones, 1976). Commonly used designations for infection with this organism are dermatophilosis and cutaneous streptothricosis. Mycotic dermatitis (a misnomer) and lumpy wool are used to describe infection of wooled areas of the skin in sheep. When the skin of the lower limbs of sheep is involved, the condition is termed strawberry footrot.

Although the disease affects animals of all ages, it is more prevalent and often more severe in young animals. Damage to the skin predisposes to infection with *D. congolensis*. Zoospores are most often transmitted by direct contact with infected animals. In endemic tropical regions, the prevalence and severity of dermatophilosis correlates with infestation with *Amblyomma variegatum* (Morrow *et al.*, 1989). A number of blood-sucking insects may also be important in disease transmission in the tropics. Economic loss derives from damage to hides and fleece. Human skin infections, occasionally acquired through close contact with infected animals, are rare (Stewart, 1972).

Clinical signs

Lesion distribution usually correlates with those areas of skin predisposed to infection. Heavy prolonged rainfall in association with warm environmental temperatures can result in lesions predominantly affecting the dorsum of farm animals. Trauma to the face and limbs of animals grazing in thorny scrub can predispose to lesions in these sites. Early lesions present as papules and are often detectable only by palpation. As lesions progress, serous exudate causes matting of hairs giving them a tufted appearance. Lesions may coalesce to form irregular elevated crusty scabs. Tufts of hair can be readily plucked from the lesion along with adherent scab material and underlying exudate. Scab formation tends to be more pronounced in cattle and sheep than in horses.

Localized infections are usually of little consequence.

Lesions may resolve spontaneously within a few weeks, particularly in dry conditions. In severe infections, lesions may be extensive and deaths may occasionally occur particularly in calves and lambs. Rarely, oral lesions result in depression, difficulty with eating and loss of condition.

Diagnosis

Diagnosis is based on the clinical appearance of lesions and demonstration of *D. congolensis* in scabs. Isolation of the organism is confirmatory.

Treatment

Parenterally administered antibiotics such as long-acting oxytetracycline are usually effective. Alternatively, high doses of penicillin-streptomycin combinations on three consecutive days may be used. For treatment to be effective, satisfactory epidermal concentrations of the antibiotics are required. The outcome of treatment is influenced by the severity and extent of lesions. Topical treatments are ineffective.

Control

Control measures vary with geographical location and climatic factors; they are based on minimizing the effects of predisposing factors and early treatment of clinical cases.

- Clinically affected animals should be isolated and treated promptly.
- Shelter can be provided during periods of prolonged rainfall.
- Grazing areas should be cleared of thorny scrub.
- Tick infestation must be reduced by dipping or spraying with acaracides at weekly intervals and by elimination of tick habitats.
- Prophylactic use of long-acting tetracyclines may be required in endemic regions.
- Control of intercurrent diseases reduces the severity of dermatophilosis.

References

Biberstein, E.L., Jang, S.S. and Hirsh, D.C. (1985). *Nocardia asteroides* infection in horses: A review. *Journal of the American Veterinary Medical Association*, **186**, 273–277.

Deem, R.L., Beaman, B.L. and Gershwin, M.E. (1982). Adoptive transfer of immunity to *Nocardia asteroides* in nude mice. *Infection and Immunity*, **38**, 914–920.

Hoyles, L., Falsen, E., Foster, G., Pascual, C., Greko, C. and Collins, M.D. (2000). *Actinomyces canis* sp. nov. isolated from dogs. *International Journal of Systematic and Evolutionary Microbiology*, **50**, 1547–1551.

Jones, R.T. (1976). Subcutaneous infection with *Dermatophilus congolensis* in a cat. *Journal of Comparative Pathology*, **86**, 415–421.

Koehne, G. (1981). *Nocardia asteroides* abortion in swine.

Journal of the American Veterinary Medical Association, **179**, 478–479.

Lawson, P.A., Falsen, E., Akervall, E., Vandamme, P. and Collins, M.D. (1997). Characterization of some *Actinomyces*-like isolates from human clinical specimens: reclassification of *Actinomyces suis* (Soltys and Spratling) as *Actinobaculum suis* comb. nov. and description of *Actinobaculum schaalii* sp. nov. *International Journal of Systematic Bacteriology*, **47**, 899–903.

Morrow, A.N., Heron, I.D., Walker, A.R. and Robinson, J.L. (1989). *Amblyomma variegatum* ticks and the occurrence of bovine streptothricosis in Antigua. *Journal of Veterinary Medicine B*, **36**, 241–249.

Okewole, A.A., Odeyemi, P.S., Ocholi, R.A., Irokanulo, E.A., Haruna, E.S. and Oyetunde, I.L. (1989). *Actinomyces viscosus* from a case of abortion in a Friesian heifer. *Veterinary Record*, **124**, 464.

Palmer, N.C., Kierstead, M. and Wilson, R.W. (1979). Abortion in swine associated with *Actinomyces* spp. *Canadian Veterinary Journal*, **20**, 199.

Specht, T.E., Breuhaus, B.A., Manning, T.O., Miller, R.T. and Cochrane, R.B. (1991). Skin pustules and nodules caused by *Actinomyces viscosus* in a horse. *Journal of the American Veterinary Medical Association*, **198**, 457–459.

Stewart, G.H. (1972). Dermatophilosis: a skin disease of animals and man. *Veterinary Record*, **91**, 537–544 and 555–561.

Wallace, R.J., Brown, B.A., Tsukamura, M., Brown, J.M. and Onyi, G.O. (1991). Clinical and laboratory features of *Nocardia nova*. *Journal of Clinical Microbiology*, **29**, 2407–2411.

Further reading

Ellis, T.M., Masters, A.M., Sutherland, S.S., Carson, J.M. and Gregory, A.R. (1993). Variation in cultural, morphological, biochemical properties and infectivity of Australian isolates of *Dermatophilus congolensis*. *Veterinary Microbiology*, **38**, 81–102.

Kirpensteijn, J. and Fingland, R.B. (1992). Cutaneous actinomycosis and nocardiosis in dogs: 48 cases (1980–1990). *Journal of the American Veterinary Medical Association*, **201**, 917–920.

Chapter 13

Listeria species

Most *Listeria* species are small, Gram-positive cocco-bacillary rods, up to 2 μm in length (Fig. 13.1). They are catalase-positive, oxidase-negative, motile, facultative anaerobes. The genus is composed of six species, three of which are pathogenic. *Listeria monocytogenes*, the most important of these pathogens, has been implicated world-wide in diseases of many animal species and humans. It was first isolated from laboratory rabbits with septicaemia and monocytosis (Murray *et al.*, 1926). The organism can grow over a wide temperature range from 4°C to 45°C and can tolerate pH values between 5.5 and 9.6. The other two pathogens, *L. ivanovii* and *L. innocua*, are less frequently implicated in diseases of animals. The clinical manifestations of infections with *Listeria* species are summarized in Table 13.1.

Usual habitat

Listeria species can replicate in the environment. They are widely distributed and can be recovered from herbage, faeces of healthy animals, sewage effluent and bodies of fresh water.

Differentiation of *Listeria* species

The pattern of haemolysis on sheep blood agar, CAMP tests and acid production from a short range of sugars are useful differentiating laboratory methods for *Listeria*

Key points

- Small, Gram-positive rods
- Grow on non-enriched media
- Tolerates wide temperature and pH ranges
- Small haemolytic colonies on blood agar
- Facultative anaerobes, catalase-positive, oxidase-negative
- Tumbling motility at 25°C
- Aesculin hydrolysed
- Environmental saprophytes
- Outbreaks of listeriosis often related to silage feeding

---

species (Table 13.2). The colonies are small, smooth and transparent after incubation for 24 hours.

- Commercially-available biochemical test kits can be used to distinguish *Listeria* species.
- Sixteen serotypes, based on cell wall and flagellar antigens, are recognized (Low *et al.*, 1993).
- Phage typing is reproducible and discriminating but its diagnostic applications are limited.
- A chemiluminescent DNA probe assay is available for rapid and specific identification of *L. monocytogenes* from colonies on primary isolation plates (Okwumabua *et al.*, 1992).
- DNA fingerprinting methods are currently used in reference laboratories.

Pathogenesis and pathogenicity

Infection with *L. monocytogenes* usually follows ingestion of contaminated feed and may result in septicaemia, encephalitis or abortion. Organisms probably penetrate the M cells in Peyer's patches in the intestine. Spread occurs via lymph and blood to various tissues. In pregnant animals, infection results in transplacental transmission. There is evidence that the organism can invade through breaks in the oral or nasal mucosa. From this site, migration in cranial nerves is thought to be the main route

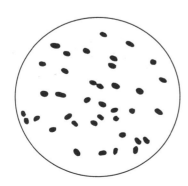

Figure 13.1 The typical coccobacillary form of *Listeria monocytogenes* from an actively-growing culture.

Table 13.1 Clinical manifestations of infections with *Listeria* species in domestic animals.

Species	Hosts	Forms of disease
Listeria monocytogenes	Sheep, cattle, goats	Encephalitis (neural form) Abortion Septicaemia Endophthalmitis (ocular form)
	Cattle	Mastitis (rare)
	Dogs, cats, horses	Abortion, encephalitis (rare)
	Pig	Abortion, septicaemia, encephalitis
	Birds	Septicaemia
L. ivanovii	Sheep, cattle	Abortion
L. innocua	Sheep	Meningoencephalitis (rare)

of infection in neural listeriosis. Lesions in the brain stem, often unilateral, are composed of microabscesses and perivascular lymphocytic cuffs.

Listeria monocytogenes has the ability to invade both phagocytic and non-phagocytic cells, to survive and replicate intracellularly and to transfer from cell-to-cell without exposure to humoral defence mechanisms. Specific surface proteins, internalins, facilitate both the adherence of organisms to host membranes and their subsequent uptake. Virulent strains also possess a cytolytic toxin, listeriolysin, which destroys the membranes of phagocytic vacuoles allowing listeria to escape into the cytoplasm. In the cytoplasm, the organisms utilize cellular microfilaments to generate tail-like structures which confer motility. The motile listeria contact the internal surface of the cytoplasmic membrane and induce pseudopod-like projections. These projections containing the bacteria are taken up by adjacent cells. The

entire process is then repeated following replication of listeria in newly-infected cells (Chakraborty and Wehland, 1997).

Clinical infections

Infections with *L. monocytogenes* have been recorded in more than 40 species of domestic and wild animals. Sporadic abortions in sheep and cattle have been attributed to infection with *L. ivanovii*. *Listeria innocua* has been implicated in a case of ovine meningoencephalitis (Walker *et al.*, 1994). The forms of listeriosis which occur in domestic animals are listed in Table 13.1.

Listeriosis in ruminants

Listeriosis in ruminants may present as encephalitis, abortion, septicaemia or endophthalmitis. Usually only one form of the disease occurs in a group of affected animals. Septicaemia, often encountered in newborn piglets, foals, cage birds and poultry, can also occur in adult sheep.

Although *L. monocytogenes* is widely distributed in the environment, outbreaks of listeriosis tend to be seasonal in European countries and to affect silage-fed animals in late pregnancy. *Listeria monocytogenes* can replicate in the surface layers of poor-quality silage with pH values above 5.5. In such circumstances, listerial numbers may reach 10^7 colony-forming units kg^{-1} of silage. In good quality silage, multiplication of the organisms is inhibited by the acid produced by fermentation. Susceptibility to infection with *L. monocytogenes* has been attributed to decreased cell-mediated immunity associated with advanced pregnancy.

Clinical signs

The incubation period of neural listeriosis (circling disease) ranges from 14 to 40 days. Dullness, circling and tilting of the head, are common clinical signs. Unilateral

Table 13.2 Laboratory methods for differentiating *Listeria* species.

Listeria species	Haemolysis on sheep blood agar	CAMP test		Acid production from sugars		
		S. aureus	*R. equi*	D-mannitol	L-rhamnose	D-xylose
L. monocytogenes	+	+	−	−	+	−
L. ivanovii	++	−	+	−	−	+
L. innocua	−	−	−	−	v	−
L. seeligeri	+	+	−	−	−	+
L. welshimeri	−	−	−	−	v	+
L. grayi	−	−	−	+	v	−

v variable reactions

facial paralysis results in drooling of saliva and drooping of the eyelid and ear. Exposure keratitis may occur in some cases. Body temperature may be elevated in the early stages of the disease. In sheep and goats, recumbency and death may follow within a few days of the emergence of clinical signs. The duration of illness is usually longer in cattle. Abortion, without evidence of systemic illness may occur up to 12 days after infection. Septicaemic listeriosis, with a short incubation period of 2 to 3 days, is most commonly encountered in lambs although it may occur occasionally in pregnant sheep. In cattle and sheep, keratoconjunctivitis and iritis (ocular listeriosis) are localized, often unilateral and have been attributed to direct contact with contaminated silage.

Diagnosis
- Characteristic neurological signs or abortion in association with silage feeding may suggest listeriosis.
- Appropriate specimens for laboratory examination depend on the form of the disease:
  — Cerebrospinal fluid (CSF) and tissue from the medulla and pons of animals with neurological signs should be sampled. Fresh tissue is required for isolation of organisms and fixed tissue for histopathological examination.
  — Specimens from cases of abortion should include cotyledons, foetal abomasal contents and uterine discharges.
  — Suitable samples from septicaemic cases include fresh liver or spleen and blood.
- Smears from cotyledons or from liver lesions may reveal Gram-positive coccobacillary bacteria.
- Immunofluorescence using monoclonal antibodies may facilitate a rapid diagnosis.
- Histological examination of brain tissue reveals microabscesses and heavy perivascular mononuclear cuffing in the medulla and elsewhere in the brain stem.
- White cell numbers exceeding $1.2 \times 10^7 L^{-1}$ and a protein concentration of greater than $0.4 gL^{-1}$ in CSF are found in neural listeriosis.
- Isolation methods:
  — Specimens from cases of abortion and septicaemia can be inoculated directly onto blood, selective blood and MacConkey agars. The plates are incubated aerobically at 37°C for 24 to 48 hours.
  — A cold-enrichment procedure is necessary for isolating the organism from brain tissue. Small pieces of medulla are homogenized and a 10% suspension is made in nutrient broth. The suspension is held at 4°C in a refrigerator and subcultured weekly onto blood agar for up to 12 weeks.
- Identification criteria for *L. monocytogenes* isolates:
  — Colonies are small, smooth and flat with a blue-green colour when illuminated obliquely. Rough variants occur infrequently. Individual colonies are usually surrounded by a narrow zone of complete haemolysis.
  — Catalase test is positive, distinguishing this organism from streptococci and *Arcanobacterium pyogenes* which have similar colonies but are catalase-negative.
  — CAMP test is positive with *Staphylococcus aureus* but not with *Rhododoccus equi* (Table 13.2).
  — Aesculin is hydrolysed.
  — Isolates incubated in broth at 25°C for 2 to 4 hours exhibit a characteristic tumbling motility.
  — Most isolates of animal origin are virulent, a characteristic which can be confirmed by animal inoculation. Instillation of a drop of broth culture into the eye of a rabbit induces keratoconjunctivitis (Anton test).

Treatment
Ruminants in the early stages of septicaemic listeriosis respond to systemic therapy with ampicillin or amoxicillin. Response to antibiotic therapy may be poor in neural listeriosis although prolonged high doses of ampicillin or amoxicillin combined with an aminoglycoside may be effective. Ocular listeriosis requires treatment with antibiotics and corticosteroids injected sub-conjunctivally.

Control
- Poor-quality silage should not be fed to pregnant ruminants. Silage feeding should be discontinued if an outbreak of listeriosis is confirmed.
- Feeding methods which minimize direct ocular contact with silage should be implemented.
- Vaccination with killed vaccines, which do not induce an effective cell-mediated response, is not protective because *L. monocytogenes* is an intracellular pathogen. Live, attenuated vaccines, which are available in some countries, are reported to reduce the prevalence of listeriosis in sheep (Gudding *et al.*, 1989).

Human listeriosis

If normal healthy adults acquire infection, the disease usually presents as a mild febrile illness resembling influenza. Papular lesions on the hands and arms, principally in veterinarians and farmers, can result from contact with infective material. Infection with *L. monocytogenes* can lead to abortion in pregnant women and can be life-threatening in neonates, the elderly and in immunosuppressed individuals.

Human infections usually result from consumption of contaminated food such as raw milk, soft cheeses, coleslaw and uncooked vegetables. *Listeria monoctogenes* may survive pasteurization because of its intracellular localization and tolerance to heat. Direct transfer from infected animals to humans is uncommon and is of little consequence in healthy, non-pregnant individuals.

References

Chakraborty, T. and Wehland, J. (1997). The host cell infected with *Listeria monocytogenes*. In *Host response to intracellular pathogens*. Ed. S.H.E. Kaufmann. Springer, New York. pp. 271–290.

Gudding, R., Nesse, L.L. and Gronstol, H. (1989). Immunization against infections caused by *Listeria monocytogenes* in sheep. *Veterinary Record*, **125**, 111–114.

Low, J.C., Wright, F., McLauchlin, J. and Donachie, W. (1993). Serotyping and distribution of *Listeria* isolates from cases of ovine listeriosis. *Veterinary Record*, **133**, 165–166.

Murray, E.G.D., Webb, R.A. and Swann, M.B.R. (1926). A disease of rabbits characterised by a large mononuclear leucocytosis caused by a hitherto undescribed bacillus *Bacterium monocytogenes*. *Journal of Pathology and Bacteriology*, **29**, 407–439.

Okwumabua, O., Swaminathan, B., Edmonds, P., Wenger, J., Hogan, J. and Alden, M. (1992). Evaluation of a chemiluminescent DNA probe assay for the rapid confirmation of *Listeria monocytogenes*. *Research in Microbiology*, **143**, 183–189.

Walker, J.K., Morgan, J.H., McLauchlin, J., Grant, K.A. and Shallcross, J.A. (1994). *Listeria innocua* isolated from a case of ovine meningoencephalitis. *Veterinary Microbiology*, **42**, 245–253.

Further reading

Low, J.C. and Donachie, W. (1997). A review of *Listeria monocytogenes* and listeriosis. *Veterinary Journal*, **153**, 9–29.

Chapter 14

Erysipelothrix rhusiopathiae

Erysipelothrix rhusiopathiae is a non-motile, Gram-positive, facultative anaerobe. It is catalase-negative, oxidase-negative, resistant to high salt concentrations and grows in the temperature range 5°C to 42°C and in the pH range of 6.7 to 9.2. Isolates from animals with acute infections form smooth colonies while isolates from chronically infected animals form rough colonies. Smears from smooth colonies yield slender rods (0.2 to 0.4 x 0.8 to 2.5 μm) whereas rough colonies are usually composed of short filaments which decolourize readily (Fig. 14.1). The bacterium grows on nutrient agar but growth is improved in media containing blood or serum.

Erysipelothrix rhusiopathiae causes erysipelas in pigs and turkeys worldwide. Sheep and other domestic animals are occasionally infected. The bacterium also causes erysipeloid, a localized cellulitis, in humans. The disease conditions associated with infection in domestic species are listed in Box 14.1.

Recently, several serotypes of *E. rhusiopathiae* have been reclassified as a new species, *E. tonsillarum*, using DNA-DNA hybridization studies (Takahashi *et al.*, 1992). This species appears to be non-pathogenic for pigs but causes endocarditis in dogs (Eriksen *et al.*, 1987).

Usual habitat

It is claimed that up to 50% of healthy pigs harbour *E. rhusiopathiae* in tonsillar tissues. Carrier pigs excrete the organism in faeces and in oronasal secretions. The bacterium has also been isolated from sheep, cattle, horses,

---

Key points

- Gram-positive, small rods (smooth form) or filaments (rough form)
- Growth on non-enriched media
- Small colonies, with incomplete haemolysis in 48 hours
- Growth over wide temperature and pH ranges
- Catalase-negative
- Coagulase-positive
- Non-motile, oxidase-negative, facultative anaerobe
- H_2S formed along stab line in TSI agar
- Found in porcine tonsils
- Causes swine erysipelas and turkey erysipelas

---

dogs, cats, poultry and from 50 species of wild mammals and over 30 species of wild birds. Although soil and surface water can become contaminated with *E. rhusiopathiae*, survival time in soil probably does not exceed 35 days under optimal conditions. The bacterium is often present in the slime layer of fish, a potential source of human infection.

Definitive identification of *Erysipelothrix rhusiopathiae*

- Colonial morphology and haemolytic activity
  Non-haemolytic, pin-point colonies appear after incubation for 24 hours and, after 48 hours, a narrow zone of greenish, incomplete haemolysis develops around the colonies. At this stage differences in colony morphology are evident. Smooth colonies are up to 1.5 mm in diameter, convex and circular with even edges while rough colonies are slightly larger, flat and opaque with irregular edges. A 'bottle-brush' type of growth is characteristic of rough isolates when they are stab-inoculated into nutrient gelatin and incubated at room temperature for up to 5 days.
- Biochemical reactions
  Commercially-available biochemical test kits can be used for definitive identification. Reactions for

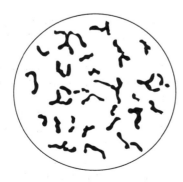

Figure 14.1 Filaments of *Erysipelothrix rhusiopathiae* from a chronic lesion, showing morphological variation.

presumptive identification include:
— Catalase-negative
— Coagulase-positive (Tesh and Wood, 1988). Few pathogens produce this enzyme apart from some staphylococci (*see* Chapter 8).
— H_2S production is detected by a thin, black central line in triple sugar iron (TSI) agar when this medium is stab-inoculated.
• Serotyping for epidemiological studies
A heat-stable peptidoglycan extracted from the cell wall is used for serotyping in precipitation reactions. Twenty-three serotypes have been identified. Some isolates are non-typable. In affected pigs, the serotypes most commonly involved are 1a, 1b and 2.
• Virulence testing in laboratory animals
Isolates of *E. rhusiopathiae* vary considerably in virulence. If necessary, the virulence can be confirmed by intraperitoneal inoculation of mice or pigeons.
• A PCR-based method for the detection of virulent *E. rhusiopathiae* isolates has been developed (Shimoji *et al.*, 1998).

Pathogenesis and pathogenicity

Infection is usually acquired by ingestion of material contaminated by pig faeces. Entry may occur through the tonsils, skin or mucous membranes. Virulence factors include a capsule which protects the organism against phagocytosis, the ability to adhere to endothelial cells and the production of neuraminidase, an enzyme which may enhance cell penetration.

In the septicaemic form of the disease, vascular damage is characterized by swelling of endothelial cells, adherence of monocytes to vascular walls and widespread hyaline microthrombus formation. Localization of the bacteria in joint synovia and on heart valves during haematogenous spread, accounts for the development of chronic lesions at these sites. Long-term articular damage may result from an immune response to persistent bacterial antigens. Viable *E. rhusiopathiae* are rarely isolated from chronically affected joints.

Clinical infections

Infections with *E. rhusiopathiae* are encountered in pigs, turkeys and sheep (Box 14.1). Other domestic animals are occasionally affected.

Swine erysipelas

Subclinically-infected carrier pigs are the main reservoir of infection. Pigs with acute disease excrete large numbers of organisms in faeces. Infection is usually acquired through ingestion of contaminated food or water and less commonly through minor skin abrasions. The frequency of disease outbreaks in free-range pigs may be reduced by keeping

---

Box 14.1 Clinical manifestations of *Erysipelothrix rhusiopathiae* infection in domestic animals.

• Pigs (swine erysipelas)
— septicaemia
— 'diamond skin' lesions
— chronic arthritis
— chronic valvular endocarditis
— abortion
• Sheep
— polyarthritis in lambs
— post-dipping lameness
— pneumonia
— valvular endocarditis
• Turkeys (turkey erysipelas)
— septicaemia
— arthritis
— valvular endocarditis

---

them on concrete.

The susceptibility of individual pigs and the virulence of the *E. rhusiopathiae* strain, both of which are highly variable, determine the course and outcome of infection. Pigs under 3 months of age are normally protected by maternally-derived antibodies while animals over 3 years of age usually have acquired a protective active immunity through exposure to strains of low virulence. Factors which may predispose to disease development include changes in diet, extreme ambient temperatures and fatigue.

Clinical signs
Swine erysipelas can occur in four forms. The septicaemic and cutaneous ('diamond') forms are acute while arthritis and vegetative endocarditis are chronic forms of the disease. Chronic arthritis has the most significant negative impact on productivity.

Septicaemia occurs after an incubation period of 2 to 3 days. During an outbreak of acute disease, some pigs may be found dead and others are febrile, depressed and walk with a stiff, stilted gait or remain recumbent. Mortality may be high in some outbreaks. Pregnant sows with the septicaemic form may abort.

In the diamond-skin form, systemic signs are less severe and mortality rates are much lower than in animals with septicaemia. Pigs are febrile and cutaneous lesions progress from small, light pink or purple, raised areas to more extensive and characteristic diamond-shaped erythematous plaques. Some of these lesions resolve within one week; others become necrotic and may slough.

Arthritis which is commonly encountered in older pigs can present as stiffness, lameness or reluctance to bear weight on affected limbs. Joint lesions, which may be initially mild, can progress to erosion of articular cartilage with eventual fibrosis and ankylosis. In vegetative endocarditis, the least common form, wart-like thrombotic masses are present, usually on the mitral valves. Many affected animals are asymptomatic but some may develop congestive heart failure or die suddenly if stressed by physical exertion or by pregnancy.

Diagnosis
- Diamond-shaped skin lesions are pathognomonic.
- Specimens for laboratory examination include blood for haemoculture and postmortem specimens of liver, spleen, heart valves or synovial tissues. Organisms are rarely recovered from skin lesions or chronically affected joints.
- Microscopic examination of specimens from acutely affected animals may reveal slender Gram-positive rods. Filamentous forms may be demonstrable in smears from chronic valvular lesions (Fig. 14.1).
- Blood and MacConkey agar plates, inoculated with specimen material are incubated aerobically at 37°C for 24–48 hours. Selective media, containing either sodium azide (0.1%) or crystal violet (0.001%), may be used for contaminated samples.
- Identification criteria for isolates:
  — Colonial morphology after incubation for 48 hours
  — Absence of growth on MacConkey agar
  — Appearance in Gram-stained smears from colonies
  — Negative catalase test
  — Coagulase production
  — H_2S production in TSI agar slants
  — Biochemical test profile.
- Serological tests are not applicable for diagnosis.

Treatment
Both penicillin and tetracyclines are effective for treatment. Hyperimmune serum can be used concurrently with antibiotic therapy. When chronic lesions have developed, antibiotic therapy is ineffective.

Control
- Hygiene and management practices should be evaluated and, where necessary, brought to a satisfactory standard.
- Chronically affected animals should be culled.
- Affected pigs should be isolated.
- Both live attenuated and inactivated vaccines are available. Attenuated vaccines can be given orally, systemically or by aerosol. They should not be administered to animals receiving antibiotic therapy.

Turkey erysipelas

Birds of all ages are susceptible. Toms may excrete the organisms in their semen and turkey hens may die suddenly within 4 to 5 days of artificial insemination. The disease usually occurs as a septicaemia and mortality rates may be high. Dark-coloured, swollen snoods are

characteristic of the disease. Postmortem findings include enlarged friable livers and spleens. Chronically affected birds may exhibit arthritis and vegetative endocarditis and they gradually lose weight and become emaciated. Vaccination with an inactivated vaccine stimulates protective immunity.

Infections in sheep

Non-suppurative polyarthritis of lambs may result from entry of organisms through the navel or, more commonly, through docking or castration wounds. Post-dipping lameness, which affects older lambs and adult sheep, is due to cellulitis and laminitis. The organism enters through skin abrasions in the region of the hoof from heavily contaminated dipping solutions. Valvular endocarditis and pneumonia in ewes, associated with *E. rhusiopathiae*, have also been reported (Griffiths *et al.*, 1991).

Human erysipeloid

Many human infections with *E. rhusiopathiae* are occupational in origin. Workers engaged in the fish and poultry industries and other agriculturally-based occupations may be at risk of acquiring infection. Organisms enter through minor skin abrasions causing a localized cellulitis referred to as erysipeloid (Mutalib *et al.*, 1993). Rarely, extension by haematogenous spread in untreated patients can lead to joint and heart involvement.

References

Eriksen, K., Fossum, K., Gamlem, H., Grondalen, J., Kucsera, G. and Ulstein, T. (1987). Endocarditis in two dogs caused by *Erysipelothrix rhusiopathiae*. *Journal of Small Animal Practice*, **28**, 117–123.

Griffiths, I.B., Done, S.H. and Readman, S. (1991). Erysipelothrix pneumonia in sheep. *Veterinary Record*, **128**, 382–383.

Mutalib, A.A., King, J.M. and McDonough, P.L. (1993). Erysipelas in caged laying chicken and suspected erysipeloid in animal caretakers. *Journal of Veterinary Diagnostic Investigation*, **5**, 198–201.

Shimoji, Y., Mori, Y., Hyakutake, K., Sekizaki, T. and Yokomizo, Y. (1998). Use of an enrichment broth-PCR 3: combination assay for rapid diagnosis of swine erysipelas. *Journal of Clinical Microbiology*, **36**, 86–89.

Takahashi, T., Fujisawa, T., Tamura, Y., Suzuki, S., Muramatsu, M., Sawada, T., Benno, Y. and Mitsuoka, T. (1992). DNA relatedness among *Erysipelothrix rhusiopathiae* strains representing all twenty-three serovars and *Erysipelothrix tonsillarum*. *International Journal of Systematic Bacteriology*, **42**, 469–473.

Tesh, M.J. and Wood, R.L. (1988). Detection of coagulase activity in *Erysipelothrix rhusiopathiae*. *Journal of Clinical Microbiology*, **26**, 1058–1060.

Further reading

Wood, R.L. (1992). Erysipelas. In: *Diseases of Swine*, Seventh Edition. Eds. A.D. Leman, B.E. Straw, W.L. Mengeling, S. D'Allaire and D.J. Taylor. Iowa State University Press, Ames, Iowa. pp. 475–486.

Chapter 15

Bacillus species

Most *Bacillus* species are large, Gram-positive, endospore-producing rods up to 10.0 μm in length. A few non-pathogenic species are Gram-negative, and organisms in smears prepared from old cultures decolourize readily. In smears from tissues or cultures, cells occur singly, in pairs or in long chains (Fig. 15.1). The genus is comprised of more than 50 species with diverse characteristics. *Bacillus* species are catalase-positive, aerobic or facultatively anaerobic and, with the exception of *Bacillus anthracis* and *B. mycoides*, motile. Most species are saprophytes with no pathogenic potential. However, they often contaminate clinical specimens and laboratory media. *Bacillus anthracis* is the most important pathogen in the group. The name *Clostridium piliforme* has been proposed for *Bacillus piliformis*, the agent of Tyzzer's disease (Duncan *et al.*, 1993).

> **Key points**
> - Large, Gram-positive rods
> - Endospores produced
> - Aerobes or facultative anaerobes
> - Growth on non-enriched media
> - Most species motile, catalase-positive and oxidase-negative
> - Majority are non-pathogenic environmental organisms
> - *Bacillus anthracis* causes anthrax
> - *Bacillus licheniformis* is implicated in sporadic abortions in cattle and sheep

Usual habitat

Bacillus species are widely distributed in the environment mainly because they produce highly resistant endospores. In soil, endospores of *B.anthracis* can survive for more than 50 years. Some *Bacillus* species can tolerate extremely adverse conditions such as desiccation and high temperatures.

Differentiation of *Bacillus* species

The ability to grow aerobically and to produce catalase distinguishes *Bacillus* species from the clostridia, which

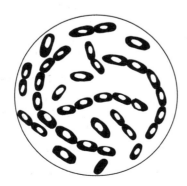

Figure 15.1 Rods of *Bacillus* species in chain formation. Endospores appear as unstained areas within the cells.

are also Gram-positive, endospore-forming rods. Differentiation of *Bacillus* species is largely based on colonial characteristics and biochemical tests. Many species, including *B. anthracis*, do not produce capsules when grown on laboratory media.

- Colonial characteristics of *Bacillus* species which are pathogenic for animals and man:
  - *Bacillus anthracis* colonies are up to 5 mm in diameter, flat, dry, greyish and with a 'ground glass'appearance after incubation for 48 hours. At low magnification, curled outgrowths from the edge of the colony impart a characteristic, 'medusa head' appearance. Rarely, isolates are weakly haemolytic.
  - *Bacillus cereus* colonies are similar to those of *B. anthracis* but are slightly larger with a greenish tinge. The majority of strains produce a wide zone of complete haemolysis around the colonies. Because they have some similar characteristics, *B. anthracis* and *B. cereus* require careful differentiation (Table 15.1).
  - *Bacillus licheniformis* colonies are dull, rough, wrinkled and strongly adherent to the agar. Characteristic hair-like outgrowths are produced from streaks of the organisms on agar media. Colonies become brown with age. The name of this

Table 15.1 Differentiating features of *Bacillus anthracis* and *B. cereus*.

Feature	B. anthracis	B. cereus
Motility	Non-motile	Motile
Appearance on sheep blood agar	Non-haemolytic	Haemolytic
Susceptibility to penicillin (10 unit disc)	Susceptible	Resistant
Lecithinase activity on egg yolk agar	Weak and slow	Strong and rapid
Effect of gamma phage	Lysis	Lysis rare
Pathogenicity for animals (application to scarified area at tail base of mouse)	Death in 24 to 48 hours	No effect

species derives from the similarity of its colonies to lichen.
- Commercial biochemical test kits for confirming the identity of *Bacillus* species are available.

Clinical infections

The major disease conditions caused by bacteria in this group are listed in Table 15.2. Anthrax is the most important of these diseases. *Bacillus licheniformis* is an emerging pathogen in the group as a cause of abortion in cattle and sheep. *Bacillus cereus* is important in human food poisoning and is associated with rare cases of mastitis in cows.

Infections with *Bacillus licheniformis*

Bacillus licheniformis, an organism widespread in the environment and associated with food spoilage, has recently been recognized as a cause of abortion in cattle and sheep. On some farms in Britain, multiple bovine abortions have been attributed to infection with *B. licheniformis* and an association with the feeding of silage or mouldy hay has been suggested. Because this organism is ubiquitous, it is only of diagnostic significance when isolated in heavy, pure culture from foetal abomasal contents.

Anthrax

Anthrax is a severe disease which affects virtually all mammalian species including humans. The disease, which occurs worldwide, is endemic in some countries and in defined regions of other countries. Ruminants are highly susceptible, often developing a rapidly fatal septicaemic form of the disease. Pigs and horses are moderately susceptible to infection, while carnivores are comparatively resistant. Birds are almost totally resistant to infection, a characteristic attributed to their relatively high body temperatures.

Epidemiology

Endospore formation is the most important factor in the persistence and spread of anthrax. The endospores of *B. anthracis* can survive for decades in soil. It has been suggested that, in some geographically defined regions, germination of spores with multiplication of vegetative cells may occur in the soil for short periods at ambient temperatures above 15°C. Soils in such regions are alkaline, rich in calcium and nitrogen and have a high moisture content. Such soil conditions also favour spore survival. Outbreaks of anthrax in herbivores can occur when pastures are contaminated by spores originating from buried carcases. Spores may be brought to the surface by flooding, excavation, subsidence, or by the activity of earthworms. Flooding may also concentrate spores in particular locations (Dragon and Rennie, 1995).

Sporadic outbreaks of the disease have been associated with the importation of contaminated meat-and-bone meal, fertilizers of animal origin and hides. Infection is usually acquired by ingestion of spores and, less commonly, by inhalation or through skin abrasions. Although carnivores are comparatively resistant to infection, the ingestion of large numbers of *B. anthracis* from an anthrax carcase can produce disease.

Table 15.2 Clinical manifestations of diseases caused by *Bacillus anthracis* and other *Bacillus* species.

Bacillus species	Susceptible animals	Clinical manifestations
B. anthracis	Cattle, sheep	Fatal peracute or acute septicaemic anthrax
	Pigs	Subacute anthrax with oedematous swelling in pharyngeal region; an intestinal form with higher mortality is less common
	Horses	Subacute anthrax with localized oedema; septicaemia with colic and enteritis sometimes occurs
	Humans	Skin, pulmonary and intestinal forms of anthrax are recorded in man periodically
B. cereus	Cattle	Mastitis (rare)
	Humans	Food poisoning, eye infections
B. licheniformis	Cattle, sheep	Sporadic abortion
B. larvae	Bees	American foulbrood

Pathogenesis and pathogenicity

The virulence of *B. anthracis* derives from the presence of a capsule and the ability to produce a complex toxin. Both virulence factors are encoded by plasmids and are required for disease production. The expression of virulence factors is regulated by host temperature and carbon dioxide concentration. The capsule, composed of poly-D-glutamic acid, inhibits phagocytosis. The complex toxin consists of three antigenic components: protective antigen, oedema factor and lethal factor. Individually each factor lacks toxic activity in experimental animals, although protective antigen induces antibodies which confer partial immunity. Protective antigen acts as the binding moiety for both oedema factor and lethal factor. Oedema factor is a calmodulin-dependent adenylate cyclase and, once it has entered cells following binding to protective antigen, causes increased levels of cyclic AMP. The resultant upset in water homeostasis causes the fluid accumulation seen in clinical disease. Neutrophils are the principal target of oedema factor which severely inhibits their function. Lethal toxin consists of lethal factor, a zinc metallo-protease and protective antigen which acts as the binding domain as for oedema factor. It stimulates macrophages to release cytokines, specifically TNF alpha and interleukin-1 beta. In naturally-occurring disease, local effects of the complex toxin include swelling and darkening of tissues due to oedema and necrosis. When septicaemia occurs, increased vascular permeability and extensive haemorrhage lead to shock and death.

Clinical signs and pathology

The incubation period of anthrax ranges from hours to days. The clinical presentation and pathological changes vary with the species affected, the challenge dose and the route of infection.

In cattle and sheep the disease is usually septicaemic and rapidly fatal. Although most animals are found dead without premonitory signs, pyrexia with temperatures up to 42°C (108°F), depression, congested mucosae and petechiae may be observed antemortem. Animals which survive for more than one day may abort or display subcutaneous oedema and dysentery. In cattle, post-mortem findings include rapid bloating, incomplete rigor mortis, widespread ecchymotic haemorrhages and oedema, dark unclotted blood and blood-stained fluid in body cavities. An extremely large soft spleen is characteristic of the disease in cattle. Splenomegaly and oedema are less prominent postmortem features in affected sheep, which are reported to be more susceptible than cattle and succumb more rapidly.

In pigs, infection generally results in oedematous swelling of the throat and head along with regional lymphadenitis. If oedema in the laryngeal region does not interfere with breathing, affected pigs may survive. Intestinal involvement manifests clinically as dysentery due to multifocal, haemorrhagic enteric lesions. Mortality rates may be high.

The clinical course of anthrax in horses is often prolonged for several days. Following introduction of spores into abrasions, extensive subcutaneous oedema of the thorax, abdomen or legs may develop. Swelling of the pharynx, similar to that in pigs, has been described. Less commonly, colic and dysentery due to severe haemorrhagic enteritis, may result from ingestion of spores. If septicaemia occurs, extensive ecchymoses and splenomegaly are found at postmortem.

In dogs, which are rarely affected, the course of the disease and pathological changes resemble those observed in affected pigs.

Diagnosis

- Carcases of animals which have died from anthrax are bloated, putrify rapidly and do not exhibit rigor mortis. Dark, unclotted blood may issue from the mouth, nostrils and anus. The carcases of such animals should not be opened because this will facilitate sporulation, with the risk of long-term environmental contamination.
- Peripheral blood from the tail vein of ruminants or peritoneal fluid from pigs should be collected into a sterile syringe. Cotton wool soaked in 70% alcohol should be applied to the site after collection to minimize leakage of contaminated blood or fluid. Thin smears of blood or fluid, stained with polychrome methylene blue, reveal chains of square-ended, blue-staining rods surrounded by pink capsules (Fig. 15.2). The amount of capsular material diminishes with time after the death of the animal.
- Blood and MacConkey agars are inoculated with the suspect specimens and incubated aerobically at 37°C for 24 to 48 hours.
- Identification criteria for isolates:
  — Colonial morphology
  — Microscopic appearance in a Gram-stained smear
  — Absence of growth on MacConkey agar
  — Cultural features and, if necessary, pathogenicity

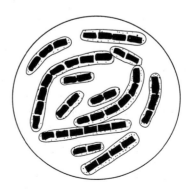

Figure 15.2 Numerous chains of *Bacillus anthracis* as they appear in a thin blood smear. When stained with polychrome methylene blue, the blue-staining organisms are surrounded by pink capsules (M'Fadyean reaction).

tests in laboratory animals (Table 15.1).
— Biochemical test profile

- The Ascoli test is a thermoprecipitation test designed to detect antigens of *B. anthracis* in biological materials such as hides. Homogenized material is boiled and clarified by filtration. The filtrate is used as the source of antigen in ring precipitation or gel diffusion tests with *B. anthracis* antiserum. This test lacks specificity because *B. anthracis* shares thermostable antigens with other *Bacillus* species.

- Agar gel immunodiffusion, complement fixation, ELISA and immunofluorescence tests have been evaluated for the diagnosis of anthrax, but they are either too insensitive or lack the required specificity for routine use.

- New molecular diagnostic methods based on the use of PCR to amplify specific virulence plasmid markers are being developed.

Treatment

If administered early in the course of the disease, high doses of penicillin G or oxytetracycline may prove effective.

Control

Suspected cases of anthrax must be reported immediately to appropriate regulatory authorities. Control measures should be designed to take account of the prevalence of disease in a particular country or geographical region.

- In endemic regions:
  — Annual vaccination, particularly of cattle and sheep, is advisable. The Sterne strain spore vaccine should be given about 1 month before anticipated outbreaks. The spores in this live vaccine convert to non-encapsulated avirulent vegetative organisms.
  — Chemoprophylaxis, employing long-acting penicillin, should be considered when outbreaks threaten valuable livestock.
  — A killed vaccine is available for humans who may be exposed to infection in the course of their work.

- In non-endemic regions following a disease outbreak:
  — Movement of animals, their waste products, feed and bedding from affected and adjacent premises must be prohibited.
  — Personnel implementing control measures should wear protective clothing and footwear which must be disinfected before leaving the affected farm.
  — Foot-baths containing sporicidal disinfectant (5% formalin, or 3% peracetic acid) should be placed at entrances to affected farms.
  — Contaminated buildings should be sealed and fumigated with formaldehyde before bedding is removed. Following removal of bedding and loose fittings, all drains should be blocked and the building should be sprayed with 5% formalin which should be left to act for at least 10 hours before final washing.
  — Immediate disposal of carcases, bedding, manure, fodder and other contaminated material is mandatory. Carcases should be incinerated or buried deeply away from water courses. Contaminated material and equipment must be disinfected with 10% formalin or, if appropriate, incinerated.
  — Scavanger animals should not be allowed access to suspect carcases and insect activity should be minimized by application of insecticides on and around carcases.
  — In-contact animals should be isolated and kept under close observation for at least 2 weeks.

Anthrax in humans

Three main forms of the disease occur in man. Cutaneous anthrax (malignant pustule) is the result of endospores entering abraded skin. This localized lesion can progress to septicaemia if not treated. Pulmonary anthrax ('wool-sorters' disease') follows inhalation of spores while intestinal anthrax results from ingestion of infective material. The disease may prove fatal in the absence of early treatment.

References

Dragon, D.C. and Rennie, R.P. (1995). The ecology of anthrax spores: tough but not invincible. *Canadian Veterinary Journal*, **36**, 295–301.

Duncan, J.A., Carman, R.J., Olsen, G.J. and Wilson, K.H. (1993). The agent of Tyzzer's disease is a *Clostridium* species. *Clinical Infectious Diseases*, **16** (supplement 4), 422.

Further reading

Dixon, T.C., Meselson, M., Guillemin, J. and Hanna, P.C. (1999). Anthrax. *New England Journal of Medicine*, **341**, 815–826.

Turnbull, P.C.B., Bell, R.H.V., Saigawa, K., Munyenyembe, F.E.C., Mulenga, C.K. and Makala, L.H.C. (1991). Anthrax in wildlife in the Luangwa Valley, Zambia. *Veterinary Record*, **128**, 399–403.

Watson, A. and Keir, D. (1994). Information on which to base assessments of risk from environments contaminated with anthrax spores. *Epidemiology and Infection*, **113**, 479–490.

Williams, D.R., Rees, G.B. and Rogers, M.E. (1992). Observations on an outbreak of anthrax in pigs in north Wales. *Veterinary Record*, **131**, 363–366.

Chapter 16

Clostridium species

The clostridia are large Gram-positive bacteria which are fermentative, catalase-negative and oxidase-negative, and require enriched media for growth. They are straight or slightly curved rods and the majority are motile by flagella which are peritrichous. *Clostridium* species produce endospores which usually cause bulging of mother cells (Fig. 16.1). The size, shape and location of endospores can be used for species differentiation. Although most pathogenic clostridial species are strict anaerobes, some are comparatively aerotolerant. Clostridia occur worldwide and particular species may be associated with defined geographical regions. Recent changes in the nomenclature of some species are indicated in Table 16.1.

Although more than 100 clostridial species are recognised, less than 20 are pathogenic. These can be grouped in four categories, three based on toxin activity and tissues affected and the fourth containing pathogens of lesser importance (Fig. 16.2). *Clostridium tetani* and *C. botulinum*, the neurotoxic clostridia, affect neuromuscular function without inducing observable tissue damage. In contrast, histotoxic clostridia produce relatively localized lesions in tissues such as muscle and liver, and may subsequently cause toxaemia. *Clostridium perfringens*

> **Key points**
> - Large, Gram-positive rods
> - Endospores produced
> - Anaerobic, catalase- and oxidase-negative
> - Motile (except *C. perfringens*)
> - Enriched media required for growth
> - Colonies of *C. perfringens* surrounded by zones of double haemolysis
> - Present in soil, in alimentary tracts of animals and in faeces
> - Pathogens can be grouped according to the mode and sites of action of their potent exotoxins:
>   —neurotoxic clostridia
>   —histotoxic clostridia
>   —enteropathogenic and enterotoxaemia-producing clostridia
> - Produce diverse forms of disease in many animal species

types A to E, important members of the third category, produce inflammatory lesions in the gastrointestinal tract along with enterotoxaemia. Clostridia in the fourth category are associated with sporadic diseases, usually affecting individual animals.

Usual habitat

Clostridia are saprophytes which are found in soil, freshwater or marine sediments with suitably low redox potentials. They constitute part of the normal intestinal flora and some may be sequestered as endospores in muscle or liver. Sequestered endospores, if activated, may produce disease.

Specimen collection and cultural requirements

To ensure survival of these fastidious anaerobes, special methods are required for collection and processing of specimens.

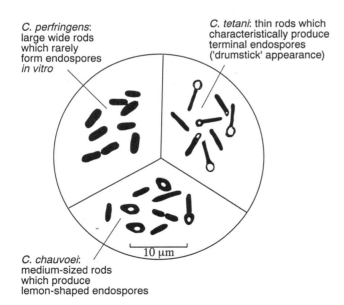

C. perfringens: large wide rods which rarely form endospores *in vitro*

C. tetani: thin rods which characteristically produce terminal endospores ('drumstick' appearance)

C. chauvoei: medium-sized rods which produce lemon-shaped endospores

10 μm

Figure 16.1 Characteristic morphology of some clostridial species.

Table 16.1 Nomenclature changes of some *Clostridium* species.

Present name	Former name
Clostridium perfringens	*Clostridium welchii*
Clostridium argentiense	*Clostridium botulinum* type G
Clostridium haemolyticum	*Clostridium novyi* type D
Clostridium novyi	*Clostridium oedematiens*
Clostridium piliforme	*Bacillus piliformis*

- Unless specimens are taken from live or recently dead animals, postmortem clostridial invaders may rapidly spread from the intestine into tissues leading to difficulty with the interpretation of laboratory results.
- Blocks of tissue or fluids from affected animals should be placed in anaerobic transport media for transfer to the laboratory. Specimens must be cultured promptly after collection.
- Blood agar enriched with yeast extract, vitamin K and haemin is suitable for the culture of clostridia. Media should be freshly prepared or pre-reduced to ensure absence of oxygen.
- Suitable atmospheric requirements are provided by culturing in anaerobic jars containing hydrogen supplemented with 5 to 10% carbon dioxide to enhance growth. Some vegetative clostridia if exposed to the air for more than 15 minutes may not survive.

Differentiation of clostridia

Laboratory procedures for differentiating most clostridia include colonial morphology, biochemical tests, toxin neutralization methods and gas-liquid-chromatography for profiling organic acids.

- Colonial morphology is of limited value for differentiating most clostridial species. However, colonies of *C. perfringens* are surrounded by a characteristic double-zone of haemolysis.
- Miniaturized commercial kits are available for biochemical identification.
- Specific toxins can be identified in body fluids or in intestinal contents by toxin neutralization or protection tests in laboratory rodents, usually mice.
- Fluorescent antibody techniques are widely used for the rapid identification of histotoxic clostridia in lesions.
- Immunoassay methods such as ELISA can be used for toxin detection. The polymerase chain reaction can be employed to detect genes coding for toxin production of isolates of *C. botulinum*. These tests have now replaced many of the mouse bioassay tests but have not yet been developed for the detection of all toxins.

Clinical conditions caused by neurotoxic clostridia

The neurotoxic clostridia, *C. tetani* and *C. botulinum*, produce their effects by elaborating potent neurotoxins. The neurotoxin of *C. tetani* is produced by organisms replicating locally in damaged tissues. Absorbed toxin exerts its effect on synaptic junctions remote from the site of toxin production. The neurotoxin of *C. botulinum* is usually produced by organisms replicating in decaying organic matter or in the anaerobic conditions in contaminated cans of meat or vegetables. When absorbed from the gastrointestinal tract into the bloodstream, the toxin affects the functioning of neuromuscular junctions. Some features of the neurotoxins of *C. tetani* and *C. botulinum* are presented in Table 16.2.

Tetanus

Tetanus is an acute potentially fatal intoxication which

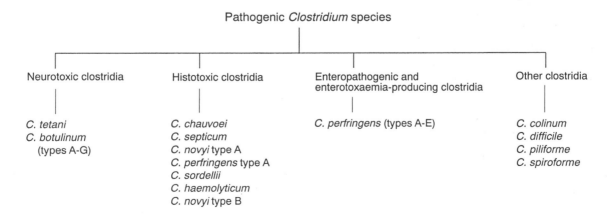

Figure 16.2 Pathogenic *Clostridium* species of veterinary importance.

Table 16.2 Production, mode of action and effects of the neuro-toxins of *Clostridium tetani* and *C. botulinum*.

Feature of neuro-toxin	*Clostridium tetani*	*Clostridium botulinum*
Site of production	In wounds	In carcases, decaying vegetation, canned foods. Occasionally in wounds or in intestine (toxico-infections)
Genes which regulate production	In plasmids	Usually in genome (in bacteriophages for types C and D)
Antigenic type	One antigenic type (tetanospas-min)	Eight antigenically distinct toxins, types A to G
Mode of action	Synaptic inhibition	Inhibition of neuro-muscular transmission
Clinical effect	Muscular spasms	Flaccid paralysis

affects many species including humans. However, species susceptibility to toxin varies considerably. Horses and man are highly susceptible, ruminants and pigs moderately so, and carnivores are comparatively resistant. Poultry are not susceptible to tetanus.

Clostridium tetani, the aetiological agent, is a straight, slender anaerobic Gram-positive rod. Spherical endospores, which are terminal and bulge mother cells, impart a characteristic 'drumstick' appearance to sporulated organisms (Fig. 16.1). The endospores are resistant to chemicals and boiling but are killed by autoclaving at 121°C for 15 minutes. *Clostridium tetani* has a swarming growth and is haemolytic on blood agar due to the production of tetanolysin. Ten serological types of *C. tetani* can be distinguished by their flagellar antigens. The neurotoxin, tetanospasmin, is antigenically uniform irrespective of serotype, and antibodies induced by the neurotoxin of any one of the serotypes neutralize the neurotoxins produced by the others.

Infection occurs when endospores are introduced into traumatized tissue from soil or faeces. Common sites of infection include deep penetrating wounds in the horse, castration and docking wounds in sheep, abrasions associated with dystocia in cows and ewes, and the umbilical tissues in all young animals. The presence of necrotic tissue, foreign bodies and contaminating facultative anaerobes in wounds may create the anaerobic conditions in which *C. tetani* spores can germinate. The clostridial organisms may replicate more readily in the tissues when the haemolytic toxin, tetanolysin, is released. Vegetative bacteria multiplying in necrotic tissues produce the potent tetanospasmin which is responsible for the clinical signs of tetanus.

Pathogenesis

Structurally, tetanus toxin consists of two chains joined by a disulphide bridge. The light chain is the toxic moiety and the heavy chain is responsible for receptor binding and internalization of the toxin. The neurotoxin binds irreversibly to ganglioside receptors on motor neuron terminals and is transported to the nerve cell body and its dendritic processes in the central nervous system in toxin-containing vesicles, by retrograde intra-axonal flow. Toxin is transferred trans-synaptically to its site of action in the terminals of inhibitory neurons, where it blocks pre-synaptic transmission of inhibitory signals (Sanford, 1995). It does this by hydrolysis of synaptobrevins, protein components of vesicles containing neurotransmitters. Because release of inhibitory neurotransmitters is prevented, spastic paralysis results. Toxin can also be blood-borne, especially when produced in large amounts and can then bind to motor terminals throughout the body prior to transfer to the central nervous system. Bound toxin is not neutralized by antitoxin.

Clinical signs

The incubation period of tetanus is usually between 5 and 10 days but may extend to three weeks. When the development of clinical signs is delayed, the wound at the site of infection may have healed and the condition is then referred to as latent tetanus. The clinical effects of the neurotoxin are similar in all domestic animals. However, the nature and severity of the clinical signs are dependent on the anatomical site of the replicating bacteria, the amount of toxin produced and species susceptibility. Wounds on or near the head are usually associated with a shorter incubation period and an increased tendency to generalized tetanus. Localized tetanus, which usually affects less susceptible species such as dogs, presents as stiffness and spasm of muscles close to the site of injury as a result of the effect of toxin on local nerve endings.

Clinical signs include stiffness, localized spasms, altered heart and respiratory rates, dysphagia and altered facial expression. Comparatively mild tactile or auditory stimuli may precipitate tonic contraction of muscles. Spasm of mastigatory muscles may lead to 'lockjaw'. Generalized muscle stiffness can result in a 'saw-horse' stance especially in horses. Animals which recover from tetanus are not necessarily immune because the amount of toxin which can induce clinical disease is usually below the threshold required to stimulate the production of neutralizing antibodies.

Diagnostic procedures

The diagnosis of tetanus is usually presumptive and is based on the clinical signs and a history of recent trauma in unvaccinated animals.

• Differentiation from strychnine poisoning is necessary, particularly in dogs.

- Gram-stained smears prepared from material from lesions may reveal the characteristic 'drumstick' forms of *C. tetani* (Fig. 16.1).
- Anaerobic culture of *C. tetani* from necrotic wound tissue may be attempted but is often unsuccessful.
- Serum from affected animals may be used to demonstrate circulating neurotoxin, using mouse inoculation.

Treatment

- Antitoxin should be administered promptly, either intravenously or into the subarachnoid space, on three consecutive days to neutralize unbound toxin.
- Toxoid may be given subcutaneously to promote an active immune response even in those animals which have received antitoxin.
- Large doses of penicillin are administered intramuscularly or intravenously to kill toxin-producing vegetative cells of *C. tetani* in the lesion.
- Surgical debridement of wounds and removal of foreign bodies, followed by flushing with hydrogen peroxide, produces aerobic conditions which help to inhibit bacterial replication at the site of injury.
- Affected animals should be housed in a quiet dark environment. Fluid replacement therapy, sedatives, muscle relaxants and good nursing can minimize clinical discomfort and maintain vital functions.

Control

- Farm animals should be vaccinated routinely with tetanus toxoid. A booster dose of vaccine may be advisable if a vaccinated animal sustains a deep wound.
- In horses, prompt surgical debridement of wounds is desirable.
- Unvaccinated animals, which have sustained deep wounds or which are presented for surgery, should be given antitoxin. This passive protection usually lasts about three weeks.

Botulism

Botulism is a serious, potentially fatal intoxication usually acquired by ingestion of pre-formed toxin. *Clostridium botulinum*, the aetiological agent, is an anaerobic Gram-positive rod which produces oval, subterminal endospores. The endospores of *C. botulinum* are distributed in soils and aquatic environments worldwide. Eight types of *Clostridium botulinum* are recognized on the basis of the toxins (A, B, C_α, C_β, D, E, F, G) which they produce. These neurotoxins, which are inactivated by boiling for up to 20 minutes, induce similar clinical signs but differ in their antigenicity and potency. Some *C. botulinum* types are confined to particular geographical regions. Germination of endospores, with growth of vegetative cells and toxin production, occurs in anaerobic locations such as rotting carcases, decaying vegetation and contaminated canned foods. Toxico-infectious botulism,

an uncommon form of the disease, occurs when spores germinate in wounds or in the intestinal tract. Intestinal toxico-infectious botulism has been recorded in foals (shaker-foal syndrome), pups (Farrow *et al.*, 1983), broiler chickens and turkey poults.

Clostridium botulinum types C and D cause most outbreaks of botulism in domestic animals. Outbreaks of disease occur most commonly in waterfowl, cattle, horses, sheep, mink, poultry and farmed fish. Pigs and dogs are relatively resistant to the neurotoxins and botulism is rare in domestic cats. Botulism in cattle has been associated with ingestion of poultry carcases present in ensiled poultry litter used as bedding or spread on pasture (McLoughlin *et al.*, 1988). Poor quality baled silage and silage or hay containing rodent carcases have been linked to outbreaks of botulism in horses and ruminants. Pica, arising from starvation or phosphorus deficiency in herbivores on ranches in South Africa, USA and Australia, may induce affected animals to chew bones or carcases containing botulinum toxin. The resultant botulism is known as lamsiekte in South Africa, bulbar paralysis in Australia and loin disease in the USA. Contaminated raw meat and carcases are often sources of toxin for carnivores. Waterfowl and other birds can acquire toxin from dead invertebrates, decaying vegetation or from the

Table 16.3 Toxins of *Clostridium botulinum*.

Toxin	Source	Susceptible species
Type A	Meat, canned products Toxico-infection Meat, carcases	Humans Infants Mink, dogs, pigs
Type B	Meat, canned products Toxico-infection Toxico-infection	Humans Infants Foals (up to two months of age)
Type C	Dead invertebrates, maggots, rotting vegetation and carcases of poultry	Waterfowl, poultry
	Ensiled poultry litter, baled silage (poor quality), hay or silage contaminated with rodent carcases	Cattle, sheep, horses
	Meat, especially chicken carcases	Dogs, mink, lions, monkeys
Type D	Carcases, bones Feed contaminated with carcases	Cattle, sheep Horses
Type E	Dead invertebrates, sludge in earth-bottomed ponds Fish	Farmed fish Fish-eating birds, humans
Type F	Meat, fish	Humans
Type G	Soil-contaminated food	Humans (in Argentina)

consumption of maggots containing toxin (Harihan and Mitchell, 1977; Quinn and Crinion, 1984). The usual sources of the toxins of *C. botulinum* types A-G for susceptible species are summarized in Table 16.3.

Pathogenesis

The neurotoxins of *C. botulinum* are the most potent biological toxins known. Preformed toxin in food, absorbed from the gastrointestinal tract, circulates in the bloodstream and acts at the neuromuscular junctions of cholinergic nerves and at peripheral autonomic synapses. Its structure is similar to that of tetanus toxin and it binds to receptors on nerve endings and enters cells during acetylcholine release. As with tetanus toxin, hydrolysis of synaptobrevins causes irreversible interference with the release of the transmitter, acetylcholine in this instance, resulting in flaccid paralysis. Death results from paralysis of respiratory muscles. The difference between the effects of tetanus and botulinum toxins is due to their different sites of action. Tetanus toxin travels up the nerve axon to the ventral horn whereas botulinum toxin remains at the neuromuscular junction.

Ingested spores of *C. botulinum* are normally excreted in the faeces. In toxico-infectious botulism, however, germination of spores in the intestine, results in toxin production by the vegetative organisms. The factors which predispose to toxico-infectious botulism are not known. The shaker-foal syndrome, a form of toxico-infectious botulism in foals up to two months of age, has been attributed to the impact of stress on the dam leading to increased corticosteroid levels in the milk (Swerczek, 1980).

Clinical signs

The clinical signs of botulism, which develop 3 to 17 days after ingestion of toxin, are similar in all species. Dilated pupils, dry mucous membranes, decreased salivation, tongue flaccidity and dysphagia are features of the disease in farm animals. Incoordination and knuckling of the fetlocks is followed by flaccid paralysis and recumbency. Paralysis of respiratory muscles leads to abdominal breathing. Body temperature remains normal and affected animals are alert. Death may occur within days of the emergence of clinical signs. In birds, there is progressive flaccid paralysis which initially affects legs and wings. Paralysis of muscles of the neck (limberneck) is evident only in long-necked species.

Diagnostic procedures

Suspect carcases and material should be handled with caution as large amounts of potent neurotoxin may be present.

- Clinical signs and a history of access to contaminated food may suggest botulism as the cause of an outbreak of an ill-defined neurological disease.

- Confirmation requires the demonstration of toxin in the serum of affected animals. The traditional method for demonstrating toxin is by mouse inoculation. Injected mice develop a characteristic 'wasp-waist' appearance, a consequence of abdominal breathing following paralysis of respiratory muscles. Serum collected from dead animals is unsuitable for mouse inoculation.
- The polymerase chain reaction and nucleic acid probe-based methods have been used for the detection of *C. botulinum* toxin genes. Immunological methods using ELISA or chemiluminescent assays are sensitive and specific procedures for toxin detection.
- Toxin neutralization tests in mice, using monovalent antitoxins, can be employed to identify the specific toxin involved if required.
- Sera should be collected from a number of affected animals because failure to demonstrate toxin in individual animals does not exclude botulism.
- Identification of the toxin in feedstuffs may be of value in epidemiological studies.

Treatment

- If available, polyvalent antiserum is effective in neutralizing unbound toxin early in the course of disease. Cost and availability limit the extent to which it can be used therapeutically.
- Therapeutic agents such as tetraethylamide and guanidine hydrochloride, which enhance transmitter release at neuromuscular junctions, may be of value when given intravenously.
- Mildly affected animals often recover over a period of weeks without therapy.
- Good nursing should complement the therapeutic regime.

Control

- Vaccination of cattle with toxoid may be indicated in endemic regions in South Africa and Australia. Routine vaccination of farmed mink and foxes may be advisable.
- Suspect foodstuffs should not be fed to domestic animals.
- Where feasible, provision of a balanced diet prevents pica in herbivores when grazing on ranges during periods of drought.

Clinical conditions caused by histotoxic clostridia

The histotoxic clostridia produce a variety of lesions in domestic animals (Table 16.4). The exotoxins elaborated by replicating bacteria induce both local tissue necrosis and systemic effects which may be lethal. Some histotoxic clostridia are present in the tissues as latent spores which can germinate and produce specific clinical diseases. These include *C. chauvoei* and occasionally *C. septicum* in muscle tissue, and *C. novyi* type B and *C. haemolyticum* in the liver. Histotoxic clostridia introduced into wounds, often as mixed infections, can cause malignant oedema and gas gangrene. The clostridial species involved include *C. chauvoei*, *C. septicum*, *C. novyi* type A, *C. perfringens* type A and, occasionally, *C. sordellii*.

The abomasitis caused by *C. septicum* in sheep (braxy) is an example of a local histotoxic effect.

Usual habitats

Endospores of histotoxic clostridia are widely distributed in the environment and can persist for long periods in soil. The endospores of particular clostridial species are often found in certain localities and in well-defined geographical regions.

Pathogenesis

It is probable that the majority of ingested endospores are excreted in the faeces but some may leave the intestine and become distributed in the tissues where they remain dormant. The sequence of events which lead to endospore distribution in tissues is unclear. Spores originating in the intestinal lumen may be transported to the tissues in phagocytes. Tissue injury leading to reduced oxygen tension is required for spore germination and replication of vegetative bacteria. Local necrosis produced by the exotoxins of the replicating bacteria allows further proliferation of the organisms in the tissues with extension of the necrotizing process. Endogenous infections which include blackleg, infectious necrotic hepatitis and bacillary haemoglobinuria result from activation of dormant spores in muscle or liver.

The exogenous infections, malignant oedema and gas gangrene, result from the introduction of clostridial organisms into wounds. The anaerobic environment in necrotic tissue is conducive to replication of the clostridia, which are often present together with facultative anaerobes in mixed infections. Extension of local tissue destruction results from exotoxin production. The generalized clinical signs in both exogenous and endogenous clostridial infections are manifestations of toxaemia. The major toxins produced by the histotoxic clostridia are listed in Table 16.4.

Clinical infections

The clinical infections produced by histotoxic clostridia include blackleg, malignant oedema, gas gangrene, braxy, infectious necrotic hepatitis and bacillary haemoglobinuria. These disease conditions tend to recur on certain farms in the absence of suitable vaccination programmes.

Table 16.4 Histotoxic clostridia, their major toxins and the diseases produced in domestic animals.

| *Clostridium* species | Disease | Toxin | |
		Name	Biological activity
C. chauvoei	Blackleg in cattle and sheep	α	Lethal, haemolytic, necrotizing
		β	Deoxyribonuclease
		γ	Hyaluronidase
		δ	Oxygen-labile haemolysin
C. septicum	Malignant oedema in cattle, pigs and sheep	α	Lethal, haemolytic, necrotizing
	Abomasitis in sheep (braxy) and occasionally in calves	β	Deoxyribonuclease
		γ	Hyaluronidase
		δ	Oxygen-labile haemolysin
C. novyi type A	'Big head' in young rams	α	Necrotizing, lethal
	Wound infections		
C. perfringens type A	Necrotic enteritis in chickens	α	Haemolytic, necrotizing, lethal, lecithinase
	Necrotizing enterocolitis in pigs		
	Gas gangrene		
C. sordellii	Myositis in cattle, sheep and horses	α	Lecithinase
	Abomasitis in lambs	β	Oedema-producing lethal factor
C. novyi type B	Infectious necrotic hepatitis (black disease) in sheep	α	Necrotizing, lethal
	and occasionally in cattle	β	Necrotizing, haemolytic, lethal, lecithinase
C. haemolyticum	Bacillary haemoglobinuria in cattle and occasionally in sheep	β	Necrotizing, haemolytic, lethal, lecithinase

Histotoxic clostridial infection should be considered when individual animals die suddenly. Gross postmortem findings may further indicate clostridial involvement.

Blackleg

Blackleg, an acute disease of cattle and sheep caused by *C. chauvoei,* occurs worldwide. In cattle, the disease is most often encountered in young thriving animals from 3 months to 2 years of age and infection is usually endogenous, the latent spores in muscle becoming activated through traumatic injury. The disease may affect sheep of any age and, in many instances, exogenous infection occurs through skin wounds. In both cattle and sheep, gangrenous cellulitis and myositis caused by exotoxins produced by the replicating organisms usually lead to rapid death. The large muscle masses of the limbs, back and neck are frequently affected. Skeletal muscle damage is manifest by lameness, swelling and crepitation due to gas accumulation. Lesions in the muscles of the tongue and throat may produce dyspnoea. Myocardial and diaphragmatic lesions may cause sudden death without premonitory signs. Fluorescent antibody techniques applied to specimens from lesions are rapid and sensitive confirmatory methods.

Malignant oedema and gas gangrene

Malignant oedema and gas gangrene are exogenous, necrotizing, soft tissue infections. The bacteria most commonly implicated are *C. septicum* in malignant oedema and *C. perfringens* type A in gas gangrene. However *C. novyi* type A, *C. chauvoei* and, rarely, *C. sordellii* have also been incriminated either alone or in association with other clostridial species. Other aerobic and anaerobic opportunistic invaders may also be present in the lesions. Infection can follow contamination of wounds, parturition injuries or injection sites. Tissue devitalization associated with trauma provides the low redox potential, the alkaline pH and the protein breakdown products required for clostridial proliferation.

Malignant oedema manifests as cellulitis with minimal gangrene and gas formation. Tissue swelling due to oedema, and coldness and discolouration of the overlying skin are obvious clinical features. Generalized signs of toxaemia include depression and prostration. Death may follow rapidly when lesions are extensive.

Gas gangrene is characterized by extensive bacterial invasion of damaged muscle tissue. Gas production is detectable clinically as subcutaneous crepitation. The clinical features of toxaemia in gas gangrene are similar to those encountered in malignant oedema.

In rams, clostridial infection of head wounds caused by fighting, is termed 'big head'. There is oedematous swelling of subcutaneous tissues of the head, neck and cranial thorax. Death may be rapid. The clinical signs are attributed to the necrotizing lethal α toxin of *C. novyi* type A.

Braxy

Braxy, an abomasitis of sheep, is caused by the exotoxins of *C. septicum.* The disease, which occurs in winter during periods of heavy frost or snow, has been recorded in parts of northern Europe and occasionally elsewhere in the world. It has been suggested that ingestion of frozen herbage may cause local devitalization of abomasal tissue at its point of contact with the rumen, allowing invasion by *C. septicum.* The course of the disease is rapid and most animals die without premonitory signs. Anorexia, depression and fever may be evident immediately before death. *Clostridium septicum* may be demonstrated in specimens from the abomasal lesion by the fluorescent antibody technique.

Infectious necrotic hepatitis

Infectious necrotic hepatitis (black disease) is an acute disease affecting sheep and occasionally cattle. Rare cases have been described in horses and pigs. The hepatic necrosis is caused by exotoxins of *C. novyi* type B replicating in liver tissue which has been damaged by immature *Fasciola hepatica* or other migrating parasites. Although the condition is considered to be endogenous, it is possible that the migrating flukes may carry the bacteria or their spores to the liver. Death is rapid with no premonitory signs and the disease requires differentiation from acute fascioliasis. The term 'black disease' relates to the dark discolouration of the skin caused by the marked subcutaneous venous congestion observed at postmortem examination. The fluorescent antibody technique may be used to demonstrate *C. novyi* type B in specimens from liver lesions.

Bacillary haemoglobinuria

Bacillary haemoglobinuria occurs primarily in cattle and occasionally in sheep. In this endogenous infection with *C. haemolyticum*, the clostridial endospores are dormant in the liver, probably in Kupffer cells. As in infectious necrotic hepatitis, the main factor which facilitates spore germination and clostridial replication is fluke migration. The β toxin, a lecithinase, produced by vegetative cells, causes intravascular haemolysis in addition to hepatic necrosis. Haemoglobinuria, a major clinical feature of the disease, is a consequence of extensive red cell destruction. The aetiological agent may be demonstrated in specimens from hepatic lesions by the fluorescent antibody technique.

Diagnostic procedures

- Histotoxic clostridia contributing to these conditions

can be identified by fluorescent antibody techniques.

- *Clostridium perfringens* is cultured anaerobically on blood agar at 37°C for 48 hours.
- Colonies of *C. perfringens* type A are up to 5 mm in diameter, circular, flat, greyish and surrounded by a zone of double haemolysis (Fig. 16.3).
- A positive CAMP test occurs with *Streptococcus agalactiae*. A diffusible factor produced by *S. agalactiae* enhances the partial haemolysis of the alpha toxin of *C. perfringens*. The pattern of haemolysis is similar to that observed in the *S. agalactiae* reaction with the beta haemolysin of *Staphylococcus aureus* (*see* Fig. 9.4).
- The Nagler reaction, a plate neutralization test, identifies the alpha toxin of *C. perfringens,* which has lecithinase activity (Fig. 16.4).
- A PCR-based method for the identification of *C. chauvoei* from clinical material has been described (Kuhnert *et al.*, 1997).

Treatment and control of histotoxic clostridial diseases

- Because the pathogenesis of the diseases caused by the histotoxic clostridia is similar, the procedures relevant to their treatment and control are also similar.
- Although treatment is usually ineffective, penicillin or broad-spectrum antibiotics administered to animals early in the disease may be of value.
- Vaccination, usually with bacterin and toxoid components in adjuvant, is the most effective method for preventing these diseases. Multicomponent vaccines which induce protection against several pathogenic clostridial species may be required on some farms. Animals should be vaccinated at three months of age and given a booster injection approximately three weeks later. Annual revaccination is recommended.

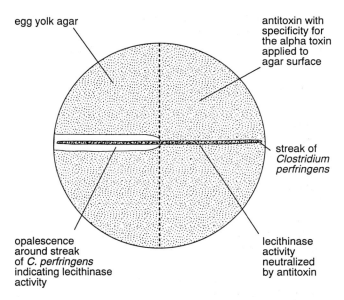

Figure 16.4 Nagler reaction produced by *Clostridium perfringens* growing on egg yolk agar. Antitoxin with specificity for the alpha toxin is applied to the surface of one half of an egg yolk agar plate and allowed to dry. *Clostridium perfringens* is streaked across the plate which is incubated anaerobically at 37°C for 24 hours. Although the organism grows on both halves of the plate, lecithinase activity is evident only on the half without antitoxin.

Enteropathogenic and enterotoxaemia-producing clostridia

Clostridia which produce enterotoxaemia and enteropathy replicate in the intestinal tract and elaborate toxins which produce both localized and generalized effects. *Clostridium perfringens* types B, C and D are of particular significance in domestic animals. Factors which predispose to clostridial proliferation in the intestine include inappropriate husbandry methods, sudden dietary changes and local environmental influences.

Usual habitat

Clostridium perfringens is found in soil, in faeces, and in the intestinal tracts of animals and man. *Clostridium perfringens* types B, C and D may survive in soil as spores for several months. *Clostridium perfringens* type A, which constitutes part of the normal intestinal flora, is widely distributed in soil.

Pathogenesis and pathogenicity

Clostridium perfringens types A to E produce a number of potent, immunologically distinct exotoxins which cause the local and systemic effects encountered in enterotoxaemias. The pattern of toxin production varies with

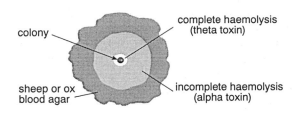

Figure 16.3 Double haemolysis on blood agar around a colony of *Clostridium perfringens*.

each *C. perfringens* type and determines the clinical syndrome observed. The toxins produced by *C. perfringens* types A to E, their biological activities and associated diseases are presented in Table 16.5. A range of minor toxins, some of which may enhance virulence, is also recognized. These include two haemolysins (δ and θ), a collagenase (κ) and a hyaluronidase (μ).

Predisposing intestinal and dietary factors allow opportunistic overgrowth of *C. perfringens* in sheep (Box 16.1). Sustained high levels of clostridial exotoxins are usually required for the development of systemic clinical signs.

Clinical infections

The diseases associated with *C. perfringens* types A to E are listed in Table 16.5. Although *C. perfringens* type A is primarily associated with gas gangrene in humans and domestic animals and with food poisoning in humans, it has also been implicated in necrotizing enterocolitis in suckling and feeder pigs, necrotic enteritis in broiler chickens, canine haemorrhagic gastroenteritis and typhlocolitis in horses. *Clostridium perfringens* type E causes enteritis in rabbits and occasionally haemorrhagic enteritis in calves. In sheep, *C. perfringens*, types B, C and D cause lamb dysentery, 'struck' and pulpy kidney respectively. *Clostridium perfringens* type C causes haemorrhagic enteritis in neonatal piglets. In other species, comparable diseases are periodically described.

Lamb dysentery

Lamb dysentery, caused by *C. perfringens* type B, has been reported in parts of Europe and South Africa. Morbidity in flock outbreaks can be up to 30% with high mortality rates. Affected lambs, usually in the first week of life, may show abdominal distension, pain and blood-stained faeces. Many die suddenly without premonitory signs. The high susceptibility of this age group can be attributed to the absence of microbial competition and low proteolytic activity in the neonatal intestine (Box 16.1). In the absence of proteolytic activity, the β toxin retains its potency and produces disease. At postmortem, extensive haemorrhagic enteritis with areas of ulceration in the small intestine is present. Increased capillary permeability induced by the toxin results in fluid accumulation in the peritoneal cavity and in the pericardial sac.

Pulpy kidney disease

This disease, caused by *C. perfringens* type D, occurs in sheep worldwide. The condition is also described as 'over-eating disease' because gorging on a high grain diet or on succulent pasture predisposes to its development (Box 16.1). Ingestion of excessive quantities of food leads to 'carry-over' of partially digested food from the rumen into the intestine. The high starch content in the partially digested food is a suitable substrate for rapid clostridial proliferation. Sustained production of ε toxin, which exists as a prototoxin and requires activation by proteolytic

Table 16.5 Types of *Clostridium perfringens* and their major toxins.

Clostridium perfringens	Disease	Toxin	
		Name	Biological activity
Type A	Necrotic enteritis in chickens Necrotizing enterocolitis in pigs, Canine haemorrhagic gastroenteritis	α (significant toxin) Enterotoxin	Lecithinase Cytotoxic
Type B	Lamb dysentery Haemorrhagic enteritis in calves and foals	α β (significant toxin) ε (exists as a prototoxin and requires activation by proteolytic enzymes)	Lecithinase Lethal, necrotizing Increases intestinal and capillary permeability, lethal
Type C	'Struck' in adult sheep Sudden death in goats and feedlot cattle Necrotic enteritis in chickens Haemorrhagic enteritis in neonatal piglets	α β (significant toxin) Enterotoxin	Lecithinase Lethal, necrotizing Cytotoxic
Type D	Pulpy kidney in sheep Enterotoxaemia in calves, adult goats and kids	α ε (significant toxin, exists as a prototoxin and requires activation by proteolytic enzymes)	Lecithinase Increases intestinal and capillary permeability, lethal
Type E	Haemorrhagic enteritis in calves Enteritis in rabbits	α ι (significant toxin)	Lecithinase Lethal

Box 16.1 Factors which predispose to the development of enterotoxaemias associated with *Clostridium perfringens* in sheep.

- Low proteolytic activity in the neonatal intestine:
  — Presence of trypsin inhibitors in colostrum
  — Low level of pancreatic secretion
- Incomplete establishment of normal intestinal flora in neonates
- Dietary influences in older animals:
  — Abrupt change to a rich diet
  — Gorging on energy-rich diet
  — Intestinal hypomotility, a consequence of overeating

enzymes, leads to toxaemia and the development of clinical signs.

Thriving lambs from 3 to 10 weeks of age are commonly affected. The course of the disease is usually short and lambs are often found dead. Clinical signs include dullness, opisthotonos, convulsions and terminal coma. Central nervous system signs such as blindness and head pressing may be present in subacute disease. Bloating may be evident in the later stages of illness. Hyperglycaemia and glycosuria are constant features of the disease. Affected adult sheep, which have survived for several days, may exhibit diarrhoea and staggering.

In acute disease, the only postmortem findings may be scattered hyperaemic areas in the intestines and fluid accumulation in the pericardial sac. Rapid kidney autolysis which leads to pulpy cortical softening is a typical postmortem finding. Focal symmetrical encephalomalacia, a manifestation of the subacute effects of ε toxin on the vasculature, is characterized by symmetrical haemorrhagic lesions in the basal ganglia and midbrain.

Clostridium perfringens type C infection in sheep

Infection with *C. perfringens* type C causes 'struck', an acute enterotoxaemia in adult sheep in defined geographical regions such as the Romney Marsh district in England. The disease, which occurs in sheep at pasture, manifests as sudden death although some animals may be found in terminal convulsions. The β toxin plays the major role in the pathogenesis of the disease. Postmortem findings include jejunal ulceration, patchy hyperaemia in the small intestine and accumulation of fluid in the peritoneal cavity along with congestion of peritoneal vessels and petechial haemorrhages.

Haemorrhagic enteritis in piglets

This peracute enterotoxaemia caused by *C. perfringens* type C has been described worldwide in newborn piglets.

Often, entire litters are affected with mortality rates up to 80%. Infection is probably acquired from the sow's faeces. Poor husbandry may be a predisposing factor in some outbreaks.

The clinical course of the disease is short, death occurring within 24 hours of onset. Older piglets up to 2 weeks of age, which are occasionally affected, develop a more chronic form of the disease. The clinical signs include dullness, anorexia and, terminally, blood-stained faeces and perianal hyperaemia. Necrosis of the intestinal mucosa and blood-stained contents are present at postmortem examination. The lesions are usually found in the terminal small intestine, caecum and colon. Excess serosanguineous fluid is present in the pleural and peritoneal cavities.

Necrotic enteritis of chickens

Necrotic enteritis, caused by *C. perfringens* types A or C, primarily affects broilers up to 12 weeks of age. It is an acute enterotoxaemia characterized by sudden onset and high mortality. Confluent necrotic areas in the mucosa of the small intestine are found postmortem. Dietary changes, intestinal hypomotility and mucosal damage caused by coccidia and other enteric pathogens may predispose to the development of disease.

Infections caused by *C. perfringens* types B, C and D in other species

Enterotoxaemias caused by *C. perfringens* type B have been recorded in newborn foals, calves and in adult goats. In these species the condition is rapidly fatal and severe haemorrhagic enteritis is a common postmortem finding.

Clostridium perfringens type C has been associated with a disease in feedlot cattle similar to 'struck' in adult sheep. In calves, lambs and foals, infections with *C. perfringens* type C result in acute enterotoxaemia along with a haemorrhagic enteritis resembling that produced by the infection in newborn piglets.

Enterotoxaemia caused by *C. perfringens* type D has been reported in kids and adult goats. The clinical and pathological features of acute disease in kids are similar to those of pulpy kidney disease in lambs. Subacute forms of the disease are also described, but focal symmetrical encephalomalacia has not been recorded in goats.

Diagnostic procedures

- Sudden deaths in groups of unvaccinated animals on farms where outbreaks of clostridial enterotoxaemias have previously been recorded may suggest the involvement of *C. perfringens* types B, C or D.
- In recently-dead animals, postmortem findings may be of value. The presence of focal symmetrical encephalomalacia is indicative of *C. perfringens* type D

involvement (Buxton *et al.,* 1978).
- Direct smears from the mucosa or contents of the small intestine of recently-dead animals, which contain large numbers of thick Gram-positive rods, are consistent with clostridial enterotoxaemia.
- Glycosuria is a constant finding in pulpy kidney disease.
- Toxin neutralization tests using mouse and guinea-pig inoculation can definitively identify the toxins of *C. perfringens* present in the intestinal contents of recently-dead animals. Because of the lability of some of these toxins, particularly the β toxin, failure to demonstrate their presence in intestinal contents does not necessarily exclude a diagnosis of clostridial entero-toxaemia. The supernatant from centrifuged ileal contents is generally used for the test. Antitoxins with specificity for each *C. perfringens* type are added to supernatant fluid to produce a mixture of 3 parts test fluid to 1 part known antitoxin. Saline added to super-natant is used as a positive control for the presence of toxin. To allow neutralization of toxin, each mixture is held at room temperature for 1 hour before intravenous injection into mice or intradermal injection into guinea-pigs. It is usual to inject 0.3 ml of the mixture into mice and 0.2 ml into guinea-pigs. The pattern of cross-neu-tralization observed in the mouse or guinea-pig tests indicates the specific *C. perfringens* type which is the cause of the enterotoxaemia (Table 16.6).
- ELISA can be used as an alternative to *in vivo* assays for demonstrating toxin in intestinal contents (Songer, 1997). The sensitivity and specificity of ELISA for detection of *C. perfringens* toxins approaches that of mouse or guinea-pig inoculation methods.

Treatment and control

- Hyperimmune serum, if available, may be of value in some instances. Because of the acute nature of the disease antibiotic therapy, although sometimes used, is generally ineffective.
- Vaccination is the principal control method. Ewes should be vaccinated with toxoid six weeks before lambing to ensure passive protection for lambs up to eight weeks of age. Ewes being vaccinated for the first time should be given two doses of vaccine one month apart. Annual revaccination is recommended.
- For the prevention of pulpy kidney disease, lambs should be vaccinated with toxoid before they are two months old and a booster injection should be given one month later.
- Sudden dietary changes and other factors predisposing to enterotoxaemias should be avoided (Box 16.1).

Other clostridia occasionally involved in diseases of animals

This diverse group of clostridia is comprised of organisms which produce sporadic disease problems in domestic animals.

Clostridium piliforme

Clostridium piliforme, a spore-forming, filamentous Gram-negative intracellular pathogen is an atypical member of the clostridia. It has not been cultured on artificial media and grows only in tissue culture or in fertile eggs. Although originally named *Bacillus piliformis*, DNA sequencing demonstrated its relatedness to the clostridia (Duncan *et al.*, 1993).

Infection with *C. piliforme*, Tyzzer's disease, results in severe hepatic necrosis. The condition was originally

Table 16.6 Toxin neutralization tests, in mice or guinea-pigs, for identifying the types of *Clostridium perfringens* implicated in entero-toxaemias.

Antitoxin (specificity)	Test result				
	Toxins identified in intestinal contents				
	α	α, β, ε	α, β	α, ε	α, ι
Type A (anti-α)	–	D	D	D	D
Type B (anti-α, β, ε)	–	–	–	–	D
Type C (anti-α, β)	–	D	–	D	D
Type D (anti-α, ε)	–	D	D	–	D
Type E (anti-α, ι)	–	D	D	D	–

D   death of mouse or dermal necrosis in guinea-pig because toxins are not neutralized
–   mouse or guinea-pig unaffected; toxins neutralized

described in mice and other laboratory animals (Sparrow and Naylor, 1978). It has been sporadically reported in foals and rarely in calves, dogs and cats. Stress or immunosuppression may predispose to infection.

Affected foals are usually under 6 weeks of age and many are found comatose or dead. The incubation period, following oral infection, is up to 7 days. Clinical signs include depression, anorexia, fever, jaundice and diarrhoea. Hepatomegaly with extensive areas of necrosis is the principal postmortem finding. Diagnosis is based on the histological demonstration of the organisms in hepatocytes using the Warthin-Starry silver impregnation technique. Because of the acute nature of the disease, specific therapy is not applicable.

Clostridium difficile

Clostridium difficile has been reported in dogs with chronic diarrhoea (Berry and Levett, 1986) and in haemorrhagic enterocolitis in new born foals (Jones *et al.*, 1988). It may be associated with acute colitis in adult horses following antibiotic therapy or grain overload.

Clostridium colinum

Clostridium colinum has been implicated in enteritis in quails (quail disease), chickens, turkeys, pheasants and grouse. The organism is shed in the faeces of clinically affected and carrier birds. Mortality may approach 100% in susceptible quail but is usually less than 10% in chickens. Intestinal ulceration and, in some instances, hepatic necrosis are present at postmortem examination.

Antibiotics are used therapeutically in drinking water or in feed. Contaminated litter should be removed regularly as part of a control programme.

Clostridium spiroforme

Clostridium spiroforme, a clostridial organism with atypical coiled morphology, has been implicated in spontaneous and antibiotic-induced enteritis in rabbits. This enterotoxaemia-like condition may be fatal within 48 hours. Predisposing factors include oral administration of antibiotics and low fibre diets. Antibiotic administration adversely affects the intestinal flora of the rabbit which is composed predominantly of Gram-positive bacteria. A toxin elaborated by *C. spiroforme* is neutralized by antitoxin to the ι toxin of *C. perfringen*s type E (Borriello and Carman, 1983).

References

Berry, A.P. and Levett, P.N. (1986). Chronic diarrhoea in dogs associated with *Clostridium difficile* infection. *Veterinary Record*, **118**, 102-103.

Borriello, S.P. and Carman, R.J. (1983). Association of an iota-like toxin and *Clostridium spiroforme* with both spontaneous and antibiotic-associated diarrhoea and colitis in rabbits. *Journal of Clinical Microbiology*, **17**, 414-418.

Buxton, D., Linklater, K.A. and Dyson, D.A. (1978). Pulpy kidney disease and its diagnosis by histological examination. *Veterinary Record*, **102**, 241.

Duncan, A.J., Carman, R.J., Olsen, G.J. and Wilson, K.H. (1993). The agent of Tyzzer's disease is a *Clostridium* species. *Clinical Infectious Diseases*, **16** (Suppl. 4), 422.

Farrow. B.R.H., Murrell, W.G., Revington, M.L., Stewart, B.J. and Zuber, R.M. (1983). Type C botulism in young dogs. *Australian Veterinary Journal*, **60**, 374-377.

Harihan, H. and Mitchell, W.R. (1977). Type C botulism: the agent, host spectrum and environment. *Veterinary Bulletin*, **47**, 95-103.

Jones, R.L., Adney, W.S., Alexander, A.F., Shideler, R.K., Traub-Dargatz, J.L. (1988). Haemorrhagic necrotizing enterocolitis associated with *Clostridium difficile* infection in four foals. *Journal of the American Veterinary Medical Association*, **193**, 76-79.

Kuhnert, P., Krampe, M., Capaul, S.E., Frey, J. and Nicolet, J. (1997). Identification of *Clostridium chauvoei* in cultures and clinical material from blackleg using PCR. *Veterinary Microbiology*, **51**, 291-298.

McLoughlin, M.F., McIlray, S.G. and Neill, S.D. (1988). A major outbreak of botulism in cattle being fed ensiled poultry litter. *Veterinary Record*, **122**, 579-581.

Quinn, P.J. and Crinion, R.A.P. (1984). A two year study of botulism in gulls in the vicinity of Dublin Bay. *Irish Veterinary Journal*, **38**, 214-219.

Sanford, J.P. (1995). Tetanus - forgotten but not gone. *New England Journal of Medicine*, **332**, 812-813.

Songer, J.G. (1997). Clostridial diseases of animals. In *The Clostridia : molecular biology and pathogenesis*. Eds. J. Rood, B.A. McClane, J.G. Songer and R.W. Titball. Academic Press, San Diego. pp. 153-182.

Sparrow, S. and Naylor, P. (1978). Naturally occurring Tyzzer's disease in guinea pigs. *Veterinary Record*, **102**, 288.

Swerczek, T.W. (1980). Toxicoinfectious botulism in foals and adult horses. *Journal of the American Veterinary Medical Association*, **176**, 217-220.

Further reading

Bagadi, H.O. (1974). Infectious necrotic hepatitis (black disease) of sheep. *Veterinary Bulletin*, **44**, 385–388.

Gay, C.C., Lording, P.M., McNeil, P. and Richards, W.P.C. (1980). Infectious necrotic hepatitis (black disease) in a horse. *Equine Veterinary Journal*, **12**, 26–27.

Hatheway, C.L. and Johnson, E.A. (1998). *Clostridium*: the spore-bearing anaerobes. In *Topley and Wilson's Microbiology and Microbial Infections*. Volume. 2. Eds. L. Collier, A. Balows and M. Sussman. Arnold, London. pp. 733-782.

Jones, T. (1996). Botulism. *In Practice*, **18**, 312–313.

Lee, E.A. and Jones, B.R. (1996). Localized tetanus in two cats after ovario-hysterectomy. *New Zealand Veterinary Journal*, **44**, 105–108.

Lewis, C.J. and Naylor, R. (1996). Sudden death in lambs associated with *Clostridium sordellii* infection, *Veterinary Record*, **138**, 262.

Niilo, L. (1980). *Clostridium perfringens* in animal disease: a review of current knowledge. *Canadian Veterinary Journal*, **21**, 141–148.

Niilo, L. (1988). *Clostridium perfringens* type C enterotoxaemia. *Canadian Veterinary Journal*, **29**, 658-664.

Pearce, O. (1994). Treatment of equine tetanus. *In Practice*, **16**, 322–325.

Popoff, M.R. (1984). Bacteriological examination in enterotoxaemia of sheep and lambs. *Veterinary Record*, **114**, 324.

Rood, J.I., McClane, B.A., Songer, J.G. and Titball, R.W. (1997). *The Clostridia: Molecular Biology and Pathogenesis*. Academic Press, San Diego.

Chapter 17

Mycobacterium species

Mycobacteria are aerobic, non-spore-forming, non-motile, rod shaped, acid-fast bacilli. Individual species differ in size; the rods of *Mycobacterium bovis* and *M. avium* subsp. *avium* are slender and up to 4 μm in length, whereas those of *M. avium* subsp. *paratuberculosis* are broad and are usually less than 2 μm long.

Although mycobacteria are cytochemically Gram-positive, the high lipid and mycolic acid content of their cell walls prevents uptake of the dyes employed in the Gram stain. The cell wall lipids bind carbol fuchsin which is not removed by the acid-alcohol decolourizer used in the Ziehl-Neelsen (ZN) staining method. Bacilli, which stain red by this method, are called acid-fast or ZN-positive.

The mycobacteria include diverse species ranging from environmental saprophytes and opportunistic invaders to obligate pathogens.

Although some pathogenic mycobacteria exhibit a particular host preference, they can occasionally infect other species (Table 17.1). Mycobacterial diseases in domestic animals are usually chronic and progressive. The closely-related members of the *M. tuberculosis* complex (*M. tuberculosis*, *M. bovis* and *M. africanum*), cause tuberculosis in humans.

Key points

- Acid-fast (ZN-positive) rods
- Cell walls rich in complex lipids and waxes containing mycolic acids
- Complex egg-enriched media required for growth of pathogenic species
- Aerobic, non-motile, non-spore-forming
- Genus includes obligate pathogens, opportunistic pathogens and saprophytes
- Pathogenic species grow slowly, colonies visible after several weeks
- Some mycobacteria produce carotenoid pigments
- Resistant to chemical disinfectants and environmental influences but susceptible to heat treatment (pasteurization)
- Multiply intracellulary and cause chronic, granulomatous infections
- Major diseases include tuberculosis, Johne's disease and feline leprosy

---

Usual habitat

Lipid-rich walls render mycobacteria hydrophobic and resistant to adverse environmental influences. Environmental mycobacteria are found in soil, on vegetation and in water. Obligate pathogens, shed by infected animals, can also survive in the environment for extended periods (Morris *et al.*, 1994).

Differentiation of pathogenic mycobacteria

The ZN staining method is used to differentiate mycobacteria from other bacteria. Differentiation of pathogenic mycobacteria relies on cultural characteristics, biochemical tests, animal inoculation, chromatographic analyses and molecular techniques. In addition, mycobacteria associated with opportunistic infections can be differentiated on the basis of pigment production, optimal incubation temperature and growth rate (Table 17.2).

- Safety precautions, including the use of a biohazard cabinet, must be implemented when working with material containing mycobacteria.
- Pathogenic mycobacteria grow slowly and colonies are not evident until cultures have been incubated for at least three weeks. In contrast, the colonies of rapidly growing saprophytes are visible within days.
- *Mycobacterium bovis*, *M. tuberculosis* and *M. avium* subsp. *paratuberculosis* have an optimal incubation temperature of 37°C. Mycobacteria belonging to the *M. avium* complex grow in the temperature range of 37 to 43°C.
- Cultural features:
  — Pathogenic species of mycobacteria can be distinguished by their colonial appearance on egg-based media.
  — The influence of glycerol and sodium pyruvate on growth rate is used to differentiate pathogenic species.
  — Supplementation of media with mycobactin is

Table 17.1 Mycobacteria which are pathogenic for animals and man.

Mycobacterium species	Main hosts	Species occasionally infected	Disease
M. tuberculosis[a]	Man, captive primates	Dogs, cattle, psittacine birds, canaries	Tuberculosis (worldwide)
M. bovis	Cattle	Deer, badgers, possums, man, cats, other mammalian species	Tuberculosis
M. africanum	Man		Tuberculosis (regions in Africa)
M. avium complex[a]	Most avian species except psittacines	Pigs, cattle	Tuberculosis
M. microti	Voles	Occasionally other mammalian species	Tuberculosis
M. marinum	Fish	Man, aquatic mammals, amphibians	Tuberculosis
M. leprae	Man	Armadillos, chimpanzees	Leprosy
M. lepraemurium	Rats, mice	Cats	Rat leprosy, feline leprosy
M. avium subsp. paratuberculosis	Cattle, sheep, goats, deer	Other ruminants	Paratuberculosis (Johne's disease)
Unspecified acid-fast bacteria[a]	Cattle		Associated with skin tuberculosis
M. senegalense, M. farcinogenes	Cattle		Implicated in bovine farcy

a cattle infected with these mycobacteria often exhibit sensitivity to tuberculin

required for *M. avium* subsp. *paratuberculosis*. Mycobactin is extracted from laboratory-maintained, rare, non-mycobactin-dependent isolates of *M. avium* subsp. *paratuberculosis*.

- Biochemical differentiation, based on specific test methods, aids in the identification of *M. tuberculosis*, *M. bovis* and *M. avium*. Some mycobacterial isolates cannot be assigned to a given species using biochemical differentiation as their biochemical profiles are difficult to interpret (Gunn-Moore *et al.*, 1996).
- Guinea-pig and rabbit inoculation was used in the past to differentiate *M. tuberculosis* from *M. bovis* and *M. avium*. Guinea-pigs are highly susceptible to infection with *M. tuberculosis* and *M. bovis*. Rabbits are highly susceptible to infections with *M. bovis* and *M. avium*.
- Chromatographic analyses of the lipid composition of some mycobacterial species are used in specialized laboratories.
- Pigment production and photoreactivity for opportunistic mycobacteria:
  — Non-chromogens produce colonies devoid of orange, carotenoid pigments.
  — Photochromogens, when cultured in the dark, produce non-pigmented colonies which become pigmented after a period of exposure to light.
  — Scotochromogens produce pigment when cultured in the dark or in light.

- Molecular techniques:
  — DNA probes, complementary to species-specific sequences of rRNA, are commercially available for the *M. tuberculosis* complex, the *M. avium* complex and *M. kansasii*.
  — Nucleic acid amplification procedures, including the polymerase chain reaction, are being developed as sensitive and rapid methods for the detection of mycobacteria in tissue samples (Aranaz *et al.*, 1996).
  — DNA restriction endonuclease analyses (DNA fingerprinting) are used in epidemiological studies (Collins *et al.*, 1994).

Clinical infections

The diseases caused by pathogenic mycobacteria are presented in Table 17.1. The major pathogenic *Mycobacterium* species which affect domestic animals exhibit a considerable degree of host specificity although they can produce sporadic disease in a number of other hosts.

Diseases in domestic animals caused by mycobacteria include tuberculosis in avian and mammalian species, paratuberculosis in ruminants and feline leprosy. Two other clinical conditions, skin tuberculosis and bovine farcy are associated with the presence of acid-fast bacteria in lesions. In skin tuberculosis of cattle, nodular lesions

Table 17.2 Clinical significance, growth characteristics and biochemical differentiation of pathogenic mycobacteria.

	M. tuberculosis	M. bovis	M. avium complex	M. avium subsp. paratuberculosis
Significance of infection	Important in man and occasionally in dogs	Important in cattle and occasionally in other domestic animals and man	Important in free-range domestic poultry, opportunistic infections in man and domestic animals	Important in cattle and other ruminants
Cultural characteristics and requirements				
Growth rate	Slow (3-8 weeks)	Slow (3-8 weeks)	Slow (2-6 weeks)	Very slow (up to 16 weeks)
Optimal incubation temperature	37°C	37°C	37-43°C	37°C
Atmospheric requirements	Aerobic	Aerobic	Aerobic	Aerobic
Colonial features	Rough, buff, difficult to break apart	Cream-coloured, raised with central roughness, break apart easily	Sticky, off-white, break apart easily	Small, hemispherical; some pigmented
Essential growth supplement	None	None	None	Mycobactin
Effect of added glycerol	Enhanced growth (eugonic)	Growth inhibited (dysgonic)	Enhanced growth (eugonic)	
Effect of added sodium pyruvate	No effect	Enhanced growth	No effect	
Biochemical differentiation				
Niacin accumulation	+	−	−	
Pyrazinamidase production	+	−	+	
Nitrate reduction	+	−	−	
Susceptibility to TCH (10 μg/ml)[a]	Resistant	Susceptible	Resistant	

a   TCH, Thiophen-2-carboxylic acid hydrazine

are located along the course of lymphatics in the limbs. Unspecified acid-fast bacilli have been demonstrated in these lesions. *Mycobacterium senegalense* and *M. farcinogenes* have been isolated from the lesions of bovine farcy. Their aetiological role in this condition, however, is uncertain.

Granulomatous lesions which develop following opportunistic infections with environmental saprophytic mycobacteria are encountered occasionally in domestic animals. These saprophytic mycobacteria are grouped on the basis of pigment production and growth rate (Box 17.1). Members of the *M. avium* complex are grouped with those which produce opportunistic infection because they are occasionally involved in mammalian infections.

Tuberculosis in cattle

Bovine tuberculosis, caused by *M. bovis,* occurs worldwide. Because of the zoonotic implications of the disease and production losses due to its chronic progressive nature, eradication programmes have been introduced in many countries. When eradication programmes are successful, infections in cattle caused by members of the *M. avium* complex and by other saprophytic mycobacteria are occasionally encountered. The incidence of human infection with *M. bovis* has been reduced to low levels in countries where tuberculosis eradication programmes have been implemented in cattle. In addition, pasteurization of milk has eliminated exposure of humans to infection from dairy products. Cross-infection with *M. tuberculosis* from infected humans has been recorded on rare occasions in cattle.

Epidemiology

Although *M. bovis* can survive for several months in the environment, transmission is mainly through aerosols generated by infected cattle. Dairy cattle in particular are at risk because husbandry methods allow close contact between animals at milking and when housed during winter months. Calves can become infected by ingesting contaminated milk and ingestion is the probable route of transmission to pigs and cats. Wildlife reservoirs of *M. bovis* are major sources of infection for grazing cattle in some countries. They include the badger in Europe, the brush-tailed possum in New Zealand and the Cape buffalo and other ruminants in Africa. Deer, both wild and farmed, are particularly susceptible and may act as reservoirs of infection for cattle.

Pathogenesis and pathogenicity

The virulence of *M. bovis* relates to its ability to survive and multiply in host macrophages (Fig. 17.1). Specific toxic factors, contributing to virulence, have not been identified. The macrophage accumulation at the primary site of infection is initially a response to the foreign body effect of waxes and lipids in the mycobacterial cell wall. Survival within the cytoplasm of macrophages is promoted by interference with phagosome-lysosome fusion and failure of lysosomal digestion. Bacilli released from dead macrophages are engulfed by surrounding viable phagocytes. Migration of macrophages containing viable mycobacteria can disseminate infection.

The complex lipid and waxy composition of the mycobacterial cell wall contributes not only to virulence

but also, in association with tuberculoproteins, to the immunogenicity on which the development of the host responses and the lesions depends. With the development of cell-mediated immunity some weeks after infection, macrophage recruitment accelerates under the influence of cytokines produced by T lymphocytes sensitized to tuberculoprotein. In addition, these macrophages become activated through cytokine stimulation and proliferate. The gradual accumulation of macrophages in the lesion and the formation of a granulomatous response lead to the development of a tubercle, the typical host response in the delayed-type hypersensitivity to mycobacterial infections (Fig. 17.2).

Clinical signs and pathology

Clinical signs are evident only in advanced disease and cattle with extensive lesions can appear to be in good health. Loss of condition may become evident as the disease progresses. In advanced pulmonary tuberculosis, animals may eventually develop a cough and intermittent pyrexia. Involvement of mammary tissue may result in marked induration of affected quarters, often accompanied by supramammary lymph node enlargement. Tuberculous mastitis facilitates spread of infection to calves and cats, and is of major public health importance.

In the early stages of the disease, lesions may be difficult to detect at postmortem examination. These small lesions are composed of aggregates of macrophages, termed epithelioid cells. Multinucleate Langhans' giant cells, formed from the fusion of macrophages, may also be present. In older lesions, fibroplasia produces early capsule formation and there is central caseous necrosis, detectable grossly as yellowish cheesy material. The characteristic histological appearance of a typical tubercle is illustrated in Figure 17.2.

Diagnostic procedures

- The tuberculin test, based on a delayed-type hypersensitivity to mycobacterial tuberculoprotein, is the standard antemortem test in cattle. The test can be adapted for use in pigs and farmed deer. Reactivity in cattle is usually detectable 30-50 days after infection (Monaghan *et al.*, 1994). Tuberculin, prepared from mycobacteria and called purified protein derivative (PPD), is injected intradermally to detect sensitization. Two main methods of tuberculin testing are employed:
—In the single intradermal (caudal fold) test, 0.1 ml of bovine PPD is injected intradermally into the caudal fold of the tail. The injection site is examined 72 hours later and a positive reaction is characterized by a hard or oedematous swelling.
—In the comparative intradermal test, 0.1 ml of avian PPD and 0.1 ml of bovine PPD are injected intradermally into separate clipped sites on the side of the neck about 12 cm apart. Skin thickness at the injection sites is measured with calipers before injection

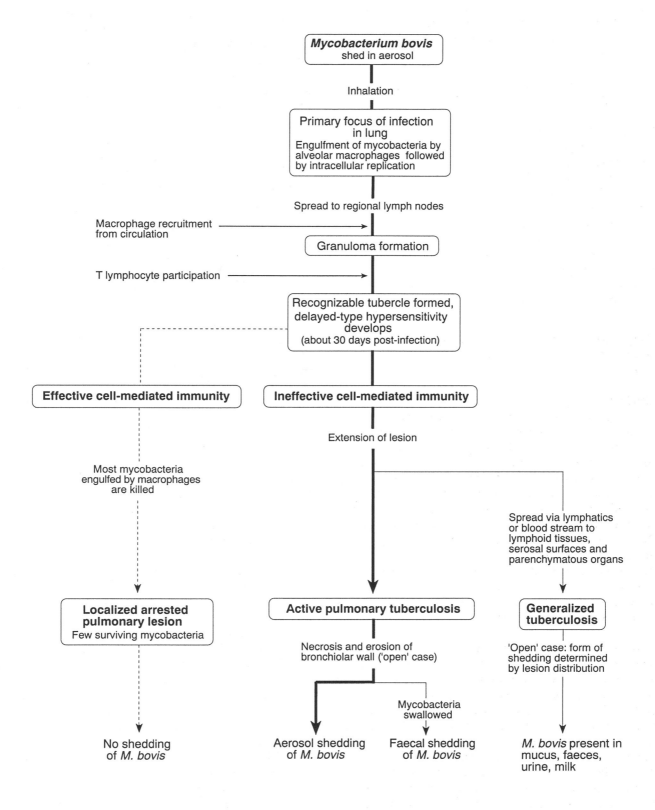

Figure 17.1 The possible consequences of *Mycobacterium bovis* infection in cattle, acquired via aerosols.

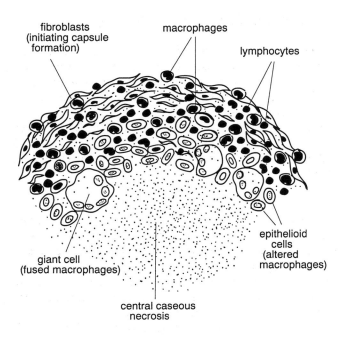

Figure 17.2 Microscopic appearance of part of a typical bovine tuberculous lesion. The tubercle consists of a peripheral zone of mononuclear cells, fibroblasts and giant cells with central caseous necrosis.

of tuberculins and after 72 hours. An increase in skin thickness at the injection site of bovine PPD which exceeds that at the avian PPD injection site by 4 mm or more is interpreted as evidence of infection and the animal is termed a reactor.

- False positive reactions which occur in the tuberculin test may be attributed to sensitization to mycobacteria other than *M. bovis*.
- False negative test results may be recorded:
  — Cattle tested before delayed-type hypersensitivity to tuberculoproteins develops (at about 30 days post-infection) do not react.
  — In some cattle an unresponsive state, referred to as anergy, may accompany advanced tuberculosis. The mechanisms involved are incompletely understood.
  — A transient desensitization may follow injection of tuberculin. Reactivity usually returns within 60 days.
  — Cows may be unresponsive to the tuberculin test during the early postpartum period.
- Blood-based tests which have been developed for use in conjunction with the tuberculin test include:
  — Gamma interferon assay
  — ELISA for detecting circulating antibodies
  — Lymphocyte transformation and related assays
- Specimens suitable for laboratory examination include lymph nodes, tissue lesions, aspirates and milk.
- The low numbers of mycobacteria present in bovine lesions can render visual confirmation difficult using

the ZN stain. In contrast, large numbers of acid-fast bacilli are usually present in smears of specimens from deer and badgers (Fig. 17.3).

- Stained tissue sections usually reveal typical patterns of tubercle formation (Fig. 17.2).
- Isolation of *M. bovis* requires:
  — Decontamination of specimens to eliminate fast-growing contaminating bacteria. Ground-up specimens are treated for up to 30 minutes with 2-4% sodium hydroxide or 5% oxalic acid, followed by neutralization of the alkali or acid. Centrifugation is used to concentrate the mycobacteria and the supernatant fluid is discarded.
  — Slants of Lowenstein-Jensen medium, without glycerol and containing 0.4% sodium pyruvate, are inoculated with the centrifuged deposit and incubated aerobically at 37°C for up to 8 weeks.
- Identification criteria for isolates:
  — Growth rate and colonial appearance
  — Positive ZN-staining of bacilli in smears from colonies
  — Biochemical profile (Table 17.2)
  — Analytical and molecular techniques
- Commercially-available, rapid, automated systems can be used for isolating pathogenic mycobacteria of the *M. tuberculosis* complex (Yearsley *et al.*, 1998).

Control

- Treatment and vaccination are inappropriate in control programmes for cattle.
- In many countries, tuberculin testing followed by isolation and slaughter of reactors has been implemented as the basis of national eradication schemes.
- Routine meat inspection forms part of the surveillance programme for bovine tuberculosis in many countries.
- Wildlife reservoirs such as badgers and possums are major obstacles to disease eradication in some

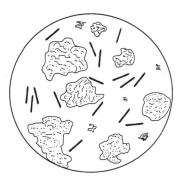

Figure 17.3 Thin rods of *Mycobacterium bovis* as they appear in a smear from a tuberculous lesion from deer or badgers. Organisms are sparse in lesions from cattle. Using the Ziehl-Neelsen method, the mycobacteria stain red (acid-fast) and other lesion material stains blue.

countries. Effective measures for dealing with infected wildlife species have not been described.

Tuberculosis in poultry and other avian species

Avian tuberculosis, which occurs worldwide, is usually caused by members of the *M. avium* complex, serotypes 1 to 3. The disease is encountered most often in free-range adult birds. Bacilli, excreted in the faeces of birds with advanced lesions, can survive for long periods in soil.

Non-specific clinical signs including dullness, emaciation and lameness develop in affected birds only when the disease is at an advanced stage. At postmortem examination, granulomatous lesions are characteristically present in the liver, spleen, bone marrow and intestines. Diagnosis is based on the postmortem findings and on the demonstration of large numbers of ZN-positive bacilli in smears from lesions. Antemortem diagnosis of avian tuberculosis in free-range poultry is based on tuberculin testing, using avian PPD injected into the skin of a wattle. *M. tuberculosis* occasionally infects parrots and canaries and *M. genavense* has been isolated from pet birds (Hoop *et al.*, 1993).

Members of the *M. avium* complex cause opportunistic infections in immunocompromized humans. Rare cases of generalized disease in cats, dogs and horses caused by members of the complex have been reported. Pigs infected through the ingestion of uncooked swill contaminated with *M. avium* often develop small tubercles in the retropharyngeal, submaxillary and cervical lymph nodes.

Feline leprosy

It is generally considered that feline leprosy, a cutaneous disease of worldwide distribution, is caused by *M. lepraemurium*, the aetiological agent of rat leprosy. Sporadic transmission of the organism to cats probably occurs through bites from infected rodents, the wildlife reservoirs. Nodular lesions, involving subcutaneous tissues, may be solitary or multiple and are usually confined to the head region or the limbs. The nodules, which are fleshy and freely movable, tend to ulcerate. Large numbers of ZN-positive bacilli are present in smears from the lesions. Histopathological examination demonstrates many infiltrating macrophages which contain densely-packed mycobacteria.

Mycobacterium lepraemurium, a slow-growing fastidious organism, requires a specially formulated culture medium for growth. It does not appear to be infectious for other species of domestic animals or for humans. Diagnosis is based on the histopathological features of the lesions and negative cultural results for *M. bovis* and opportunistic mycobacteria, which can also cause granulomatous dermatitis in cats. Surgical excision of lesions is the preferred treatment.

Paratuberculosis (Johne's disease)

Paratuberculosis is a chronic, contagious, invariably fatal enteritis which can affect domestic and wild ruminants. The aetiological agent, *M. avium* subsp. *paratuberculosis*, is an acid-fast organism formerly referred to as *Mycobacterium johnei*.

Uncertainty exists regarding an association between infection with *M. avium* subsp. *paratuberculosis* and Crohn's disease, a chronic enteritis in humans (Thompson, 1994).

Epidemiology
The epidemiology of the disease has been studied in cattle and the pattern of infection and spread in other species is assumed to be similar. Infection is acquired by calves at an early age through ingestion of organisms shed in the faeces of infected animals. *Mycobacterium avium* subsp. *paratuberculosis* may remain viable in the environment for up to one year under suitable conditions.

Shedding of *M. avium* subsp. *paratuberculosis* in milk has been recorded (Taylor *et al.*, 1981). Although the organism has been isolated from the genital organs and semen of infected bulls (Larsen *et al.*, 1981), venereal transmission is unimportant epidemiologically. *In utero* transmission has been reported but is probably insignificant as a mode of spread (Seitz *et al.*, 1989). In a survey of wild rabbits in Scotland, 67% were infected with *M. avium* subsp. *paratuberculosis* (Greig *et al.*, 1997). However, it has not been determined if the strain infecting rabbits is infectious for domestic ruminants.

Calves under one month of age are particularly susceptible to infection and more likely to develop clinical disease than animals infected later in life. The incubation period of paratuberculosis is protracted and variable. Clinical disease is rarely encountered in cattle under 2 years of age. Signs of disease do not develop in all infected animals; some become subclinical carriers and shed mycobacteria intermittently in their faeces.

Pathogenesis and pathogenicity
Mycobacterium avium subsp. *paratuberculosis* is an intracellular pathogen and cell-mediated reactions are mainly responsible for the enteric lesions. Ingested mycobacteria, engulfed by macrophages in which they survive and replicate, are found initially in Peyer's patches. As the disease progresses, an immune-mediated granulomatous reaction develops, with marked lymphocyte and macrophage accumulation in the lamina propria and submucosa. The resulting enteropathy leads to loss of plasma proteins and malabsorption of nutrients and water. The macrophages in the intestinal wall and in the regional lymph nodes contain large numbers of mycobacteria.

Clinical signs and pathology
Clinical signs develop in most ruminant species after a

prolonged subclinical phase of infection. Affected cattle are usually more than 2 years of age when signs are first observed. The disease is clinically evident only in mature sheep and goats. Clinical signs may develop rapidly in farmed deer and may be evident by one year of age.

The main clinical feature in cattle is diarrhoea, initially intermittent but becoming persistent and profuse. Progressive weight loss results without loss of appetite, and affected animals seldom survive for more than a year after initial detection.

In sheep and goats, diarrhoea is less marked and may be absent. In some infected deer, there may be rapid weight loss and sudden onset of diarrhoea with death in two to three weeks. In others, extreme emaciation may develop over a period of months without evidence of diarrhoea (Gilmour and Nyange, 1989).

In cattle, the mucosa of affected areas of the terminal small intestine and the large intestine is usually thickened and folded into transverse corrugations. The mesenteric and ileocaecal lymph nodes are enlarged and oedematous. Thickening of the intestinal mucosa is less marked in sheep, and necrosis and caseation may be present in the regional lymph nodes. Lesions in deer are similar to those in sheep.

Diagnosis

- Paratuberculosis requires differentiation from other chronic wasting diseases in ruminants.
- Specimens for direct microscopy from live animals include scrapings or pinch biopsies from the rectum. Faeces may be submitted for culture and serum for serological tests.
- Postmortem specimens for histopathological examination from cattle include tissue from affected regions of the intestines and from regional lymph nodes.
- Specimens for microscopical examination should be stained by the ZN technique (Fig. 17.4).
- Isolation of *M. avium* subsp. *paratuberculosis* from faeces or tissues is a sensitive diagnostic procedure but it is difficult and time-consuming. After decontamination of the specimen with 0.3% benzalkonium chloride and concentration by centrifugation, slants of Herrold's egg-yolk medium with and without mycobactin are inoculated with the deposit. Slants are incubated aerobically at 37°C for up to 16 weeks and examined weekly for evidence of growth.
- Identification criteria for isolates:
  — Colonies less than 1 mm in diameter, usually colourless and hemispherical appear in 5-16 weeks. Isolates from sheep may be pigmented.
  — Smears from colonies are ZN-positive.
  — Medium containing mycobactin supports growth.
- Serological tests:
  — Complement fixation tests have been used but are laborious and relatively insensitive.
  — The agar-gel immunodiffusion test has low

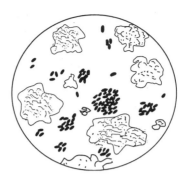

Figure 17.4 Clusters of *Mycobacterium paratuberculosis* in a rectal scraping from a cow with Johne's disease. Using the Ziehl-Neelsen method, the short mycobacterial rods, present in clumps, stain red (acid-fast). Faecal and rectal debris stain blue.

sensitivity but may be useful for confirming clinical infection.
  — ELISA, using serum absorbed with a suspension of *M. phlei* to enhance specificity, is a reliable diagnostic test which may detect subclinically-infected animals.
- Cell-mediated responses:
  — Johnin, the counterpart of tuberculin PPD, may be used as a field test. The preparation is inoculated intradermally or intravenously into cattle. The reliability of the test is questionable and, in addition, it may sensitize cattle to tuberculin.
  — The gamma interferon assay is being evaluated but is expensive.
  — Assays based on lymphocyte stimulation appear to be of limited value and are infrequently used.
- DNA probes, which are highly sensitive, are being used to detect *M. avium* subsp. *paratuberculosis* in faeces.

Control

- Animals with clinical signs suggestive of paratuberculosis should be isolated. If the condition is confirmed, affected animals should be slaughtered promptly as they shed large numbers of mycobacteria which can contaminate buildings and pasture.
- Detection and elimination of subclinically affected animals is challenging for clinicians and laboratory staff. Testing should be carried out on a herd or flock basis. Subclinical excretors may be detected by faecal culture at intervals of six months or by detection of *M. avium* subsp. *paratuberculosis* in faeces using DNA probes. Serology, using the absorbed ELISA, may detect subclinical infection.
- In problem herds, appropriate hygiene and husbandry measures should be instituted to prevent infection of young susceptible animals. Calves should be separated from their dams at birth and raised on pasteurized milk. They should remain isolated from the herd until 2 years of age.

- Inactivated adjuvanted vaccines are available. In cattle, vaccination may reduce the number of clinical cases but cannot be relied on to eliminate the disease from a herd. Because vaccinated animals usually become sensitized to tuberculin, vaccine use in some countries is subject to regulatory control. Vaccination may prevent infection in sheep (Cranwell, 1993).

References

Aranaz, A., Liebana, E., Pickering, X., Novoa, C., Mateos, A. and Dominguez, L. (1996). Use of polymerase chain reaction in the diagnosis of tuberculosis in cats and dogs. *Veterinary Record*, **138**, 276–280.

Collins, D.M., deLisle, G.W., Collins, J.D. and Costello, E. (1994). DNA restriction fragment typing of *Mycobacterium bovis* isolates from cattle and badgers in Ireland. *Veterinary Record*, **134**, 681–682.

Cranwell, M.P. (1993). Control of Johne's disease in a flock of sheep by vaccination. *Veterinary Record*, **133**, 219–220.

Gilmour, N. and Nyange, J. (1989). Paratuberculosis (Johne's disease) in deer. *In Practice*, **11**, 193–196.

Greig, A., Stevenson, K., Perez, V., Pirie, A.A., Grant, J.M. and Sharp, J.M. (1997). Paratuberculosis in wild rabbits (*Oryctolagus cuniculus*). *Veterinary Record*, **140**, 141–143.

Gunn-Moore, D.A, Jenkins, P.A. and Lucke, V.M. (1996). Feline tuberculosis : a literature review and discussion of 19 cases caused by an unusual mycobacterial variant. *Veterinary Record,* **138**, 53-58.

Hoop, R.K., Bottger, E.C., Ossent, P. and Salfinger, M. (1993). Mycobacteriosis due to *Mycobacterium genavense* in six pet birds. *Journal of Clinical Microbiology*, **31**, 990–993.

Larsen, A.B., Stalheim, H.V., Hughes, D.E., Appell, L.H., Richards, W.D. and Himes, E.M. (1981). *Mycobacterium paratuberculosis* in semen and genital organs of a semen-donor bull. *Journal of the American Veterinary Medical Association*, **179**, 169–171.

Monaghan, M.L., Doherty, M.L., Collins, J.D., Kazda, J.F. and Quinn, P.J. (1994). The tuberculin test. *Veterinary Microbiology,* **40**, 111–124.

Morris, R.S., Pfeiffer, D.U. and Jackson, R. (1994). The epidemiology of *Mycobacterium bovis* infections. *Veterinary Microbiology*, **40**, 153–177.

Runyon, E.H. (1959). Anonymous mycobacteria in pulmonary disease. *Medical Clinics of North America*, **43**, 273–290.

Seitz, S.E., Heider, L.E., Hueston, W.D., Bech-Neilsen, S., Rings, M. and Spangler, L. (1989). Bovine fetal infection with *Mycobacterium paratuberculosis*. *Journal of the American Veterinary Medical Association*, **194**, 1423–1426.

Taylor, T.K., Wilks, C.R. and McQueen, D.S. (1981). Isolation of *Mycobacterium paratuberculosis* from the milk of a cow with Johne's disease. *Veterinary Record*, **109**, 532–533.

Thompson, D.E. (1994). The role of mycobacteria in Crohn's disease. *Journal of Medical Microbiology*, **41**, 74–94.

Yearsley, D., O'Rourke, J., O'Brien, T. and Egan, J. (1998). Comparison of three methods for the isolation of mycobacteria from bovine tissue lesions. *Veterinary Record*, **143**, 480–481.

Further reading

Alfredson, S. and Saxegaard, F. (1992). An outbreak of tuberculosis in pigs and cattle caused by *Mycobacterium africanum*. *Veterinary Record*, **131**, 51–53.

Griffin, J.F.T. and Buchan, G.S. (1994). Aetiology, pathogenesis and diagnosis of *Mycobacterium bovis* in deer. *Veterinary Microbiology*, **40**, 193–205.

Jackson, R. (1991). *Symposium on tuberculosis. Publication No. 132. Veterinary Continuing Education*, Massey University, Palmerston North, New Zealand.

Neill, S.D., Pollock, J.M., Bryson, D.B. and Hanna, J. (1994). Pathogenesis of *Mycobacterium bovis* in cattle. *Veterinary Microbiology*, **40**, 41–52.

Pollock, J.M., Girvin, R.M., Lightboy, K.A., Clements, R.A., Neill, S.D., Buddle, B.M. and Anderson, P. (2000). Assesment of defined antigens for the diagnosis of bovine tuberculosis in skin test-reactor cattle. *Veterinary Record*, **146**, 659–665.

Thoen, C.O. and Karlson, A.G. (1991). Tuberculosis. In *Diseases of Poultry*. Eds. B.W. Calnek, H.J. Barnes, C.W. Beard, W.M. Reid and H.W. Yoder. Ninth Edition. Iowa State Press, Ames, Iowa. pp. 172–185.

Thorel, M-F, Krichevsky, M. and Levy-Frebault, V.V. (1990). Numerical taxonomy of mycobactin-dependent mycobacteria, emended description of *Mycobacterium avium* and description of *Mycobacterium avium* subsp. nov., *Mycobacterium avium* subsp. *paratuberculosis* subsp. nov. and *Mycobacterium avium* subsp. *silvaticum* subsp. nov. *International Journal of Systematic Bacteriology*, **40**, 254–260.

Chapter 18

Enterobacteriaceae

Bacteria belonging to the family *Enterobacteriaceae* are Gram-negative rods up to 3 μm in length (Fig. 18.1) which ferment glucose and a wide range of other sugars, and are oxidase-negative. They are catalase-positive, non-spore-forming facultative anaerobes which grow well on MacConkey agar because they are not inhibited by the bile salts in the medium. These enteric organisms reduce nitrates to nitrites and some species, notably *Escherichia coli*, ferment lactose. The motile enterobacteria have peritrichous flagella. The family contains more than 28 genera and over 80 species. Less than half of the genera are of veterinary importance (Fig 18.2). The term 'coliform', formerly only used to describe enterobacteria capable of fermenting lactose, is now sometimes used to describe other members of the family.

Enterobacteria can be arbitrarily grouped in three categories: major pathogens, opportunistic pathogens and non-pathogens. Those without pathogenic significance for animals, such as *Hafnia* and *Erwinia*, can be isolated from faeces and the environment and may contaminate clinical specimens. Opportunistic pathogens occasionally cause clinical disease in locations other than the alimentary tract. The major animal pathogens *E. coli*, *Salmonella* species and *Yersinia* species can cause both enteric and systemic disease.

Key points
- Gram-negative rods
- Growth on non-enriched media
- Oxidase-negative
- Facultative anaerobes, catalase-positive
- Most are motile by peritrichous flagella
- Ferment glucose, reduce nitrate to nitrite
- Enteric bacteria which tolerate bile salts in MacConkey agar
- Cause a variety of clinical infections
- Major enteric and systemic pathogens:
  —*Escherichia coli*
  —*Salmonella* serotypes
  —*Yersinia* species
- Opportunistic pathogens:
  —*Proteus* species
  —*Enterobacter* species
  —*Klebsiella* species
  —Some other members of the *Enterobacteriaceae*

Usual habitat

Bacteria belonging to the *Enterobacteriaceae* have a worldwide distribution, inhabit the intestinal tract of animals and man and contaminate vegetation, soil and water.

Differentiation of the *Enterobacteriaceae*

Gram-negative rods which are oxidase-negative, facultative anaerobes and grow on MacConkey agar, are presumed to be members of the *Enterobacteriaceae*. The main criteria for differentiating pathogenic members are presented in Table 18.1. Few enterobacteria, apart from some strains of *E. coli*, produce haemolysis on blood agar.

- Lactose fermentation in MacConkey agar:
  — The colonies of lactose fermenters and the surrounding medium are pink due to acid production from lactose.
  — The colonies of non-lactose fermenters and the surrounding medium have a pale appearance and are alkaline due to utilization of peptones in the medium.

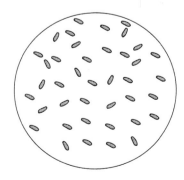

Figure 18.1 Medium-sized rods of members of the *Enterobacteriaceae*, morphologically indistinguishable from some other Gram-negative organisms.

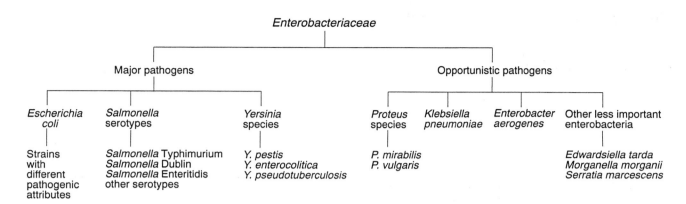

Figure 18.2 Members of the *Enterobacteriaceae* of veterinary importance.

Table 18.1 The clinical relevance, growth characteristics and biochemical reactions of members of the *Enterobacteriaceae* which are of veterinary importance.

	Escherichia coli	*Salmonella* serotypes	*Yersinia* species	*Proteus* species	*Enterobacter aerogenes*	*Klebsiella pneumoniae*
Clinical importance	Major pathogen	Major pathogens	Major pathogens	Opportunistic pathogens	Opportunistic pathogen	Opportunistic pathogen
Cultural characteristics	Some strains haemolytic	–	–	Swarming growth[a]	Mucoid	Mucoid
Motility at 30°C	Motile	Motile	Motile[b]	Motile	Motile	Non-motile
Lactose fermentation	+	–	–	–	+	+
IMViC tests						
Indole production	+	–	v	±[c]	–	–
Methyl red test	+	+	+	+	–	–
Voges-Proskauer test	–	–	–	v	+	+
Citrate utilization test	–	+	–	v	+	+
H_2S production in TSI agar	–	+	–	+	–	–
Lysine decarboxylase	+	+	–	–	+	+
Urease activity	–	–	+[b]	+	–	+

a   when cultured on non-inhibitory medium
b   except *Y. pestis*

c   *P. vulgaris* +; *P. mirabilis* –
v   reaction varies with individual species

- Reactions on selective/indicator media:
  - A number of media, commonly including brilliant green (BG) agar and xylose-lysine-deoxycholate (XLD) agar are used to differentiate salmonellae from other enteropathogens. On BG agar, salmonella colonies and the surrounding medium show a red alkaline reaction. On XLD medium the colonies of most salmonella serotypes are red (alkaline reaction) with black centres due to hydrogen sulphide (H_2S) production.
  - Eosin-methylene blue (EMB) agar is used for identifying *E. coli*. The colonies of some isolates have a metallic sheen, a feature unique to *E. coli*.
- Colonial morphology:
  - Mucoid colonies are typical of *Klebsiella* and *Enterobacter* species while rare isolates of *E. coli* are mucoid.
  - *Proteus* species produce characteristic swarming on non-inhibitory media, such as blood agar.
  - *Serratia marcescens* is unique among the opportunistic pathogens in its ability to produce red pigment.
- Reactions in triple sugar iron (TSI) agar:

  This is a non-inhibitory indicator medium used primarily to confirm that colonies isolated on BG or XLD media are those of salmonellae. Other members of the *Enterobacteriaceae* isolated on BG or XLD media can be differentiated by their reactions in TSI. Triple sugar iron agar contains 0.1% glucose, 1% lactose and 1% sucrose and chemicals to indicate H_2S production. Phenol red is used as an indicator for pH change (red at pH 8.2, yellow at pH 6.4). A black precipitate of ferrous sulphide is indicative of H_2S production. An inoculum from a single isolated colony of the organism under test is stab-inoculated with a straight wire into the butt of the TSI agar and, on withdrawal, the slant surface is inoculated. The loosely-capped tube is incubated for 18 hours at 37°C. The reactions in this medium of the more important members of the *Enterobacteriaceae* are presented in Table 18.2.
- Additional biochemical tests:
  - The lysine decarboxylase production test is used to distinguish *Proteus* species from *Salmonella* species as these organisms have similar reactions in TSI agar. *Proteus* species are negative in the test, whereas *Salmonella* species invariably produce the enzyme. Production of lysine decarboxylase is indicated by a purple colour of the liquid medium; in a negative test the medium is a yellow colour.
  - Urease production distinguishes *Proteus* species from *Salmonella* species. *Proteus* species produce urease whereas *Salmonella* species do not.
  - The IMViC (indole production, methyl red test, Voges-Proskauer test, citrate utilization) tests are a group of biochemical reactions used to differentiate

Table 18.2 Reactions of the *Enterobacteriaceae* of veterinary importance in triple sugar iron (TSI) agar[a].

Species	pH change[c] Slant	pH change[c] Butt	H_2S production
Salmonella serotypes[b]	Red	Yellow	+[d]
Proteus mirabilis	Red	Yellow	+
P. vulgaris	Yellow	Yellow	+
Escherichia coli	Yellow	Yellow	−
Yersinia enterocolitica	Yellow	Yellow	−
Y. pseudotuberculosis and *Y. pestis*	Red	Yellow	−
Enterobacter aerogenes	Yellow	Yellow	−
Klebsiella pneumoniae	Yellow	Yellow	−

a   the majority of strains give the reactions indicated
b   *Salmonella* serotypes and *Proteus* species can be differentiated by lysine decarboxylase production and urease activity (see Table 18.1)
c   red, alkaline; yellow, acid
d   exceptions include *S. cholerasuis*

E. coli from other lactose fermenters (Table 18.1).
  - Tests for motility allow differentiation of *Klebsiella* species (non-motile) from *Enterobacter* species (motile). Both species produce similar mucoid colonies which are difficult to distinguish (Table 18.1).
- Commercial biochemical tests:

  A number of commercial biochemical test systems are available for differentiating enterobacteria. Some of these systems incorporate a wide range of biochemical tests and results can be matched against computer-generated numerical profiles to identify isolates to a species level.
- Serotyping of *E. coli*, *Salmonella* and *Yersinia* species:

  Slide agglutination tests with antisera are used to detect O (somatic) and H (flagellar) antigens in all three species and sometimes detection of K (capsular) antigens is carried out (Fig. 18.3). Serotyping allows identification of the organisms involved in disease outbreaks and has applications in epidemiological investigations.
- Molecular techniques, usually based on nucleic acid analyses, are used in reference laboratories for differentiating enterobacteria.

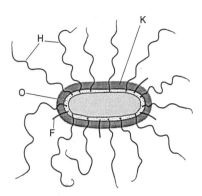

Figure 18.3 Schematic diagram of a typical member of the *Enterobacteriaceae* indicating the K (capsular), O (somatic), F (fimbrial) and H (flagellar) antigens used for serotyping isolates.

Escherichia coli

Escherichia coli is usually motile with peritrichous flagella and often fimbriate. This lactose fermenter produces pink colonies on MacConkey agar and has characteristic biochemical reactions in IMViC tests (Table 18.1). Some strains produce colonies with a metallic sheen when grown on eosin-methylene blue agar. Haemolytic activity on blood agar is a characteristic of certain strains of *E. coli*.

Somatic (O), flagellar (H) and sometimes capsular (K) antigens are used for serotyping *E. coli* . The somatic antigens are lipopolysaccharide in nature and located at the surface of the cell wall. The specificity of these antigens is determined by carbohydrate side chains. The flagellar antigens are protein in nature and the capsular antigens are composed of polysaccharides. Proteinaceous fimbrial (F) antigens act as adhesins facilitating attachment to mucosal surfaces.

Colonization of the mammalian intestinal tract by *E. coli* from environmental sources occurs shortly after birth. These organisms persist as important members of the normal flora of the intestine throughout life. Most strains of *E. coli* are of low virulence but may cause opportunistic infections in extra-intestinal locations such as the mammary gland and urinary tract. Pathogenic strains of *E. coli* possess virulence factors which allow them to colonize mucosal surfaces and subsequently produce disease. Predisposing factors which permit colonization and render animals susceptible to the development of clinical disease include age, immune status, nature of diet and heavy exposure to pathogenic strains.

The main categories of pathogenic strains of *E. coli* and their clinical effects are presented in Fig. 18.4. Not all strains conform strictly to these categories and some may exhibit pathogenic effects typical of more than one strain.

In recent years, *E. coli* O157:H7 has emerged as a major food-borne, zoonotic pathogen in humans, responsible for the haemorrhagic colitis-haemolytic uraemic syndrome.

Pathogenesis and pathogenicity

The virulence factors of pathogenic strains of *E. coli* include capsules, endotoxin, structures responsible for colonization, enterotoxins and other secreted substances.

- Capsular polysaccharides, which are produced by some *E. coli* strains, interfere with the phagocytic uptake of these organisms. Capsular material, which is weakly antigenic, also interferes with the antibacterial effectiveness of the complement system.
- Endotoxin, a lipopolysaccharide (LPS) component of the cell wall of Gram-negative organisms, is released on death of the bacteria. It is composed of a lipid A moiety, core polysaccharide and specific side chains. The role of LPS in disease production includes pyrogenic activity, endothelial damage leading to disseminated intravascular coagulation, and endotoxic shock. These effects are of greatest significance in septicaemic disease.
- Fimbrial adhesins which are present on many enterotoxigenic strains of *E. coli* allow attachment to mucosal surfaces in the small intestine and in the lower urinary tract. Firm attachment to the mucosa facilitates colonization by diminishing the expulsive effects of peristalsis and the flushing effect of urine. Many fimbrial adhesins have been identified. The most significant adhesins in strains of *E. coli* producing disease in domestic animals are K88 (F4), K99 (F5), 987P (F6) and F41. Originally, some of the fimbrial adhesins were mistakenly thought to be capsular (K) antigens and fimbriae were formerly known as pili (987P). The most common adhesin present in strains of *E. coli* infecting pigs is K88. The K99 and F41 adhesins occur in calves and K99 in lambs. The numbers of receptors for K88 adhesins on pig enterocytes are genetically determined and decline with age. Although neonatal piglets are susceptible to strains of *E. coli* bearing 987P adhesins, resistance to colonization develops by three weeks of age. Both K88 and K99 adhesins are encoded by plasmids.
- An adhesin, termed intimin, appears to be necessary for the binding of enteropathogenic *E. coli* (EPEC) to enterocytes.
- The pathological effects of infection with pathogenic *E. coli*, other than those attributed to endotoxin, derive mainly from the production of enterotoxins, verotoxins or cytotoxic necrotizing factors (Fig. 18.4). Unlike enterotoxins which affect only the functional activity of enterocytes, verotoxins and cytotoxic necrotizing

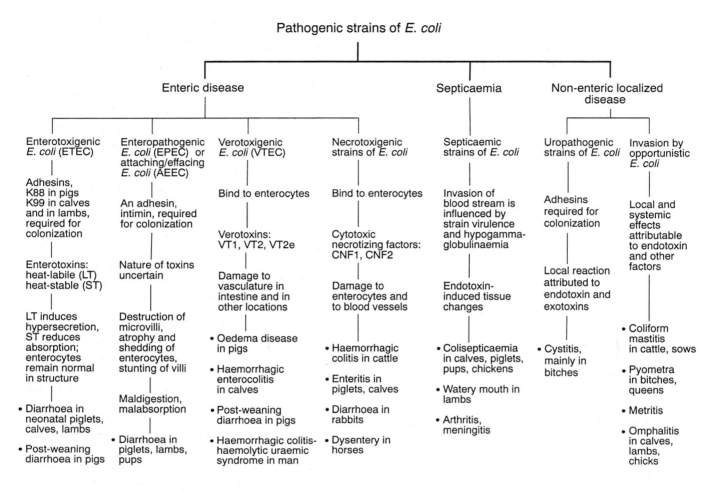

Figure 18.4 An outline of the pathogenic strains of *Escherichia coli*, their virulence factors and diseases which they produce.

factors can produce demonstrable cell damage at their sites of action.

— Two types of enterotoxins, heat labile (LT) and heat-stable (ST) have been identified. Each type of enterotoxin has two subgroups. Many strains of enterotoxigenic *E. coli* (ETEC) from pigs produce LT1 which induces hypersecretion of fluid into the intestine through stimulation of adenylate cyclase activity. Most ETEC isolates which produce LT1 also possess K88 adhesins. A second heat-labile toxin, LT2, has been demonstrated in some ETEC strains isolated from cattle. One of the heat-stable enterotoxin subgroups, STa, has been identified in strains of ETEC isolated from porcine, bovine, ovine and human specimens. This toxin induces increased guanylate cyclase activity in enterocytes and the resultant increase in intracellular guanosine monophosphate stimulates fluid and electrolyte secretion into the small intestine and inhibits fluid absorption from the intestine. The precise cytotoxic effect of the other heat-stable enterotoxin, STb, is not known.

— Verotoxins (VT) are similar structurally, functionally and antigenically to the Shiga toxin of *Shigella dysenteriae*. These toxins are heat-labile and lethal for cultured Vero cells. Verotoxigenic *E. coli* (VTEC) colonizing the intestines can damage enterocytes and, when verotoxin is absorbed into the bloodstream, it exerts a deleterious effect on endothelial cells in relatively defined anatomical locations such as the central nervous system in pigs. Verotoxins inhibit protein synthesis in eukaryotic cells but the relatively greater degree of damage induced in certain tissues may relate to differences in receptors for these toxins. Vascular damage can lead to oedema, haemorrhage and thrombosis. The vero-toxin VT2e is implicated in oedema disease of pigs.

— Two types of cytotoxic necrotizing factors, CNF1 and CNF2, have been demonstrated in extracts of strains of *E. coli* isolated from cases of diarrhoea, septicaemia and urinary tract infections in animals and man. It is known that CNF1 is encoded chromosomally whereas CNF2 is encoded by a trans-missible plasmid known as Vir. Although these toxins have been shown to induce pathological changes in laboratory animals and tissue culture, the role of CNF-producing *E. coli* in naturally-occurring disease is still uncertain.

- Alpha-haemolysin, although often a useful marker for virulence in certain strains of *E. coli*, does not appear to contribute directly to their virulence but is closely linked with the expression of other virulence factors. Haemolysin production is often a feature of strains of *E. coli* isolated from pigs with oedema disease and diarrhoea. It has been suggested that the action of α-haemolysin may increase the availability of iron for invading organisms.
- Siderophores, iron-binding molecules such as aerobactin and enterobactin, are synthesized by certain pathogenic strains of *E. coli*. When available iron levels in the tissues are low, these iron-binding molecules may contribute to bacterial survival.
- Pathogenic *E. coli* strains which lack defined virulence factors:
  — Formerly the term enteropathogenic *E. coli* (EPEC) was used to denote all pathogenic strains. More recently the term has been used as a synonym for attaching/effacing *E. coli* (AEEC) strains.
  — Although verotoxins are produced by many strains of attaching/effacing *E. coli* (AEEC), these toxins are apparently not directly involved in the pathogenesis of the enteric lesions (Hall *et al.*, 1988). After attaching to enterocytes, AEEC isolates produce effacement of microvilli, premature enterocyte exfoliation and villous distortion. Epithelial erosion may result in dysentery (Wray *et al.*, 1989).
  — The term enterohaemorrhagic *E. coli* is applied to strains such as O157:H7 which cause dysentery in humans.

Clinical infections

The main categories of disease produced by pathogenic strains of *E. coli* are indicated in Fig. 18.4. Clinical infections in young animals may be limited to the intestines (enteric colibacillosis, neonatal diarrhoea), or may manifest as septicaemia (colisepticaemia, systemic colibacillosis) or toxaemia (colibacillary toxaemia). In older pigs, post-weaning enteritis and oedema disease are manifestations of toxaemia. Non-enteric localized infections in adult animals, many due to opportunistic invasion, can involve the urinary tract, mammary glands and uterus.

Enteric colibacillosis

Enteric colibacillosis affects primarily new-born calves, lambs and piglets. Oral infection with a pathogenic strain of *E. coli*, colonization of the intestine and toxin production are prerequisites for the development of this condition. The incidence and severity of the disease increases under intensive systems of management. This may reflect

heavy exposure of young animals to pathogenic strains of *E. coli* as a result of build-up of infection in the environment. Factors which may predispose young farm animals to infection by strains of pathogenic *E. coli* are summarized in Box 18.1. Enterotoxigenic strains of ETEC, possessing fimbrial adhesins such as K88 and K99, are of particular importance in neonatal diarrhoea. These strains colonize the distal small intestine by attaching to receptors which are present on the enterocytes of neonates. They produce enterotoxins (LT and STa) which stimulate hypersecretory diarrhoea and interfere with fluid absorption without major morphologically-detectable damage to enterocytes. In contrast, necrosis of enterocytes with stunting and fusion of villi are features of enteric colibacillosis caused by strains of attaching/effacing *E. coli* (AEEC), which colonize the lower small intestine and the colon. These strains induce diarrhoea through maldigestion and malabsorption of nutrients in the small intestine and by reducing the absorptive capacity of the colonic mucosa.

In enteric colibacillosis in calves, diarrhoea develops within the first few days of birth. Faecal consistency is somewhat variable. In some cases faeces are profuse and watery, in others they are pasty, white or yellowish and rancid. This rancid faecal material may accumulate on the tail and hind limbs. Depression becomes marked as dehydration and acidosis develop. Mildly affected animals may recover spontaneously. Untreated severely affected calves die within a few days.

Piglets may succumb to enteric colibacillosis within 24 hours of birth. Often, an entire litter is affected and, as the disease progresses, piglets refuse to suck. A profuse watery diarrhoea rapidly leads to dehydration, weakness and death. Although enteric colibacillosis occasionally

---

> *Box 18.1*. Factors which may predispose young farm animals to infection with pathogenic *Escherichia coli* strains
>
> - Insufficient or no colostral immunity
> - Build-up of pathogenic *E. coli* strains
> - Overcrowding and poor hygiene, facilitating increased transmission of organisms
> - Normal flora of neonates not fully established
> - Naive immune system in neonates
> - Receptors for ETEC adhesins are present only during first week of life in calves
> - Pigs retain receptors for some adhesins past weaning age (post-weaning diarrhoea)
> - Digestive tract of young pigs equipped only for easily digested foods. Accumulation of undigested and unabsorbed nutrients encourages replication of *E. coli*
> - Stress factors such as cold ambient temperatures and frequent mixing of animals

affects lambs, the septicaemic form of the disease is more common.

Colisepticaemia

Systemic infections with *E. coli* are relatively frequent in calves, lambs and poultry. Septicaemic strains of *E. coli* have special attributes for resisting host defence mechanisms. They invade the bloodstream following infection of the intestines, lungs or umbilical tissues (navel ill).

Septicaemic spread throughout the body commonly occurs in calves with low levels of maternally-derived antibodies, and the severity of the disease corresponds to the degree of hypogammaglobulinaemia (Penhale *et al.*, 1970). Colisepticaemia often presents as an acute fatal disease with many of the clinical signs attributable to the action of endotoxin. Pyrexia, depression, weakness and tachycardia, with or without diarrhoea, are early signs of the disease. Hypothermia and prostration precede death which may occur within 24 hours. Meningitis and pneumonia are commonly encountered in affected calves and lambs. Post-septicaemic localization in the joints of calves and lambs results in arthritis with swelling, pain, lameness and stiff gait.

Watery mouth occurs in lambs up to 3 days of age and has been associated with systemic invasion by *E. coli* (King and Hodgson, 1991; Sargison *et al.*, 1997). It is characterised by severe depression, loss of appetite, profuse salivation and abdominal distension. The condition is encountered in lambs born in confined lambing areas. Morbidity rates may exceed 20% and mortality in affected lambs is high, many dying within 24 hours of clinical onset. Death is attributable to endotoxic shock.

In poultry, airsacculitis and pericarditis may develop following septicaemia. Coligranuloma (Hjärre's disease) is characterized by chronic inflammatory changes which are encountered at postmortem in laying hens and resemble tuberculous lesions.

Oedema disease of pigs

Oedema disease is a toxaemia which usually occurs 1 to 2 weeks after weaning in rapidly-growing pigs. The aetiology of the disease is complex with nutritional and environmental changes and other stress factors contributing to its development. A limited number of haemolytic *E. coli* serotypes have been isolated from the intestinal tract in cases of the disease. These non-invasive strains replicate in the tract and produce a verotoxin (VT2e) which is absorbed into the bloodstream and damages endothelial cells with consequent perivascular oedema.

The onset of oedema disease is sudden with some animals found dead without showing clinical signs. Characteristic signs include posterior paresis, muscular

tremors and oedema of the eyelids and the front of the face. The squeal may be hoarse due to laryngeal oedema. The faeces are usually firm. Flaccid paralysis precedes death which typically occurs within 36 hours of the onset of clinical signs. Animals which recover frequently have residual neurological dysfunction. The characteristic post-mortem lesions are oedema of the greater curvature of the stomach and the mesentery of the colon. Perivascular oedema in the central nervous system, detectable on histological examination, accounts for the neurological dysfunction. Cerebrospinal angiopathy, in which there is marked fibrinoid necrosis in vessel walls, may develop in animals surviving acute disease.

Post-weaning diarrhoea of pigs

This condition occurs within a week or two after weaning, often following changes in feeding regimens or in management and with possible involvement of rotaviruses. The majority of outbreaks are associated with ETEC strains. Clinical signs vary from an afebrile disease with inappetence to watery diarrhoea in severe cases. Diarrhoea and purplish discolouration of areas of the skin are often observed. Some animals may die suddenly (van Béers-Schreurs *et al.*, 1992). Occasionally VTEC strains are implicated in the condition.

Coliform mastitis

Infection of the mammary glands of cows and sows by members of the *Enterobacteriaceae*, including *E. coli*, occurs opportunistically. In dairy cows, the source of infection is faecal contamination of the skin of the mammary gland and relaxation of the teat sphincter following milking increases vulnerability to infection. Cows with low somatic cell counts are particularly susceptible to infection. No specific serotypes of *E. coli* have been linked with this form of mastitis. The acute form of the disease is characterized by endotoxaemia and can be life-threatening. Peracute disease may be fatal in 24 to 48 hours. Affected animals are severely depressed with drooping ears and sunken eyes. Mammary secretions are watery and contain white flecks.

Urogenital tract infections

Opportunistic ascending infections of the urinary tract by certain uropathogenic strains of *E. coli* result in cystitis especially in bitches. These strains possess virulence factors such as fimbriae which facilitate mucosal colonization.

Invasion of hyperplastic endometrium by opportunistic strains of *E. coli* is a critical factor in the pathogenesis of canine pyometra. Prostatitis in dogs is also associated with invasion of opportunistic *E. coli* strains.

Diagnostic procedures

The age and species of the affected animal, the clinical signs and the duration of illness may suggest the type of infection and the category of disease. The history, progress of the disease and the system or organ affected influence the selection of specimens, the laboratory procedures for diagnosis and appropriate treatment and control measures.

- Suitable specimens include faecal samples from animals with enteric disease, tissue specimens from cases of septicaemia, mastitic milk, samples of mid-stream urine and cervical swabs from suspected cases of pyometra or metritis.
- Specimens cultured on blood and MacConkey agar are incubated aerobically at 37°C for 24 to 48 hours.
- Identification criteria for isolates:
  — On blood agar the colonies are greyish, round and shiny with a characterisitic smell. Colonies may be haemolytic or non-haemolytic.
  — On MacConkey agar colonies are bright pink.
  — IMViC tests can be used for confirmation (Table 18.1).
  — The colonies of some *E. coli* strains have a metallic sheen on EMB agar.
  — A full biochemical profile may be necessary to identify isolates from coliform mastitis or cystitis.
  — Some serotypes are found in association with certain disease conditions. Slide agglutination tests for O and H antigens are employed for serotype identification.
- In suspected cases of colisepticaemia, isolation of the organism in pure culture from the blood or from parenchymatous organs is considered confirmatory.
- When enterotoxigenic strains of *E. coli* are suspected, the presence of either enterotoxins or fimbrial antigens can be confirmed by immunological methods or molecular techniques such as the polymerase chain rection.
  — Enterotoxins in the small intestine can be detected, using methods employing monoclonal antibodies (Carroll *et al.*, 1990). Some of these reagents are available commercially.
  — For expression of fimbrial antigens, isolates should be subcultured on Minca medium. Fimbrial antigens can be identified using ELISA or latex agglutination (Thorns *et al.*, 1989).
  — DNA probes specific for genes encoding heat-labile and heat-stable enterotoxins may be used to identify enterotoxigenic strains of *E. coli*.
- The toxins produced by verotoxigenic and necro-toxigenic strains can be detected by Vero cell assay (Wray *et al.*, 1993).
- Molecular methods based on the detection of genes encoding toxins are also used.

Treatment

The nature and duration of therapeutic measures are determined by the severity and duration of the disease process.

- In calves with neonatal diarrhoea, milk should be withdrawn and replaced by fluids containing electrolytes. Milk feeding can be resumed gradually when clinical improvement is evident. Severely dehydrated calves require parenteral fluid replacement therapy.
- Calves with hypogammaglobulinaemia can be given bovine gammaglobulin intravenously.
- In most domestic species, enteric diseases may be treated by oral administration of antimicrobial compounds which are active in the gastrointestinal tract. Systemic and localized infections require parenteral administration of therapeutic agents. Treatment should be based on susceptibility testing of isolates.
- Because of the extensive local tissue damage, intrammammary treatment of coliform mastitis is often of limited value. Therapy is aimed at counteracting shock and eliminating toxic material from the mammary gland by constant stripping of the affected quarters.

Control

- Newborn animals should receive ample amounts of colostrum shortly after birth. Colostral antibodies can prevent colonization of the intestine by pathogenic *E. coli*. Absorption of gammaglobulin from the intestine declines progressively after birth and is negligible by 36 hours.
- A clean, warm environment should be provided for newborn animals.
- Dietary regimes may contribute to the development of oedema disease and other post-weaning conditions. New feed should be introduced gradually.
- Vaccination is of value for a limited number of the diseases caused by *E. coli*. Vaccination methods used for prevention of enteric disease in piglets and calves include:
  — Commercially available killed vaccines containing prevalent pathogenic *E. coli* serotypes can be given to pregnant sows. Alternatively, autogenous, killed vaccines prepared from strains of *E. coli* implicated in disease outbreaks on a farm can be used.
  — Vaccination of pregnant cows with purified *E. coli* K99 fimbrial or whole-cell preparations, often combined with rotavirus antigen, can be used to enhance colostral protection (Snodgrass, 1986).

Salmonella serotypes

Salmonellae are usually motile and do not ferment lactose (Table 18.1). Rarely, lactose-fermenting strains are encountered. The genus *Salmonella* contains more than 2,400 serotypes. Serotyping is based on the Kaufmann and White schema in which somatic (O) and flagellar (H) antigens are identified. Occasionally, capsular (Vi) antigens may be detected. In a modification of this scheme, two species are proposed, *S. enterica* and *S. bongori*. *Salmonella enterica* has been divided into six subspecies (Le Minor and Popoff, 1987; Reeves *et al.*, 1989). The majority of salmonellae of veterinary importance belong to *S. enterica* subspecies *enterica*. The subspecies are further qualified by the serotype to give a final designation such as *S. enterica* subspecies *enterica* serotype Typhimurium. This nomenclature is now being used by the majority of bacteriologists and is adhered to throughout this book.

Salmonella serotypes occur worldwide and infect many mammals, birds and reptiles and are mainly excreted in faeces. Ingestion is the main route of infection in salmonellosis although it can also occur through the mucosae of the upper respiratory tract and conjunctiva (Fox and Gallus, 1977). Organisms may be present in water, soil, animal feeds, raw meat and offal and in vegetable material. The source of environmental contamination is invariably faeces. In poultry, some serotypes such as *Salmonella* Enteritidis infect the ovaries, and the organisms can be isolated from eggs. Salmonellae can survive in damp shaded soil for up to 9 months (Carter *et al.*, 1979).

Pathogenesis and pathogenicity

Although many aspects of the pathogenesis of salmonellosis are poorly understood, particularly the relationship between salmonella toxins and cell damage, some of the general features associated with virulence are known. The virulence of salmonellae relates to their ability to invade host cells, replicate in them and resist both digestion by phagocytes and destruction by the complement components of the plasma. Following adherence, probably through fimbrial attachment, to the surface of intestinal mucosal cells, the bacteria induce ruffling of cell membranes (Salyers and Whitt, 1994). The ruffles facilitate uptake of the bacteria in membrane-bound vesicles, which often coalesce. The organisms replicate in these vesicles and are eventually released from the cells, which sustain only mild or transient damage. The complex invasion process is mediated by the products of a number of chromosomal genes, whereas growth within host cells depends on the presence of virulence plasmids.

Resistance to digestion by phagocytes and to the lethal action of complement components facilitates the spread of organisms within the host. The toxic oxidative effects of free radicals produced by phagocytes are minimized by bacterial catalase and superoxide dismutase activities. Resistance to killing by complement is partially dependent on the length of O antigen chains of lipopolysaccharide (LPS). Long chains of LPS prevent the complement components of the membrane attack complex from interacting with and damaging the bacterial cell membrane (Salyers and Whitt, 1994). The LPS is also responsible for the endotoxic effects of infection with salmonellae. It may contribute to the local inflammatory response which damages intestinal epithelial cells and results in the development of diarrhoea. Bacterial cell wall LPS also mediates the endotoxic shock which may accompany septicaemic salmonellosis.

Clinical infections

Salmonellosis is of common occurrence in domestic animals and the consequences of infection range from subclinical carrier status to acute fatal septicaemia. Some *Salmonella* serotypes such as *Salmonella* Pullorum and *Salmonella* Gallinarum in poultry, *Salmonella* Choleraesuis in pigs and *Salmonella* Dublin in cattle are relatively host-specific. In contrast, *Salmonella* Typhimurium has a comparatively wide host range. It is recognised that healthy adult carnivores are innately resistant to salmonellosis.

Salmonellae often localize in the mucosae of the ileum, caecum and colon, and in the mesenteric lymph nodes of infected animals. Although most organisms are cleared from the tissues by host defense mechanisms, subclinical infection may persist with shedding of small numbers of salmonellae in the faeces. Latent infections, in which salmonellae are present in the gall bladder but are not excreted, also occur. Clinical disease may develop from subclinical and latent infections if affected animals are stressed. The stress factors which have been most often associated with the development of clinical salmonellosis are listed in Box 18.2. Some of these factors such as transportation and overcrowding have proved to be significant in outbreaks of the disease in young animals and in adult sheep and horses. Salmonellosis in adult cattle is usually sporadic and is also often associated with stress.

Other factors which determine the clinical outcome of infection include the number of salmonellae ingested, the virulence of the infecting serotype or strain and the

---

> *Box 18.2* Stress factors which may activate latent or subclinical salmonellosis.
>
> - Intercurrent infections
> - Transportation
> - Overcrowding
> - Pregnancy
> - Extreme ambient temperatures
> - Water deprivation
> - Oral antimicrobial therapy
> - Sudden changes in rations altering the intestinal flora
> - Surgical procedures requiring general anaesthesia

Table 18.3 *Salmonella* serotypes of clinical importance and the consequences of infection.

Salmonella serotype	Hosts	Consequences of infection
Salmonella Typhimurium	Many animal species	Enterocolitis and septicaemia
	Humans	Food poisoning
Salmonella Dublin	Cattle	Many disease conditions
	Sheep, horses, dogs	Enterocolitis and septicaemia
Salmonella Choleraesuis	Pigs	Enterocolitis and septicaemia
Salmonella Pullorum	Chicks	Pullorum disease (bacillary white diarrhoea)
Salmonella Gallinarum	Adult birds	Fowl typhoid
Salmonella Arizonae	Turkeys	Arizona or paracolon infection
Salmonella Enteritidis	Poultry	Often subclinical in poultry
	Many other species	Clinical disease in mammals
	Humans	Food poisoning
Salmonella Brandenburg	Sheep	Abortion

susceptibility of the host. Host susceptibility may be related to immunological status, genetic make-up or age. Young and debilitated or aged animals are particularly susceptible and may develop the septicaemic form of the disease.

In most animal species, both enteric and septicaemic forms of salmonellosis are recorded. A number of serotypes have been associated with abortion in farm animals, often without other obvious clinical signs in dams. The *Salmonella* serotypes of importance in domestic animals and the consequences of infection are indicated in Table 18.3. *Salmonella* Dublin causes a variety of clinical effects in cattle (Table 18.4). Terminal dry gangrene and bone lesions are common manifestations in chronic infections with *Salmonella* Dublin in calves (Gitter *et al.*, 1978).

Enteric salmonellosis

Enterocolitis caused by salmonella organisms can affect most species of farm animals, irrespective of age. Acute disease is characterized by fever, depression, anorexia and profuse foul-smelling diarrhoea often containing blood, mucus and epithelial casts. Dehydration and weight loss follow and pregnant animals may abort. Severely affected young animals become recumbent and may die within a few days of acquiring infection. On farms with endemic salmonellosis, the milder clinical signs often observed may be attributed to the influence of acquired immunity. Chronic enterocolitis can follow acute salmonellosis in pigs, cattle and horses. Intermittent fever, soft faeces and gradual weight loss, leading to emaciation, are common features of this condition.

Septicaemic salmonellosis

The septicaemic form can occur in all age groups but is most common in calves, in neonatal foals and in pigs less than four months of age. Onset of clinical disease is sudden with high fever, depression and recumbency. If treatment is delayed, many young animals with septicaemic salmonellosis die within 48 hours. Surviving animals can develop persistent diarrhoea, arthritis, meningitis or pneumonia.

In pigs with septicaemic *Salmonella* Choleraesuis infection, there is a characteristic bluish discolouration of the ears and snout. Intercurrent viral infections often predispose to severe clinical forms of the disease. The close clinical and pathological relationships which have been recognized in animals infected with *Salmonella* Choleraesuis ('hog-cholera bacillus') and classical swine fever virus, either jointly or separately, exemplify both the importance of intercurrent infections and the difficulty of clinically distinguishing the diseases caused by these agents.

Salmonellosis in poultry

Salmonella Pullorum, *Salmonella* Gallinarum and *Salmonella* Enteritidis can infect the ovaries of hens and be transmitted through eggs. The presence of *Salmonella* Enteritidis in undercooked egg dishes may result in human food poisoning (Cooper, 1994).

Pullorum disease or bacillary white diarrhoea (*Salmonella* Pullorum) infects young chicks and turkey poults up to 2 to 3 weeks of age. The mortality rate is high and affected birds huddle under a heat source and are anorexic, depressed and have whitish faecal pasting around their vents. Characteristic lesions include whitish nodes throughout the lungs and focal necrosis of liver and spleen.

Fowl typhoid (*Salmonella* Gallinarum) can produce lesions in young chicks and poults similar to those of pullorum disease. However, in countries where fowl typhoid is endemic, a septicaemic disease of adult birds occurs, often resulting in sudden deaths. Characteristic findings include an enlarged, friable, bile-stained liver and enlarged spleen. As *Salmonella* Pullorum and *Salmonella* Gallinarum possess similar somatic antigens (Table 18.5), both have been eradicated from many countries by a serological testing and slaughter policy for pullorum disease.

Paratyphoid is a name given to infections of poultry by non-host-adapted salmonellae such as *Salmonella*

Table 18.4 Infection with *Salmonella* Dublin in cattle.

Outcome of infection/age group	Comments
Subclinical faecal excretors/all ages	Probable outcome of most infections. Small numbers of salmonellae excreted intermittently in faeces.
Latent carriers/all ages	Salmonella present in gall bladder. No excretion of organisms.
Acute or chronic enteric disease/all ages	Enterocolitis with foul-smelling diarrhoea containing blood, mucus and epithelial shreds or casts.
Septicaemia/all ages	Potentially fatal disease with fever and depression. Diarrhoea or dysentery may be present. Dramatic drop in milk production in dairy cows. Calves surviving acute disease may develop arthritis (joint ill), meningitis or pneumonia.
Abortion	A common cause of abortion in some European countries. No signs of illness may be evident.
Joint ill/calves	May follow septicaemia or umbilical infection.
Osteomyelitis/young animals	Often involves the cervical vertebrae or bones of the distal limb. In cervical osteomyelitis, nervous signs relate to spinal cord compression.
Terminal dry gangrene/calves	Disseminated intravascular coagulation due to endotoxaemia results in local ischaemia and gangrene of distal parts of hind limbs, ears and tail.

Enteritidis and *Salmonella* Typhimurium. These infections are often subclinical in laying birds.

Diagnostic procedures

- A history of previous outbreaks of the disease on the premises, the age group affected and the clinical picture may suggest salmonellosis.
- At postmortem, enterocolitis with blood-stained luminal contents and enlarged mesenteric lymph nodes are commonly observed.
- Laboratory confirmation is required. Specimens for submission should include faeces and blood from live animals. Intestinal contents and samples from tissue lesions should be submitted from dead animals and abomasal contents from aborted foetuses.
- Isolation of salmonellae from blood or parenchymatous organs is deemed to be confirmatory for septicaemic salmonellosis.
- A heavy growth of salmonellae on plates directly inoculated with faeces, intestinal contents or foetal abomasal contents strongly suggests the aetiological involvement

of the pathogen. Recovery of small numbers of salmonellae from faeces is usually indicative of a carrier state.
- Specimens should be cultured directly onto BG and XLD agars and also added to selenite F, Rappaport or tetrathionate broth for enrichment and subsequent subculture (Fig. 18.5). The plates and enrichment broth are incubated aerobically at 37°C for up to 48 hours. Subcultures are made from the enrichment broth at 24 and 48 hours.
- Identification criteria for isolates:
  — On brilliant green agar, colonies and medium are red indicating alkalinity. On XLD agar, colonies are red (alkaline) with a black centre, indicating H_2S production.
  — Suspicious colonies, subcultured from the selective media into TSI agar and lysine decarboxylase broth, should be examined after incubation for 18 hours at 37°C to establish their biochemical identity as salmonellae (Tables 18.1 and 18.2).
  — If reactions in TSI agar and lysine decarboxylase broth are inconclusive, a biochemical profile using a battery of biochemical tests may allow definitive identification.
  — The isolates from the TSI agar slant are confirmed as salmonellae using commercially available antisera for O and H antigens in a slide agglutination test. Serotypes with O antigens in common are assigned to a serogroup (Table 18.5).
  — Serotypes which have flagellar (H) antigens in two phases, phase 1 (specific) and phase 2 (non-specific), are termed diphasic. The antigens in both phases must be determined. The majority of organisms in these serotypes usually possess H antigens in a single phase and are agglutinated by the appropriate antiserum. However, a minority of bacteria, invariably present in the alternative phase, can be selected by a procedure referred to as 'phase changing' (Fig. 18.6). When the alternative phase is isolated, the antigenic formula used for serotyping can be completed.
  — Biotyping is required for serotypes which are antigenically indistinguishable such as *Salmonella* Pullorum and *Salmonella* Gallinarum (Table 18.6).
- Phage typing is used in epidemiological studies to identify isolates with specific characteristics such as multiple resistance to antibiotics and enhanced virulence. Examples of important phage types are *Salmonella* Typhimurium DT (definitive type) 104 which exhibits multiple resistance to antibiotics and *Salmonella* Enteritidis PT (phage type) 4 which is found in poultry products and is a common cause of food poisoning in humans.
- Serological tests such as ELISA and agglutination techniques are of greatest value when used on a herd or flock basis. A rising antibody titre using paired serum

Table 18.5 Somatic and flagellar antigens and the serogroups of selected *Salmonella* serotypes.

Serotype	Serogroup	Somatic (O) antigens	Flagellar (H) antigens	
			Phase 1	Phase 2
Salmonella Typhimurium	B	1, 4, [5], 12	i	1, 2
Salmonella Choleraesuis	C$_1$	6, 7	c	1, 5
Salmonella Choleraesuis biotype *Kunzendorf*	C$_1$	6, 7	[c]	1, 5
Salmonella Enteritidis	D$_1$	1, 9, 12	g, m	[1, 7]
Salmonella Dublin	D$_1$	1, 9, 12, [Vi]	g, p	–
Salmonella Gallinarum	D$_1$	1, 9, 12	–	–
Salmonella Pullorum	D$_1$	9, 12	–	–
Salmonella Anatum	E$_1$	3, 10	e, h	1,6

1 presence dependent on phage conversion
Vi capsular antigen
[ ] antigen may be present or absent

samples is indicative of active infection.

- DNA probes can be used to screen large numbers of faecal samples for salmonellae (Maddox and Fales, 1991).

Treatment

- Antibiotic therapy should be based on results of susceptibility testing because R-plasmids coding for multiple resistance are comparatively common in salmonellae.
- Oral antimicrobial therapy should be used judiciously for treating enteric salmonellosis because it may disturb the normal intestinal flora, extend the duration of salmonella excretion and increase the probability of drug resistance developing. In the septicaemic form of the disease, intravenous antibiotic therapy must be used.
- Fluid and electrolyte replacement therapy is required to counteract dehydration and shock.

Control

Control is based on reducing the risk of exposure to infection. Intensively-reared, food-producing animals are more likely to acquire infection and are also a major source of human infection (Cooper, 1994).

- Measures for excluding infection from a herd or flock free of salmonellosis:
  — A closed-herd policy should be implemented when feasible.
  — Animals should be purchased from reliable sources and remain isolated until negative for salmonellae on three consecutive samplings.
  — Steps should be taken to prevent contamination of

foodstuffs and water. In this context, rodent control is important.
  — Protective clothing and footwear should be worn by personnel entering hatcheries and minimal disease pig units.
- Measures for reducing environmental contamination:
  — Effective routine cleaning and disinfection of buildings and equipment is essential.
  — Overstocking and overcrowding should be avoided.
  — Slurry should be spread on arable land where possible. An interval of at least two months should elapse before grazing commences on pastures following the application of slurry.
  — The continuous use of paddocks for susceptible animals should be avoided.

Table 18.6 Differentiation of the biotypes of *Salmonella* Pullorum and *Salmonella* Gallinarum.

	Salmonella **Pullorum**	*Salmonella* **Gallinarum**
Glucose (gas)	+	–
Dulcitol	–	+
Maltose	–	+
Ornithine decarboxylase	+	–
Rhamnose	+	–
Motility	–	–

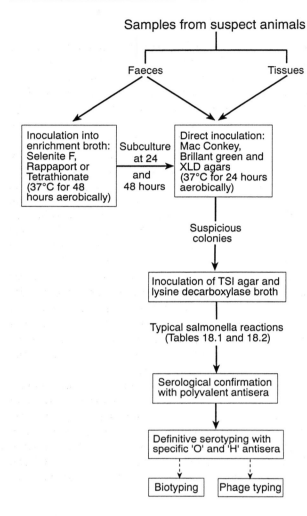

Figure 18.5 Procedures for the isolation and identification of *Salmonella* serotypes from clinical specimens.

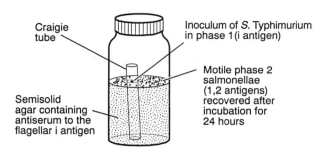

Figure 18.6 The Craigie tube method for 'phase-changing' salmonella isolates. The biphasic organism, *Salmonella* Typhimurium illustrates the principle of the method. In phase 1 this bacterium has flagellar i antigens. The organism is inoculated into a Craigie tube placed in semi-solid agar containing antiserum to the flagellar i antigen and incubated aerobically at 37°C for 24 hours. Salmonellae in phase 1 are agglutinated by the antiserum and immobilized. Those in phase 2 with flagellar 1, 2 antigens are not immobilized. The motile phase 2 organisms which move out from the bottom of the Craigie tube can be sampled at the agar surface.

- Strategies for enhancing resistance and reducing the likelihood of clinical disease:
  - Vaccination procedures are used in cattle, sheep, poultry and pigs. Modified live vaccines which stimulate humoral immunity and cell-mediated immunity are preferable to bacterins. Modern molecular techniques are likely to lead to the development of more effective vaccines (Cooper, 1994; Lax *et al.*, 1995).
  - The impact of stress factors (Box 18.2) should be reduced by appropriate decisions relating to management of animals and surgical or therapeutic intervention.
  - Feeding of antimicrobial drugs either for prophylaxis or growth promotion should be avoided where possible.
- Measures for controlling an outbreak of salmonellosis:
  - Detection and elimination of the source of infection is essential.
  - Clinically affected animals should be isolated.

- Movement of animals, vehicles and humans should be curtailed.
- Foot baths containing suitable disinfectant, such as 3% iodophor, should be placed at strategic locations to limit spread of salmonellae.
- Careful disposal of contaminated carcases and bedding is mandatory.
- Contaminated buildings and utensils should be thoroughly cleaned and disinfected. The choice of disinfectant is determined by the size and cleanliness of the building and the nature of the utensils. A 3% concentration of sodium hypochlorite or iodophors is suitable for clean surfaces. Phenolic disinfectants are suitable for buildings with residual organic matter. Fumigation with formaldehyde is the most effective method for disinfecting poultry houses.
- Herd vaccination may be of value for limiting the spread of infection during outbreaks of disease in cattle (Wray, 1991).
- Humans working with clinically affected animals should be aware of the risk of acquiring infection.

Yersinia species

Yersinia species are non-lactose fermenters and, with the exception of *Y. pestis* are motile (Table 18.1). Although there are more than 10 *Yersinia* species, only *Y. pestis, Y. enterocolitica* and *Y. pseudotuberculosis* are pathogenic for animals and man (Table 18.7). *Yersinia ruckeri* causes perioral haemorrhagic inflammation in some species of fish. Growth of yersiniae tends to be less rapid than other members of the *Enterobacteriaceae*. They character-

Table 18.7 The consequences of infection with *Yersinia* species.

Yersinia species	Hosts	Consequences of infection
Y. enterocolitica	Pigs, other domestic animals, wildlife	Subclinical enteric infections, occasionally enteritis
	Ewes	Sporadic abortion
	Humans	Gastroenterocolitis
Y. pseudotuberculosis	Farmed deer, sheep, goats, cattle, buffaloes, pigs	Enteritis in young animals, subclinical infections common in older animals, mesenteric lymphadenitis
	Cattle, sheep, goats	Sporadic abortion
	Guinea-pigs, other laboratory animals	Focal hepatic necrosis, septicaemia
	Caged birds	Septicaemia
	Humans	Enterocolitis, mesenteric lymphadenitis
Y. pestis	Humans	Bubonic and pneumonic plague
	Rodents	Sylvatic plague
	Cats	Feline plague

istically demonstrate bipolar staining in Giemsa-stained smears from animal tissues.

Serotyping and biotyping methods are used for identifying pathogenic yersiniae. Of the ten serotypes of *Y. pseudotuberculosis*, serotypes I, II and III contain the majority of pathogenic isolates. There are five biotypes and more than 50 serotypes of *Y. enterocolitica*. Somatic antigens 2, 3, 5, 8 and 9 are present in isolates from clinical infections caused by this species. Serotype O:9 is of particular importance because it shares common antigens with *Brucella* species and it may induce false-positive reactions in brucella agglutination tests.

Yersinia pseudotuberculosis and *Y. enterocolitica* are found in the intestinal tract of a wide range of wild mammals, birds and domestic animals. All these animals may be reservoirs of infection. Many avian species may act as amplifier hosts and may also transfer the organisms mechanically (Cork *et al.*, 1995). Both organisms can grow in a wide temperature range (5 to 42°C) and survive for long periods in cool wet conditions.

In endemic areas, wild rodents are important reservoirs of *Y. pestis*. Fleas, especially *Xenopsylla cheopis*, the Oriental rat flea, transmit the infection to man and other animals.

Pathogenesis and pathogenicity

Pathogenic yersiniae are facultative intracellular organisms which possess plasmid and chromosomal encoded virulence factors, many of which are required for survival and multiplication in macrophages. *Yersinia pseudotuberculosis* and *Y. enterocolitica* are less virulent than *Y. pestis* and rarely produce generalized infections. The pathogenetic mechanisms in enteric disease caused by *Y. enterocolitica* and *Y. pseudotuberculosis* are incompletely understood. It is probable that both organisms gain entry to the mucosa through M cells of Peyer's patches. Adhesion to and subsequent invasion through these cells are facilitated by factors such as invasin and adhesion/invasion proteins which have an affinity for integrins on cell surfaces. Once in the mucosa, the bacteria are engulfed by macrophages in which they survive and are transported to the mesenteric lymph nodes (Brubaker, 1991). Replication in the nodes follows with the development of necrotic lesions and neutrophil infiltration. Survival of *Y. pseudotuberculosis* and *Y. enterocolitica* is enhanced by antiphagocytic proteins secreted by the organisms which interfere with the normal functioning of neutrophils in the host.

Yersinia pestis is more invasive than *Y. pseudotuberculosis* and *Y. enterocolitica* and possesses additional virulence factors. These include an antiphagocytic protein capsule (Fraction 1) and a plasminogen activator which aids systemic spread. Endotoxin, with properties similar to the endotoxin produced by other members of the *Enterobacteriaceae*, also contributes to the pathogenesis of disease.

Clinical infections

Yersinia pseudotuberculosis causes enteric infections, in a wide variety of wild and domestic animals which are often subclinical. The septicaemic form of disease, known as pseudotuberculosis, can occur in laboratory rodents and aviary birds. Sporadic abortions caused by *Y. pseudotuberculosis* have been reported in cattle (Jerrett and Slee, 1989), sheep (Otter, 1996) and goats (Witte and Collins, 1985).

Wild and domestic animals may act as reservoirs of *Yersinia enterocolitica* which is primarily a human enteric pathogen. The pig is the natural reservoir for *Y. enterocolitica* serotype O3 biotype 4, which is an important pathogen in humans. Rare cases of enteric disease, precipitated by stress, may be encountered in pigs, farmed deer, goats and lambs. *Yersinia enterocolitica* has been implicated in sporadic ovine abortion (Corbel *et al.*, 1990).

Yersinia pestis, the cause of human bubonic plague ('black death'), can infect both dogs and cats in endemic areas. Cats, which are particularly susceptible, may be a source of infection for owners and attending veterinarians (Kaufmann *et al.*, 1981).

Enteric yersiniosis

Enteritis caused by *Y. pseudotuberculosis* is relatively common in young farmed deer in New Zealand and Australia (Henderson 1983; Jerrett *et al.*, 1990). Outbreaks of the disease have been reported also in buffaloes in Brazil (Riet-Correa *et al.*, 1990). Enteric disease has been reported in sheep, goats and cattle under one year of age. Subclinical infection in many species is common and clinical disease may be precipitated in the winter months by stress factors such as poor nutrition, weaning, transportation and cold wet conditions. There may be prolonged survival of *Y. pseudotuberculosis* on pasture in cold wet weather, facilitating faecal-oral transmission.

Enteritis in young deer and lambs is characterized by profuse watery diarrhoea, sometimes blood-stained, which may be rapidly fatal if untreated. The luminal contents of the small and large intestine are watery and mucosal hyperaemia is evident at postmortem examination. Severely affected animals may show mucosal ulceration. The mesenteric lymph nodes are often enlarged and oedematous and scattered pale necrotic foci may be present in the liver.

A clinically similar but less severe enterocolitis caused by *Y. enterocolitica* has been described in young ruminants.

Diagnosis

- The species and age group affected, especially during cold wet spells of weather, may suggest yersiniosis.
- Histological examination of intestinal lesions may reveal clusters of organisms in microabscesses within the mucosa.
- Confirmation requires isolation and identification of *Y. pseudotuberculosis* or, occasionally, *Y. enterocolitica*:
  - Samples from tissues can be plated directly onto blood and MacConkey agars and incubated aerobically at 37°C for up to 72 hours.
  - Faecal samples may be plated directly onto special selective media.
  - A cold enrichment procedure may facilitate recovery of yersiniae from faeces especially if they are present in low mumbers. A 5% suspension of faeces in phosphate buffered saline, held at 4°C for three weeks, is subcultured weekly onto MacConkey agar.
- Serotyping may be necessary to establish whether the isolates belong to known pathogenic serotypes.

Treatment and control

- Fluid replacement therapy together with broad spectrum antimicrobial treatment should be initiated promptly in young animals.
- A formalin-killed *Y. pseudotuberculosis* vaccine composed of serotypes I, II and III, administered in two doses three weeks apart has been shown to decrease the occurrence of clinical disease in young deer.
- Stressful conditions should, where practicable, be mimimized.

Septicaemic yersiniosis

Septicaemia, caused by *Y. pseudotuberculosis* occurs in birds kept in cages or aviaries. It is presumed that infection is acquired through contact with the faeces of wild birds or rodents, or through the feeding of contaminated leafy plants. In aviaries, overcrowding may predispose to the development of disease. Infected birds may die suddenly. Some may display ruffling of feathers and listlessness shortly before death. Pin-point white necrotic foci are present in the liver at postmortem. Confirmation is based on the isolation and identification of *Y. pseudotuberculosis* from the liver and other internal organs.

Treatment is seldom feasible due to the acute nature of the disease. Control should be aimed at preventing faecal contamination of food and water by wild birds and rodents.

Pseudotuberculosis in laboratory animals

Infection with *Y. pseudotuberculosis* in colonies of guinea-pigs or rodents is usually introduced through faecal contamination of food by wild rodents. Diarrhoea and gradual weight loss leading to emaciation and death are the signs most often observed in affected animals. Some animals may die suddenly from septicaemia.

At postmortem examination, numerous white necrotic lesions are present in the liver. Affected mesenteric lymph nodes are enlarged and may show caseous necrosis.

Treatment is usually not desirable because some animals in the colony may become carriers and the organism is zoonotic. Depopulation, disinfection and restocking are the preferred control measures. Exclusion of wild rodents is an essential step in preventing infection with *Y. pseudotuberculosis*.

Feline plague

Cats usually acquire infection with *Y. pestis* by ingestion of infected rodents. Three clinical forms of the disease are recognized: bubonic, septicaemic and pneumonic. The most common form of the disease is characterized by enlarged lymph nodes (buboes) associated with lymphatic drainage from the site of infection. Clinical signs include fever, depression and anorexia. Affected superficial lymph nodes may rupture, discharging serosanguineous fluid or pus. Septicaemia may occur without lymphadenopathy and is potentially fatal. Pneumonic lesions may result from haematogenous spread.

Cats with pneumonic lesions are a potential source of human infection through aerosol generation and should be euthanized. Human infection can also be acquired through cat scratches and bites and possibly through the bites of fleas from infected cats. Care should be taken when handling infected animals.

Diagnosis
- Lymphadenopathy and severe depression in cats in endemic areas may suggest feline plague.
- Specimens from suspect cases should be sent to specialized reference laboratories. Suitable specimens include pus, blood and lymph node aspirates.
- Giemsa-stained smears from abscesses or lymph node aspirates may reveal large numbers of bipolar-staining rods.
- Direct fluorescent antibody tests are carried out in reference laboratories.
- A passive haemagglutination test, using Fraction 1A antigen, can be used on paired serum samples taken two weeks apart from suspect cats. A substantial increase in the antibody level is usually indicative of active infection.

Treatment and control
- Cats with suspected plague should be kept in isolation and immediately treated for fleas to prevent those handling the animal becoming exposed to flea bites. The bubonic form of the disease may respond to parenterally administered tetracyclines or chloramphenicol. Multidrug resistance, mediated by a transferable plasmid, has been reported recently in *Y. pestis* (Galimand *et al.*, 1997).
- In endemic areas, dogs and cats should be routinely treated for fleas.
- Rodent control measures should be implemented after flea control procedures are in place.

Opportunistic pathogens

This group of enterobacteria, which rarely cause enteric disease in domestic animals, are sometimes involved in localized opportunistic infections in diverse anatomical locations. Faecal contamination of the environment accounts for widespread distribution of the organisms and contributes to the occurrence of opportunistic infection. Predisposing factors include intercurrent infection, tissue devitalization and the inherent vulnerability of certain organs.

These opportunistic invaders have characteristics which may allow them to circumvent host defence mechanisms and colonize and survive in affected organs. *Klebsiella pneumoniae* and *Enterobacter* species produce abundant capsular material which may inhibit phagocytosis and enhance intracellular survival. Adhesins are of particular importance in those bacteria which colonize the lower urinary tract. Siderophores produced by some

Table 18.8 Opportunistic pathogens in the *Enterobacteriaceae* and their associated clinical conditions.

Bacterial species	Clinical conditions
Edwardsiella tarda	Diarrhoea; wound infections in some animal species (rare)
Enterobacter aerogenes	Coliform mastitis in cows and sows
Klebsiella pneumoniae	Coliform mastitis in cows; endometritis in mares; pneumonia in calves and foals; urinary tract infections in dogs
Morganella morganii subsp. *morganii*	Ear and urinary tract infections in dogs and cats (uncommon)
Proteus mirabilis and *P. vulgaris*	Urinary tract infections in dogs and horses; associated with otitis externa in dogs
Serratia marcescens	Bovine mastitis (uncommon); septicaemia in chickens (rare)

opportunistic pathogens, contribute to bacterial survival when the supply of available iron in tissues is limited. Some toxic effects of these opportunistic pathogens are attributable to release of endotoxin from dead bacteria. This can induce local and systemic changes which include inflammatory responses, pyrexia, endothelial damage and microthrombosis.

Clinical infections

The clinical conditions arising from infections with opportunistic members of the *Enterobacteriaceae* are presented in Table 18.8. *Klebsiella pneumoniae* and *Enterobacter aerogenes* are two opportunistic pathogens commonly encountered in coliform mastitis of dairy cattle. These organisms usually gain entry to the mammary gland from contaminated environmental sources. Sawdust used for bedding, for example, may be the source of infection in coliform mastitis caused by *Klebsiella pneumoniae*. This bacterium is also reported to be one of the commonest causes of metritis in mares and its presence on the preputial sheath of stallions suggests the possibility of venereal transmission. *Proteus* species and *Klebsiella* species cause infections of the lower urinary tract in dogs. *Proteus* species are often implicated in otitis externa in dogs and sometimes in cats. A variety of factors may predispose to this infection (*see* Chapter 40).

The other opportunistic pathogens in this group *Edwardsiella tarda*, *Morganella morganii* subsp. *morganii* and *Serratia marcescens* are rarely associated with clinical disease in domestic animals.

Diagnostic procedures

When opportunistic pathogens are involved in a disease

process, clinical signs are non-specific.

- Specimens for examination should be collected from the infected organ.
- Blood agar and MacConkey agar inoculated with the specimens are cultured aerobically at 37°C for 24 to 48 hours.
- Identification criteria for isolates:
  — Gram-negative rods
  — Oxidase-negative, catalase-positive
  — Growth and appearance on MacConkey agar
  — Colonial appearance on blood agar
  — Appropriate biochemical profile for presumptive or definitive identification

Treatment and control

- The type of treatment is determined by the location and severity of the infection.
- Antibiotic therapy should be based on antibiotic susceptibility testing.
- Predisposing causes and sources of infection should be identified and, if possible, eliminated.

References

Brubaker, R.R. (1991). Factors promoting acute and chronic diseases caused by yersiniae. *Clinical Microbiological Reviews*, **4**, 309–324.

Carroll, P.J., Woodward, M.J. and Wray, C. (1990). Detection of LT and ST1a toxins by latex and EIA tests. *Veterinary Record*, **127**, 335–336.

Carter, M.E., Dewes, H.B. and Griffiths, O.V. (1979). Salmonellosis in foals. *Journal of Equine Medicine and Surgery*, **3**, 78–83.

Cooper, G.L. (1994). Salmonellosis – infections in man and chicken: pathogenesis and the development of live vaccines – a review. *Veterinary Bulletin*, **64**, 123–143.

Corbel, M.J. Brewer, R.A. and Hunter, D. (1990). Characterisation of *Yersinia enterocolitica* strains associated with ovine abortion. *Veterinary Record*, **127,** 526–527.

Cork, S.C., Marshall, R.B., Madie, P. and Fenwick, S.G. (1995). The role of wild birds and the environment in the epidemiology of yersiniae in New Zealand. *New Zealand Veterinary Journal*, **43**, 169–174.

Fox, J.G. and Gallus, C.B. (1977). Salmonella-associated conjunctivitis in a cat. *Journal of the American Veterinary Medical Association*, **171**, 845–847.

Galimand, M., Guiyoule, A., Gerbaud, G., Rasoamanana, B., Chanteau, S., Carniel, E. *et al.* (1997). Multidrug resistance in *Yersinia pestis* mediated by a transferable plasmid. *New England Journal of Medicine*, **337**, 677–680.

Gitter, M., Wray, C. Richardson, C. and Pepper, R.T. (1978). Chronic *Salmonella dublin* infection of calves. *British Veterinary Journal*, **134,** 113–121.

Hall, G.A., Chanter, N. and Bland, A.P. (1988). Comparison in gnotobiotic pigs of lesions caused by verotoxigenic and non-verotoxigenic *Escherichia coli*. *Veterinary Pathology*, **25**, 205–210.

Henderson, T.G. (1983). Yersiniosis in deer from the Otago-Southland region of New Zealand. *New Zealand Veterinary Journal*, **31**, 221–224.

Jerrett, I.V. and Slee, K.J. (1989). Bovine abortion associated with *Yersinia pseudotuberculosis* infection. *Veterinary Pathology*, **26**, 181–183.

Jerrett, I.V., Slee, K.J. and Robertson, B.I. (1990). Yersiniosis in farmed deer. *Australian Veterinary Journal*, **67**, 212–214.

Kaufmann, A.F., Mann, J.M., Gardiner, T.M., Heaton, F., Poland, J.D., Barnes, A.M. *et al.* (1981). Public health implications of plague in domestic cats. *Journal of the American Veterinary Medical Association*, **179**, 875–878.

King, T. and Hodgson, C. (1991). Watery mouth in lambs. *In Practice*, **13**, 23-24.

Lax, A.J., Barrow, P.A., Jones, P.W. and Wallis, T.S. (1995). Current perspectives in salmonellosis. *British Veterinary Journal*, **151**, 351–377.

LeMinor, L. and Popoff, M.Y. (1987). Designation of *Salmonella enterica* sp. nov. as the type and only species of the genus *Salmonella*. *International Journal of Systematic Bacteriology*, **37**, 465–468.

Maddox, C.W. and Fales, W.H. (1991). Use of a *Salmonella typhimurium*-derived probe in the detection of *Salmonella* sp. and in the characterization of *Salmonella cholerae-suis* virulence plasmids. *Journal of Veterinary Diagnostic Investigation*, **3**, 218–222.

Otter, A. (1996). Ovine abortion caused by *Yersinia pseudotuberculosis*. *Veterinary Record*, **138**, 143–144.

Penhale, W.J., McEwan, A.D., Fisher, E.W. and Selman, I. (1970). Quantitative studies on bovine immunoglobulins II. Plasma immunoglobulin levels in market calves and their relationship to neonatal infection. *British Veterinary Journal*, **126**, 30–37.

Reeves, M.W., Evins, G.M., Heiba, A.A., Plikaytis, B.D. and Farmer, J.J. (1989). Clonal nature of *Salmonella typhi* and its genetic relatedness to other salmonellae as shown by multilocus enzyme electrophoresis, and proposal of *Salmonella bongori* comb. nov. *Journal of Clinical Microbiology*, **27**, 313–320.

Riet-Correa, F., Gil-Turnes, C., Reyes, J.C., Schild, A.L. and Méndez, M.C. (1990). *Yersinia pseudotuberculosis* infection of buffaloes (*Bubalus bubalis*). *Journal of Veterinary Diagnostic Investigation*, **2**, 78–79.

Salyers, A.A. and Whitt, D.D. (1994). *Bacterial pathogenesis*. ASM Press, Washington, DC. pp. 229-243.

Sargison, N.D., West, D.M., Parton, K.H., Hunter, J.E. and Lumsden, J.S. (1997). A case of 'watery mouth' in a New Zealand Romney lamb. *New Zealand Veterinary Journal*, **45**, 67–68.

Snodgrass, D.R. (1986). Evaluation of a combined rotavirus and enterotoxigenic *Escherichia coli* vaccine in cattle. *Veterinary Record*, **119**, 39–43.

Thorns, C.J., Sojka, M.G. and Roeder, P.L. (1989). Detection of fimbrial adhesins of ETEC using monoclonal antibody-based latex reagents. *Veterinary Record*, **125,** 91-92.

van Béers-Schreurs, H.M.G., Vellenga, L., Wensing, Th. and Breukink, H.J. (1992). The pathogenesis of the post-weaning syndrome in weaned pigs; a review. *Veterinary Quarterly*, **14**, 29–34.

Witte, S.T. and Collins, T.C. (1985). Abortion and early neonatal death of kids attributed to intrauterine *Yersinia pseudotuberculosis* infection. *Journal of the American Veterinary Medical Association*, **187**, 834.

Wray, C. (1991). Salmonellosis in cattle. *In Practice*, **13**, 13–15.

Wray, C., McLaren, I.M. and Pearson, G.R. (1989). Occurrence of 'attaching and effacing' lesions in the small intestine of calves experimentally infected with bovine isolates of vero-cytotoxigenic *Escherichia coli*. *Veterinary Record*, **125**, 365–368.

Wray, C., McLaren, I.M. and Carroll, P.J. (1993). *Escherichia coli* isolated from farm animals in England and Wales between 1986 and 1991. *Veterinary Record*, **133,** 439–42.

Further reading

Gyles, C.L. (1994). *Escherichia coli in domestic animals and humans*. CAB International, Wallingford, England.

Sussman, M. (1997). *Escherichia coli: mechanisms of virulence*. Cambridge University Press, Cambridge.

Wray, C. and Wray, A. (2000). *Salmonella in Domestic Animals*. CABI Publishing, Wallingford, Oxford.

Chapter 19

Pseudomonas aeruginosa and *Burkholderia* species

Pseudomonas aeruginosa, Burkholderia mallei and *B. pseudomallei* are Gram-negative rods (0.5 to 1.0 x 1 to 5 μm) which are obligate aerobes and oxidize carbohydrates. Most isolates are oxidase-positive and catalase-positive. They are motile by one or more polar flagella, with the exception of *B. mallei* which is non-motile. The majority of these organisms have no special growth requirements and grow well on MacConkey agar. *Burkholderia mallei* requires 1% glycerol in media for optimal growth. *Pseudomonas aeruginosa*, characterized by the production of diffusible pigments, causes a variety of opportunistic infections in a wide range of animals. A number of other *Pseudomonas* species may be isolated from clinical specimens. *Pseudomonas fluorescens* and *P. putida* occasionally infect freshwater fish.

Burkholderia species, previously classified in the genus *Pseudomonas,* include *B. mallei*, the cause of glanders and *B. pseudomallei*, the cause of melioidosis. Both diseases are zoonoses.

> ### Key points
> - Medium-sized, Gram-negative rods
> - Obligate aerobes
> - Most isolates are oxidase-positive and catalase-positive
> - *Pseudomonas* species and *Burkholderia pseudomallei* are motile by polar flagella
> - *Burkholderia mallei* is non-motile and requires 1% glycerol in media for optimal growth
> - Diffusable pigments are produced by *P. aeroginosa*
> - *Burkholderia mallei* causes glanders
> - *Burholderia pseudomallei* causes melioidosis
> - *Pseudomonas aeruginosa* causes opportunistic infections

Usual habitat

Pseudomonas species are environmental organisms which occur worldwide in water and soil, and on plants. *Pseudomonas aeruginosa* is also found on the skin, on mucous membranes and in faeces. *Burkholderia pseudomallei*, which is found in soils, occasionally infects animals and man. Wild rodents can act as reservoirs of this organism. It is widely distributed in some tropical and subtropical regions of southeast Asia and Australia. Although *B. mallei* can survive in the environment for up to 6 weeks, its reservoir is infected *Equidae*.

Differentiation of *Pseudomonas* and *Burkholderia* species

- The comparative colonial and biochemical features of these organisms are presented in Table 19.1.
- Many *Pseudomonas* species produce pigments. *Pseudomonas aeruginosa* strains can form up to four diffusible pigments (Box 19.1). Pyocyanin, unique to this organism, is produced by most strains and specifically identifies *P. aeruginosa*. Pyocyanin-enhancing media are available for isolates which are weak pyocyanin producers. Pigment production is observed most clearly on media without dyes such as nutrient agar. Pyorubin and pyomelanin develop slowly and may be detectable only after incubation for 1 to 2 weeks. Colonies of *B. pseudomallei* and *B. mallei* become brownish with age but do not produce pigments.
- The majority of *Pseudomonas* and *Burkholderia* species are motile. Absence of motility distinguishes *B. mallei* from other members of the group.

Clinical infections

Burkholderia mallei, a major pathogen of *Equidae*, causes both acute and chronic disease. It manifests mainly as lesions in the skin and the respiratory tract. Infection with *B. pseudomallei* can cause chronic suppurative lesions in the lungs and other organs of a wide range of species. In contrast, *P. aeruginosa* is an opportunistic pathogen which may occasionally cause acute systemic disease.

Pseudomonas aeruginosa infections

Pseudomonas aeruginosa causes a wide range of opportunistic infections (Table 19.2). Although predisposing

Table 19.1 Comparative features of *Pseudomonas aeruginosa*, *Burkholderia mallei* and *Burkholderia pseudomallei*.

Feature	P. aeruginosa	B. mallei	B. pseudomallei
Colonial morphology	Large and flat with serrated edges	White and smooth becoming granular and brown with age	Ranges from smooth and mucoid to rough and dull becoming yellowish-brown with age
Haemolysis on blood agar	+[a]	−	+[a]
Diffusible pigment production	+	−	−
Colony odour	grape-like	none	musty
Growth on MacConkey agar	+	+[b]	+
Growth at 42°C	+	−	+
Motility	+	−	+
Oxidase production	+	−[c]	+
Oxidation of:			
glucose	+	+	+
lactose	−	−	+
sucrose	−	−	+[b]

a 40% of strains positive
b over 75% of strains positive
c 25% of strains negative

factors are associated with the occurrence of many of these infections, some species, such as farmed mink, appear to be particularly susceptible to the organism (Long *et al.*, 1980). Haemorrhagic pneumonia and septicaemia, caused by *P. aeruginosa*, occurs sporadically in ranched mink with mortality rates up to 50% in some outbreaks. Bovine mastitis associated with this organism (Crossman and Hutchinson, 1995) is often linked to contaminated water used for udder washing or to the insertion of contaminated intramammary antibiotic tubes. Fleece-rot of sheep, a condition associated with heavy or prolonged rainfall, has been reported from the UK and Australia. Maceration of the skin surface following water penetration of the fleece allows colonization by *P. aeruginosa*, resulting in suppurative dermatitis. The bluish-green pyocyanin pigment produced by *P. aeruginosa* discolours the wool. *Pseudomonas aeruginosa* is often found in the oral cavity of snakes and can cause necrotic stomatitis in captive reptiles kept under poor husbandry conditions.

Box 19.1 Pigments produced by *Pseudomonas aeruginosa*.

- Pyocyanin (blue green)
- Pyoverdin (greenish-yellow)
- Pyorubin (red)
- Pyomelanin (brownish-black)

Pathogenesis and pathogenicity

Pathogenic strains of *P. aeruginosa* produce a variety of toxins and enzymes which promote tissue invasion and damage. Attachment to host cells is mediated by fimbriae. Colonization and replication are aided by antiphagocytic properties of exoenzyme S, extracellular slime and outer-membrane lipopolysaccharides. Resistance to complement-mediated damage and the ability to obtain

Table 19.2 Clinical conditions arising from infection with *Pseudomonas aeruginosa*.

Host	Disease condition
Cattle	Mastitis, metritis, pneumonia, dermatitis, enteritis (calves)
Sheep	Mastitis, fleece-rot, pneumonia, otitis media
Pigs	Respiratory infections, otitis
Horses	Genital tract infections, pneumonia, ulcerative keratitis
Dogs, cats	Otitis externa, cystitis, pneumonia, ulcerative keratitis
Mink	Haemorrhagic pneumonia, septicaemia
Chinchillas	Pneumonia, septicaemia
Reptiles (captive)	Necrotic stomatitis

iron from host tissues are additional virulence factors. Tissue damage is caused by toxins such as exotoxin A, phospholipase C and proteases. Exotoxin A is a bipartite toxin with binding and active components. The active component, once internalized in a cell, blocks protein synthesis by ADP-ribosylation and elongation of Factor 2 with resultant cell death. The cytoplasmic membranes of neutrophils are damaged by a leukocidin.

Dissemination is aided by exoenzyme S and systemic toxicity is attributed to exotoxin A and endotoxin. The host defence mechanisms against *P. aeruginosa* include opsonizing antibodies and phagocytosis by macrophages.

Diagnostic procedures
- Specimens for laboratory examination include pus, respiratory aspirates, mid-stream urine, mastitic milk and ear swabs.
- Blood agar and MacConkey agar plates, inoculated with suspect material, are incubated aerobically at 37°C for 24 to 48 hours.
- Identification criteria for isolates :
  — Colonial morphology and characteristic fruity, grape-like odour
  — Pyocyanin production
  — Lactose-negative, pale colonies on MacConkey agar
  — Oxidase-positive
  — Triple sugar iron agar unchanged
  — Biochemical profile (Table 19.1)

Treatment and control
- Predisposing causes and sources of infection should be identified and, where possible, eliminated.
- *Pseudomonas aeruginosa* is extremely resistant to many antibiotics and susceptibility testing should be carried out on isolates. A combination of either gentamicin or tobramycin with either carbenicillin or ticaricillin may be effective.
- Vaccines may be required for farmed mink and chinchillas. As there are antigenic differences between strains, polyvalent or autogenous formalin-killed bacterins should be employed. Humoral antibody induced by a polyvalent exotoxin A-polysaccharide vaccine appears to be protective (Cryz *et al.*, 1987).

Glanders

Glanders, caused by *B. mallei*, is a contagious disease of *Equidae* characterized by the formation of nodules and ulcers in the respiratory tract or on the skin. Humans and carnivores are also susceptible to infection. Once world-wide in distribution, glanders has now been eradicated from most developed countries, but sporadic cases of disease occur in the Middle East, India, Pakistan and China. The disease is reported to be endemic in Mongolia.

Transmission follows ingestion of food or water contaminated by nasal discharges of infected *Equidae*. Less commonly, infection may be acquired by inhalation or through skin abrasions. An acute septicaemic form of the disease is characterized by fever, mucopurulent nasal discharge and respiratory signs. Death usually follows within a few weeks. Chronic disease is more common and presents as nasal, pulmonary and cutaneous forms, all of which may be observed in an affected animal. In the nasal form, ulcerative nodules develop on the mucosa of the nasal septum and lower part of the turbinates. A purulent, blood-stained nasal discharge and regional lymphadeno-pathy are usually present. The ulcers eventually heal leaving star-shaped scars. The respiratory form is characterized by respiratory distress and the development of tubercle-like lesions throughout the lungs. The cutaneous form, termed farcy, is a lymphangitis in which nodules occur along the course of the lymphatic vessels of the limbs. Ulcers develop and discharge a yellowish pus. Chronically affected animals may die after several months or may recover and continue to shed organisms from the respiratory tract or skin.

Carnivores may contract the disease by eating infected carcases (Galati *et al.*, 1974).

Pathogenesis
Glanders in the horse is usually a chronic, disseminated, debilitating disease but the mechanisms of pathogenicity are not known. The presence of *B. mallei* in the host gives rise to a hypersensitivity reaction, the basis of the mallein test.

Diagnostic procedures
- In regions where the disease is endemic, clinical signs may be diagnostic.
- Specimens for laboratory diagnosis should include discharges from lesions and blood for serology. Specimens must be processed in a biohazard cabinet.
- *Burkholderia mallei* grows on media containing 1% glycerol and most strains will grow on MacConkey agar. Plates are incubated aerobically at 37°C for 2 to 3 days.
- Identification criteria for isolates :
  — Colonial characteristics
  — Majority of strains grow on MacConkey agar without utilizing lactose
  — Comparatively unreactive biochemically and non-motile (Table 19.1)
- Suitable serological tests include the complement fixation test and agglutination techniques.
- The mallein test is an efficient field test both for confirmation and for screening in-contact animals. Mallein, a glycoprotein extract of *B. mallei*, is injected intradermally (0.1 ml) just below the lower eyelid. A positive reaction is indicated by local swelling and mucopurulent ocular discharge after 24 hours.

Treatment and control

* A test and slaughter policy is enforced in countries where the disease is exotic.
* In endemic areas, antibiotic therapy is inappropriate as treated animals often become subclinical carriers.
* Effective cleaning and disinfection of all contaminated areas must be carried out. Formalin (1.5%) or an iodophor (2.0%) can be used, with a contact time of 6 hours.

Melioidosis

Melioidosis, caused by *B. pseudomallei*, is endemic in tropical and subtropical regions of southeastern Asia and Australia where the organism is widely distributed in soil and water. Infection may follow ingestion, inhalation or skin contamination from environmental sources. The bacterium is an opportunistic pathogen and stress factors or immunosuppression may predispose to clinical disease. Many animal species, including humans, are susceptible and subclinical infections may occur. Because infection is usually disseminated, abscesses develop in many organs including lungs, spleen, liver, joints and central nervous system. Melioidosis is a chronic, debilitating, progressive disease, often with a long incubation period. Clinical signs, which are variable, relate to lesion severity and distribution. In horses melioidosis, which can mimic glanders, is often referred to as pseudoglanders.

Pathogenesis and pathogenicity

The pathogenesis of melioidosis is poorly understood. Extracellular products of *B. pseudomallei* such as an exotoxin, a dermonecrotic protease and a lecithinase have been implicated in disease production (Dance, 1990). Both strain virulence and host immunosuppression may influence the establishment and outcome of infection.

Diagnostic procedures

* In regions where the disease is encountered, gross pathological findings may aid diagnosis.
* Specimens for laboratory diagnosis should include pus from abscesses, affected tissues and blood for serology. A biohazard cabinet must be used for processing specimens.
* A fluorescent antibody technique for demonstrating the organism in tissue smears is available in some reference laboratories.
* Blood agar and MacConkey agar plates, inoculated with suspect material, are incubated aerobically at 37°C for 24-48 hours.

* Identification criteria for isolates :
  — Colonial morphology and characteristic musty odour
  — Lactose utilized in MacConkey agar
  — Biochemical characteristics (Table 19.1)
  — Slide agglutination test using specific antiserum
  — ELISA, complement fixation and indirect haemagglutination tests can be used for detecting serum antibodies.

Treatment and control

* Confirmation of infection followed by slaughter of infected animals is mandatory in countries where the disease is exotic.
* Treatment is expensive and unreliable. Relapses can occur after antibiotic therapy is discontinued.
* Vaccines are being developed in some countries.

References

Crossman, P.J. and Hutchinson, I. (1995). Gangrenous mastitis associated with *Pseudomonas aeruginosa*. *Veterinary Record*, **136**, 548.

Cryz, S.J., Furer, E., Sadoff, J.C. and Germanier, R. (1987). A polyvalent *Pseudomonas aeruginosa* O-polysaccharide-toxin A conjugate vaccine. *Antibiotics and Chemotherapy*, **39**, 249–255.

Dance, D.A.B. (1990). Melioidosis. *Reviews in Medical Microbiology*, **1**, 143–150.

Galati, P., Puccini, V. and Contento, F. (1974). An outbreak of glanders in lions. *Veterinary Pathology*, **11**, 445.

Long, G.G., Gallina, A.M. and Gorham, J.R. (1980). *Pseudomonas* pneumonia of mink: pathogenesis, vaccination and serological studies. *American Journal of Veterinary Research*, **41**, 1720–1725.

Further reading

Currie, B., Smith-Vaughan, H., Golledge, C., Buller, N., Sriprakash, K.S. and Kemp, D.J. (1994). *Pseudomonas pseudomallei* isolates collected over 25 years from a non-tropical endemic focus show clonality on the basis of ribotyping. *Epidemiology and Infection*, **113**, 307–312.

Dance, D.A.B., King, C., Aucken, H., Knott, C.D., West, P.G. and Pitt, T.L. (1992). An outbreak of melioidosis in imported primates in Britain. *Veterinary Record*, **130**, 525–529.

Davies, I.H. and Done, S.H. (1993). Necrotic dermatitis and otitis media associated with *Pseudomonas aeruginosa* in sheep following dipping. *Veterinary Record*, **132**, 460–461.

Pritchard, D.G. (1995). Glanders. *Equine Veterinary Education*, **7**, 29–32.

Chapter 20

Aeromonas species, *Plesiomonas shigelloides* and *Vibrio* species

Aeromonas species, *Plesiomonas shigelloides* and *Vibrio* species are Gram-negative bacteria with a number of common attributes. They are found in aquatic environments, possess some similar biochemical characteristics and morphological features, and are opportunistic pathogens of fish, reptiles and rarely mammals. *Vibrio cholerae*, an important human pathogen, produces cholera which is a severe life-threatening enteric infection.

Morphologically, *Aeromonas* and *Plesiomonas* species are straight medium-sized rods, unlike *Vibrio* species which are curved. Most members of these genera are catalase-positive, oxidase-positive, facultative anaerobes which are motile by polar flagella. The positive oxidase reaction distinguishes this group of organisms from members of the *Enterobacteriaceae*. Although *Aeromonas* species and *Plesiomonas shigelloides* grow on non-enriched media, many *Vibrio* species are halophilic. The optimal temperature for growth of some species in the group is lower than 37°C. Microaerophilic organisms, formerly classified as *Vibrio* species, are now assigned to the genus *Campylobacter*.

Usual habitat

Aeromonas species and *P. shigelloides* are found in fresh water and are present in the oral cavity and on the skin of fish and reptiles. Most *Vibrio* species are found in brackish and salt water.

Clinical infections

Members of these genera are primarily pathogens of fish and reptiles, although some species can infect mammals and birds. Infections are usually opportunistic requiring stress factors for the initiation of disease. Species which have been associated with disease processes are presented in Table 20.1. *Aeromonas hydrophila*, *P. shigelloides* and *V. metschnikovii* are the opportunistic pathogens which have been most often encountered in domestic animals and man. The main distinguishing characteristics of these three species are presented in Table 20.2.

The pathogenetic mechanisms involved in the production of disease are poorly understood. *Aeromonas hydrophila* produces adhesins and exotoxin. *Plesiomonas shigelloides*, which causes diarrhoea in humans, possesses a large

> **Key points**
> - Medium-sized Gram-negative rods, some *Vibrio* species are curved
> - Grow on non-enriched media; NaCl supplementation required for most *Vibrio* species
> - Catalase-positive, oxidase-positive, facultative anaerobes
> - Majority motile by polar flagella
> - Found in aquatic environments
> - Opportunistic pathogens of fish and reptiles and rarely of mammals

plasmid which may be associated with virulence (Herrington *et al.*, 1987).

Infections caused by *Aeromonas hydrophila*

Aeromonas hydrophila has been associated occasionally with disease conditions in domestic animals. Abortion attributed to *A. hydrophila* was recorded in cattle (Wohlgemuth *et al.*, 1972). The organism has also been isolated from a young dog with septicaemia (Pierce *et al.*, 1973). Experimentally, *A. hydrophila* produces haemorrhagic colitis in rabbits (Hibbs *et al.*, 1971). Infections caused by *Aeromonas* species in animals and man are indicated in Table 20.1.

Infections caused by *Plesiomonas shigelloides*

These infections occur most commonly in tropical and subtropical regions. The disease conditions caused by *P. shigelloides* in animals and man are listed in Table 20.1.

Infections caused by *Vibrio* species

Apart from the important human pathogen, *V. cholerae*, there are at least five other species which cause enteric infections in humans. Food poisoning caused by *Vibrio parahaemolyticus* is associated with the consumption of raw or undercooked seafoods. *Vibrio metschnikovii* causes

Table 20.1 Species of *Aeromonas, Plesiomonas, Listonella* and *Vibrio* and associated disease conditions.

Organism	Host	Disease condition
Aeromonas salmonicida	Salmonid fish Goldfish	Furunculosis 'Ulcer disease'
A. hydrophila	Amphibians Snakes (captive) Freshwater fish Cattle Young dogs Humans	'Red-leg' syndrome Ulcerative stomatitis, pneumonia, septicaemia Haemorrhagic septicaemia Abortion Septicaemia Food poisoning
Plesiomonas shigelloides	Fish, reptiles Harbour seals Humans	Septicaemia Diarrhoea Diarrhoea, neonatal meningitis
Vibrio cholerae	Humans	Cholera
V. para-haemolyticus	Humans	Food poisoning associated with seafood
V. metschnikovii	Chickens	Severe enteric disease
Listonella anguillarum	Marine fish, eels	Skin lesions, septicaemia

enteric disease in chickens. *Listonella anguillarum (Vibrio anguillarum)* and some *Vibrio* species are pathogens of fish.

Diagnostic procedures

A definitive diagnosis requires the isolation and identification of the pathogen from lesions (Table 20.2). Because of the widespread distribution of the majority of these bacteria in the environment, laboratory results should be interpreted with caution.

Treatment

Antibiotic therapy should be based on susceptibility testing of *Aeromonas* species and *P. shigelloide*s. Cephalosporins may be of therapeutic value. Gentamicin and nalidixic acid are usually effective for the treatment of infections caused by *Vibrio* species.

References

Herrington, D.A., Tzipori, S., Robins-Browne, R.M., Tall, B.D. and Levine, M.M. (1987). *In vitro* and *in vivo* pathogenicity

Table 20.2 Distinguishing characteristics of *Aeromonas hydrophila, Plesiomonas shigelloides* and *Vibrio metschnikovii.*

Characteristic	*A. hydrophila*	*P. shigelloides*	*V. metschnikovii*
Morphology	Straight rods	Straight rods	Curved rods
Motility by polar flagella	+	+	+
Oxidase production	+	+	− [a]
Catalase production	+	+	+
Haemolysis on sheep blood agar	+	−	+
Growth on MacConkey agar	+	+	−
Growth in nutrient broth with NaCl (6%)	−	−	+
Sensitivity to vibriostat (150 μg concentration)[b]	−	+	+
Reduction of nitrate to nitrite	+	+	− [a]
Lysine decarboxylase production	+	+	−
Arginine dihydrolase production	+	+	v
Ornithine decarboxylase production	−	+	−
Utilization of:			
sucrose	+	−	+
mannitol	+	−	+
inositol	−	+	v
lactose	−	−	v

a most *Vibrio* species are positive　　　b 2, 4-diamino-6, 7-diisopropylpteridine phosphate (0/129 Oxoid)　　　v variable reactions of *Plesiomonas shigelloides*. *Infection and Immunity,* **55**, 979–985.

Hibbs, C.M., Merker, J.W. and Kruckenberg, S.M. (1971). Experimental *Aeromonas hydrophila* infection in rabbits. *Cornell Veterinarian*, **61**, 380–386.

Pierce, R.L., Daley, C.A., Gates, C.E. and Wohlgemuth, K. (1973). *Aeromonas hydrophila* septicaemia in a dog. *Journal of the American Veterinary Medical Association,* **162**, 469.

Wohlgemuth, K., Pierce, R.L. and Kirkbride, C.A. (1972). Bovine abortion associated with *Aeromonas hydrophila*. *Journal of the American Veterinary Medical Association*, **160**, 1001–1002.

Further reading

Brenden, R.A., Miller, M.A. and Janda, J.M. (1988). Clinical disease spectrum and pathogenic factors associated with *Plesiomonas shigelloides* infections in humans. *Reviews of Infectious Diseases*, **10**, 303–316.

Marcus, L.C. (1971). Infectious diseases of reptiles. *Journal of the American Veterinary Medical Association*, **159**, 1626–1631.

Shotts, E.B., Gaines, J.L., Martin, L. and Prestwood, A.K. (1972). *Aeromonas*-induced deaths among fish and reptiles in a eutrophic inland lake. *Journal of the American Veterinary Medical Association*, **161**, 603–607.

Chapter 21

Actinobacillus species

Actinobacillus species are non-motile, Gram-negative rods (0.3 to 0.5 x 0.6 to 1.4 μm) which occasionally have a coccobacillary appearance. These facultative anaerobes ferment carbohydrates producing acid but not gas. Most species are urease- and oxidase-positive. Actinobacilli exhibit some host specificity and are mainly pathogens of farm animals. Species of veterinary importance are presented in Fig. 21.1.

Recent DNA hybridization and rRNA sequencing studies have led to a reappraisal of the genetic relationships between the genera *Actinobacillus*, *Pasteurella* and *Haemophilus*, which are in the family *Pasteurellaceae* (Dewhirst *et al.*, 1992). *Actinobacillus lignieresii*, *A. equuli*, *A. suis* and *A. pleuropneumoniae* are closely related, but *A. seminis*, *A. actinomycetemcomitans* and *A. capsulatus* may require reclassification.

Usual habitat

Actinobacilli are commensals on mucous membranes of animals particularly in the upper respiratory tract and oral cavity. As actinobacilli cannot survive for long in the environment, carrier animals play a major role in transmission.

Differentiation of *Actinobacillus* species

Actinobacillus species are usually distinguished by colonial characteristics and biochemical reactions (Table 21.1).

- On primary isolation on blood agar, colonies of *A. lignieresii*, *A. equuli*, and *A. suis* exhibit cohesive properties when touched with an inoculation loop.
- Growth and reactions on MacConkey agar:
  - —*A. lignieresii, A. equuli* and *A. suis* grow well on MacConkey agar. Colonies of *A. lignieresii* are initially pale turning pink after 48 hours. *Actinobacillus equuli* and *A. suis* ferment lactose, producing pink colonies.
  - —*A. pleuropneumoniae* and *A. seminis* do not grow on MacConkey agar.
- Commercially-available biochemical kits or specialized test methods can be used to differentiate *Actinobacillus* species. *Actinobacillus seminis* which is catalase-

> **Key points**
> - Medium-sized, non-motile, Gram-negative rods
> - Facultative anaerobes
> - Most species are oxidase-positive and produce urease
> - Species of veterinary importance grow on MacConkey agar, apart from *Actinobacillus pleuropneumoniae*
> - Commensals on mucous membranes
> - Produce a wide range of disease conditions in domestic animals

positive, is relatively inactive biochemically.
- Serotyping of *A. pleuropneumoniae* isolates is based on differences in capsular polysaccharide antigens and is carried out using slide agglutination or gel-diffusion tests.

Pathogenesis and pathogenicity

The virulence factors possessed by the actinobacilli are poorly defined with the exception of those associated with *A. pleuropneumoniae*, the cause of pleuropneumonia in pigs.

Clinical infections

Actinobacilli can cause a variety of infections in farm animals including 'timber (wooden) tongue' in cattle, pleuropneumonia in pigs and systemic disease in foals and piglets (Fig. 21.1).

Actinobacillosis in cattle

Actinobacillosis, a chronic pyogranulomatous inflammation of soft tissues, is most often manifest clinically in cattle as induration of the tongue, referred to as timber tongue. Potentially important lesions occur in the oesophageal groove and the retropharyngeal lymph nodes. The aetiological agent, *Actinobacillus lignieresii*, is a commensal of the oral cavity and the intestinal tract. It can

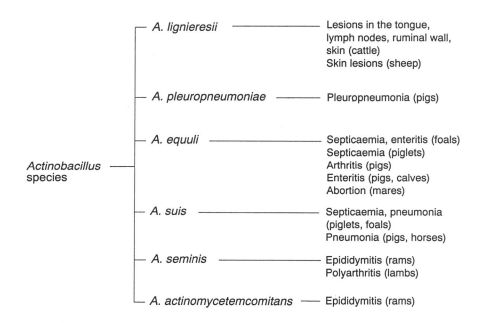

Figure 21.1 Actinobacillus species and the conditions which they cause in domestic animals.

survive for up to 5 days in hay or straw. The organisms enter tissues through erosions or lacerations in the mucosa and skin. A localized pyogranulomatous response is associated with club colonies containing the bacteria. In addition, spread through the lymphatics to the regional lymph nodes may induce pyogranulomatous lymphadenitis.

Bovine actinobacillosis is usually a sporadic disease, although herd outbreaks of limited extent can occur (Campbell *et al.*, 1975). Animals with timber tongue have difficulty in eating and drool saliva. Involvement of the tissues of the oesophageal groove can lead to intermittent tympany and enlargement of the retropharyngeal lymph nodes can cause difficulty in swallowing and stertorous breathing. Lesions of cutaneous actinobacillosis may be found on the head, thorax, flanks and upper limbs. Animals with ulcerated discharging lesions can contaminate the environment. Localized pyogranulomatous lesions in the retropharyngeal lymph nodes are often found at slaughter.

Diagnosis
- Induration of the tongue is characteristic of the disease and there may be a history of grazing rough pasture.
- Specimens for laboratory examination include pus, biopsy material and tissues from lesions at postmortem.
- Gram-negative rods are demonstrable in smears from exudates.
- Pyogranulomatous foci containing club colonies may be evident in tissue sections.
- Cultures on blood agar and MacConkey agar are incubated aerobically at 37°C for 24 to 72 hours.

- Identification criteria for isolates:
  — Small, sticky, non-haemolytic colonies on blood agar
  — Slow lactose fermentation on MacConkey agar
  — Biochemical profile (Table 21.1)

Treatment and Control
- Animals with discharging lesions should be isolated.
- Sodium iodide parenterally or potassium iodide orally is effective.
- Potentiated sulphonamides or a combination of penicillin and streptomycin are usually effective. Oral isoniazid for 30 days has been used in animals with refractory lesions.
- Rough feed or pasture which may damage the oral mucosa should be avoided.

Infections in other animals caused by *A. lignieresii*

Cutaneous actinobacillosis of sheep presents as granulomatous lesions mainly on the head without tongue involvement. Granulomatous mastitis in sows, bite wounds in dogs and glossitis in a horse have been attributed to infection with *A. lignieresii* (Baum *et al.*, 1984).

Pleuropneumonia of pigs

Pleuropneumonia, caused by *A. pleuropneumoniae*, can affect susceptible pigs of all ages and occurs in major pig-rearing regions worldwide. This highly contagious

Table 21.1 Differentiating features of *Actinobacillus* species.

Feature	A. lignieresii	A. pleuropneumoniae	A. equuli	A. suis
Haemolysis on sheep blood agar	–	+	v	+
Colony type on blood agar	Cohesive	Not cohesive	Cohesive	Cohesive
Growth on MacConkey agar	+	–	+	+
CAMP test with *S. aureus*	–	+	–	–
Oxidase production	+	v	+	+
Catalase production	+	v	v	+
Urease production	+	+	+	+
Hydrolysis of aesculin	–	–	–	+
Acid from:				
L-arabinose	v	–	–	+
lactose	+[a]	–	+	+
maltose	+	+	+	+
mannitol	+	v	+	–
melibiose	–	–	+	+
salicin	–	–	–	+
sucrose	+	+	+	+
trehalose	–	–	+	+

+   over 90% isolates positive   a   slow reaction
–   less than 10% isolates positive   v   variable reaction

disease, primarily in pigs under 6 months of age, appears to be increasing in prevalence as a consequence of intensive rearing practices.

Pathogenesis and pathogenicity

Virulence factors associated with *A. pleuropneumoniae* have been partially elucidated. Virulent strains possess capsules which are both antiphagocytic and immunogenic, whereas non-encapsulated strains are avirulent (Bertram, 1990). Fimbriae and other adhesins allow the organisms to attach to cells of the respiratory tract (Utrera and Pijoan, 1991). *Actinobacillus pleuropneumoniae* produces three related cytotoxins which belong to the repeats-in-structural-toxin (RTX) cytolysin family. These toxins act by producing pores in cell membranes. Neutrophils chemically attracted to infected lung tissue are damaged and release lytic enzymes. The sustained inflammatory response is considered to be a major factor in causing rapid tissue necrosis.

Clinical signs and epidemiology

Subclinical carrier pigs, which are encountered in unaffected populations, harbour the organisms in the respiratory tract and tonsillar tissues. Poor ventilation and sudden drops in ambient temperature seem to precipitate disease outbreaks. Aerosol transmission occurs in confined groups. In outbreaks of acute disease, some pigs may be found dead and others show dyspnoea, pyrexia, anorexia and a disinclination to move. Blood-stained froth may be present around the nose and mouth, and many pigs show cyanosis. Pregnant sows may abort. Morbidity rates can range from 30-50% and case fatality rates may reach 50%. Concurrent infections with *Pasteurella multocida* and mycoplasmas may exacerbate the condition. At post-mortem areas of consolidation and necrosis are found in the lungs along with fibrinous pleurisy. Blood-stained froth may be found in the trachea and bronchi.

Diagnosis

- There may be a history of ventilation failure or environmental temperature decrease prior to an outbreak of pulmonary disease.
- Specimens for laboratory examination should include tracheal washings or affected portions of lung tissue.
- Areas of haemorrhagic consolidation close to the main bronchi and severe fibrinous pleuritis may suggest this condition.
- Specimens, cultured on chocolate agar and blood agar,

are incubated in an atmosphere of 5-10% CO_2 at 37°C for 2 to 3 days.
- Identification criteria for isolates:
  — Small colonies surrounded by clear haemolysis
  — No growth on MacConkey agar
  — Positive CAMP test with *Staphylococcus aureus*
  — Biochemical profile (Table 21.1)
- Twelve serotypes and two biotypes are recognised (Komal and Mittal, 1990). Isolates belonging to biotype 1 require V factor (NAD) for growth whereas those belonging to biotype 2 are NAD-independent. The serotypes prevalent in a particular region should be identified prior to the implementation of vaccination programmes. Serological techniques are also used for epidemiological studies.
- Immunofluorescent techniques or PCR-based techniques may be used to demonstrate the organism in tissues.

Treatment
- As antibiotic resistance is encountered in some strains, chemotherapy should be based on the results of antibiotic susceptibility testing.
- Prophylactic administration of antibiotics to in-contact pigs may limit the severity of clinical disease.

Control
- Polyvalent bacterins may induce protective immunity but fail to prevent transmission or the development of a carrier state. A subunit vaccine containing toxoids of the three *A. pleuropneumoniae* toxins and capsular antigen has been developed (Valks *et al.*, 1996).
- Predisposing factors such as poor ventilation, chilling and overcrowding should be avoided.

Sleepy foal disease

Sleepy foal disease is an acute, potentially fatal septicaemia of newborn foals caused by *Actinobacillus equuli*. Although primarily a pathogen of foals, *A. equuli* occasionally produces disease conditions, such as abortion, septicaemia and peritonitis, in adult horses (Gay and Lording, 1980). The organism is found in the reproductive and intestinal tracts of mares. Foals can be infected *in utero* and after birth via the umbilicus. Affected foals are febrile and recumbent. Death usually occurs in 1 to 2 days. Foals which recover from the acute septicaemic phase may develop polyarthritis, nephritis, enteritis or pneumonia.

Foals dying within 24 hours of birth have petechiation on serosal surfaces and enteritis. Meningoencephalitis can be detectable histologically. Foals which survive for 1 to 3 days have typical pin-point suppurative foci in the kidneys.

Diagnosis
- History of the disease occurring on the premises in previous seasons.
- The clinical signs in a neonatal foal may suggest the disease.
- Specimens should be cultured on blood agar and MacConkey agar and incubated aerobically at 37°C for 1 to 3 days.
- Identification criteria for isolates:
  — Sticky colonies with variable haemolysis on blood agar
  — Lactose-fermenting colonies on MacConkey agar
  — Biochemical profile (Table 21.1)

Treatment and Control
Unless the disease is detected early, antimicrobial therapy is of little benefit.
- The organism is usually susceptible to streptomycin, tetracyclines and ampicillin.
- Supportive treatment includes blood transfusion and bottle-feeding with colostrum.
- Mares which have had affected foals should be monitored closely at subsequent foalings.
- Good hygiene should be observed.
- Prophylactic antibiotic therapy may be considered for newborn foals.
- No commercial vaccines are available.

Infections in other animals caused by *A. equuli*

Actinobacillus equuli occasionally produces septicaemia in neonatal pigs (Windsor, 1973). Enteritis in calves has been attributed to *A. equuli* (Osbaldiston and Walker, 1972).

Actinobacillus suis infection of piglets

Actinobacillus suis may be present in the upper respiratory tract of sows and piglets become infected by aerosols or possibly through skin abrasions. The infection occurs mainly in young pigs under 3 months of age (Sanford *et al.*, 1990). The disease is characterized by septicaemia and rapid death. Mortality may be up to 50% in some litters. Clinical signs include fever, respiratory distress, prostration and paddling of the forelimbs. Petechial and ecchymotic haemorrhages occur in many organs and there may be evidence of interstitial pneumonia, pleuritis, meningoencephalitis, myocarditis and arthritis. An unusual form of the infection in mature pigs has been reported with skin lesions resembling those of swine erysipelas (Miniats *et al.*, 1989).

Diagnosis
- Specimens from tissues, obtained at postmortem, should be cultured on blood agar and MacConkey agar and incubated at 37°C for 1 to 3 days.
- Identification criteria for isolates:

— Sticky, haemolytic colonies.

— Pink, lactose-fermenting colonies on MacConkey agar.

—Biochemical profile (Table 21.1).

Treatment and control

- Treatment should be based on antibiotic susceptibility testing of isolates. The organism is usually susceptible to ampicillin, carbenicillin, potentiated sulphonamides and tetracyclines.
- Contaminated pens should be disinfected.
- No commercial vaccines are available.

Actinobacillus suis infection in horses

Actinobacillus suis can be isolated from the upper respiratory tract of horses. Isolates from horses have sometimes been referred to as *A. suis*-like organisms. They have been associated with diseases resembling those produced by *A. equuli* in foals and occasionally in adult horses (Carman and Hodges, 1982; Nelson *et al.*, 1996).

Actinobacillus seminis infection in rams

Actinobacillus seminis is a common cause of epididymitis in young rams. The condition is endemic in New Zealand, Australia and South Africa, and has also been reported in the USA and the UK (Sponenberg *et al.*, 1982; Low *et al.*, 1995). The organism is found in the prepuce, and epididymitis occurs probably following an ascending opportunistic infection. Abscesses form in affected epididymides and there may be purulent discharge through fistulae onto the scrotal skin. Virgin rams between 4 and 8 months of age are most commonly affected.

Diagnosis

- Specimens for laboratory examination should include pus, biopsy material or tissue obtained at postmortem.
- Specimens should be cultured on blood agar and incubated aerobically at 37°C for 27 to 72 hours.
- Identification criteria for isolates:
  — Small pin-point, non-haemolytic colonies
  — No growth on MacConkey agar
  — Catalase-positive
  — Unreactive in many biochemical tests

References

Baum, K.H., Shin, S.J., Rebhun, W.C. and Pattern, V.H. (1984). Isolation of *Actinobacillus lignieresii* from enlarged tongue of a horse. *Journal of the American Veterinary Medical Association*, **185**, 792–793.

Betram, T.A. (1990). *Actinobacillus pleuropneumoniae*: molecular aspects of virulence and pulmonary injury. *Canadian Veterinary Journal*, **54**, S53–S56.

Campbell, S.G., Whitlock, R.H., Timoney, J.F. and Underwood, A.M. (1975). An unusual epizootic of actinobacillosis in dairy heifers. *Journal of the American Veterinary Medical Association*, **166**, 604–606.

Carman, M.G. and Hodges, R.T. (1982). *Actinobacillus suis* in horses. *New Zealand Veterinary Journal*, **30**, 82–84.

Dewhirst, F.E., Pasteur, B.J., Olsen, I. and Fraxser, G.J. (1992). Phylogeny of 54 representative strains of species in the family *Pasteurellaceae* as determined by comparison of 16S rRNA sequences. *Journal of Bacteriology,* **174**, 2002–2013

Gay, C.C. and Lording, P.M. (1980). Peritonitis in horses associated with *Actinobacillus equuli*. *Australian Veterinary Journal,* **56**, 296–300.

Komal, J.P.S. and Mittal, K.R. (1990). Grouping of *Actinobacillus pleuropneumoniae* strains of serotype 1 through 12 on the basis of their virulence in mice. *Veterinary Microbiology*, **25**, 229–240.

Low, J.C., Somerville, D., Mylne, M.J.A. and McKelvey, W.A.C. (1995). Prevalence of *Actinobacillus seminis* in the semen of rams in the United Kingdom. *Veterinary Record*, **136**, 268–269.

Miniats, O.P., Spinato, M.T. and Sanford, S.E. (1989). *Actinobacillus suis* septicaemia in mature swine: two outbreaks resembling erysipelas. *Canadian Veterinary Journal*, **30**, 943–947.

Nelson, K.M., Darien, B.J., Konkle, D.M. and Hartmann, F.A. (1996). *Actinobacillus suis* septicaemia in two foals. *Veterinary Record*, **138**, 39–40.

Osbaldiston, G.W. and Walker, R.D. (1972). Enteric actinobacillosis in calves. *Cornell Veterinarian*, **62**, 364–371.

Sanford, S.E., Josephson, G.K.A., Rehmtulla, A.J. and Tilker, A.M.E. (1990). *Actinobacillus suis* infection in pigs in south eastern Ontario. *Canadian Veterinary Journal*, **31**, 443–447.

Sponenberg, D.P., Carter, M.E., Carter, G.R., Cordes, D.O., Stevens, S.E. and Veit, H.P. (1982). Suppurative epididymitis in a ram infected with *Actinobacillus seminis*. *Journal of the American Veterinary Medical Association,* **182**, 990–991.

Utrera, V. and Pijoan, C. (1991). Fimbriae of *Actinobacillus pleuropneumoniae* strains isolated from pig respiratory tracts. *Veterinary Record*, **128**, 357–358.

Valks, M.M.H., Nell, T. and van den Bosch, J.F. (1996). A clinical field trial in finishing pigs to evaluate the efficacy of a new APP subunit vaccine. In *Proceedings of the 14th International Pig Veterinary Society Congress, Bologna, Italy.* 7–10 July. p. 208.

Windsor, R.S. (1973). *Actinobacillus equuli* infection in a litter of pigs and a review of previous reports on similar infections. *Veterinary Record*, **92**, 178–180.

Further reading

Burrows, L.L. and Lo, R.Y.C. (1992). Molecular characterization of an RTX toxin determinant from *Actinobacillus suis*. *Infection and Immunity*, **60**, 2166–2173.

Duff, J.P., Scott, W.A., Wilkes, M.K. and Hunt, B. (1996). Otitis in a weaned pig: a new pathological role for *Actinobacillus*

(*Haemophilus*) *pleuropneumoniae*. *Veterinary Record*, **139**, 561–563.

Habrun, B., Frey, J., Bilic, V., Nicolet, J. and Humski, A. (1998). Prevalence of serotypes and toxin types of *Actinobacillus pleuropneumoniae* in pigs in Croatia. *Veterinary Record*, **143**, 255–256.

Rycroft, A.N., Woldeselassie, A., Gordon, P.J. and Bjornson, A. (1998). Serum antibody in equine neonatal septicaemia due to *Actinobacillus equuli*. *Veterinary Record*, **143**, 254–255.

Chapter 22

Pasteurella species and *Mannheimia haemolytica*

Pasteurella and *Mannheimia* species are small (0.2 x 1-2 μm) non-motile, Gram-negative rods or coccobacilli. They are oxidase-positive facultative anaerobes, and most species are catalase-positive. Although non-enriched media will support their growth, these organisms grow best on media supplemented with blood or serum. They usually remain viable for only a few days on culture plates. Some species, such as *Mannheimia haemolytica*, *Pasteurella trehalosi* and *P. aerogenes* can tolerate the bile salts in MacConkey agar. In smears from infected tissues stained by the Giemsa method, pasteurellae exhibit bipolar staining (Fig. 22.1).

The family *Pasteurellaceae* comprises five genera, *Actinobacillus*, *Haemophilus*, *Mannheimia*, *Pasteurella* and *Lonepinella*. These genera share a number of common features and some organisms have been reclassified within these genera following deoxyribonucleic acid hybridization studies and 16S rRNA sequencing. *Pasteurella aerogenes*, *P. trehalosi* and *P. pneumotropica* are more closely related to members of the genus *Actinobacillus* than they are to other *Pasteurella* species (Mutters *et al.*, 1985). *Pasteurella trehalosi* is now used to denote *Pasteurella haemolytica* biotype T isolates while biotype A isolates of *P. haemolytica* have been allocated to a new genus and renamed *Mannheimia haemolytica* (Sneath and Stevens, 1990; Angen *et al.*, 1999). *Pasteurella multocida*, *P. trehalosi* and *M. haemolytica* are major pathogens (Table 22.1). The genera *Actinobacillus* and *Haemophilus* also contain major pathogens of

> **Key points**
> - Small Gram-negative rods
> - Optimal growth on enriched media
> - Non-motile, oxidase-positive, facultative anaerobes
> - Most species are catalase-positive
> - Some species grow on MacConkey agar
> - Bipolar staining is prominent in smears from lesions, using the Giemsa method
> - Commensals in the upper respiratory tract
> - Respiratory pathogens

domestic animals (*see* Chapters 21 and 24). Other *Pasteurella* and *Mannheimia* species which have been isolated from domestic animals and man are presented in Table 22.2.

Usual habitat

Most *Pasteurella* and *Mannheimia* species are commensals on the mucosae of the upper respiratory tract of animals. Their survival in the environment is relatively short.

Differentiation of *Pasteurella* and *Mannheimia* species

Pasteurellae and *Mannheimia* species can be distinguished by colonial and growth characteristics, and by biochemical reactions. Strains of *P. multocida* can be differentiated by serotyping and biotyping, whereas *M. haemolytica*/*P. trehalosi* strains are differentiated by serotyping.
- Colonial characteristics:
  —*P. multocida* colonies are round, greyish, shiny and non-haemolytic. Colonies of some pathogenic strains are mucoid due to the production of thick hyaluronic acid capsules. The colonies have a subtle but characteristic sweetish odour.
  —*M. haemolytica*, *M. granulomatis* and *P. trehalosi* colonies are haemolytic and odourless.
  —Colonies of the other *Pasteurella* species are round, greyish and non-haemolytic except those of

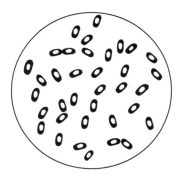

Figure 22.1 Bipolar staining of *Pasteurella* species. Bacteria in Giemsa-stained blood smears from lesions have this characteristic staining pattern.

Table 22.1 The major pathogenic *Pasteurella* and *Mannheimia* species, their principal hosts and associated diseases.

Pasteurella species	Hosts	Disease conditions
P. multocida		
type A	Cattle	Associated with bovine pneumonic pasteurellosis (shipping fever); associated with enzootic pneumonia complex of calves; mastitis (rare)
	Sheep	Pneumonia; mastitis
	Pigs	Pneumonia, atrophic rhinitis
	Poultry	Fowl cholera
	Rabbits	Snuffles
	Other animal species	Pneumonia following stress
type B	Cattle, buffaloes	Haemorrhagic septicaemia (Asia)
type D	Pigs	Atrophic rhinitis, pneumonia
type E	Cattle, buffaloes	Haemorrhagic septicaemia (Africa)
M. haemolytica (*P. haemolytica* biotype A)	Cattle	Bovine pneumonic pasteurellosis (shipping fever)
	Sheep	Septicaemia (under 3 months of age); pneumonia; gangrenous mastitis
P. trehalosi (*P. haemolytica* biotype T)	Sheep	Septicaemia (5 to 12 months of age)

P. testudinis, which are haemolytic.
- On MacConkey agar, *M. haemolytica* and *P. trehalosi* grow as pin-point, red colonies. Most pathogenic *Pasteurella* species do not grow on MacConkey agar.
- Methods for differentiating the main pathogenic *Pasteurella* and *Mannheimia* species are summarized in Table 22.3.
- *Pasteurella* and *Mannheimia* species are relatively active biochemically:
  — Reactions in conventional biochemical tests are indicated in Table 22.3.
  — Commercially-available biochemical test strips can also be used.
  — In TSI agar slopes, a yellow slant and yellow butt without H_2S production are typical.
- Serotyping of *Pasteurella* and *Mannheimia* species:
  — The types (or serogroups) of *P. multocida* are identified on the basis of differences in capsular polysaccharides (Carter, 1955) and are designated A, B, D, E and F (Table 22.1). The organisms are further subdivided into about 16 somatic types on the basis of serological differences in cell wall lipopolysaccharides (Heddleston *et al.*, 1972; Namioka and Murata, 1961). Both capsular and somatic antigens

are used to designate a specific serotype. Serological methods for establishing both the capsular and somatic types include agglutination and agar gel diffusion tests. An indirect haemagglutination test can be used for identification of capsular antigens.
  — Seventeen serotypes of *M. haemolytica/P. trehalosi* are recognised on the basis of extractable surface antigens. A passive haemagglutination procedure or a rapid plate agglutination test may be used to identify each serotype. Serotypes 3, 4, 10 and 15 are classified as *P. trehalosi*; the remaining serotypes are classified as *M. haemolytica* except serotype 11 which is reclassified as *M. glucosida*.
- Biotyping of *Pasteurella multocida* is occasionally carried out in epidemiological investigations but is not generally used for diagnosis. Three biotypes or

Table 22.2 *Pasteurella* and *Mannheimia* species of minor veterinary significance.

Pasteurella species	Hosts	Comments
P. aerogenes	Pigs	Intestinal commensal; rarely implicated in abortion
P. anatis	Ducks	Found in intestine
P. avium *P. langaaensis* (*P. langaa*) *P. volantium*	Chickens	Commensals in upper respiratory tract
P. caballi	Horses	Commensal in the upper respiratory tract; occasionally implicated in respiratory disease and peritonitis
P. canis	Dogs	Commensal in oral cavity; occasionally infects wounds
P. dagmatis	Dogs, cats	Commensal in oral cavity and nasopharynx; occasionally infects wounds
P. gallinarum	Poultry	Commensal in the upper respiratory tract; occasional low-grade infections
M. granulomatis	Cattle	Fibrogranulomatous panniculitis
P. lymphangitidis	Cattle	Lymphangitis (rare)
P. mairii	Pigs	Abortion (rare)
P. pneumotropica	Rodents	Commensal in the upper respiratory tract; sporadic cases of pneumonia and bite-wound abscess
P. stomatis	Dogs, cats	Found in respiratory tract
P. testudinis	Turtles, tortoises	Abscessation (rare)

Table 22.3 Differentiation of the main pathogenic *Pasteurella* and *Mannheimia* species.

Feature	M. haemolytica	Pasteurella species		
		P. multocida	P. trehalosi	P. pneumotropica
Haemolysis on sheep blood agar	+	−	+	−
Growth on MacConkey agar	+	−	+	v
Distinctive odour from colonies	−	+	−	−
Indole production	−	+	−	+
Catalase activity	+	+	−	+
Urease activity	−	−	−	+
Ornithine decarboxylase activity	−	+	−	+
Acid from:				
lactose	+	−	−	v
sucrose	+	+	+	+
D-trehalose	−	v	+	+
L-arabinose	−	v	−	−
maltose	+	−	+	v
D-xylose	+	v	−	v

+   most strains positive
−   most strains negative
v   variable reactions

subspecies of *P. multocida* are recognised, namely *P. multocida* subspecies *multocida*, *P. multocida* subspecies *septica* and *P. multocida* subspecies *gallicida*.

Pathogenesis and pathogenicity

Many *P. multocida* infections are endogenous. The organisms, which are normally commensals of the upper respiratory tract, may invade the tissues of immunosuppressed animals. Exogenous transmission can also occur either by direct contact or through aerosols. Factors of importance in the development of disease include adhesion of the pasteurellae to the mucosa and the avoidance of phagocytosis. Fimbriae may enhance mucosal attachment and the capsule, particularly in type A strains, has a major antiphagocytic role. In septicaemic pasteurellosis, severe endotoxaemia and disseminated intravascular coagulation cause serious illness which can prove fatal.

Four main virulence factors have been identified in strains of *M. haemolytica* and *P. trehalosi* (Confer *et al.*, 1990): fimbriae which may enhance colonization; a capsule that inhibits complement-mediated destruction of the organisms in serum; endotoxin which can alter bovine leukocyte functions and is directly toxic to bovine endothelial cells; leukotoxin, a pore-forming cytolysin that affects leukocyte and platelet functions when present at low concentrations and causes cytolysis at high concentrations. The subsequent release from damaged cells of lysosomal enzymes and inflammatory mediators, such as tumour necrosis factor-α and eicosanoids, contributes to severe tissue damage in these infections.

Diagnostic procedures

- There may be a history of exposure to stress arising from transportation or overcrowding.
- Suitable specimens for laboratory examination from live animals include tracheobronchial aspirates, nasal swabs or mastitic milk.
- Tissue or blood smears from septicaemic cases, stained by Giemsa or Leishman methods, may reveal large numbers of bipolar-staining organisms.
- Specimens should be cultured on blood agar and MacConkey agar. Plates are incubated aerobically at 37°C for 24 to 48 hours. Blood agar, supplemented with neomycin, bacitracin and actidione, can be used for the isolation of *P. multocida* from heavily contaminated specimens.
- Identification criteria for isolates:
  — Colonial characteristics
  — Growth on MacConkey agar
  — Positive oxidase test
  — Biochemical profile

Control

- Chemoprophylaxis with sulphonamides, trimethoprim, tylosin or tetracyclines in weaner, grower and sow rations could be considered.
- Improvement in husbandry must be instituted to minimize the influence of predisposing factors.
- Vaccination with a combined *B. bronchiseptica* bacterin and *P. multocida* toxoid may reduce the severity of the disease and improve growth rates (Voets *et al.*, 1992). Sows should be vaccinated at 4 and 2 weeks before farrowing and young piglets at 1 week and 4 weeks of age.

Fowl cholera

Fowl cholera is a primary avian pasteurellosis caused by *P. multocida* capsular type A. It is highly contagious and affects both domestic and wild birds. The disease usually presents as an acute septicaemia which is often fatal. Turkeys tend to be more susceptible than chickens. Postmortem lesions include haemorrhages on serous surfaces and accumulation of fluid in body cavities. In sporadic chronic cases of the disease, the signs and lesions are often related to localized infections. The wattles, sternal bursae and joints are usually swollen due to the accumulation of fibrinopurulent exudates.

In the acute septicaemic form of the disease, numerous characteristic bipolar-staining organisms can be detected in blood smears and *P. multocida* can be isolated from blood, bone marrow, liver or spleen. The bacterium may be difficult to isolate from chronic lesions.

Medication of the feed or water with sulphonamides or tetracyclines early in an outbreak of acute disease may decrease the mortality rate. Polyvalent adjuvant bacterins are widely used. Autogenous vaccines may be required if the commercial vaccines are ineffective. Modified live vaccines are available in some countries.

Snuffles in rabbits

Snuffles is a common, recurring, purulent rhinitis in rabbits which is caused by type A strains of *P. multocida*. *Bordetella bronchiseptica* infection may sometimes cause similar clinical signs. *Pasteurella multocida* is a commensal in the upper respiratory tract of healthy carrier rabbits. Clinical disease is often precipitated by stress factors such as overcrowding, chilling, transportation, concurrent infections and poor ventilation resulting in high levels of atmospheric ammonia. There is a purulent nasal discharge which cakes on the fore legs because affected rabbits paw their noses. Sneezing and coughing may be observed. Sequelae include conjunctivitis, otitis media and subcutaneous abscessation. Bronchopneumonia may develop in young rabbits. Treatment or prophylactic therapy with antibiotics may be of value. Predisposing stress factors must be eliminated. No vaccine is available.

References

Angen, O., Mutters, R., Caugant, D.A., Olsen, J.E. and Bisgaard, M. (1999). Taxonomic relationships of the [*Pasteurella*] *haemolytica* complex as evaluated by DNA-DNA hybridizations and 16S rRNA sequencing with proposal of *Mannheimia haemolytica* gen. nov., comb. nov., *Mannheimia granulomatis* comb. nov., *Mannheimia glucosida* sp. nov., *Mannheimia ruminalis* sp. nov. and *Mannheimia varigena* sp. nov. *International Journal of Systematic Bacteriology*, **49**, 67–86.

Carter, G.R. (1955). Studies on *Pasteurella multocida*. 1. A haemagglutination test for the identification of serological types. *American Journal of Veterinary Research*, **16**, 481–484.

Chanter, N., Rutter, J.M. and Luther, P.D. (1986). Rapid detection of toxigenic *Pasteurella multocida* by an agar overlay method. *Veterinary Record*, **119**, 629–630.

Confer, A.W., Panciera, R.J., Clinkenbeard, K.D. and Mosier, D.M. (1990). Molecular aspects of virulence of *Pasteurella haemolytica*. *Canadian Journal of Veterinary Research*, **54**, 548–552.

Dalgleish, R. (1990). Bovine pneumonic pasteurellosis. *In Practice*, **12**, 223–226.

De Alwis, M.C.L. (1992). Haemorrhagic septicaemia – a general review. *British Veterinary Journal*, **148**, 99–112.

Donachie, E. (2000). Bacteriology of bovine respiratory disease. *Cattle Practice*, 8, 5–7.

Faged, N.T., Neilsen, J.P. and Pedersen, K.B. (1988). Differentiation of toxigenic from non-toxigenic isolates of *Pasteurella multocida* by enzyme-linked immunosorbent assay. *Journal of Clinical Microbiology*, **26**, 1419–1420.

Heddleston, K.L., Gallagher, J.E. and Rebers, P.A. (1972). Fowl cholera: gel diffusion precipitin test for serotyping *Pasteurella multocida* from avian species. *Avian Diseases*, **16**, 925–936.

Mutters, R., Ihm, P., Pohl, S., Frederiksen, W. and Mannheim, W. (1985). Reclassification of the genus *Pasteurella* Trevison 1887 on the basis of deoxyribonucleic acid homology, with proposals for the new species *P. dagmatis*, *P. canis*, *P. stomatis*, *P. anatis* and *P. langaa*. *International Journal of Systematic Bacteriology*, **35**, 309–322.

Myint, A. and Carter, G.R. (1989). Prevention of haemorrhagic septicaemia in buffaloes and cattle with a live vaccine. *Veterinary Record*, **124**, 508–509.

Nagai, S., Someno, S. and Yagihashi, T. (1994). Differentiation of toxigenic from non-toxigenic isolates of *Pasteurella multocida* by PCR. *Journal of Clinical Microbiology*, **32**, 1004–1010.

Namioka, S. and Murata, M. (1961). Serological studies on *Pasteurella multocida*. II Characteristics of somatic (O) antigens of the organism. *Cornell Veterinarian*, **51**, 507–521.

Rutter, M. (1989). Atrophic rhinitis. *In Practice*, **11**, 74–80.

Rutter, J.M. and Luther, P.D. (1984). Cell culture assay for toxigenic *Pasteurella multocida* from atrophic rhinitis of pigs. *Veterinary Record*, **114**, 393–396.

Schreuer, D., Schuhmacher, C., Touffet, S., *et al.* (2000).

Evaluation of the efficacy of a new combined (*Pasteurella*) *Mannheimia haemolytica* serotype A1 and A6 vaccine in preruminant calves by virulent challenge. *Cattle Practice*, **8**, 9–12.

Sneath, P.H.A. and Stevens, M. (1990). *Actinobacillus rossii* sp. nov., *Actinobacillus seminis* sp. nov., nom. rev., *Pasteurella bettii* sp. nov., *Pasteurella lymphangitidis* sp. nov., *Pasteurella mairi* sp. nov. and *Pasteurella trehalosi* sp. nov. *International Journal of Systematic Bacteriology*, **40**, 148–153.

Voets, M.T., Klaassen, C.H.L., Charlier, P., Wiseman, A. and Descamps, J. (1992). Evaluation of atrophic rhinitis vaccine under controlled conditions. *Veterinary Record,* **130**, 549–553.

Further reading

DiGiacomo, R.F., Xu, Y., Allen, V., Hinton, M.H. and Pearson, G.R. (1991). Naturally acquired *Pasteurella multocida* infection in rabbits: clinicopathological aspects. *Canadian Journal of Veterinary Research*, **55**, 234–238.

Goodwin, R.F.W., Chanter, N. and Rutter, J.M. (1990). Screening pig herds for toxigenic *Pasteurella multocida* and turbinate damage in a health scheme for atrophic rhinitis. *Veterinary Record*, **127**, 83–86.

Gonzales, C.T. and Maheswaran, S.K. (1993). The role of induced virulence factors produced by *Pasteurella haemolytica* in the pathogenesis of bovine pneumonic pasteurellosis: review and hypothesis. *British Veterinary Journal*, **149**, 183–193.

Holst, E., Rollof, J., Larsson, L. and Nielsen, J.P. (1992). Characterization and distribution of *Pasteurella* species recovered from infected humans. *Journal of Clinical Microbiology*, **30**, 2984–2987.

Riet-Correa, F., Mendez, M.C., Schild, A.L., Ribeiro, G.A. and Almeida, S.M. (1992). Bovine focal proliferative fibrogranulomatous panniculitis (Lechiguana) associated with *Pasteurella granulomatis*. *Veterinary Pathology*, **29**, 93–103.

Ward, C.L., Wood, J.L.N., Houghton, S.B., Mumford, J.A. and Chanter, N. (1998). *Actinobacillus* and *Pasteurella* species isolated from horses with lower airway disease. *Veterinary Record*, **143**, 277–279.

Chapter 23

Francisella tularensis

Francisella tularensis, originally classified as a *Pasteurella* species, is a poorly staining Gram-negative rod (0.2 x 0.2-0.7 μm) which tends to have a coccobacillary appearance. It is an obligate aerobe, non-motile, oxidase-negative and weakly catalase-positive. This fastidious organism requires the addition of cysteine or cystine to blood agar for growth. It does not grow on MacConkey agar.

Francisella tularensis has a high lipid content and virulent isolates from infected animals produce capsules. Highly virulent type A strains, *F. tularensis* subspecies *tularensis* (formerly subsp. *nearctica*), occur only in North America. Less virulent type B strains, *F. tularensis* subspecies *holarctica* (formerly subsp. *palaearctica*) which are assigned to two biogroups (Pearson, 1998), are found in both Eurasia and North America (Fig. 23.1). Distinguishing features of the subspecies are presented in Table 23.1.

Two other *Francisella* species, *F. novicida* and *F. philomiragia* may be associated with human infections (Hollis *et al.*, 1989).

Usual habitat

Reservoir hosts of *F. tularensis* include lagomorphs, rodents, galliform birds and deer. *Francisella tularensis* may survive for 3-4 months in mud, water and contaminated carcasses (Rohrbach, 1988). Type A strains are associated with terrestrial animal reservoirs and type B

> **Key points**
> - Gram-negative coccobacillary rods
> - Non-motile, obligate aerobes
> - Fastidious, cysteine required for growth
> - No growth on MacConkey agar
> - Oxidase-negative, catalase-positive
> - Facultative intracellular pathogen
> - Survives in the environment for up to 4 months
> - Wildlife reservoirs and arthropods important in epidemiology
> - Causes tularaemia in animals and humans

strains are frequently linked to water-borne infections and to aquatic mammals such as beavers and muskrats.

Epidemiology

Ticks and the deerfly (*Chrysops discalis*) are important vectors in North America. The main tick species, in which *F. tularensis* can be passed trans-stadially and trans-ovarially, include *Dermacentor variabilis, D. andersoni* and *Amblyomma americanum*. At each stage of their life cycles, these ticks usually feed on vertebrate hosts different from, and larger than, the hosts parasitized at the previous stage. Direct transmission between domestic animals is uncommon.

Clinical infections

Francisella tularensis can infect wildlife species, domestic animals and humans. Fulminant disease can occur in immunosuppressed individuals. Chronic, granulomatous lesions or subclinical infections may develop. Type A strains probably account for the majority of clinical infections in domestic animals while type B strains tend to cause a comparatively mild illness which may not be evident.

Tularaemia in domestic animals

Although infection with *F. tularensis* is probably common

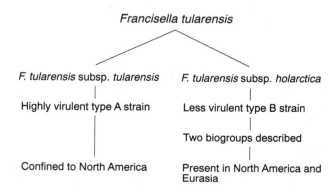

Figure 23.1 Geographical distribution and comparison of the subspecies of *Francisella tularensis*.

in domestic animals in endemic areas, outbreaks of tularaemia are relatively rare. The disease has been reported in sheep (Frank and Meinershagen, 1961), horses (Claus *et al.*, 1959) and young pigs.

Adult pigs and cattle appear to be comparatively resistant to infection. Dogs and cats may be infected and seroconvert without clinical signs of disease. In serological surveys, significant antibody titres to the pathogen were found in 6% of feral cats (McKeever *et al.*, 1958) and 48% of dogs (Schmid *et al.*, 1983).

Pathogenesis and pathology

Infection with *F. tularensis* usually occurs through skin abrasions or by arthropod bites. Animals can also acquire infection through inhalation or by ingestion. The organism is a facultative, intracellular pathogen which can survive in macrophages but not in neutrophils. In macrophages the organism inhibits phagosome/lysosome fusion and replicates in acidified phagosomes. The acidification of these vacuoles is essential for the release of iron from transferrin (Fortier *et al.*, 1995). Iron is a growth requirement for the organism.

Lymphadenitis, either local or generalized, is a constant finding and septicaemia is common. Pale necrotic foci are present in enlarged superficial lymph nodes and miliary lesions may be evident in the liver and spleen. Areas of pulmonary consolidation may also be present. Primary pulmonary lesions due to aerosol inhalation have been described in affected dogs.

Clinical signs

Outbreaks of tularaemia have been reported in sheep and other domestic animals. Transmission of infection often correlates with heavy tick infestation.

Table 23.1 Distinguishing features of *Francisella tularensis* subspecies *tularensis* and *F. tularensis* subspecies *holarctica*.

Feature	*F. tularensis* subsp. *tularensis* (type A)	*F. tularensis* subsp. *holarctica* (type B)
Pathogenicity	Classical tularaemia in animals and humans	Less serious disease in animals and humans
Reservoirs	Lagomorphs, rodents, galliform birds	Water, mud, aquatic animals
Capsule production	+	+
Cysteine required for growth	+	+
Citrulline ureidase activity	+	−
Acid from glucose	+	−

In most domestic species, the disease is characterized by fever, depression, inappetence, stiffness and other manifestations of septicaemia.

Diagnosis

- Although clinical signs are non-specific, heavy tick infestation in severely ill animals in endemic regions may indicate the presence of tularaemia.
- Suitable specimens for laboratory tests include blood for serology, scrapings from ulcers, lymph node aspirates and biopsy material or postmortem samples from affected tissues.
- Agglutination antibody titres of 1:80 or higher are presumptive evidence of infection with *F. tularensis*. A rising antibody titre is indicative of an active infection.
- A fluorescent antibody technique can be used for the identification of *F. tularensis* in tissues or exudates and from cultures.
- Isolation procedures for *F. tularensis* must be carried out in a biohazard cabinet. Special precautions should also be observed when handling suspect cases of tularaemia and during postmortem examinations.
- Glucose-cysteine-blood agar is used for culture with the addition of antibiotics when samples are contaminated. Plates are incubated aerobically at 37°C for up to 7 days.
- Identification criteria for isolates:
  — Small, grey, mucoid colonies, surrounded by a narrow zone of incomplete haemolysis, appear after incubation for 3 to 4 days.
  — Immunofluorescence can be used to confirm the identity of the pathogen in smears from the colonies.
  — A slide agglutination test can be carried out on cultures using antiserum specific to *F. tularensis*.
  — Biochemical tests for distinguishing type A strains from type B strains are carried out in reference laboratories (Table 23.1).
- Detection of *F. tularensis* in blood by polymerase chain reaction procedures has been reported (Long *et al.*, 1993).
- If samples contain few organisms, isolation in embryonated eggs or laboratory animals can be attempted.

Treatment

Effective antibiotics include amikacin, streptomycin, imipenem-cilastatin and the fluoroquinolones. A high relapse rate may occur if animals are treated with bacteriostatic antibiotics.

Control

Defined control measures are required in endemic areas as there are no commercially available vaccines for use in animals.

- Ectoparasite control is essential. Daily removal of ticks

from dogs and cats is advisable.
- Precautions should be taken to prevent contamination of food and water with infected carcasses or excreta of wildlife species.
- In endemic regions dogs and cats should be prevented from hunting wildlife species.

Tularaemia in humans

Tularaemia in humans, a serious and potentially fatal infection, often presents as a slow-healing ulcer accompanied by lymphadenopathy. Individuals particularly at risk, such as hunters, trappers, veterinarians and laboratory workers, should take precautions when handling suspect animals or materials.

A modified live vaccine is available for personnel working with *F. tularensis* in specialized laboratories.

References

Claus, K.D., Newhall, J.H. and Mee, D. (1959). Isolation of *Pasteurella tularensis* from foals. *Journal of Bacteriology*, **78**, 294–295.

Fortier, A.H., Leiby, D.A., Narayanan, R.B., Asafoadjei, E., Crawford, R.M., Nancy, C.A. and Meltzer, M.S. (1995). Growth of *Francisella tularensis* LVS in macrophages: the acidic intracellular compartment provides essential iron required for growth. *Infection and Immunity*, **63**, 1478–1483.

Frank, F.W. and Meinershagen, W.A. (1961). Tularemia epizootic in sheep. *Veterinary Medicine*, **56**, 374–378.

Hollis, D.G., Weaver, R.E., Steigerwalt, A.G., Wenger, J.D., Wayne Moss, C. and Brenner, D.J. (1989). *Francisella philomiragia* comb. nov. (formerly *Yersinia philomiragia*) and *Francisella tularensis* biogroup *novicida* (formerly *Francisella novicida*) associated with human disease. *Journal of Clinical Microbiology*, **27**, 1601–1608.

Long, G.W., Oprandy, J.J., Narayanan, R.B., Fortier, A.H., Porter, K.R. and Nacy, C.A. (1993). Detection of *Francisella tularensis* in blood by polymerase chain reaction. *Journal of Clinical Microbiology*, **31**, 152–154.

McKeever, S., Schubert, J.H. and Moody, M.D. (1958). Natural occurrence of tularemia in marsupials, carnivores, lagomorphs and large rodents in southwestern Georgia and northwestern Florida. *Journal of Infectious Diseases*, **103**, 120–126.

Pearson, A. (1998). Tularaemia. In *Zoonoses – Biology, Clinical Practice and Public Health Control*. Eds. S.R. Palmer, E.J.L. Soulsby and D.I.H. Simpson. Oxford University Press, Oxford. pp. 267–279.

Rohrbach, B.W. (1988). Zoonosis update: Tularemia. *Journal of the American Veterinary Medical Association*, **193**, 428–432.

Schmid, G.P., Kornblatt, A.N. and Connors, C.A. (1983). Clinically mild tularemia associated with tick-borne *Francisella tularensis*. *Journal of Infectious Diseases*, **148**, 63–67.

Chapter 24

Haemophilus species

Haemophilus species are small (less than 1 μm x 1 to 3 μm), Gram-negative rods, which often appear coccobacillary and may occasionally form short filaments. These motile organisms, which are facultative anaerobes with variable reactions in catalase and oxidase tests, do not grow on MacConkey agar. They are fastidious bacteria requiring one or both of the growth factors X (haemin) and V (nicotinamide adenine dinucleotide, NAD). Optimal growth occurs in an atmosphere of 5-10% CO_2 on chocolate agar which supplies both X and V factors. Small, transparent, dewdrop-like colonies are formed by most *Haemophilus* species after incubation for 48 hours. Colonies of '*H. somnus*' have a yellowish hue and some isolates are haemolytic on sheep blood agar.

The main pathogens in the genus are '*H. somnus*' in cattle and sheep, *H. parasuis* in pigs and *H. paragallinarum* which is responsible for infectious coryza of chickens (Table 24.1). Other *Haemophilus* species, which are commensals on the mucous membranes of animals, rarely cause disease (Table 24.2). The soluble antigens of *Haemophilus* species exhibit heterogenicity. More than 12 serotypes of *H. parasuis*, 15 serotypes of '*H. somnus*' and

Key points
■ Small, motile Gram-negative rods
■ Fastidious, requirement for the X and V factors in chocolate agar
■ Optimal growth in 5-10% CO_2
■ Facultative anaerobes
■ Commensals on mucous membranes of many animal species
■ Important pathogens include '*Haemophilus somnus*' (cattle) *H. parasuis* (pigs) and *H. paragallinarum* (poultry)

approximately 9 serotypes of *H. paragallinarum* have been identified.

Nucleic acid hybridization studies and the development of a sensitive porphyrin test for factor X requirement have resulted in reclassification of some species in the genus. '*Haemophilus somnus*' has been retained in the genus although it does not have a requirement for either the X or V factors. Furthermore, the name '*Haemophilus somnus*' has not been validated and has no standing in recognised nomenclature. *Haemophilus agni* and *Histophilus ovis* are now considered to be ovine strains of '*H. somnus*' (Walker *et al.*, 1985; Corbeil *et al.*, 1995).

Usual habitat

Haemophilus species are commensals on the mucous membranes of the upper respiratory tract. They are susceptible to desiccation and do not survive for long periods away from their hosts.

Differentiation of *Haemophilus* species

Haemophilus species are differentiated by requirements for X and V growth factors, by growth enhancement in an atmosphere of CO_2, by catalase and oxidase reactions and by carbohydrate utilization (Table 24.3).

- Isolation techniques
  Both X and V factors are required in media for isolation

Table 24.1 *Haemophilus* species of veterinary importance.

Haemophilus species	Hosts	Disease conditions
'*H. somnus*'	Cattle	Septicaemia, thrombotic meningoencephalitis, bronchopneumonia (in association with other pathogens), sporadic reproductive tract infections
'*H. somnus*' (ovine strains)	Sheep	Epididymitis in young rams; vulvitis, mastitis and reduced reproductive performance in ewes; septicaemia, arthritis, meningitis and pneumonia in lambs
H. parasuis	Pigs	Glasser's disease, secondary invader in respiratory disease
H. paragallinarum	Chickens Pheasants, turkeys, guinea fowl	Infectious coryza Respiratory disease

Table 24.2 *Haemophilus* species which occur as commensals in domestic animals.

Haemophilus species	Host	Comments
H. aphrophilus	Dog	Commensal of pharynx
H. felis	Cat	Commensal of nasopharynx; occasionally involved in respiratory disease
H. haemo-globinophilus	Dog	Commensal of the lower genital tract
'*H. ovis*'	Sheep	Commensal in respiratory tract; rarely implicated in broncho-pneumonia
H. paracuniculus	Rabbits	Isolated from intestines

of some *Haemophilus* species. Although '*H. somnus*' does not have an absolute requirement for these factors, its growth is enhanced by their presence. The X factor is heat stable and is present in red blood cells. The heat-labile V factor, which is also present in red blood cells, is susceptible to NADases in plasma. There are two common methods for ensuring the availability of both X and V factors in culture media:

— Chocolate agar, which supplies both factors, is prepared by heating molten blood agar in a water bath at 80°C for about 10 minutes. The chocolate-brown colour of the medium is due to lysis of the red cells. The heat-stable X factor, released from the lysed cells, is unaffected by this procedure. The V factor, which is also released from the lysed cells, tolerates a temperature of 80°C for a short period whereas the plasma NADases which degrade V factor are destroyed.

— *Staphylococcus aureus* growing on blood agar releases V factor into the medium. Colonies of *Haemophilus* species which require V factor grow close to the *S. aureus* colony, a phenomenon referred to as satellitism.

• Tests for X and V factor requirements:
— The disc method for determining X and V factor

requirements is illustrated and explained in Fig. 24.1. This test is particularly suitable for determining V factor requirement.

— The porphyrin test is a more accurate method for determining the growth requirement for X factor. The *Haemophilus* isolate is grown at 37°C for 4 hours in broth containing a porphyrin precursor. When the culture is exposed to UV light in the dark, porphyrin production is detected by a red fluorescence, indicating that the isolate does not have a requirement for the X factor.

• Biochemical reactions:
— Some biochemical tests (Table 24.3) can be carried out using conventional media. For testing carbohydrate utilization, a phenol red broth containing 1% of the sugar under test, filter-sterilized V and X factors and 1% serum is used.

— Commercially-available biochemical kits are used for testing isolates in a wider range of tests (Palladino *et al.*, 1990).

Pathogenesis and pathogenicity

Young or previously unexposed animals are particularly susceptible to infections by *Haemophilus* species. Specific-pathogen-free pigs, which do not harbour *H. parasuis* as a commensal, often develop signs of disease on primary exposure to the pathogen. Environmental stress factors appear to contribute to the development of *Haemophilus* infections. Although virulence factors have not been fully identified, endotoxin is thought to play a role in the pathogenesis of infections.

'*Haemophilus somnus*' can adhere firmly to several host cell types, including endothelial and vaginal epithelial cells. The organism is reported to cause degeneration of macrophages and it suppresses neutrophil function. Degeneration of vascular endothelial cells and transmural neutrophil infiltration are prominent findings in thrombotic meningoencephalitis (Corbeil *et al.*, 1995). Certain outer membrane proteins which confer virulence allow widespread dissemination of the bacteria in the host. Immunity to '*H. somnus*' appears to be predominantly humoral in nature (Cole *et al.*, 1992). However, phase variation in the lipopolysaccharide antigen types may influence survival and persistence in host animals.

Table 24.3 Comparative features of pathogenic *Haemophilus* species of veterinary importance.

Haemophilus species	Growth factor required	Catalase production	Oxidase production	Utilization of		
				Sucrose	Lactose	Mannitol
'*H. somnus*'	None	−	+	−	−	+
H. parasuis	Factor V	+	−	+	±	−
H. paragallinarum	Factor V	−	−	+	−	+

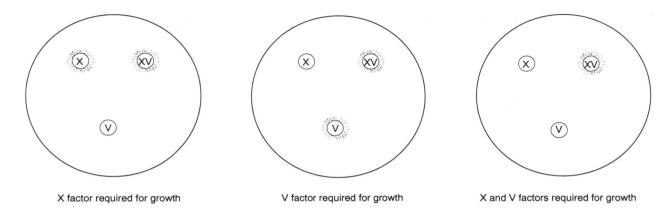

X factor required for growth   V factor required for growth   X and V factors required for growth

Figure 24.1 Disc method for determining the requirement for X and V growth factors. Isolates of *Haemophilus* species are spread over nutrient agar and discs containing X, V, and X and V factors are placed on the inoculated media. After incubation in 10% CO_2 at 37°C for 3 days, colonies of *Haemophilus* species grow around the discs supplying the growth factor required by the particular isolate.

Diagnostic procedures

- Specimens for laboratory examination depend on the clinical condition and type of lesions. *Haemophilus* species are fragile and neither refrigeration nor transport media maintain viability. Ideally, clinical specimens should be frozen in dry ice and delivered to a laboratory within 24 hours of collection.
- Either chocolate agar or blood agar inoculated with a streak of *S. aureus*, incubated under 5-10% CO_2 at 37°C for 2 to 3 days in a moist atmosphere, is used for isolation.
- Identification criteria for isolates :
  — Small, dewdrop-like colonies after 1 to 2 days
  — Enhancement of growth by CO_2
  — Requirement for X and V growth factors
  — Biochemical profile
- Although serological tests have been developed for epidemiological purposes, these tests are of little diagnostic value because *Haemophilus* species are widely distributed in animal populations.

Clinical infections

The *Haemophilus* species which are pathogenic for animals tend to be host-specific (Table 24.1). Some *Haemophilus* species of uncertain pathogenicity which are occasionally isolated from domestic animals are listed in Table 24.2.

Infections caused by '*H. somnus*' in cattle

'*Haemophilus somnus*' is part of the normal bacterial flora of the male and female bovine genital tracts. The organism can also colonize the upper respiratory tract. Environmental stress factors contribute to the development of clinical disease. '*Haemophilus somnus*' is more

resistant in the environment than most other *Haemophilus* species. It can survive in nasal discharges and blood for up to 70 days at ambient temperatures and for up to 5 days in vaginal discharges. Transmission is by direct contact or by aerosols. Serological surveys indicate that at least 25% of cattle have antibodies to '*H. somnus*' (Harris and Janzen, 1989).

Clinical signs

Because septicaemia is commonly associated with '*H. somnus*' infection, many organ systems may be involved and the resulting clinical presentation can be variable. Thrombotic meningoencephalitis (TME), a common consequence of septicaemia, is encountered sporadically in young cattle recently introduced to feedlots. Some animals may be found dead and others may present with high fever and depression, sometimes accompanied by blindness, lameness and ataxia. Sudden death due to myocarditis has also been described. Arthritis often develops in animals which survive the acute phase of the disease.

'*Haemophilus somnus*' is one of the bacterial pathogens commonly isolated from the enzootic calf pneumonia complex. Sporadic cases of abortion, endometritis, otitis and mastitis caused by '*H. somnus*' have been recorded.

Diagnosis

- Severe neurological signs in young feedlot cattle may be indicative of TME.
- Multiple foci of haemorrhagic necrosis, detectable grossly in affected brains at postmortem are consistent with TME. Vasculitis, thrombosis and haemorrhage are detectable histologically in brain, heart and other parenchymatous organs.
- Confirmation is by isolation and identification of '*H. somnus*' from cerebrospinal fluid, postmortem lesions or aborted foetuses.

Treatment and control

- Animals with clinical signs of septicaemia should be isolated and those at risk should be monitored closely to detect early signs of the disease.
- Although oxytetracycline is usually used for therapy, penicillin, erythromycin and potentiated sulphonamides are also effective.
- Commercially-available bacterins may reduce morbidity and mortality rates if administered one month before outbreaks of disease are anticipated.

Infections caused by '*Haemophilus somnus*' in sheep

Healthy sheep may carry '*H. somnus*' in the prepuce or vagina. Epididymitis in young rams, caused by '*H. somnus*' has been recorded (Lees *et al.*, 1990). Vulvitis, mastitis and reduced reproductive performance in ewes have been attributed to infection with '*H. somnus*'. The organism has also been associated with septicaemia, arthritis, meningitis and penumonia in lambs.

Glasser's disease

Glasser's disease, caused by *H. parasuis*, manifests as polyserositis and leptomeningitis usually affecting pigs from weaning up to 12 weeks of age. Some cases present as polyarthritis.

Haemophilus parasuis is part of the normal flora of the upper respiratory tract of pigs. Piglets acquire the organism from sows shortly after birth either by direct contact or through aerosols. The presence of maternally-derived antibodies prevents the development of clinical signs. However, Glasser's disease may occur sporadically in 2 to 4 week old piglets subjected to stressful environmental conditions (Smart *et al.*, 1989). Active immunity to *H. parasuis* is usually established by 7 to 8 weeks of age.

Clinical signs

The incubation period is 1 to 5 days. Clinical signs usually develop in conventionally-reared pigs 2 to 7 days following exposure to stress factors such as weaning or transportation. Anorexia, pyrexia, lameness, recumbency and convulsions are features of the disease. Cyanosis and thickening of the pinnae are often encountered. Pigs may die suddenly without showing signs of illness.

Diagnosis

- Because organisms such as *Streptococcus suis* and *Mycoplasma hyorhinis* produce clinicopathological changes similar to those of Glasser's disease, diagnosis requires isolation and identification of *H. parasuis*.
- Postmortem findings in Glasser's disease may include fibrinous polyserositis, polyarthritis and meningitis.
- Isolation and identification of *H. parasuis* from joint

fluid, heart blood, cerebrospinal fluid or postmortem tissues of a recently-dead pig is confirmatory.

Treatment and control

- Antimicrobial drugs such as tetracyclines, penicillins or potentiated sulphonamides, administered early in the course of the disease, are usually effective.
- Predisposing stress factors should be identified and, where possible, eliminated.
- Commercially-available bacterins or autogenous bacterins may stimulate protective immunity. Immunity is serotype specific.

Infectious coryza of chickens

Infectious coryza, caused by *H. paragallinarum*, affects the upper respiratory tract and paranasal sinuses of chickens. Its economic importance relates to loss of condition in broilers and reduced egg production in laying birds. Chronically ill and, occasionally, clinically normal carrier birds act as reservoirs of infection. Transmission occurs by direct contact, by aerosols or from contaminated drinking water. Chickens become susceptible at about 4 weeks after hatching and susceptibility increases with age.

Clinical signs

The mild form of disease manifests as depression, serous nasal discharge and slight facial swelling. In severe disease, swelling of one or both infraorbital sinuses is marked and oedema of the surrounding tissues may extend to the wattles. In laying birds, egg production may be severely affected.

A copious, tenacious exudate may be evident at postmortem in the infraorbital sinuses and tracheitis, bronchitis and airsacculitis may be present.

Diagnosis

- Facial swelling is a characteristic finding.
- Isolation and identification of *H. paragallinarum* from the infraorbital sinuses of several affected birds is confirmatory.
- Immunoperoxidase staining can be used to demonstrate *H. paragallinarum* in the tissues of the nasal passages and sinuses (Nakamura *et al.*, 1993).
- Serological tests such as agglutination tests, ELISA or agar gel immunodiffusion tests are used to demonstrate antibodies about 2 to 3 weeks after infection and to confirm the presence of *H. paragallinarum* in a flock.

Treatment and control

- Medication of water and feed with oxytetracycline or erythromycin should be initiated early in an outbreak of disease.
- An all-in/all-out management policy should be implemented and replacement birds should be obtained from coryza-free stock. Good management of poultry

units minimizes the risk of infection.

- Bacterins may be of value in units where the disease recurs. Vaccines should be administered about 3 weeks before outbreaks of coryza are anticipated.

References

Cole, S.P., Guiney, D.G. and Corbeil, L.B. (1992). Two linked genes for outer membrane proteins are absent in four non-disease strains of *H. somnus*. *Molecular Biology*, **6**, 1895–1902.

Corbeil, L.B., Gogolewski, R.P., Stephens, L.R. and Inzana, T.J. (1995). *Haemophilus somnus*: antigen analysis and immune responses. In *Haemophilus, Actinobacillus and Pasteurella*. Eds. W. Donachie, F.A. Lainson and J.C. Hodgson. Plenum Press, New York and London. pp. 63–73.

Harris, F.W. and Janzen, E.D. (1989). The *Haemophilus somnus* disease complex (hemophilosis): a review. *Canadian Veterinary Journal*, **30**, 816–822.

Lees, V.W., Meek, A.H. and Rosendal, S. (1990). Epidemiology of *Haemophilus somnus* in young rams. *Canadian Journal of Veterinary Research*, **54**, 331–336.

Nakamura, K., Hosoe, T., Shirai, J., Sawata, A., Tanimura, N. and Maeda, M. (1993). Lesions and immunoperoxidase localisation of *Haemophilus paragallinarum* in chickens with infectious coryza. *Veterinary Record*, **132**, 557–558.

Palladino, S., Leahy, B.J. and Newall, T.L. (1990). Comparison of the RIM-H Rapid Identification Kit with conventional tests for identification of *Haemophilus* spp. *Journal of Clinical Microbiology*, **28**, 1862–1863.

Smart, N.L., Miniats, O.P., Rosendal, S. and Friendship, R.M. (1989). Glasser's disease and prevalence of subclinical infection with *Haemophilus parsuis* in swine in southern Ontario. *Canadian Veterinary Journal*, **30**, 339–343.

Walker, R.L., Biberstein, E.L., Pritchett, R.F. and Kirkham, C. (1985). Deoxyribonucleic acid relatedness among 'Haemophilus somnus', 'Haemophilus agni', 'Histophilus ovis', 'Actinobacillus seminis' and *Haemophilus influenzae*. *International Journal of Systematic Bacteriology*, **35**, 46–49.

Further reading

Inzana, T.J., Johnson, J.L., Shell, L., Moller, K. and Kilian, M. (1992). Isolation and characterization of a newly identified *Haemophilus* species from cats : 'Haemophilus felis'. *Journal of Clinical Microbiology*, **30**, 2108–2112.

Miller, R.B., Lein, D.H., McEntee, K.E., Hall, C.E. and Shin, S. (1983). *Haemophilus somnus* infection of the reproductive tract of cattle: a review. *Journal of the American Veterinary Medical Association*, **182**, 1390–1392.

Chapter 25

Taylorella equigenitalis

This organism, *Taylorella equigenitalis*, was formerly known as *Haemophilus equigenitalis*. It is a short (0.7 x 0.7 to 1.8 μm), non-motile, Gram-negative rod, which gives positive reactions in catalase, oxidase and phosphatase tests. It is microaerophilic, slow-growing and highly fastidious, requiring chocolate agar and 5 to 10% CO_2 for optimal growth. Although the bacterium is not dependent on the X or V growth factors, availability of factor X stimulates growth. It does not grow on MacConkey agar.

Key points

- Short, non-motile Gram-negative rods
- Fastidious, optimal growth on chocolate agar
- Microaerophilic, 5-10% CO_2 required
- Positive oxidase, catalase and phosphatase tests but otherwise unreactive
- Causes contagious equine metritis

Usual habitat

The organism is found in the genital tracts of stallions, mares and foals. In stallions, *T. equigenitalis* is harboured in the urethral fossa and the pathogen localizes in the clitoral fossa of infected mares.

Clinical infections

Taylorella equigenitalis, the cause of contagious equine metritis, appears to infect only *Equidae* (Platt and Taylor, 1982).

Contagious equine metritis

Contagious equine metritis (CEM) was first reported as a clinical entity in 1977 in thoroughbreds in Britain and Ireland (Crowhurst, 1977; O'Driscoll *et al.*, 1977). Outbreaks of the disease were subsequently described in other European countries and in the USA, Australia and Japan. It is a highly contagious, localized venereal disease characterized by mucopurulent vulval discharge and temporary infertility in mares. The condition is economically important because it disrupts breeding programmes on thoroughbred stud farms.

Infected stallions and mares are the main reservoirs of infection. Transmission of the bacterium usually occurs during coitus although infection may also be introduced by contaminated instruments. It is considered that spontaneous ascending infection in mares is unlikely and that *T. equigenitalis* must be deposited in the uterus for infection to establish (Platt and Taylor, 1982). Foals born to infected dams may acquire infection *in utero* or during parturition. *Taylorella equigenitalis* has been isolated from more than 75% of the offspring of infected mares at 2 to 4 years of age (Timoney and Powell, 1982). These offspring and mares which have recovered clinically may act as sources of infection.

Pathogenesis

Pre-ejaculatory fluid and semen may be contaminated with *T. equigenitalis* from the urethral fossa. There is strong clinical and epidemiological evidence that strains differ in pathogenicity (Parlevliet *et al.*, 1997). After introduction into the uterus, pathogenic organisms replicate and induce an acute endometritis. Initially, mononuclear cell and plasma-cell infiltration predominates, a feature rarely observed in acute bacterial endometritis (Ricketts *et al.*, 1978). Later, migration of neutrophils into the uterine lumen produces a profuse mucopurulent exudate. Although the pathogen may persist in the uterus, acute endometrial changes subside within a few days.

Clinical signs

Infected stallions and a minority of infected mares remain asymptomatic. Most affected mares develop a copious mucopurulent vulval discharge without systemic disturbance within a few days of service by a carrier stallion. The discharge may continue for up to 2 weeks and affected mares remain infertile for several weeks. Some mares recover without treatment and up to 25% remain carriers (Platt and Taylor, 1982). Infection does not confer protective immunity and reinfection can occur.

Diagnostic procedures

- A copious, mucopurulent vulval discharge 2 to 7 days after service may indicate the presence of CEM.

- Specimens for bacteriology should be collected before and during the breeding season.
- Swabs from mares should be taken from the clitoral fossa and sinuses and from the endometrium at oestrus using a double-guarded swab. When taking swabs, disposable gloves should be changed between each animal.
- Foals of infected mares should be sampled before 3 months of age. Swabs should be taken from the clitoral fossa of fillies and from the penile sheath and tip of the penis in colts. Swabs from stallions and teaser stallions are taken from the urethra, urethral fossa and penile sheath in addition to pre-ejaculatory fluid.
- Swabs must be placed in Amies charcoal transport medium and reach the laboratory within 24 hours of collection. Samples should be submitted to laboratories which are officially certified by a regulatory authority.
- Chocolate agar-based media are suitable for isolation with the addition of amphotericin B, crystal violet and streptomycin. Plates with and without streptomycin should be inoculated as some isolates of *T. equigenitalis* are susceptible to this antibiotic. A medium incorporating trimethoprim and clindamycin has been developed (Timoney *et al.*, 1982). Inoculated plates are incubated under 5 to 10% CO_2 at 37°C for 4 to 7 days.
- Identification criteria for isolates:
  — Colonies, which may be visible after 48 hours, are small, smooth, yellowish-grey and have an entire edge.
  — Reactions in the catalase, oxidase and phosphatase tests are positive.
  — A slide agglutination test, using high-titred *T. equigenitalis* antiserum, can be carried out on the culture.
  — A fluorescent antibody technique, rendered specific by absorption with *Mannheimia haemolytica*, may be used.
  — A latex agglutination kit is available commercially to identify the pathogen.
- A polymerase chain reaction technique has been developed for detecting *T. equigenitalis* in specimens (Bleumink-Pluym *et al.*, 1993).
- Serological tests including the agglutination, complement fixation and ELISA tests are useful for confirming active or recent infections but do not detect asymptomatic carriers.

Treatment

Asymptomatic carriers must be treated as well as clinically affected animals. Elimination of *T. equigenitalis* from both mares and stallions can usually be accomplished by washing the external genitalia with a 2% solution of chlorhexidine combined with local application of antimicrobial drugs such as nitrofurazone ointment on a daily basis (Watson, 1997). In addition, a daily intrauterine irrigation with penicillin solution is carried out in mares for 5 to 7 days. Ablation of clitoral sinuses may be necessary in a few mares in which *T. equigenitalis* persists after treatment.

Control

- Contagious equine metritis is a notifiable disease in many countries with an advanced thoroughbred industry.
- Control regimens are based on laboratory detection of asymptomatic and clinical infections with *T. equigenitalis* in animals used for breeding.
- Appropriate, routine hygienic methods must be practiced on stud farms to prevent lateral spread of the pathogen.
- If CEM is diagnosed on stud farms, all breeding services should immediately cease.
- Animals which have been treated for CEM should be sampled to ensure bacteriological freedom from the pathogen.
- Test-mating a stallion to 2 maiden mares is a sensitive method for detecting infection. Samples from the mares are then examined bacteriologically.
- No vaccine is available for CEM.

References

Bleumink-Pluym, N.M.C., Houwers, D.J., Parlevliet, J.M. and Colenbrander, B. (1993). PCR-based detection of CEM agent. *Veterinary Record*, **133**, 375–376.

Crowhurst, R.C. (1977). Genital infection in mares. *Veterinary Record*, **100**, 476.

Fontijne, P., Ter Laak, E.A. and Hartman, E.G. (1989). *Taylorella equigenitalis* isolated from an aborted foal. *Veterinary Record*, **125**, 485.

O'Driscoll, J.G., Troy, P.T. and Geoghegan, F.J. (1977). An epidemic of venereal disease in thoroughbreds. *Veterinary Record*, **101**, 359–360.

Parlevliet, J.M., Bleumink-Pluym, N.M.C., Houwers, D.J., Remmen, J.L.A.M., Sluyter, F.J.H. and Colenbrander, B. (1997). Epidemiologic aspects of *Taylorella equigenitalis*. *Theriogenology*, **47**, 1169–1177.

Platt, H. and Taylor, C.E.D. (1982). Contagious equine metritis. In *Medical Microbiology*. Volume 1. Eds. C.S.F. Easmon and J. Jeljaszewicz. Academic Press, New York. pp. 49–96.

Ricketts, S.W., Rossdale, P.D. and Samuel, C.A. (1978). Endometrial biopsy studies of mares with contagious equine metritis 1977. *Equine Veterinary Journal*, **10**, 160–166.

Timoney, P.J. and Powell, D.G. (1982). Isolation of the contagious equine metritis organism from colts and fillies in the United Kingdom and Ireland. *Veterinary Record*, **111**, 478–482.

Timoney, P.J., Shin, S.J. and Jacobson, R.H. (1982). Improved selective medium for isolation of the contagious equine metritis organism. *Veterinary Record*, **111**, 107–108.

Watson, E.D. (1997). Swabbing protocols in screening for contagious equine metritis. *Veterinary Record*, **140**, 268–271.

Further reading

Anon (1997). Keeping CEM at bay. *Veterinary Record*, **140**, 265.

Bleumink-Pluym, N.M.C., Ter Laak, E.A. and Vander Zeijst, B.A.M. (1990). Epidemiologic study of *Taylorella equigenitalis* strains by field inversion gel electrophoresis of genome restriction endonuclease fragments. *Journal of Clinical Microbiology,* **28**, 2012–2016.

Brewer, R.A. (1983). Contagious equine metritis: A review/summary. *Veterinary Bulletin*, **53**, 881–891.

Ricketts, S.W. (1996). Contagious equine metritis (CEM). *Equine Veterinary Education*, **8**, 166–170.

Chapter 26

Bordetella bronchiseptica and *Bordetella avium*

The genus *Bordetella* contains four species, *B. pertussis*, *B. parapertussis*, *B. bronchiseptica* and *B. avium*. *Bordetella pertussis*, the type species, and *B. parapertussis* are human pathogens associated with whooping cough in children. *Bordetella bronchiseptica* infects a wide range of animal species including man, while *B. avium* is a pathogen of avian species (Table 26.1). The bordetellae are occasional pathogens which have an affinity for ciliated respiratory epithelium. *Bordetella bronchiseptica* and *B. avium* are small (0.2 to 0.5 x 0.5 to 1.5 μm), Gram-negative rods with a coccobacillary appearance. They are catalase-positive, oxidase-positive aerobes and are motile peritrichous bacteria. Because they cannot utilize carbohydrates, they derive their energy mainly from the oxidation of amino acids and have no special growth requirements. They grow on MacConkey agar.

Usual habitat

Bordetella species are commensals on the mucous membranes of the upper respiratory tract of animals. In the environment, survival time is short.

Differentiation of *Bordetella bronchiseptica* and *B. avium*

These bacteria are usually identified by growth characteristics, biochemical reactions and by their unique ability to agglutinate red blood cells (Table 26.2). *Bordetella avium* requires differentiation from *Alcaligenes faecalis*, which is non-pathogenic.

- On sheep blood agar, colonies of virulent strains, visible after incubation for 24 hours, are small, convex and smooth. Many isolates of *B. bronchiseptica* are haemolytic, unlike *B. avium*, which is non-haemolytic.
- On MacConkey agar, both *B. bronchiseptica* and *B. avium* produce pale, non-lactose-fermenting colonies.
- A selective indicator medium containing bromothymol blue as pH indicator is used for the isolation and presumptive identification of bordetellae (Smith and Baskerville, 1979).
- Miniaturized biochemical identification systems are available for these 'non-fermenting' bacteria, which do not metabolize carbohydrates.

Key points

- Small Gram-negative rods
- Growth on non-enriched media and on MacConkey agar
- Strict aerobes
- Motile, catalase-positive, oxidase-positive
- Utilize amino acids for energy
- Toxigenic strains agglutinate mammalian red blood cells
- Commensals of upper respiratory tract
- Cause respiratory disease in mammals and birds

- Haemagglutination, an attribute uncommon in bacteria, occurs with virulent isolates of both *B. bronchiseptica* and *B. avium*.

Pathogenesis and pathogenicity

The bordetellae exhibit phase changes, which correlate with virulence and are identifiable by colonial appearance. Virulence is mediated by several factors including a filamentous haemagglutinin, pertactin and fimbriae which allow attachment to the cilia of the upper respiratory tract (Table 26.3). These factors are only expressed in the virulent phase (phase 1) and are controlled by a virulence gene regulatory system. After repeated subculture, isolates change to an avirulent form (phase 4) and colonies exhibit a different morphology which reflects alterations in bacterial structure. Phases 2 and 3 are poorly defined. The tracheal cytotoxin inhibits ciliary motility and tracheo-bronchial clearance. In addition, *B. bronchiseptica* produces an adenylate cyclase-haemolysin which primarily targets phagocytic cells (Gueirard and Guiso, 1993; Harvill *et al.*, 1999). This toxin is unique as it has the features of a repeats-in-structural-toxin but with an extra domain for an adenylate cyclase enzyme (Table 26.3). Although *B. avium* lacks the filamentous haemagglutinin, the organism does produce a haemagglutinin, which specifically agglutinates guinea-pig red cells and correlates with pathogenicity for turkey poults (Gentry-Weeks *et al.*,

Table 26.1 *Bordetella* species of veterinary importance and disease conditions with which they are associated.

Bordetella species	Host	Disease conditions
B. bronchiseptica	Pigs	Atrophic rhinitis
	Dogs	Canine infectious tracheo-bronchitis
	Kittens	Pneumonia
	Horses	Respiratory infections
	Rabbits	Upper respiratory tract infection
	Laboratory rodents	Bronchopneumonia
B. avium	Turkeys	Coryza
B. parapertussis	Lambs	Pneumonia

1988). Two other toxins, dermonecrotic toxin and osteotoxin, may be of significance in atrophic rhinitis by contributing to nasal turbinate atrophy (Rutter *et al.*, 1984).

Clearance of the bacteria is mediated by locally-produced antibodies (IgA) which appear about 4 days after infection commences. Although these antibodies can block attachment of bordetellae to cilia, they are unable to remove attached bacteria. Clearance of bordetellae from the respiratory tract may require several weeks. Carrier animals, including a percentage of adults which continue to shed the organisms, represent an important source of infection.

Diagnostic procedures

- Specimens for laboratory examination include nasal swabs, tracheal aspirates and exudates.
- Bordetellae are cultured on blood agar and MacConkey agar or on selective media. Plates are incubated aerobically at 37°C for 24 to 48 hours.
- Identification criteria for isolates:
  — Colonial appearance on blood agar or selective media.
  — Growth on MacConkey agar.
  — Biochemical profile.
  — Slide haemagglutination tests correlating with the virulence of isolates.
- Serological tests which have been developed are of limited diagnostic value.

Clinical infections

Clinical signs associated with bordetellae usually relate to upper respiratory tract infection. Young animals are most susceptible and infections in adults are usually mild or subclinical. Predisposing factors such as stress or concurrent infections contribute to field outbreaks of disease. Although morbidity rates may be high, mortality

Table 26.2 Differentiating features of *Bordetella bronchiseptica*, *B. avium* and *Alcaligenes faecalis*[a].

Feature	B. bronchiseptica	B. avium	Alcaligenes faecalis
Colonial characteristics on:			
Sheep blood agar	Haemolysis	No haemolysis	No haemolysis
MacConkey agar	Pale, pinkish hue	Pale, pinkish hue	Pale
Selective medium[b]	Small, blue	Small, blue	Large, greenish
Oxidase production	+	+	+
Catalase production	+	+	+
Urease production	+	−	−
Utilization of carbon exclusively from:			
Citrate	+	+	+
Malonate	−	−	+
Nitrate reduction	+	−	−
Motility	+	+	+
Haemagglutinating activity of virulent strains	Agglutination of ovine and bovine red blood cells[c]	Agglutination of guinea-pig red blood cells[c]	−

a   an organism which may require differentiation from bordetellae but not of veterinary significance
b   Smith and Baskerville (1979)
c   suspension of 3% washed red blood cells using a slide test

Table 26.3 Virulence factors of *Bordetella bronchiseptica* and *B. avium*.

Virulence factor	Activity	*Bordetella* species	
		B. bronchiseptica	*B. avium*
Filamentous haemagglutinin	Binds to cilia	+	−
Pertactin	Binds to cells	+	+
Fimbriae	Mediate attachment to cells	+	+
Adenylate cyclase-haemolysin	Interferes with phagocytic cell function	+	−
Tracheal cytotoxin	Inhibits ciliary action, kills ciliated cells	+	+
Dermonecrotoxic toxin	Induces skin necrosis, impairs osteogenesis	+	+
Osteotoxin	Toxic for osteoblasts	+	+
Lipopolysaccharide	Stimulates cytokine release, role in disease uncertain	+	+

rates are usually low. The diseases associated with *B. bronchiseptica* and *B. avium* are summarized in Table 26.1. *Bordetella parapertussis*, a recognised human pathogen, has been isolated from lambs with chronic non-progressive pneumonia (Cullinane *et al.*, 1987). *Bordetella bronchiseptica* is implicated in a mild form of atrophic rhinitis in pigs and in canine infectious tracheobronchitis (kennel cough). Oropharyngeal swabs from healthy cats may yield *B. bronchiseptica* and severe bronchopneumonia associated with the organism has been reported in kittens (Willoughby *et al.*, 1991). *Bordetella bronchiseptica* may occasionally cause outbreaks of respiratory disease in rabbits and in laboratory rodents. *Bordetella avium* causes turkey coryza and respiratory disease in quails (Blackall and Doheny, 1987).

Canine infectious tracheobronchitis

Canine infectious tracheobronchitis, also known as kennel cough, is one of the most prevalent respiratory complexes of dogs. Although *Bordetella bronchiseptica*, canine parainfluenzavirus 2 (PI-2) and canine adenovirus 2 (CAV 2) are considered to be the most important participating pathogens, other microbial pathogens may also be involved (Box 26.1).

Transmission occurs through respiratory secretions either by direct contact or by aerosols. Mechanical transfer on footwear or clothing, on contaminated feeding utensils and on fomites can spread infection in kennels, pet shops and animal shelters. Although morbidity rates may reach 50%, mortality rates are usually low. Organisms may remain in the respiratory tract and be shed for several months after clinical recovery.

Clinical signs

Clinical signs of infection with *B. bronchiseptica* develop within 3 to 4 days of exposure and, without complications, persist for up to 14 days. They include coughing, gagging or retching and mild serous oculonasal discharge. Affected dogs usually remain active, alert and non-febrile. The disease is self-limiting unless complicated by bronchopneumonia which may develop in unvaccinated pups or in older immunosuppressed animals.

Diagnosis
- Diagnosis is based on a history of recent exposure to carrier dogs and characteristic clinical signs.
- The appropriate specimen for laboratory examination is transtracheal aspiration fluid.
- Virulent isolates of *B. bronchiseptica* haemagglutinate ovine and bovine red cells.
- Serology, in association with vaccination history, may be of value for determining the involvement of respiratory viruses.

Treatment
- Dogs with mild clinical signs do not require specific therapy.
- If coughing persists for more than 2 weeks or if bronchopneumonia is present, antibiotic therapy may be required. Amoxicillin has proved effective in field trials (Thursfield *et al.*, 1991). Tetracyclines and fluoroquinolones may also be effective (Bemis, 1992).

Box 26.1 Microbial pathogens implicated in canine infectious tracheobronchitis (kennel cough).

- *Bordetella bronchiseptica*
- Canine adenovirus 2
- Canine parainfluenzavirus 2
- Canine distemper virus
- Canine adenovirus 1
- Canine herpesvirus 1
- Reoviruses 1, 2 and 3
- *Mycoplasma* species

Control

- Affected dogs should be isolated immediately.
- If predisposing factors are identified, they should be corrected.
- Intranasal vaccines containing *B. bronchiseptica* and PI-2 antigens induce local protective immunity and are not affected by maternal antibodies. Modified live *B. bronchiseptica* vaccines decrease the severity of clinical signs but may not prevent infection. Modified live vaccines are available for many of the viruses associated with respiratory disease in dogs.

Bordetella bronchiseptica and the development of atrophic rhinitis

Toxigenic strains of *B. bronchiseptica* are widely distributed in pig herds. They can cause turbinate hypoplasia without distortion of the snout in young piglets under 4 weeks of age. In uncomplicated infections, pigs reach slaughter age with relatively minor change in the turbinate bones (Rutter, 1989). However, the infection with *B. bronchiseptica* may facilitate colonization by toxigenic *Pasteurella multocida* type D with the subsequent development of severe atrophic rhinitis and distortion of the snout. Factors such as overstocking and poor ventilation can contribute to the development of atrophic rhinitis. The most severe form of the disease results from concurrent infection with *B. bronchiseptica* and *P. multocida* (Pedersen *et al.*, 1988).

Turkey coryza

Turkey coryza, caused by *B. avium*, is a highly contagious upper respiratory tract disease of poults with high morbidity and low mortality. Infection is spread through direct contact, by aerosols and from environmental sources. Mucus accumulates in the nares with swelling in the submaxillary sinuses. Beak-breathing, excessive lacrimation and sneezing may be evident. Infection with *B. avium* predisposes to secondary infections with bacteria such as *Escherichia coli*. Once *E. coli* becomes established, a more serious disease with high mortality can develop.

Diagnosis

- Clinical signs and gross pathological features may be indicative of the disease.
- Isolation and identification of *B. avium* from sinus and tracheal exudates is confirmatory.
- Virulent isolates agglutinate guinea-pig red blood cells.
- Microagglutination and ELISA techniques may be of diagnostic value.

Treatment and control

- Broad spectrum antibiotics early in the course of disease may be beneficial.
- Commercially-available bacterins and modified live vaccines may be used in susceptible flocks.
- Thorough cleaning and disinfection of turkey houses after an outbreak of disease are essential for the elimination of *B. avium*.

References

Bemis, D.A. (1992). *Bordetella* and mycoplasma respiratory infections in dogs and cats. *Veterinary Clinics of North America: Small Animal Practice,* **22**, 1173–1186.

Blackall, P.J. and Doheny, C.M. (1987). Isolation and characterisation of *Bordetella avium* and related species and an evaluation of their role in respiratory disease in poultry. *Australian Veterinary Journal,* **64**, 235–239.

Cullinane, L.C., Alley, M.R., Marshall, R.B. and Manktelow, B.W. (1987). *Bordetella parapertussis* from lambs. *New Zealand Veterinary Journal,* **35**, 175.

Gentry-Weeks, C.R., Cookson, B.T., Goldman, W.E., Rimler, R.B., Porter, S.B. and Curtiss, R. (1988). Dermonecrotic toxin and tracheal cytotoxin, putative virulence factors of *Bordetella avium. Infection and Immunity,* **56**, 1698–1707.

Gueirard, P. and Guiso, N. (1993). Virulence of *Bordetella bronchiseptica*: role of adenylate cyclase-haemolysin. *Infection and Immunity,* **61**, 4072–4078.

Harvill, E.T., Cotter, P.A., Yuk, M.H. and Miller, J.F. (1999). Probing the function of *Bordetella bronchiseptica* adenylate cyclase toxin by manipulating host immunity. *Infection and Immunity,* **67**, 1493–1500.

Pedersen, K.B., Nielsen, J.P., Foged, N.T., Elling, F., Nielsen, N.C. and Willeberg, P. (1988). Atrophic rhinitis in pigs: proposal for a revised definition. *Veterinary Record,* **122**, 190–191.

Rutter, M. (1989). Atrophic rhinitis. *In Practice,* **11**, 74-80.

Rutter, J.M., Taylor, R.J., Crighton, W.G., Robertson, I.B. and Benson, J.A. (1984). Epidemiological study of *Pasteurella multocida* and *Bordetella bronchiseptica* in atrophic rhinitis. *Veterinary Record,* **115**, 615–619.

Smith, I.M. and Baskerville, A.J. (1979). A selective medium facilitating the isolation and recognition of *Bordetella bronchiseptica* in pigs. *Research in Veterinary Science,* **27**, 187–192.

Thursfield, M.B., Aitken, C.G.G. and Muirhead, R.H. (1991). A field investigation of kennel cough: efficacy of different treatments. *Journal of Small Animal Practice,* **32**, 455–459.

Willoughby, K., Dawson, S., Jones, R.C., Symons, M., Daykin, J., Payne-Johnson, C. *et al.* (1991). Isolation of *B. bronchiseptica* from kittens with pneumonia in a breeding cattery. *Veterinary Record,* **129**, 407–408.

Further reading

Iversen, A.L., Lee, M.H. and Manniche, N.E. (1998). Seroprevalence of antibodies to *Bordetella bronchiseptica* in cats in the Copenhagen area of Denmark. *Veterinary Record,* **143**, 592.

Chapter 27

Moraxella bovis

Moraxella bovis occurs as short (1.0 to 1.5 x 1.5 to 2.5 μm), plump Gram-negative rods or, occasionally, cocci which typically occur in pairs (Fig. 27.1). This organism is non-motile, aerobic and usually catalase-positive and oxidase-positive. Although proteolytic, it is unable to utilize sugars. Growth, which is enhanced by the addition of blood or serum to media, does not occur on MacConkey agar. Virulent strains, when isolated from cases of infectious bovine keratoconjunctivitis, are fimbriate, haemolytic and grow into the agar. Species, other than *M. bovis*, which are periodically isolated from clinical specimens, are generally regarded as non-pathogenic.

Usual habitat

Moraxella bovis is found on mucous membranes of carrier cattle. The organism is susceptible to desiccation and is short-lived in the environment. It can survive for up to 72 hours in the salivary organs and on the body surface of flies, which can act as vectors.

Clinical infections

Moraxella bovis causes infectious bovine keratoconjunctivitis, an important ocular disease of cattle which occurs worldwide. Variants of *M. bovis* have been isolated from horses with conjunctivitis. (Hughes and Pugh, 1970).

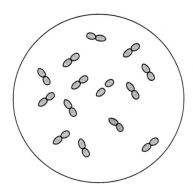

Figure 27.1 Short, plump rods of *Moraxella bovis*, characteristically occurring in pairs.

> **Key points**
> - Short Gram-negative rods, usually in pairs
> - Optimal growth on enriched media
> - Aerobic, non-motile
> - Usually catalase- and oxidase-positive
> - Proteolytic, unreactive with sugar substrates
> - Virulent strains are fimbriated and haemolytic
> - Susceptible to desiccation
> - Found on mucous membranes of carrier cattle
> - Causes infectious bovine keratoconjunctivitis

Infectious bovine keratoconjunctivitis

Infectious bovine keratoconjunctivitis (IBK), sometimes referred to as 'pink-eye' or New Forest disease, is a highly contagious condition affecting the superficial structures of the eyes, usually in animals under 2 years of age. The disease causes economic losses arising from decreased weight gain in beef breeds, loss of milk production, short-term disruption of breeding programmes and treatment costs.

There appears to be an age-related immunity, probably as a result of previous exposure. Asymptomatic carrier animals harbour *M. bovis* in the nasolacrimal ducts, nasopharynx and vagina (Ruehl *et al.*, 1993). Transmission can occur by direct contact, by aerosols and through flies acting as vectors. Factors which predispose to IBK are presented in Table 27.1.

Pathogenesis and pathogenicity

The virulence of *M. bovis* is attributed to fimbriae, which allow adherence of the organisms to the cornea, circumventing the protective effects of lacrimal secretions and blinking. Two types of fimbriae are recognized, namely, Q fimbriae (pili) which are specific for colonization and I fimbriae which allow local persistence of infection (Ruehl *et al.*, 1993). Fimbrial antigens stimulate type-specific protective immunity.

During bacterial replication, haemolysin and other lytic enzymes such as fibrolysin, phosphatase, hyaluronidase

Table 27.1 Factors which may exacerbate or predispose to outbreaks of infectious bovine keratoconjunctivitis.

Factor	Comments
Age	Young cattle less than 2 years of age are particularly susceptible to infection
Breed	*Bos taurus* breeds appear to be more susceptible than *Bos indicus* breeds
Fly activity	Flies can act as vectors of *Moraxella bovis*
Ocular irritants	Dust, tall grasses, grass seeds, wind, ultraviolet light and cold ambient temperatures may predispose to disease
Concurrent infections	Infection with bovine herpesvirus 1 or *Thelazia* species may exacerbate infectious bovine keratoconjunctivitis
Vitamin deficiency	A deficiency of vitamin A may predispose to disease

and aminopeptidase are produced. Lipopolysaccharides, associated with O antigens, also appear to play a role in virulence (DeBower and Thompson, 1997). The haemolysin is a calcium-dependent, pore-forming cytolysin which damages the cell membranes of neutrophils (Clinkenbeard and Thiessen, 1991). Release of hydrolytic enzymes from neutrophils on the corneal surface contributes to breakdown of its collagen matrix.

Strains which lack either haemolysin or fimbriae are avirulent. Isolates from carrier animals are often non-haemolytic and non-fimbriate but reversion to virulence can occur. It has been suggested that the deficiency of lysozyme in the lacrimal secretions of cattle may account for their susceptibility to *M. bovis* (Punch and Slatter, 1984).

Clinical signs
Infectious bovine keratoconjunctivitis initially manifests as blepharospasm, conjunctivitis and lacrimation. Progression of the condition through keratitis to corneal ulceration, opacity and abscessation may occasionally lead to panophthalmitis and permanent blindness (Punch and Slatter, 1984). Following ulceration, vascularization extends from the limbus and stromal oedema develops. There may be weakening of the cornea with the development of coning. In most mild cases, the cornea heals within a few weeks although there may be permanent scarring of the structure.

Some carrier animals may exhibit persistent lacrimation. Following infection with a virulent strain of *M. bovis*, neutralizing antibodies develop which are active against haemolysin produced by other strains. In contrast, antibodies which block fimbrial-mediated adherence are type-specific and exposure to *M. bovis* possessing a different fimbrial type may result in disease (Moore and Rutter, 1989).

Diagnostic procedures
- The disease characteristically affects a number of animals in a herd.
- Lacrimal secretion is the most suitable specimen for laboratory examination. Because *M. bovis* is extremely susceptible to desiccation, specimens must be processed promptly. For transportation, swabs of lacrimal secretions should be placed in 1 to 2 ml of sterile water. Ideally, specimens should be cultured within 2 hours of collection.
- A fluorescent antibody technique for demonstrating *M. bovis* in smears from lacrimal secretions is available.
- Specimens should be cultured on blood agar and MacConkey agar and incubated aerobically at 37°C for 48 to 72 hours.
- Identification criteria for isolates:
  — Round, small, shiny, friable, colonies appear after 48 hours. Colonies of virulent strains are surrounded by a zone of complete haemolysis and are embedded in the agar.
  — No growth occurs on MacConkey agar.
  — Cultures of virulent strains autoagglutinate in saline.
  — Smears from colonies reveal short Gram-negative rods in pairs (Fig. 27.1).
  — Reactions in the catalase and oxidase tests are positive. A Loeffler's serum slope may be pitted after 10 days.
- Fimbriate isolates can be assigned to 7 serogroups (Moore and Lepper, 1991).

Treatment
Antimicrobial therapy should be administered subconjunctivally or topically early in the disease (George, 1990; DeBower and Thompson, 1997).

Control
- Fimbriae-derived bacterins which are available commercially in some countries are of uncertain efficacy (Smith *et al.*, 1990).
- Management-related methods are important in the control of IBK. These include isolation of affected animals, reduction of exposure to mechanical irritants, the use of insecticidal ear tags and the control of concurrent diseases, such as infectious bovine rhinotracheitis or *Thelazia* infestation.
- The prophylactic use of intramuscular oxytetracycline can be considered for animals at risk.
- Animals which are blind should be housed.
- Vitamin A supplementation may be beneficial.

References

Clinkenbeard, K.D. and Thiessen, A.E. (1991). Mechanism of action of *Moraxella bovis* haemolysin. *Infection and Immunity*, **59**, 1148–1152.

DeBower, D. and Thompson, J.R. (1997). Infectious bovine keratoconjunctivitis. *Iowa State University Veterinarian*, **59**, 20–24.

George, L.W. (1990) Antibiotic treatment of infectious bovine keratoconjunctivitis. *Cornell Veterinarian*, **80**, 229–235.

Hughes, D.E. and Pugh, G.W. (1970). Isolation and description of a *Moraxella* from horses with conjunctivitis. *American Journal of Veterinary Research*, **31**, 457–462.

Moore, L.J. and Lepper, A.W.D. (1991). A unified serotyping scheme for *Moraxella bovis*. *Veterinary Microbiology*, **29**, 75–83.

Moore, L.J. and Rutter, J.M. (1989). Attachment of *Moraxella bovis* to calf corneal cells and inhibition by antiserum. *Australian Veterinary Journal*, **66**, 39–42.

Punch, P.I. and Slatter, D.M. (1984). A review of infectious bovine keratoconjunctivitis. *Veterinary Bulletin*, **54**, 193–207.

Ruehl, W.W., Marrs, C.F., George, L., Banks, S.J.M. and Schoolnik, G.K. (1993). Infection rates, disease frequency, pilin gene rearrangement, and pilin expression in calves inoculated with *Moraxella bovis* pilin-specific isogenic variants. *American Journal of Veterinary Research*, **54**, 248–253.

Smith, P.C., Blankenship, T., Hoover, T.R., Powe, M.C. and Wright, J.C. (1990). Effectiveness of two commercial infectious bovine keratoconjunctivitis vaccines. *American Journal of Veterinary Research*, **51**, 1147–1150.

Chapter 28

Brucella species

Brucella species are small (0.6 x 0.6 to 1.5 μm), non-motile, coccobacillary, Gram-negative bacteria. As they are not decolourized by 0.5% acetic acid in the modified Ziehl-Neelsen (MZN) staining technique, they are classed as MZN-positive. In MZN-stained smears of body fluids or tissues, they characteristically appear as clusters of red coccobacilli (Fig. 28.1). For taxonomic purposes, all *Brucella* species should be classified as *Brucella melitensis* as DNA hybridization studies have shown that the genus contains only one species. For practical reasons, however, it is permissible to use the names of brucellae formerly regarded as species, a procedure adhered to in this textbook. *Brucella* species are aerobic, capnophilic and catalase-positive. Apart from *B. ovis* and *B. neotomae*, they are oxidase-positive. All *Brucella* species are urease-positive except *B. ovis*. *Brucella ovis* and some biotypes of *B. abortus* require 5 to 10% CO_2 for primary isolation. Moreover, the growth of other *Brucella* species is enhanced in an atmosphere of CO_2. Media enriched with blood or serum are required for culturing *B. abortus* biotype 2 and *B. ovis*. Recently, brucellae have been detected in sea-mammals (Ross *et al.*, 1994). The hosts and clinical significance of *Brucella* species are presented in Table 28.1.

Key points

- Small Gram-negative coccobacilli
- Stain red using the modified Ziehl-Neelsen method
- Aerobic and capnophilic
- Non-motile, catalase-positive
- Most isolates are oxidase-positive
- Urease-positive
- Intracellular pathogens
- Target reproductive organs of certain species
- Some species cause undulant fever in humans

Usual habitat

As a general rule, brucellae have a predilection for both female and male reproductive organs in sexually mature animals and each *Brucella* species tends to infect a particular animal species. Infected animals serve as reservoirs of infection which often persists indefinitely. Organisms, shed by infected animals, can remain viable in a moist environment for many months.

Differentiation of *Brucella* species

Brucella species are differentiated by colonial appearance, biochemical tests, specific cultural requirements and growth inhibition by dyes (Table 28.2). In addition, agglutination with monospecific sera and susceptibility to bacteriophages are employed for definitive identification.

- On primary isolation, colonies of *B. abortus*, *B. melitensis* and *B. suis* occur in smooth forms, and are small, glistening, bluish and translucent after incubation for 3 to 5 days. Colonies become opaque with age. In contrast, primary isolates of *B. ovis* and *B. canis* always occur in rough forms. These rough colonies are dull, yellowish, opaque and friable. Brucellae are non-haemolytic on blood agar.
- Slide agglutination tests with monospecific antisera are used to detect the presence of important surface antigens, *abortus* antigen A and *melitensis* antigen M. The R antigen, a feature of the rough brucellae *B. ovis*

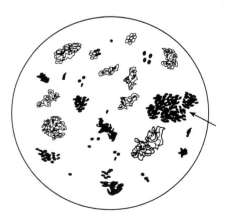

Figure 28.1 Clusters of *Brucella abortus* as they appear in a smear from a cotyledon of a cow with brucellosis. Using the modified Ziehl-Neelsen method, the small coccobacillary cells, present in clumps, stain red (arrow). Cellular debris and other bacterial cells stain blue.

Table 28.1 *Brucella* species, their host range and the clinical significance of infection.

Brucella species	Usual host/clinical significance	Species occasionally infected/ clinical significance
B. abortus	Cattle/abortion, orchitis	Sheep, goats, pigs/sporadic abortion Horses/bursitis Humans/intermittent fever, systemic disease
B. melitensis	Goats, sheep/ abortion, orchitis, arthritis	Cattle/sporadic abortion, brucellae in milk Humans/Malta fever, severe systemic disease
B. suis	Pigs/abortion, orchitis, arthritis, spondylitis, infertility	Humans/intermittent fever, systemic disease
B. ovis	Sheep/epididymitis in rams, sporadic abortion in ewes	
B. canis	Dogs/abortion, epididymitis, disco-spondylitis, sterility in male dogs	Humans/mild systemic disease
B. neotomae	Desert wood rat/not isolated from domestic animals	

and *B. canis*, can be detected by anti-R serum.
- Isolates of *B. abortus* are lysed by a specific bacteriophage (Tbilisi phage) at routine test dilution.
- If other tests give equivocal results, oxidative metabolic rates on selective substrates can be conducted in reference laboratories.

Pathogenesis and pathogenicity

The establishment and outcome of infection with brucellae depend on the number of infecting organisms and their

virulence and also on host susceptibility (Price *et al.*, 1990). Brucellae, which lack the major outer-membrane lipopolysaccharide, produce rough colonies and are less virulent than those derived from smooth colonies (Roop *et al.*, 1991). Although smooth and rough organisms can enter host cells, rough forms are usually eliminated unlike smooth forms which may persist and multiply. Virulent brucellae, when engulfed by phagocytes on mucous membranes, are transported to regional lymph nodes. Brucellae persist within macrophages but not within neutrophils. Inhibition of phagosome-lysosome function is a major mechanism for intracellular survival and an important determinant of bacterial virulence. However, many of the mechanisms used by brucellae to survive within macrophages are not fully elucidated. Various stress proteins are thought to allow the organisms to adapt to harsh conditions encountered within macrophages (Rafie-Kolpin *et al.*, 1996; Robertson and Roop, 1999). In addition, superoxide dismutase and catalase production may play a role in resistance to oxidative killing. Intermittent bacteraemia results in spread and localization in the reproductive organs and associated glands in sexually mature animals. Erythritol, a polyhydric alcohol which acts as a growth factor for brucellae, is present in high concentrations in the placentae of cattle, sheep, goats and pigs. This growth factor is also found in other organs such as the mammary gland and epididymis, which are targets for brucellae. In chronic brucellosis, organisms may localize in joints or intervertebral discs.

Diagnostic procedures

The diagnosis of brucellosis depends on serological testing and on the isolation and identification of the infecting *Brucella* species. Care should be taken during collection and transportation of specimens, which should be processed in a biohazard cabinet.

- Specimens for laboratory examination should relate to the specific clinical condition encountered.
- MZN-stained smears from specimens, particularly

Table 28.2 Characteristics of *Brucella* species of veterinary importance.

Brucella species	Number of biotypes	Requirement for CO_2	Production of H_2S	Urease activity	Growth in media containing	
					Thionin (20 μg/ml)	Basic fuchsin (20 μg/ml)
B. abortus	7	v	v	+	v	v
B. melitensis	3	−	−	v	+	+
B. suis	5	−	v	+	+	v
B. ovis	1	+	−	−	+	−
B. canis	1	−	−	+	+	−

v variable reactions related to different biotypes

cotyledons, foetal abomasal contents and uterine discharges, often reveal characteristic MZN-positive coccobacilli. In specimens containing cells, the organisms appear in clusters (Fig. 28.1).

- The polymerase chain reaction can be used to detect brucellae in tissues (Fekete *et al.*, 1992).
- A nutritious medium such as Columbia agar, supplemented with 5% serum and appropriate antimicrobial agents, is used for isolation. Plates are incubated at 37°C in 5 to 10% CO_2 for up to 5 days. Although CO_2 is a specific requirement for individual species, the majority of brucellae are capnophilic.
- Serological testing is used for international trade and for identifying infected herds or flocks and individual animals in national eradication schemes (Table 28.3). Brucellae share antigens with some other Gram-negative bacteria such as *Yersinia enterocolitica* serotype O:9 (Hilbink *et al.*, 1995), and consequently cross-reactions can occur in agglutination tests.

Clinical infections

Although each *Brucella* species has its own natural host, *B. abortus*, *B. melitensis* and biotypes of *B. suis* can infect animals other than their preferred hosts (Table 28.1).

Table 28.3 Tests used for the diagnosis of bovine brucellosis using milk or serum.

Test	Comments
Brucella milk ring test	Conducted on bulk milk samples for monitoring infections in dairy herds. Sensitive but may not be reliable in large herds
Rose-Bengal plate test	Useful screening test. Antigen suspension is adjusted to pH 3.6, allowing agglutination by IgG1 antibodies. Qualitative test only, positive results require confirmation by CFT or ELISA
Complement-fixation test (CFT)	Widely accepted confirmatory test for individual animals
Indirect ELISA	Reliable screening and confirmatory test
Competitive ELISA (using monoclonal antibodies)	Recently developed test with high specificity; capable of detecting all immunoglobulin classes and can be used to differentiate infected animals from S19-vaccinated cattle
Serum agglutination test (SAT)	A tube agglutination test which lacks specificity and sensitivity; IgG1 antibodies may not be detected, leading to false-negative results
Antiglobulin test	Sensitive test for detecting non-agglutinating antibodies not detected by the SAT

Bovine brucellosis

Bovine brucellosis, caused by *B. abortus* and formerly worldwide in distribution, has been eradicated or reduced to a low prevalence in many countries through national eradication programmes. Although acquired most often by ingestion, infection can occasionally follow venereal contact, penetration through skin abrasions, inhalation or transplacental transmission (Fig. 28.2). Abortion storms may be encountered in herds with a high percentage of susceptible pregnant cows. Abortion usually occurs after the fifth month of gestation and subsequent pregnancies are usually carried to term. Large numbers of brucellae are excreted in foetal fluids for about 2 to 4 weeks following an abortion and at subsequent parturitions, although infected calves appear normal. Infection in calves is of limited duration in contrast to cows in which infection of the mammary glands and associated lymph nodes persists for many years. Brucellae may be excreted intermittently in milk for a number of years. In bulls, the structures targeted include seminal vesicles, ampullae, testicles and epididymides. In tropical countries, hygromas involving the limb joints are often observed when the disease is endemic in a herd.

In affected herds, brucellosis can result in decreased fertility, reduced milk production, abortions in susceptible replacement animals and testicular degeneration in bulls. Abortion is a consequence of placentitis involving both cotyledons and intercotyledonary tissues. In the bull, necrotizing orchitis occasionally results in localized fibrotic lesions.

Diagnosis

- Clinical signs are not specific although abortions in first-calf heifers and replacement animals may suggest the presence of the disease.
- Clusters of MZN-positive coccobacilli may be evident in smears of cotyledons and MZN-positive organisms may also be detected in foetal abomasal contents and uterine discharges.
- Isolation and identification of *B. abortus* is confirmatory.
- Identification criteria for isolates:
  — Colonial appearance
  — MZN-positive organisms
  — Bacterial cell agglutination with a high-titred antiserum
  — Rapid urease activity
  — Biotyping using tests and other features indicated in Table 28.2
- A range of serological tests, varying in sensitivity and specificity, is available for the identification of infected animals (Table 28.3).
- Brucellin, an extract of *B. abortus*, has been used for intradermal testing (Worthington *et al.*, 1993).
- Molecular methods, such as PCR-based techniques, for

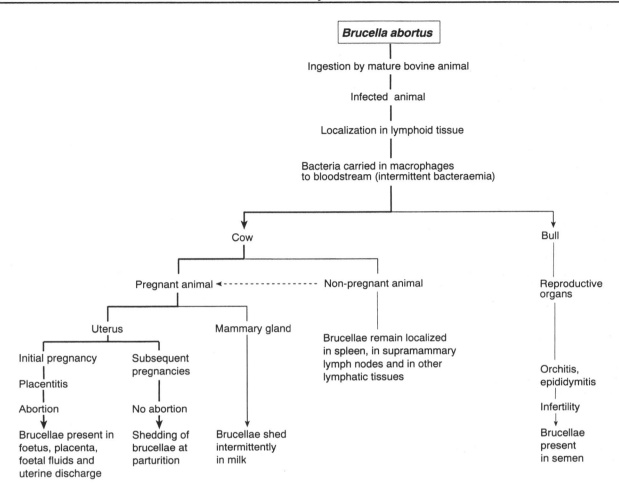

Figure 28.2 The progression of infection with *Brucella abortus* in mature susceptible cattle.

the detection of brucellae in tissues and fluids have been described.

Treatment and control
- Treatment of cattle with brucellosis is not practical.
- National eradication schemes are based on the detection and slaughter of infected cattle.
- Vaccination of young heifers, a strategic measure during the early years of eradication schemes, is discontinued when the prevalence of brucellosis reaches low levels. Immunity in brucellosis is predominantly cell-mediated. Three types of vaccines are used in cattle, attenuated strain 19 (S19) vaccine, adjuvanted 45/20 vaccine and the more recent RB51 vaccine:
  — S19 vaccine is administered to female calves up to 5 months of age. Vaccination of mature animals leads to persistent antibody titres.
  — 45/20 bacterin, although less effective, has been used in some national eradication schemes. Even when administered to adult animals, this vaccine does not induce persistent antibody titres.
  — RB51 strain is a stable, rough mutant which induces good protection against abortion and does not result

in serological responses detectable in tests used in conventional brucellosis surveillance programmes.

Caprine and ovine brucellosis

Caprine and ovine brucellosis, caused by *B. melitensis*, are most commonly encountered in countries around the Mediterranean littoral and in the Middle East, central Asia and parts of South America. Goats, in which the disease is more severe and protracted, tend to be more susceptible to infection than sheep. The clinical disease resembles brucellosis in cattle in many respects. Clinical features include high abortion rates in susceptible populations, orchitis in male animals, arthritis and hygromas. Infection resulting in abortion may not induce a protective immunity.

Diagnosis is based on clinical signs, direct examination of MZN-stained smears of fluids or tissues, isolation and identification of *B. melitensis* and serological testing. Intradermal brucellin tests are used for surveillance of unvaccinated flocks and herds. In countries where the disease is exotic, a test and slaughter policy is usually implemented. Test and slaughter policies can also reduce the prevalence of disease in endemic areas. The Rose-Bengal agglutination test and the complement fixation test are the most widely used methods for detecting infection with *B. melitensis*. An enzyme-linked immunosorbent assay is being developed. The modified live *B. melitensis* Rev. 1 strain, administered by the subcutaneous or conjunctival routes, is used for vaccination of kids and lambs up to 6 months of age.

Ovine epididymitis caused by *B. ovis*

Brucella ovis produces an infection in sheep which is chacterized by epididymitis in rams and placentitis in ewes. The infection was first recorded in New Zealand and Australia and is now established in many other sheep-rearing regions, including some European countries. The consequences of infection include reduced fertility in rams, sporadic abortion in ewes and increased perinatal mortality. Both ram-to-ram and ram-to-ewe venereal transmission occurs. Few of the ewes served by an infected ram develop disease. There is a relatively long latent period in rams following infection. *Brucella ovis* may be present in semen about 5 weeks after infection and epididymal lesions can be detected by palpation at about 9 weeks. In countries where the disease is endemic, pre-mating checks on rams include serological testing and scrotal palpation. Chronically-affected rams often have unilateral or bilateral testicular atrophy with swelling and hardening of the epididymis. The most efficient and widely-used serological tests for *B. ovis* are the agar gel immunodiffusion test, the complement fixation test and the indirect ELISA. An immunoblotting technique can also be used as a confirmatory diagnostic test (Kittelberger *et al.*, 1997). *Brucella ovis* can be isolated from semen. Young rams may be vaccinated with the *B. melitensis* Rev. 1 vaccine or with *B. ovis* bacterin.

Porcine brucellosis

Porcine brucellosis, caused by *B. suis*, occurs occasionally in the USA but is more prevalent in Latin America and Asia. There is a prolonged bacteraemia and the disease is manifest as chronic inflammatory lesions in the reproductive organs of sows and boars. Lesions may also be found in bones and joints. Infection is acquired by ingestion or by coitus and may be self-limiting in some animals. Clinical signs in sows include abortion, stillbirths, neonatal mortality and temporary sterility. Boars excreting brucellae in semen may either be clinically normal or present with testicular abnormalities. Associated sterility may be temporary or permanent. Lameness, incoordination and posterior paralysis are manifestations of joint or bone involvement. The Rose-Bengal plate agglutination test and the indirect ELISA are the most reliable

serological methods for the diagnosis of porcine brucellosis. A test and slaughter policy is the main control measure in countries where the disease is exotic. A modified live *B. suis* vaccine is used for the vaccination of pigs in south China. *Brucella suis* biotype 2 infects wild hares in parts of Europe and these animals may act as a source of infection for pigs. Brucella suis biotype 4 can infect reindeer and caribou in Northern Canada, Alaska and Siberia.

Canine brucellosis

Canine brucellosis, caused by *B. canis*, has been recorded in the USA, Japan and Central and South America. However, the distribution of the disease may be more extensive than currently recognized because of difficulties with diagnosis. As *Brucella canis* is permanently in the rough form, it is of comparatively low virulence causing relatively mild and asymptomatic infections. In breeding establishments infection may manifest clinically as abortions, decreased fertility, reduced litter sizes and neonatal mortality. Most bitches, which have aborted, subsequently have normal gestations. In male dogs, the main clinical feature of the disease is infertility often associated with orchitis and epididymitis. Infertility may be permanent and dogs with chronic infections are often aspermic. Rarely, discospondylitis may result in lameness and paresis or paralysis. A rapid slide agglutination test kit containing 2-mercaptoethanol is used as a screening test. Confirmatory tests include a tube agglutination test, ELISA and an agar gel immunodiffusion test. Treatment, which should be confined to animals not intended for breeding, may be successful early in the course of the disease. A combination of a tetracycline and an aminoglycoside may be effective (Nicoletti and Chase, 1987). Neutering infected animals reduces the risk of transmission. No commercial vaccine is available and control is based on routine serological testing and removal of infected animals from breeding programmes.

Brucellosis in humans

Humans are susceptible to infection with *B. abortus*, *B. suis*, *B. melitensis* and, rarely, with *B. canis*. Transmission to humans occurs through contact with secretions or excretions of infected animals. Routes of entry include skin abrasions, inhalation and ingestion. Raw milk and dairy produce made with unpasteurized milk are important sources of infection. Laboratory accidents account for some human infections. Brucellosis in humans, known as undulant fever, presents as fluctuating pyrexia, malaise, fatigue and muscle and joint pains. Abortion is not a feature of human infection. Osteomyelitis is the most common complication. Severe infections occur with *B. melitensis* (Malta fever) and *B. suis* biotypes 1 and 2. Human infections due to

B. abortus are moderately severe whereas those caused by *B. canis* are usually mild. Antimicrobial therapy should be administered early in an infection. Humans can develop a severe hypersensitivity reaction following infection or after accidental inoculation with attenuated vaccinal strains.

References

Fekete, A., Bantle, J.A. and Halling, S.M. (1992). Detection of *Brucella* by polymerase chain reaction in bovine foetal and maternal tissues. *Journal of Veterinary Diagnostic Investigation*, **4**, 79–83.

Hilbink, F., Fenwick, S.G., Thompson, E.J., Kittelberger, R., Penrose, M. and Ross, G.P. (1995). Non-specific seroreactions against *Brucella abortus* in ruminants in New Zealand and the presence of *Yersinia enterocolitica* O:9. *New Zealand Veterinary Journal*, **43**, 175–178.

Kittelberger, R., Diack, D.S., Ross, G.P. and Reichel, M.P. (1997). An improved immunoblotting technique for the serodiagnosis of *Brucella ovis* infections. *New Zealand Veterinary Journal*, **45**, 75–77.

Nicoletti, P. and Chase, A. (1987). The use of antibiotics to control canine brucellosis. *Compendium on Continuing Education for the Practicing Veterinarian*, **9**, 1063–1066.

Price, R.E., Templeton, J.W., Smith, R. and Adams, L.G. (1990). Ability of mononuclear phagocytes from cattle naturally resistant or susceptible to brucellosis to control in vitro intracellular survival of *Brucella abortus*. *Infection and Immunity*, **58**, 879–886.

Rafie-Kolpin, M., Essenberg, R.C. and Wyckoff, J.H. III (1996). Identification and comparison of macrophage-induced proteins and proteins induced under various stress conditions in *Brucella abortus*. *Infection and Immunity*, **64**, 5274–5283.

Robertson, G.T. and Roop, R.M. II (1999). The *Brucella abortus* host factor 1 (HF-1) protein contributes to stress resistance during stationary phase and is a major determinant of virulence in mice. *Molecular Microbiology*, **34**, 690–700.

Roop, R.M., Jeffers, G., Bagchi, T., Walker, J., Enright, F.M. and Schurig, G.G. (1991). Experimental infection of goat foetuses *in utero* with a stable rough mutant of *Brucella abortus*. *Research in Veterinary Science*, **51**, 123–127.

Ross, H.M., Foster, G., Reid, R.J., Jahans, K.L. and MacMillan, A.P. (1994). *Brucella* species infection in sea-mammals. *Veterinary Record*, **134**, 359.

Worthington, R.W, Weddell, W. and Neilson, F.J.A. (1993). A practical method for the production of *Brucella* skin test antigen. *New Zealand Veterinary Journal*, **41**, 7-11.

Further reading

Bracewell, C.D. and Corbel, M.J. (1980). An association between arthritis and persistent serological reactions to *Brucella abortus* in cattle from apparently brucellosis-free herds. *Veterinary Record*, **106**, 99.

Chapter 29

Campylobacter species

Campylobacter species are slender, curved motile Gram-negative rods (0.2 to 0.5 μm wide) with polar flagella. Daughter cells which remain joined have a characteristic gull-winged appearance and long spirals formed by joined cells also occur (Fig. 29.1). These microaerophilic organisms grow best on enriched media in an atmosphere of increased CO_2 and decreased oxygen tension. Many *Campylobacter* species grow on MacConkey agar. They are non-fermentative and oxidase-positive and have variable catalase reactions.

Campylobacter species are found in the intestinal and genital tracts of domestic animals and are widely distributed geographically. The principal disease conditions associated with infection are either intestinal, presenting as diarrhoea, or genital, causing infertility or abortion. *Campylobacter* species were previously classified in the genus *Vibrio*, and the term 'vibriosis' has been retained for some of the disease conditions which they cause. Three species, namely *C. fetus* subspecies *venerealis*, *C. fetus* subspecies *fetus* and *C. jejuni* subspecies *jejuni* (hereafter referred to as *C. jejuni*) are recognized pathogens of veterinary importance (Fig. 29.2). A number of other species, some of which have been assigned to the genus *Arcobacter*, have been isolated from domestic animals and from humans (Table 29.1). The pathogenicity of these species has not been clearly established.

> **Key points**
> - Slender, curved Gram-negative rods in gull-winged shapes and spiral forms
> - Motile, microaerophilic
> - Most species grow on MacConkey agar
> - Enhanced growth on enriched media
> - Non-fermentative, oxidase-positive with variable catalase reactions
> - Commensals of the intestinal tract and sometimes of the reproductive tract
> - Pathogens in the reproductive and intestinal tracts

Usual habitat

Many *Campylobacter* species are commensals in the intestinal tracts of warm-blooded animals. *Campylobacter jejuni* and *C. lari* (formerly *C. laridis*) colonize the intestines of birds, which can result in faecal contamination of water courses and stored food. A number of *Campylobacter* species are excreted in the faeces of pigs. *Campylobacter fetus* subspecies *venerealis* appears to be adapted principally to bovine preputial mucosa.

Differentiation of *Campylobacter* species

Campylobacter species are strictly microaerophilic, requiring an atmosphere of 5 to 10% oxygen and 1 to 10% CO_2 for growth. A selective enriched medium such as Skirrow agar is usually used for primary isolation (Terzolo *et al.*, 1991). Differentiation of isolates is based on colonial morphology and certain cultural, biochemical and antibiotic-susceptibility characteristics.

- Colonial morphology:
  - *Campylobacter fetus* subspecies *venerealis* and *C. fetus* subspecies *fetus* have small, round, smooth, translucent colonies with a dewdrop appearance.
  - *Campylobacter jejuni* produces small, flat, grey colonies with a spreading, watery appearance.
  - Colonies of some *Campylobacter* species, which

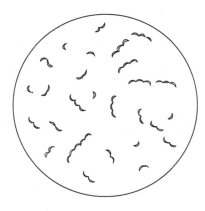

Figure 29.1 Slender curved rods of *Campylobacter* species. Characteristic gull-winged and spiral forms are shown.

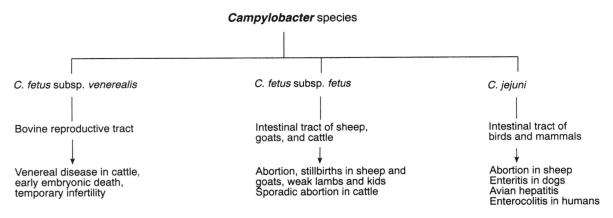

Figure 29.2 Pathogenic *Campylobacter* species, their usual habitats and the possible consequences of infection.

Table 29.1 *Campylobacter* and *Arcobacter* species of uncertain pathogenicity.

Microorganism	Host	Comments
Campylobacter coli	Pigs Humans	Present in intestine Causes enterocolitis
C. helveticus	Dogs, cats	Present in faeces
C. hyoileri	Pigs	Present in faeces
C. hyointestinalis	Pigs	Present in faeces
C. lari	Dogs, birds, other animals Humans	Present in faeces May cause enteritis
C. jejuni subsp. *doylei*	Humans	Isolated from clinical specimens
C. mucosalis	Pigs	Present in faeces
C. sputorum biovar *sputorum*	Cattle, sheep Humans	Present in genital tract Isolated from faeces and gingivae
C. sputorum biovar *fecalis*	Sheep, cattle Cattle	Present in intestinal and genital tracts Isolated from cases of bovine digital dermatitis
C. upsaliensis	Dogs Humans	Present in faeces and associated with diarrhoea May cause diarrhoea in children
Arcobacter butzleri	Humans Cattle, pigs	May cause diarrhoea Implicated in abortion
A. cryaerophilus	Many species Sheep, horses Cattle	Isolated from faeces Isolated from normal and aborted foetuses Mastitis (rare)
A. skirrowii	Cattle Cattle, sheep, pigs	Present in prepuce Isolated from aborted foetuses

may contaminate clinical specimens, can be slightly pigmented.

- Because *Campylobacter* species do not ferment carbohydrates, other metabolic activities of these organisms must be used for identification. Differentiating characteristics of the main animal pathogens and some commonly isolated commensals are presented in Table 29.2.

Pathogenesis and pathogenicity

Campylobacter fetus subspecies *venerealis* and *C. fetus* subspecies *fetus* are structurally unusual in that they possess a microcapsule or S layer, which consists of high-molecular-weight proteins arranged in a lattice formation. This S layer confers resistance to serum-mediated destruction and phagocytosis (Blaser and Pei, 1993) and enhances survival in the genital tract. Virulence factors attributed to *C. jejuni* include soluble components with enterotoxin-like activity and poorly defined mechanisms for attaching to and invading host enterocytes. The contribution of heat-stable endotoxin to the pathogenesis of campylobacteriosis is uncertain.

Diagnostic procedures

Details of the diagnostic methods for individual clinical conditions are presented in relevant sections.

- Irrespective of the source of specimens for bacterial isolation, certain general principles relating to culture techniques apply. *Campylobacter* species require microaerophilic conditions for growth, usually supplied by commercially-available generator envelopes which deliver 6% oxygen, 10% carbon dioxide and 84% nitrogen. Although most pathogenic species grow optimally at 37°C, *C. jejuni* requires up to 5 days at 42°C for optimum growth.
- Smears from cultures and from clinical specimens should be stained with dilute carbol fuchsin (DCF) for 4 minutes. This method stains the organisms more

Table 29.2 Differentiating characteristics of *Campylobacter* species.

Campylobacter species	Catalase production	Growth at 25°C	Growth at 42°C	Growth in 1% glycine	Growth in 3.5% NaCl	Production of H_2S[a]	Susceptibility to Nalidixic acid[b]	Susceptibility to Cephalothin[b]
C. fetus subsp. *venerealis*	+	+	−	−	−	−	R	S
C. fetus subsp. *fetus*	+	+	−	+	−	+	V	S
C. jejuni subsp. *jejuni*	+	−	+	+	−	+	S	R
C. lari	+	−	+	+	−	+	R	R
C. coli	+	−	+	+	−	+	S	R
C. hyointestinalis	+	+	+	+	−	+	R	S
C. mucosalis	−	−	+	+	−	+	R	S
C. sputorum biovar *sputorum*	−	−	+	+	+	+	R	S

a lead acetate method of detection	R resistant
b 30 µg discs	S susceptible
+ most strains positive	V variable
− most strains negative	

intensely than the Gram method.
- Identification criteria for isolates:
  — Growth only under microaerophilic conditions
  — Colonial morphology
  — Cell morphology in smears stained with DCF or by immunofluorescence
  — Metabolic characteristics and antibiotic susceptibility pattern.

Clinical infections

The most important consequences of infections with organisms in this group are infertility in cattle due to *C. fetus* subspecies *venerealis* and abortion in ewes caused either by *C. fetus* subspecies *fetus* or by *C. jejuni* (Fig. 29.2).

Bovine genital campylobacteriosis

Campylobacter fetus subspecies *venerealis*, the principal cause of bovine genital campylobacteriosis, is transmitted during coitus to susceptible cows by asymptomatic carrier bulls. The bacteria survive in the glandular crypts of the prepuce and bulls may remain infected indefinitely. The disease is characterized by temporary infertility associated with early embryonic death, return to oestrus at irregular periods (Fig. 29.3) and, occasionally, by sporadic abortion. About one-third of infected cows become carriers. *Campylobacter fetus* subspecies *venerealis* persists in the vagina of carrier cows, a feature attributed to antigenic shifts in the immunodominant antigens of the S layer

proteins. Extension of infection to the uterus with the development of endometritis and salpingitis can occur during the progestational phase of the oestrus cycle when both the numbers and the activity of neutrophils decline. The infertile period following uterine invasion can last for 3 to 5 months, after which natural immunity may develop. IgA antibodies, which predominate in the vagina, limit spread of the infection. IgG antibodies produced in the uterus opsonize the pathogens, facilitating phagocytosis by neutrophils and mononuclear cells (Fig. 29.3). This natural immunity may last for up to 4 years.

Campylobacter fetus subspecies *fetus*, an enteric organism acquired by ingestion, can cause sporadic abortions in cows.

Diagnosis
- Investigation of the breeding records and vaccination history of an affected herd may suggest campylobacteriosis.
- *Campylobacter* species can be detected by the fluorescent antibody technique in sheath washings from bulls or cervicovaginal mucus from cows.
- Isolation and identification of *C. fetus* subspecies *venerealis* from preputial or vaginal mucus is confirmatory. Specimens of mucus should be placed in special transport medium (Lander, 1990).
- Vaginal mucus agglutination test detects about 50% of infected, infertile cows on a herd basis.
- An ELISA can be used to demonstrate IgA antibodies in vaginal mucus after an abortion (Hum *et al.*, 1991).
- A polymerase chain reaction has been developed as a

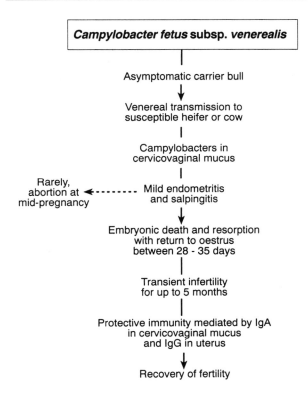

Figure 29.3 The role of *Campylobacter fetus* subsp. *venerealis* in infertility in cattle.

rapid screening test for the detection of *C. fetus* subspecies *venerealis* in bull's semen (Eaglesome *et al.*, 1995).

- Infertility due to *C. fetus* subspecies *venerealis* must be differentiated from other causes of infertility in cows.
- *Campylobacter sputorum* biovar *sputorum*, a commensal which is sometimes isolated from preputial washings, is of no clinical significance in cattle.

Treatment and control
- Dihydrostreptomycin, administered either systemically or topically into the prepuce, is used for treating bulls.
- Intrauterine administration of dihydrostreptomycin can be used therapeutically.
- Vaccination with bacterins in an oil emulsion adjuvant is used therapeutically and prophylactically in problem herds.

Ovine genital campylobacteriosis

Campylobacteriosis in ewes may be caused by either *C. fetus* subspecies *fetus* or *C. jejuni*. The disease is worldwide in distribution and is one of the most common causes of ovine abortion in some countries (Anon., 1997). *Campylobacter fetus* subspecies *fetus* is found in the faeces of cattle and sheep and *C. jejuni* may be present in the faeces of a wide range of birds and mammals. Transmission of both of these organisms is by the faecal-oral route. During pregnancy, localization in the uterus of susceptible ewes may occur following bacteraemia. The subsequent necrotic placentitis may result in abortion late in pregnancy, stillborn lambs or weak lambs. Round, necrotic lesions up to 2 cm in diameter with pale raised rims and dark depressed centres are evident on the liver surface in some aborted lambs. Aborting ewes are major sources of infection for susceptible animals in a flock. Up to 20% of ewes in a susceptible flock may abort. Recovered ewes are immune for at least 3 years and flock fertility in subsequent breeding seasons is usually good.

Diagnosis
- Typical hepatic lesions in aborted lambs are pathognomonic.
- A presumptive diagnosis is made by demonstrating the organisms in foetal abomasal contents or birth fluids.
- Isolation and identification of *C. fetus* subsecies *fetus* or *C. jejuni* is confirmatory.
- These pathogens should be differentiated from other causes of abortion in ewes (*see* Chapter 78).

Treatment and control
- Aborting ewes should be isolated and placentae and aborted foetuses promptly removed. The remainder of the flock should be moved to clean pasture.
- Vaccination of ewes with a *C. fetus* subspecies *fetus* bacterin, after confirmation of the disease in a flock, is reported to reduce the number of abortions (Gumbrell *et al.*, 1996).
- Routine vaccination of ewes with a bacterin is usually carried out immediately before or after mating, with a booster after the second month of gestation and annually thereafter. There is no cross-protection between *C. fetus* subspecies *fetus* and *C. jejuni*.
- Chlortetracycline administered daily in feed has been used to control outbreaks of abortion.

Intestinal campylobacteriosis in dogs

Diarrhoea in dogs and other domestic animals has been attributed to infection with *Campylobacter* species, particularly *C. jejuni*. Confirmation is difficult because healthy animals may shed *Campylobacter* species in their faeces. However, the presence of large numbers of campylobacter-like organisms in DCF-stained faecal smears or rectal scrapings from dogs with diarrhoea may be indicative of infection. *Campylobacter* species may contribute to the severity of enteric disease in dogs infected with other enteropathogens such as enteric viruses, *Giardia* species and helminths. Young, debilitated or immunosuppressed animals are particularly at risk. Enrofloxacin is usually effective in eliminating faecal shedding of *Campylobacter* species. Dogs shedding *C. jejuni* are a potential source of human infection.

Avian vibrionic hepatitis

Birds commonly harbour *C. jejuni* in their intestinal tracts and shed the organisms in their faeces. Chicks acquire infection from feed, water and litter when they are first introduced into contaminated premises. Infection in chickens and turkeys is usually asymptomatic and its principal importance is as a source of infection for humans following carcase contamination at slaughter. Outbreaks of disease, which are uncommon, are characterized by a substantial drop in egg production in the flock. Severely affected birds are listless and lose condition. There may be haemorrhage and multifocal necrosis in livers. A presumptive diagnosis is made by demonstrating curved rods with darting motility in bile, using phase contrast microscopy. Dihydrostreptomycin sulphate should be administered in the food early in an outbreak of disease.

Intestinal campylobacteriosis in humans

Campylobacter jejuni is the main cause of human intestinal campylobacteriosis and *Campylobacter* infection is the most frequent cause of food poisoning in many countries. *Campylobacter coli* and *C. lari* are sometimes implicated. These zoonotic infections are usually food-borne. Poultry meat is a major source of human infection. Fever, abdominal pain and diarrhoea, sometimes with blood, are the most common manifestations of this enteric infection. In addition, antimicrobial resistance in campylobacters, particularly to fluoroquinolones, is a major public health concern.

References

Anon, (1997). Sheep abortions: analysis of trends in 1996/97. *Veterinary Record*, **141**, 321.

Blaser, M.J. and Pei, Z. (1993). Pathogenesis of *Campylobacter fetus* infections: critical role of high-molecular-weight S-layer proteins in virulence. *Journal of Infectious Diseases*, **167**, 372–377.

Eaglesome, M.D., Sampath, M.J. and Garcia, M.M. (1995). A detection assay for *Campylobacter fetus* in bovine semen by restriction analysis of PCR amplified DNA. *Veterinary Research Communications*, **19**, 253–263.

Gumbrell, R.C., Saville, D.J. and Graham, C.F. (1996). Tactical control of *Campylobacter* abortion outbreaks with a bacterin. *New Zealand Veterinary Journal*, **44**, 61–63.

Hum, S., Stephens, L.R. and Quinn, C. (1991). Diagnosis by ELISA of bovine abortion due to *Campylobacter fetus*. *Australian Veterinary Journal*, **68**, 272–275.

Lander, K.P. (1990). The development of a transport and enriched medium for *Campylobacter fetus*. *British Veterinary Journal*, **146**, 327–333.

Terzolo, H.R., Paolicchi, F.A., Moreira, A.R. and Homse, A. (1991). Skirrow agar for simultaneous isolation of *Brucella* and *Campylobacter* species. *Veterinary Record*, **129**, 531–532.

Further reading

Altekruse, S.F., Swerdlow, D.L. and Stern, N.J. (1998). *Campylobacter jejuni*. *Veterinary Clinics of North America: Food Animal Practice*, **14**, 31–40.

Vandamme, P., Vancanneyt, M., Pot, B., Mels, L., Hoste, B., Dewettinck, D. *et al.* (1992). Polyphasic taxonomic study of the emended genus *Arcobacter* with *Arcobacter butzleri* comb. nov. and *Arcobacter skirrowii* sp. nov., an aerotolerant bacterium isolated from veterinary specimens. *International Journal of Systematic Bacteriology*, **42**, 344–356.

Chapter 30

Lawsonia intracellularis

This slender, curved, Gram-negative rod, *Lawsonia intracellularis*, has not been grown in cell-free media. It is a campylobacter-like organism, which was formerly referred to as ileal symbiont intracellularis. This microaerophilic, obligate intracellular pathogen is aetiologically implicated in porcine proliferative enteropathy (McOrist *et al.*, 1995). It has been cultured in enterocyte cell lines (Lawson *et al.*, 1993).

> **Key points**
> - Curved, Gram-negative rods
> - Obligate intracellular pathogens
> - Microaerophilic
> - No growth on inert media
> - Growth in tissue culture prepared from enterocytes
> - Implicated in porcine proliferative enteropathy

Usual habitat

Lawsonia intracellularis grows intracellularly in pig enterocytes and infected animals excrete small numbers in their faeces (Smith and McOrist, 1997). Although organisms resembling *L. intracellularis* have been identified in mice, it has not been established that bacteria from this source can infect pigs.

Pathogenesis and pathogenicity

Lawsonia intracellularis has an affinity for porcine enterocytes, its site of replication. Infection induces enterocyte proliferation with the development of adenomatous and inflammatory lesions in the terminal ileum, caecum and colon. This proliferative enteropathy can be reproduced experimentally by oral dosing of conventional specific-pathogen-free pigs with the pathogen. Gnotobiotic pigs, which are devoid of intestinal flora, do not develop the disease when dosed with *L. intracellularis* unless they are pre-dosed with porcine intestinal flora. There appears to be a synergistic interaction between *L. intracellularis* and common intestinal organisms such as *Escherichia coli*, *Clostridium* species and *Bacteroides* species. These organisms probably produce the correct oxygen tension and other conditions necessary for the colonization and proliferation of *L. intracellularis* (McOrist *et al.*, 1994).

Porcine proliferative enteropathy

This enteric disease occurs in weaned pigs, 6 to 12 weeks of age, and is characterized by proliferative and inflammatory changes in the terminal small intestine and large intestine. Clinical signs range from chronic intermittent diarrhoea with reduction in weight gains to acute haemorrhagic enteropathy. Although sudden deaths may occur in severely affected pigs, most animals with the milder form of the disease recover without treatment.

Lesions in the ileum, caecum and colon include thickening of the wall, mucosal necrosis and, in severe cases, clotted blood in the lumen. Enlargement of the mesenteric lymph nodes is a feature of the disease.

Diagnosis
- Clinical signs and gross pathological findings may be sufficient for a presumptive diagnosis.
- *Lawsonia intracellularis* can be demonstrated in faeces or ileal mucosa by immunofluorescence or by the polymerase chain reaction technique.
- The organism can be demonstrated in sections from lesions by silver-impregnation stains or by immunostaining.
- *Lawsonia intracellularis* can be cultured only in enterocyte cell lines.

Treatment and control
- Antimicrobial agents such as tylosin or tiamulin may be used prophylactically or therapeutically in feed or water.
- Zinc bacitracin incorporated into feed has been reported to be effective in reducing the prevalence of intestinal lesions (Kyriakis *et al.*, 1996).
- Thorough cleaning and disinfection of contaminated premises should be carried out at the end of each production cycle.

Veterinary Microbiology and Microbial Disease

References

Kyriakis, S.C., Tsinas, A., Lekkas, S., Sarris, K. and Bourtzi-Hatzopoulou, E. (1996). Clinical evaluation of in-feed zinc bacitracin for the control of porcine intestinal adenomatosis in growing/fattening pigs. *Veterinary Record*, **138**, 489–492.

Lawson, G.H.K., McOrist, S., Jasmi, S. and Mackie, R.A. (1993). Intracellular bacteria of proliferative enteropathy: cultivation and maintenance in vitro. *Journal of Clinical Microbiology*, **31**, 1136–1142.

McOrist, S., Mackie, R.A., Neef, N., Aitken, I. and Lawson, G.H.K. (1994). Synergism of ileal symbiont intracellularis and gut bacteria in the reproduction of porcine proliferative enteropathy. *Veterinary Record*, **134**, 331–332.

McOrist, S., Gebhart, C.J., Boid, R. and Barns, S.M. (1995). Characterization of *Lawsonia intracellularis* gen. nov., sp. nov., the obligately intracellular bacterium of porcine proliferative enteropathy. *International Journal of Systematic Bacteriology*, **45**, 820–825.

Smith, S.H. and McOrist, S. (1997). Development of persistent intestinal infection and excretion of *Lawsonia intracellularis* by piglets. *Research in Veterinary Science*, **62**, 6–10.

Further reading

McOrist, S., Smith, S.H. and Green, L.E. (1997). Estimate of direct financial losses due to porcine proliferative enteropathy. *Veterinary Record*, **140**, 579–581.

Knittel, J.P., Schwartz, K.J. and McOrist, S. (1997). Diagnosis of porcine proliferative enteritis. *Compendium on Continuing Education for the Practicing Veterinarian*, **19**, Sup. S26–S29, S35.

Chapter 31

Spirochaetes

The order *Spirochaetales* contains two families, *Leptospiraceae* and *Spirochaetaceae* (Fig. 31.1). It comprises spiral or helical bacteria (spirochaetes) which share some unique morphological and functional features. Members of the order are motile by means of endoflagella which are located within the periplasm (Fig. 31.2). The pathogens in the family *Leptospiraceae* belong to the genus *Leptospira*. The genera *Borrelia*, *Brachyspira* and *Treponema* in the family *Spirochaetaceae* contain significant animal and human pathogens. There are some non-pathogenic genera in each family.

Pathogenic spirochaetes are difficult to culture; many require specialized media and some require liquid media. Organisms in the group are classified on the basis of genetic relatedness. Serological methods are used for epidemiological investigations and clinical diagnosis.

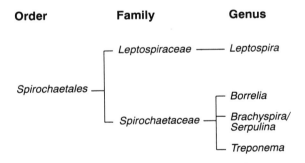

Figure 31.1 Classification of spirochaetes of veterinary importance.

Key points

- Spiral motile bacteria with endoflagella
- Labile in the environment and sensitive to desiccation
- Although Gram-negative, many stain poorly using conventional methods
- Some grow only in liquid media; most require specialized media
- Many produce zoonotic infections
- *Leptospira* species
  —Found in aquatic environments
  —Produce systemic infections in many species
  —Shed in urine of affected species
  —Cultured in liquid media aerobically at 30°C
  —Dark-field microscopy, silver staining and immunofluorescence used for recognition
- *Borrelia* species
  —Transmission by arthropod vectors
  —Cause systemic infections in many species
  —Grow slowly in specialized culture media at 30-35°C, in microaerophilic conditions
  —Culture of borreliae from infected animal is confirmatory
- *Brachyspira / Serpulina* species
  —Intestinal spirochaetes; some are important enteropathogens of pigs
  —Can be demonstrated in stained faecal smears or in silver-stained histopathological sections
  —Diagnosis confirmed by culture on selective blood agar anaerobically at 42°C

Leptospira species

Members of this species (leptospires) are motile helical bacteria (0.1 x 6 to 12 μm) with hook-shaped ends (Fig. 31.3). Although cytochemically Gram-negative, they do not stain well with conventional bacteriological dyes and are usually visualized using dark-field microscopy. Silver impregnation and immunological staining techniques are used to demonstrate leptospires in tissues. Leptospirosis, which can affect all domestic animals and humans, ranges in severity from mild infections of the urinary or genital systems to serious systemic disease (Table 31.1).

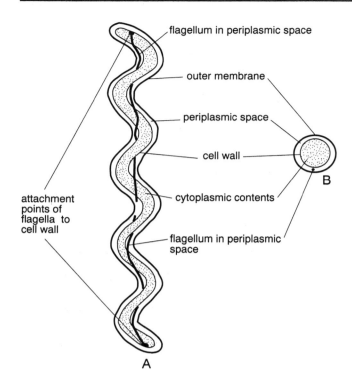

Figure 31.2 Diagrammatic illustration of a typical spirochaete indicating important structural features (A) and their relationships in cross section (B). The flagella, which are attached to the cell wall at each end of the organism, do not usually overlap.

Usual habitat

Leptospires can survive in ponds, rivers, surface waters, moist soil and mud when environmental temperatures are warm. Pathogenic leptospires can persist in the renal tubules or in the genital tract of carrier animals. Although indirect transmission can occur when environmental conditions are favourable, these fragile organisms are transmitted most effectively by direct contact.

Differentiation of *Leptospira* species

Formerly, leptospires were differentiated by serological reactions and two species were recognized, *L. interrogans* containing pathogens and *L. biflexa* containing saprophytes. Leptospiral species (genospecies) are now classified by DNA homology and, within each species, various serovars are recognized on the basis of serological reactions (Ellis, 1995). Currently, *L. borgpetersenii*, *L. fainei*, *L. inadai*, *L. interrogans* sensu stricto, *L. kirschneri*, *L. meyeri*, *L. noguchii*, *L. santarosai* and *L. weilii* are recognized as pathogenic species. A new species, *L. alexanderi*, has been described recently but its pathogenicity is uncertain (Brenner *et al.*, 1999). Currently more than 250 serovars in 23 serogroups are defined (Yasuda *et al.*, 1987; Perolat *et al.*, 1998). Cross-absorption of rabbit antisera against defined serovars is

used to determine the serovar of an isolate. Serovars with antigens in common belong to the same serogroup. Serologically similar leptospires may belong to different species. Serovar *hardjo*, for example, belongs to two species, *L. borgpetersenii* and *L. interrogans*, because common surface antigens are shared by these two genetically distinct organisms.

Epidemiology

Although leptospires are found worldwide, some serovars appear to have a limited geographical distribution. In addition, most serovars are associated with a particular host species, their maintenance host. Disease is frequently mild or subclinical in these highly susceptible maintenance hosts and is often followed by prolonged excretion of leptospires in urine. Maintenance hosts are the main source of environmental contamination and of natural transmission to other animal species which are termed incidental hosts. Incidental host species usually exhibit low susceptibility to infection, develop severe disease and are inefficient transmitters of leptospires to other animals. The maintenance hosts and the commonly infected incidental hosts of some serovars of *L. interrogans* are presented in Table 31.2. Genetic factors may account for differences observed in the severity of infection in different host species.

Pathogenesis and pathogenicity

The pathogenicity of leptospires relates to the virulence of the infecting serovar and the susceptibility of the host species. Although disease may be severe in immature maintenance hosts, serious disease occurs most commonly in incidental hosts. There is limited information on virulence factors and mechanisms of disease production. Leptospires invade tissues through moist, softened skin or through mucous membranes; motility may aid tissue invasion. They spread throughout the body via the blood

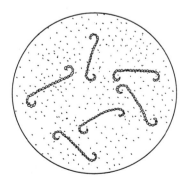

Figure 31.3 The appearance of leptospires when examined by dark-field microscopy. Their helical structure, which imparts a cord-like appearance, and their hooked ends differentiate these slender motile bacteria from most pathogenic microorganisms.

Table 31.1 Serovars of *Leptospira interrogans* which cause leptospirosis in domestic animals.

Serovar	Hosts	Clinical conditions
Leptospira borgpetersenii serovar *hardjo* *L. interrogans* serovar *hardjo*	Cattle, sheep	Abortions, stillbirths, agalactia
	Humans	Influenza-like illness; occasionally liver or kidney disease
L. borgpetersenii serovar *tarassovi*	Pigs	Reproductive failure, abortions, stillbirths
L. interrogans serovar *bratislava*	Pigs, horses, dogs	Reproductive failure, abortions, stillbirths
L. interrogans serovar *canicola*	Dogs	Acute nephritis in pups. Chronic renal disease in adult animals
	Pigs	Abortions and stillbirths. Renal disease in young pigs
L. interrogans serovar *grippotyphosa*	Cattle, pigs, dogs	Septicaemic disease in young animals; abortion
L. interrogans serovar *icterohaemorrhagiae*	Cattle, sheep, pigs	Acute septicaemic disease in calves, piglets and lambs; abortions
	Dogs, humans	Peracute haemorrhagic disease; acute hepatitis with jaundice
L. interrogans serovar *pomona*	Cattle, sheep	Acute haemolytic disease in calves and lambs; abortions
	Pigs	Reproductive failure; septicaemia in piglets
	Horses	Abortions, periodic ophthalmia

stream but, following the appearance of antibodies at about 10 days after infection, they are cleared from the circulation. Some organisms may evade the immune response and persist in the body, principally in the renal tubules but also in the uterus, eye or meninges. There is evidence that leptospiral chemotaxis for haemoglobin may be involved in the initiation of infection (Yuri *et al.*, 1993). Leptospires can evade phagocytosis in the bloodstream, possibly by inducing macrophage apoptosis (Merien *et al.*, 1997). It has been suggested that, following attachment to host cells, the organisms gain entry by receptor-mediated endocytosis (Merien *et al.*, 1997). In susceptible animals,

Table 31.2 Maintenance and incidental hosts for important serovars of *Leptospira interrogans*.

Serovar	Maintenance hosts	Incidental hosts
bratislava	Pigs, hedgehogs	Horses, dogs
canicola	Dogs	Pigs, cattle
grippotyphosa	Rodents	Cattle, pigs, horses, dogs
hardjo	Cattle, (sheep occasionally)	Humans
icterohaemorrhagiae	Brown rat	Domestic animals, humans
pomona	Pigs, cattle	Sheep, horses, dogs

damage to red cell membranes and to endothelial cells along with hepatocellular injury produces haemolytic anaemia, jaundice, haemoglobinuria and haemorrhage, associated with acute leptospirosis.

Diagnostic procedures

- Diagnosis of leptospirosis in maintenance hosts usually requires screening of a defined population.
- Clinical signs, together with a history suggestive of exposure to contaminated urine, may suggest acute leptospirosis.
- Organisms may be detected in fresh urine by dark-field microscopy, but this technique is relatively insensitive.
- Leptospires may be isolated from the blood during the first seven to ten days of infection and from urine approximately two weeks after initial infection either by culture in liquid medium or by animal inoculation. Slow-growing serovars such as *hardjo* may require incubation for six months in liquid media at 30°C. Commonly, EMJH (Ellinghausen, McCullough, Johnson and Harris) medium based on 1% bovine serum albumin and Tween 80, is used for isolation.
- Isolates should be identified using DNA profiles and serology.
- Fluorescent antibody procedures are often used for the demonstration of leptospires in tissues. Suitable tissues include kidney, liver and lung. Silver impregnation techniques can also be used for demonstration of leptospires.

- DNA hybridization, PCR, magnetic immunocapture PCR and immunomagnetic antigen capture systems have also been developed for the demonstration of leptospiral infection in tissues and urine.
- The standard serological reference test, the microscopic agglutination test, is potentially hazardous because it involves mixing live culture growing in liquid medium with equal volumes of doubling dilutions of test serum. Titres in excess of 1:400 or a four-fold rise in the titre in paired samples are diagnostically significant when accompanied by clinical signs consistent with leptospirosis. Serological diagnosis of host-adapted leptospirosis is difficult as titres may be decreasing or absent when clinical signs are observed. Some host-adapted serovars, notably *hardjo* in cattle, may elicit a poor immune response with the result that infection and prolonged urinary excretion occur without significant titres developing.
- A number of ELISA tests, developed in certain countries, are based on the predominant serovars occurring in those countries.

Clinical infections

The disease conditions associated with leptospiral infections in domestic animals are presented in Table 31.1.

Leptospirosis in cattle and sheep

Cattle are maintenance hosts for *L. borgpetersenii* serovar *hardjo* and there is increasing evidence that this serovar is also host-adapted for sheep (Cousins *et al.*, 1989). *Leptospira interrogans* serovar *hardjo* is also host-adapted for cattle. Although *L. interrogans* serovar *hardjo* appears to cause only sporadic cases of disease in cattle, it may be more virulent than *L. borgpetersenii* serovar *hardjo* (Ellis *et al.*, 1988). Susceptible replacement heifers, reared separately and introduced into an infected dairy herd for the first time at calving, may develop acute disease with pyrexia and agalactia affecting all quarters. Infection may also result in abortions and stillbirths. If management practices allow exposure to infection and the subsequent development of immunity before breeding age, reproductive problems may not develop. Agalactia caused by leptospiral infection can be confirmed by demonstrating a rising antibody titre in paired serum samples. Infection with serovar *hardjo* in sheep, particularly in intensively managed lowland flocks, can cause abortions and agalactia. Dihydrostreptomycin or amoxycillin can be used for reducing or eliminating urinary excretion of the organisms. Both monovalent and multivalent inactivated vaccines, which are commercially available, may not always be effective. Serovars incorporated into vaccines should be those which are associated with disease in a particular region. Infection with serovars *pomona*, *grippotyphosa*, and *icterohaemorrhagiae* can cause serious

disease, particularly in calves and lambs. Infection is usually accompanied by pyrexia, haemoglobinuria, jaundice and anorexia. Extensive renal damage with resultant uraemia often precedes death. Vaccination is used for control of serovar *pomona* which is an important cause of bovine abortion in some countries.

Leptospirosis in horses

Although serological evidence of leptospiral infection is common in horses, clinical disease is infrequent. Infection with serovar *bratislava*, which has been associated with abortions and stillbirths in horses, may be maintained in the equine species. Clinical disease most often results from incidental infection with serovar *pomona*, although other serovars have been implicated. Signs include abortion in mares and renal disease in young horses. An immune-mediated anterior uveitis (periodic ophthalmia, 'moon blindness') may be a manifestation of chronic leptospirosis in horses. Cross-reactions between leptospiral antigens and proteins from the cornea and lens suggest that autoimmune mechanisms may be involved (Parma *et al.*, 1992). Leptospiral vaccines are not currently licensed for use in horses.

Leptospirosis in pigs

Acute leptospirosis in pigs is usually caused by rodent-adapted serovars such as *icterohaemorrhagiae* and *copenhagenii*. These serovars cause serious, sometimes fatal, disease in young pigs with signs similar to those of acute leptospirosis in other species. In many parts of the world, the principal host-adapted serovar is *pomona*. Pigs subclinically infected with *pomona* may shed leptospires in their urine for extended periods. Infection can result in reproductive failure including abortions and stillbirths. Pigs also serve as maintenance hosts for serovars *tarassovi* and *bratislava*, which may also cause reproductive failure.

Leptospirosis in dogs and cats

The serovars associated with leptospirosis in dogs are *canicola* and *icterohaemorrhagiae*. The widespread use of vaccines incorporating these serovars has resulted in serovars *grippotyphosa* and *pomona* emerging as important canine pathogens (Rentko *et al.*, 1992). Serovar *canicola*, which is host-adapted for dogs, causes severe renal disease in pups. In animals which survive the acute phase, a chronic uraemic syndrome may subsequently develop. Incidental canine infections, usually caused by *icterohaemorrhagiae* are characterized by acute haemorrhagic disease or subacute hepatic and renal failure. In incidental canine infections due to serovars other than *icterohaemorrhagiae* or *copenhagenii*, signs of renal involvement usually predominate. It is considered that serovar *bratislava*, which has been associated with abortion and infertility, is becoming adapted to dogs which may act as maintenance hosts. Bacterins which contain only serovars *icterohaemorrhagiae* and *canicola* do not provide immunity against other serovars. Although clinical leptospirosis is uncommon in cats, infections with a number of serovars have been reported (Agunloye and Nash, 1996).

Public health aspects

Leptospirosis is an occupational disease of abattoir workers, dairy and pig farmers, veterinary surgeons and those engaged in manual work related to sewage and drainage.

Borrelia species

Borreliae, which are longer and wider than other spirochaetes, have a similar helical shape (Fig. 31.4). In addition to a linear chromosome, which is unique among bacteria, borreliae possess linear and circular plasmids. Although these spirochaetes can cause disease in animals and humans, subclinical infections are also common. Borreliae are transmitted by arthropod vectors. *Borrelia* species of importance in animals, their arthropod vectors, and the diseases which they cause are summarized in Table 31.3.

Usual habitat

Borreliae are obligate parasites in a variety of vertebrate hosts. Although these organisms persist in the environment for short periods, they depend on vertebrate reservoir hosts and arthropod vectors for long-term survival.

Differentiation of *Borrelia* species

Borreliae can be differentiated from other spirochaetes by their morphology, by the low guanine and cytosine content of their genomic DNA and by ecological, cultural and biochemical characteristics. Identification of *Borrelia*

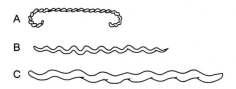

Figure 31.4 Spirochaetes of veterinary importance illustrating differences in size and shape: A, *Leptospira*; B, *Brachyspira*; C, *Borrelia*.

species depends mainly on genetic analysis. At least nine genospecies or genomic groups of *B. burgdorferi* sensu lato, have been identified using DNA-DNA hybridization, 16S rRNA sequencing and other molecular techniques.

Clinical infections

The species of particular veterinary importance are *B. burgdorferi* sensu lato, the cause of Lyme disease in animals and humans, and *B. anserina* which causes avian borreliosis. The significance of two other species, *B. theileri* and *B. coriaceae*, as animal pathogens, is uncertain.

Lyme disease

This condition, also known as Lyme borreliosis, was first identified in 1975 following investigation of a cluster of arthritis cases in children near the town of Old Lyme, Connecticut. The causative agent, a spirochaete, was named *Borrelia burgdorferi*. Several genospecies of *B. burgdorferi* have subsequently been identified in the USA and Europe. Although *B. burgdorferi* sensu stricto is the principal genotype isolated in the USA, genetic diversity among isolates has been documented (Oliver, 1996). The recognized species and genomic groups of *B. burgdorferi* sensu lato are presented in Box 31.1.

Epidemiology

Lyme disease has been reported in humans, dogs, horses and cattle, and infection has been documented in sheep.

Table 31.3 Tick vectors and natural hosts of *Borrelia* species and associated clinical conditions.

Species	Vector	Host	Clinical conditions
B. burgdorferi sensu lato	*Ixodes* species	Rodents	Arthritic, neurological and cardiac disease in dogs and occasionally in horses, cattle, sheep and humans
B. anserina	*Argas* species	Birds	Fever, weight loss and anaemia in domestic poultry
B. theileri	Many species of ticks	Cattle, sheep, horses	Mild febrile disease with anaemia
B. coriaceae	*Ornithodoros* species	Cattle, deer	Associated with epizootic bovine abortion in USA

Box 31.1 Currently recognized species and genomic groups within *Borrelia burgdorferi* sensu lato.

- *B. afzelii*
- *B. andersonii*
- *B. burgdorferi* sensu stricto
- *B. garinii*
- *B. japonica*
- *B. lusitaniae*
- *B. tanukii*
- *B. turdi*
- *B. valaisiana*
- *B. bissettii*
- Genomic group 25015

Ticks are the only competent vectors of *B. burgdorferi* sensu lato. Infection is usually acquired by larval stages of ticks feeding on small rodents. A variety of small wild animals including mice, voles, hedgehogs, lizards and birds can act as reservoir hosts. The spirochaetes persist through nymphal and adult stages of ticks which transmit infection while feeding. Adult ticks feed preferentially on large mammals such as deer and sheep, which are maintenance hosts for the tick population but are unsuitable reservoirs for *B. burgdorferi* sensu lato. The persistence of these pathogenic bacteria in a region is dependent on the presence of suitable reservoir hosts for borreliae and maintenance hosts for ticks. The most common tick vector for *B. burgdorferi* sensu lato in Europe is *Ixodes ricinus*; in central and eastern USA it is *I. scapularis*; on the west coast of the USA, it is *I. pacificus*, and in Eurasia it is *I. persulcatus*. The relationships between *B. burgdorferi* sensu lato, its hosts and tick vectors are shown in Fig. 31.5. Transovarial transmission of the spirochaete in the tick, which may occur infrequently, is not epidemiologically important. Occasional transmission of borreliae from infected incidental hosts to uninfected ticks may occur.

Although *B. burgdorferi* sensu lato has been demonstrated in the urine of dogs and horses, infected urine is an unlikely source of infection.

Pathogenesis

Transmission of *B. burgdorferi* sensu lato occurs when an infected tick feeds on a susceptible animal. Prior to feeding, the spirochaetes are restricted to the midgut of the ticks and, following ingestion of blood, they are found in the salivary glands. Following ingestion of blood by the tick, a change occurs in the expression of the outer surface protein (Osp) of the borreliae. This change in Osp expression from OspA to OspC appears to be essential for virulence (Fingerle *et al.*, 1995).

After entering the bloodstream of a susceptible host, borreliae multiply and are disseminated throughout the body. Organisms may be demonstrated in joints, brain, nerves, eyes and heart. Whether disease is caused by active infection or by host immune responses to the organism is unclear. Recent studies suggest that persistent infection, leading to the induction of cytokines, contributes to the development of lesions (Roberts *et al.*, 1998; Sprenger *et al.*, 1997; Straubinger *et al.*, 1997). There may be an association between different genotypes of *B. burgdorferi* and particular clinical syndromes in humans (van Dam *et al.*, 1993).

Clinical signs

Most infections are subclinical. Serological surveys demonstrate that exposure is common in both animal and human populations in endemic areas (Santino *et al.*, 1997).

The clinical manifestations of Lyme disease relate mainly to the sites of localization of the organisms. Clinical disease is reported frequently in dogs. Signs include fever, lethargy, arthritis and evidence of cardiac, renal or neurological disturbance. In the USA, arthritis is a common finding whereas neurological disturbance is the most frequent clinical feature in Europe and Japan. The clinical signs in horses are similar to those in dogs and include lameness, uveitis, nephritis, hepatitis and encephalitis. Lameness in cattle and sheep associated with *B. burgdorferi* sensu lato infection has been reported.

Diagnosis

Laboratory confirmation of Lyme disease may prove difficult because the spirochaetes may be present in low numbers in specimens from clinically affected animals. In addition, the organism is fastidious in its cultural requirements.

- A history of exposure to tick infestation in an endemic area in association with characteristic clinical signs may suggest Lyme disease.
- Rising antibody titres to *B. burgdorferi* sensu lato along with typical clinical signs are indicative of disease. Because subclinical infections are common in endemic areas, high titres alone are not confirmatory. The ELISA is extensively used for antibody detection; Western immunoblotting is sometimes used for confirmation of ELISA results.
- Immunofluorescence assays may also be used but, in common with ELISA, the results of these methods may be difficult to interpret.
- Culture of borreliae from clinically affected animals is confirmatory. Cultures in Barbour-Stoenner-Kelly medium should be incubated for six weeks under microaerophilic conditions and should be carried out in specialized laboratories.
- Low numbers of borreliae can be detected in samples by PCR techniques. These techniques can also be used for identifying genospecies and for epidemiological investigations (Kurtenbach *et al.*, 1998).

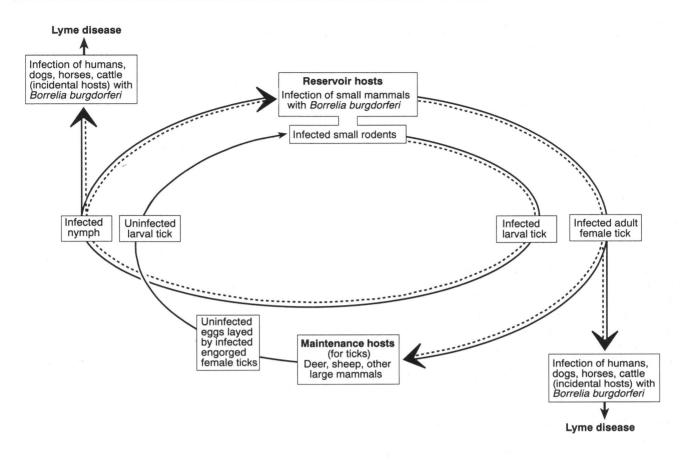

Figure 31.5 The transmission of *Borrelia burgdorferi* sensu lato (broken line) to humans and animals by different stages of *Ixodes* ticks (solid line). The occurrence of Lyme disease, which is often seasonal, relates to periods of tick activity.

Treatment and control

- Acute Lyme disease responds to treatment with amoxycillin and oxytetracycline. In chronic disease, prolonged or repeated courses of treatment may be required.
- Acaricidal sprays, baths or dips should be used to control tick infestation. Where feasible, tick habitats such as rough brush and scrub should be cleared.
- Prompt removal of ticks from companion animals may prevent infection. However, because some tick species can transmit spirochaetes shortly after attachment, it cannot be assumed that daily removal of ticks will prevent infection (Korenberg and Moskvitina, 1996).
- A number of vaccines, including whole cell bacterins and a recombinant subunit vaccine, are commercially available for use in dogs.

Public health aspects

Lyme disease is an important tick-borne infection of humans. Clinical signs include skin rash localized at the site of tick attachment followed, in the absence of treatment, by arthritis, muscle pains, and cardiac and neurological abnormalities. Infection is often acquired by walking in endemic areas during periods of tick activity. Dogs,

cats and farm animals may act as transport hosts for infected ticks thereby exposing humans to the risk of infection.

Avian spirochaetosis

This acute disease of birds, caused by *Borrelia anserina*, can result in significant economic loss in flocks in tropical and subtropical regions where the disease is endemic. Chickens, turkeys, pheasants, ducks and geese are susceptible to infection. Soft ticks of the genus *Argas* frequently transmit the disease. However, when there is contact between susceptible birds and infected material such as blood, tissues or excreta, transmission may occur. Because *B. anserina* survives poorly in the environment and for a limited time in infected birds, *Argas* ticks are important reservoirs of the organisms. The borreliae survive trans-stadial moulting in ticks and can be transmitted transovarially between tick generations. Outbreaks of avian spirochaetosis coincide with periods of peak tick activity during warm, humid seasons. Morbidity and mortality are low in flocks continually exposed to infection. The disease is characterized by fever, marked anaemia and weight loss. Paralysis may develop as the disease progresses. Immunity, which follows recovery, is serotype specific. Several serotypes may be present in a particular region.

Diagnosis can be confirmed by demonstration of the spirochaetes in buffy coat smears using dark-field microscopy. Blood or tissue smears can also be examined using immunofluorescence. Giemsa-stained smears or silver impregnation techniques can be used to demonstrate the borreliae in tissues. The organisms are usually isolated by inoculating embryonated eggs or young chicks with infected blood or homogenized tissues. Treatment with antibiotics is effective. Inactivated vaccines and tick eradication are the main control measures.

Brachyspira and *Serpulina* species

Five genospecies of intestinal spirochaetes have been isolated from pigs namely *Brachyspira hyodysenteriae*, *B. pilosicoli*, *B. innocens*, *Serpulina intermedia* and *S. murdochii*. The genera *Serpulina* and *Brachyspira* were recently combined (Ochiai *et al.*, 1997). These anaerobic spirochaetes have six to fourteen spirals and are 0.1 to 0.5 μm in width (Fig 31.4).

Usual habitat

Pathogenic *Brachyspira* species are found in the intestinal tract of both clinically affected and normal pigs. Carrier pigs can shed *B. hyodysenteriae* for up to three months and are the principal source of infection for healthy pigs.

Differentiation of *Brachyspira* species

The differentiation of *B. hyodysenteriae* from other intestinal spirochaetes is based on its pattern of haemolysis on blood agar. Tests for detecting indole production or the hydrolysis of hippurate are also useful diagnostically (Table 31.4). Restriction endonuclease analysis, restriction fragment length polymorphism, ribotyping using 16S rRNA analysis, PCR-based assays and multilocus enzyme electrophoresis have been developed both for differentiating species and for distinguishing strains of organisms within species. *Brachyspira hyodysenteriae* isolates can also be allocated to several serogroups and serotypes.

Pathogenesis

Most information on the pathogenesis of *Brachyspira* species derives from studies of *B. hyodysenteriae*. Motility in mucus is an essential virulence factor of this organism; mutant strains with altered motility are less capable of colonizing the pig intestine (Kennedy *et al.*, 1997). Colonization may be enhanced by factors in mucus with chemotactic activity for the organisms. Factors with

Table 31.4 Laboratory differentiation of *Brachyspira* species isolated from pigs.

Species	Laboratory tests		
	Haemolysis	Indole spot test	Hippurate hydrolysis
B. hyodysenteriae	Strong	+	–
B. pilosicoli	Weak	–	+
B. innocens	Weak	–	–

such chemotactic activities have been demonstrated *in vitro* (Kennedy and Yancey, 1996). Haemolytic activity, demonstrated *in vitro*, correlates with pathogenicity and three genes encoding haemolytic and cytotoxic activity have been cloned and sequenced (Muir *et al.*, 1992; ter Huurne *et al.*, 1994).

The pathogenesis of infection with *B. pilosicoli* differs from that of *B. hyodysenteriae* in that attachment of the spirochaetes to the intestinal mucosa appears to be important. Attachment of *B. pilosicoli* to the epithelial cells of the colonic mucosa leads to disruption of function with resultant cell shedding and oedema.

Clinical infections

Infections with *Brachyspira* species are of importance in pigs. *Brachyspira hyodysenteriae*, the cause of swine dysentery, and *B. pilosicoli*, the cause of porcine intestinal spirochaetosis, are recognized pathogens. There is evidence that *Serpulina intermedia* may be associated with porcine spirochaetal colitis, but this has not been confirmed experimentally. Pigs acquire infection through exposure to contaminated faeces. The disease usually spreads slowly through a herd, affecting only one or two pens at a time. Dogs, rats, mice and flies may act as transport hosts for the spirochaetes. Mice populations can maintain *B. hyodysenteriae*. Although strains of *B. pilosicoli* have been found in many species including humans, dogs, chickens and pheasants, cross-infection between species has not been clearly demonstrated. *Brachyspira* species can survive in the environment for limited periods only if protected from desiccation. *Brachyspira hyodysenteriae* can persist for several weeks in moist faeces and for at least three days in slurry.

Clinical signs

The pathogenic *Brachyspira* and *Serpulina* species and the clinical conditions associated with infection are presented in Table 31.5. Infection with *B. hyodysenteriae* causes dysentery which is most often encountered in weaned pigs from six to twelve weeks of age. Affected pigs lose

Table 31.5 Clinical conditions associated with infection caused by *Brachyspira/Serpulina* species.

Species	Clinical conditions
B. hyodysenteriae	Swine dysentery
B. pilosicoli	Intestinal spirochaetosis of pigs, dogs, birds and humans
S. intermedia	Implicated in porcine spirochaetal colitis

condition and become emaciated. Appetite is decreased and thirst may be evident. During recovery, there may be large amounts of mucus in the faeces. Although mortality is low, reduced weight gains due to poor food conversion cause major economic loss.

Brachyspira pilosicoli was identified in 1996 as the cause of porcine intestinal spirochaetosis (Trott *et al.*, 1996). Previously, enteric disease had been produced experimentally by infecting pigs with a weakly-haemolytic spirochaete (Taylor *et al.*, 1980). The clinical signs in porcine intestinal spirochaetosis are similar to those of swine dysentery but are less severe. Diarrhoea contains mucus rather than blood. Reduced feed conversion efficiency with poor weight gains have a major effect on production.

Diagnosis

- History, clinical signs and gross lesions may indicate swine dysentery.
- Blood agar with added antibiotics is used for the culture of *Brachyspira* species. Cultures are incubated anaerobically at 42°C for at least three days. Complete haemolysis is present around colonies of *B. hyodysenteriae*; other enteric spirochaetes are weakly haemolytic (Table 31.4).
- Definitive identification can be made using immunofluorescence, DNA probes or biochemical tests (Table 31.4).
- Serological tests such as ELISA can be used to investigate infection in herds.
- PCR-based techniques have been developed and may be useful for laboratory confirmation.

Treatment and control

Medication of drinking water is a useful method of treatment. Drugs commonly used include tiamulin, lincomycin and the nitroimidazoles. Improved hygiene, medication of feed and alteration of the diet may assist in controlling infection. Depopulation, thorough cleaning and disinfection of premises and strict rodent control are required for eradication of the disease.

References

Agunloye, C.A. and Nash, A.S. (1996). Investigation of possible leptospiral infection in cats in Scotland. *Journal of Small Animal Practice,* **37**, 126–129.

Brenner, D.J., Kaufmann, A.F., Sulzer, K.R., Steigerwalt, A.G., Rogers, F.C. and Weyant, R.S. (1999). Further determination of DNA relatedness between serogroups and serovars in the family *Leptospiraceae* with a proposal for *Leptospira alexanderi* sp. nov. and four new *Leptospira* genomospecies. *International Journal of Systematic Bacteriology,* **49**, 839–858.

Cousins, D.V., Ellis, T.M., Parkinson, J. and McGlashen, C.H. (1989). Evidence for sheep as a maintenance host for *Leptospira interrogans* serovar *hardjo*. *Veterinary Record,* **124**, 123–124.

Ellis, W.A. (1995). International Committee on Systematic Bacteriology. Subcommittee on the Taxonomy of *Leptospira*. Minutes of the Meetings, 1 and 2 July 1994, Prague, Czech Republic. *International Journal of Systematic Bacteriology,* **45**, 872–874.

Ellis, W.A., Thiermann, A.B., Montgomery, J., Handsaker, A., Winter, P.J. and Marshall, R.B. (1988). Restriction endonuclease analysis of *Leptospira interrogans* serovar *hardjo* isolates from cattle. *Research in Veterinary Science,* **44**, 375–379.

Fingerle, V., Hauser, U., Liegl, G., Petko, B., Preac-Mursic V. and Wilske, B. (1995). Expression of outer surface proteins A and C of *Borrelia burgdorferi* in *Ixodes ricinus*. *Journal of Clinical Microbiology,* **33**, 1867–1869.

Kennedy, M.J. and Yancey, R.J. (1996). Motility and chemotaxis in *Serpulina hyodysenteriae*. *Veterinary Microbiology,* **49**, 21–30.

Kennedy, M.J. Rosey, E.L. and Yancey, R.J. (1997). Characterization of flaA- and flaB- mutants of *Serpulina hyodysenteriae*: both flagellin subunits, FlaA and FlaB, are necessary for full motility and intestinal colonization. *FEMS. Microbiology Letters,* **153**, 119–128.

Korenberg, E.I. and Moskvitina, G.G. (1996). Interrelationships between different *Borrelia* genospecies and their principal vectors. *Journal of Vector Ecology,* **21**, 178–185.

Kurtenbach, K., Peacey, M., Rijpkema, S.G.T., Hoodless, A.N. and Nuttall, P.A. (1998). Differential transmission of the genospecies of *Borrelia burgdorferi* sensu lato by game birds and small rodents in England. *Applied and Environmental Microbiology,* **64**, 1169–1174.

Merien, F., Baranton, G. and Perolat, P. (1997). Invasion of Vero cells and induction of apoptosis in macrophages by pathogenic *Leptospira interrogans* are correlated with virulence. *Infection and Immunity,* **65**, 729-738.

Muir, S., Koopman, M.B.H., Libby, S.J., Joens, L.A., Heffron, F. and Kusters, J.G. (1992). Cloning and expression of a *Serpulina* (*Treponema*) *hyodysenteriae* haemolysin gene. *Infection and Immunity,* **60**, 4095–4099.

Ochiai, S., Adachi, Y. and Mori, K. (1997). Unification of the genera *Serpulina* and *Brachyspira*, and proposals of

Brachyspira hyodysenteriae comb. nov., *Brachyspira innocens* comb. nov. and *Brachyspira pilosicoli* comb. nov. *Microbiology and Immunology*, **41**, 445–452.

Oliver, J.H. Jr. (1996). Lyme borreliosis in the southern United States: A review (1996). *Journal of Parasitology*, **82**, 926–935.

Parma A.E., Cerone, S.I. and Sansinanea, S.A. (1992). Biochemical analysis by SDS-PAGE and western blotting of the antigenic relationship between *Leptospira* and equine ocular tissues. *Veterinary Immunology and Immunopathology*, **33**, 179–185.

Perolat, P., Chappel, R.J., Adler, B., Baranton, G., Bulach, D.M., Billinghurst, M.L., Letocart, M., Merien, F. and Serrano, M.S. (1998). *Leptospira fainei* sp. nov., isolated from pigs in Australia. *International Journal of Systematic Bacteriology*, **48**, 851–858.

Rentko, V.T., Clark, N., Ross, L.A. and Schelling, S. (1992). Canine Leptopirosis: A retrospective study of 17 cases. *Journal of Veterinary Internal Medicine*, **6**, 235–244.

Roberts, E.D., Bohn, R.P., Lowrie, R.C. Jr., Habicht, G., Katona, L., Piesman, J. and Philipp, M.T. (1998). Pathogenesis of Lyme neuroborreliosis in the Rhesus monkey: The early disseminated and chronic phases of disease in the peripheral nervous system. *Journal of Infectious Diseases*, **178**, 722–732.

Santino, I., Dastoli, R., Sessa, R. and del Piano, M. (1997). Geographical incidence of infection with *Borrelia burgdorferi* in Europe. *Panminerva Medica*, **39**, 208–214.

Sprenger, H., Krause, A., Kaufman, A., Priem, S., Fabian, D., Burmester, G.R., Gemsa, D. and Rittig, M.G. (1997). *Borrelia burgdorferi* induces chemokines in human monocytes. *Infection and Immunity*, **65**, 4384–4388.

Straubinger, R.K., Straubinger, A.F., Harter, L., Jacobson, R.H., Chang, Y-F., Summers, B., Erb, H.N. and Appel, M.J.G. (1997). *Borrelia burgdorferi* migrates into joint capsules and causes an up-regulation of interleukin-8 in synovial membranes of dogs experimentally infected with ticks. *Infection and Immunity*, **65**, 1273–1285.

Taylor, D.J., Simmons, J.R. and Laird, H.M. (1980). Production of diarrhoea and dysentery in pigs by feeding pure cultures of a spirochaete differing from *Treponema hyodysenteriae*. *Veterinary Record*, **106**, 326–332.

ter Huurne, A.A.H.M., Muir, S., van Houten, M. *et al.* Characterization of three putative *Serpulina hyodysenteriae* haemolysins. *Microbiological Pathogenesis*, **16**, 269–282.

Trott, D.J., Stanton, T.B., Jensen, N.S., *et al.* (1996). *Serpulina pilosicoli* sp. nov., the agent of porcine intestinal spirochaetosis. *International Journal of Systematic Bacteriology*, **46**, 206–215.

van Dam, A.P., Kuiper, H., Vos, K., *et al.* (1993). Different genospecies of *Borrelia burgdorferi* are associated with distinct clinical manifestations of Lyme borreliosis. *Clinical Infectious Diseases*, **17**, 708–717.

Yasuda, P.H., Steigerwalt, A.G., Sulzer, K.R., Kaufmann, A.F., Rogers, F. and Brenner, D.J. (1987). Deoxyribonucleic acid relatedness between serogroups and serovars in the family *Leptospiraceae* with proposals for seven new *Leptospira* species. *International Journal of Systematic Bacteriology*, **37**, 407–415.

Yuri, K., Takamoto, Y., Okada, M., *et al.* (1993). Chemotaxis of leptospires to hemoglobin in relation to virulence. *Infection and Immunity*, **61**, 2270–2272.

Further reading

Hampson, D.J., Ateyo, R.F. and Combs, B.G. (1997). Swine dysentery. In *Intestinal spirochaetes in domestic animals and humans*. Eds. D.J. Taylor, D.J. Trott, D.J. Hampson, and T.B. Stanton. CAB International, Wallingford, U.K. pp. 175–209.

Hubbard, M.J., Cann, K.J. and Baker. A.S. (1998). Lyme borreliosis: a tick-borne spirochaetal disease. *Reviews in Medical Microbiology*, **9**, 99–107.

Steere, A.C. (2001). Medical progress: Lyme disease. New England Journal of Medicine, **345**, 115–125.

Taylor, D.J. and Trott, D.J. (1997). Porcine intestinal spirochaetosis and spirochaetal colitis. Eds. D.J. Taylor, D.J. Trott, D.J. Hampson and T.B. Stanton. In *Intestinal spirochaetes in domestic animals and humans*. Eds. D.J. Taylor, D.J. Trott, D.J. Hampson, and T.B. Stanton. CAB International, Wallingford, U.K. pp. 211–241.

ter Huurne, A.A.H.M. and Gaastra, W. (1995). Swine dysentery: more unknown than known. *Veterinary Microbiology*, **46**, 347–360.

Chapter 32

Pathogenic anaerobic non-spore-forming Gram-negative bacteria

Many non-spore-forming, anaerobic, Gram-negative bacteria cause opportunistic mixed infections, often in association with facultative anaerobes. Synergistic interactions between the organisms in these mixed infections are common. *Fusobacterium* species and bacteria formerly referred to as *Bacteroides* species account for more than 50% of the anaerobic organisms isolated from these infections. Recent taxonomic changes to members of the genus *Bacteroides* are presented in Box 32.1.

Usual habitat

Non-spore-forming, Gram-negative anaerobes are often found on mucous membranes, particularly in the digestive tract, of animals and man. They are excreted in the faeces and they can survive for short periods in the environment. *Dichelobacter nodosus*, a primary pathogen of the epidermal tissues of the hoof region of ruminants, survives for less than 4 days in mud.

Diagnostic procedures

- In order to ensure that isolates of anaerobes are aetiologically significant, specimens for isolation procedures should be obtained by direct sampling from discharges or lesions and by suprapubic puncture in urinary infections.
- Specimens should be processed promptly after collection. Commercial kits and transport media are available for specimens from suspected anaerobic infections. In the core of a tissue specimen over 2 cm³, an anaerobic microenvironment is usually maintained. Samples of fluid in a syringe remain suitable for

---

Key points

- Gram-negative, anaerobic bacteria
- Endospores not produced
- Enriched media required for growth
- Majority are commensals on mucosal surfaces, principally in the alimentary tract
- Opportunistic pathogens
- Synergism with other bacteria in mixed infections
- *Dichelobacter nodosus* produces foot rot in sheep in association with other pathogens

---

anaerobic culture if air is expelled from the syringe and the needle is plugged.

- Anaerobic jars with an atmosphere of hydrogen and 10% CO_2 are used for incubating cultures at 37°C for up to 7 days.
- Enriched blood agars for the isolation of anaerobes are supplemented with 5 to 10% ruminant red cells, yeast extract, vitamin K and haemin. Selective media can be prepared by adding appropriate antimicrobial agents. Media must be pre-reduced by storing them in an anaerobic atmosphere for at least 6 hours before inoculation.
- Liquid media, such as cooked meat broth or thioglycollate medium supplemented with vitamin K and haemin, are useful for subculturing but are unsuitable for primary isolation.
- Special selective media are required for the isolation of *Dichelobacter nodosus* from ruminant footrot (Skerman, 1989). In some media formulations, powdered ovine hoof is added to promote enhanced growth.

Differentiation of the non-spore-forming Gram-negative anaerobes

Non-spore-forming Gram-negative anaerobes are differentiated on the basis of bacterial morphology, colonial appearance, antibiotic susceptibility testing and fatty acid production.

- Rods of *Dichelobacter nodosus* are thick, straight or

Box 32.1 Current nomenclature of organisms formerly classified as *Bacteroides* species.

- *Dichelobacter nodosus* (*Bacteroides nodosus*)
- *Prevotella heparinolytica* (*B. heparinolyticus*)
- *Prevotella melaninogenica* (*B. melaninogenicus*)
- *Porphyromonas asaccharolytica* (*B. asaccharolyticus*)
- *Porphyromonas levii* (*B. levii* or *B. melaninogenicus* subsp. *levii*)

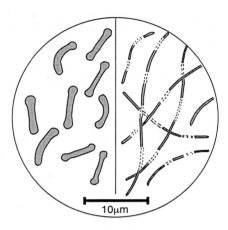

Figure 32.1 Straight or curved rods of *Dichelobacter nodosus* (left) showing characterisitic swellings at one or both ends and slender, non-branching filaments of *Fusobacterium necrophorum* which tend to stain irregularly.

slightly curved, up to 6 μm long and bulging at one or both ends. *Fusobacterum necrophorum* has irregularly staining, long, non-branching filamentous forms (Fig. 32.1).

- Colonies of Gram-negative anaerobes usually have a foetid or putrid odour due to volatile fatty acid production.
  - The appearance of *Dichelobacter nodosus* colonies is variable (Stewart *et al.*, 1986). Colonies of virulent strains from lesions of ovine footrot usually have a dark central zone, a pale granular middle zone and a spreading irregular periphery with a ground glass appearance.
  - Colonies of *Fusobacterium necrophorum* colonies are grey, round and shiny. Some isolates are haemolytic.
  - Colonies of many *Prevotella* species and *Porphyromonas* species which become darkly pigmented after incubation for 5 days may appear red under UV light.

- Antibiotic susceptibility testing, biochemical tests and gas liquid chromatography are used for more accurate identification of species.
- Methods for detecting virulent strains of *D. nodusus*, reviewed by Liu and Yong (1997), include:
  - Electrophoretic zymogram to determine proteolytic isoenzyme patterns.
  - ELISA using monoclonal antibodies.
  - Polymerase chain reaction techniques

Pathogenesis and pathogenicity

Non-spore-forming anaerobes usually exert pathogenic effects when anatomical barriers are breached allowing invasion of underlying tissues. They replicate only at low or negative reduction potentials (*Eh*). Most of those involved in opportunistic infections produce superoxide dismutase which allows them to survive in oxygenated tissues until the *Eh* reaches levels favouring their growth. Tissue trauma and necrosis followed by multiplication of facultatively anaerobic bacteria can lower *Eh* levels to a range suitable for the proliferation of non-spore-forming anaerobes. Most infections involving these organisms are mixed. Two or more bacterial species, interacting synergistically, may produce lesions which the individual organisms cannot. A relevant example of this type of synergism is the production by *Arcanobacterium pyogenes* of a heat-labile factor which stimulates *F. necrophorum* replication (Smith *et al.*, 1989). In turn, *F. necrophorum* produces a leukotoxin which correlates with the strain virulence and aids survival of *A. pyogenes* (Emery *et al.*, 1984). Synergism between *F. necrophorum* and *Dichelobacter nodosus* is important in the pathogenesis of ruminant pedal lesions (Fig. 32.2). In this instance, *F. necrophorum* facilitates tissue invasion by *D. nodosus* and is itself stimulated by a growth factor elaborated by *D. nodosus*.

Three biotypes of *F. necrophorum* are recognised. Biotype A, designated *F. necrophorum* subspecies *necrophorum* has greater haemolytic activity and is more

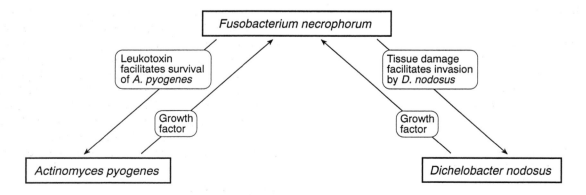

Figure 32.2 The synergistic interaction of *Fusobacterium necrophorum* with *Arcanobacterium pyogenes* and with *Dichelobacter nodosus* in the development and progression of foot lesions in ruminants.

virulent than biotype B, *F. necrophorum* subspecies *funduliforme*. Biotype C, reclassified as *F. pseudonecrophorum* appears to be non-pathogenic. Characteristics of *D. nodosus* which correlate with its ability to damage tissues include the production of thermostable proteases and elastase and the presence of agarolytic activity on agar-based media containing powdered hoof.

Clinical infections

The non-spore-forming, Gram-negative anaerobic bacteria which have been implicated in infections in domestic animals are listed in Box 32.2. *Brachyspira hyodysenteriae* is discussed in Chapter 31.

Fusobacterium necrophorum is considered to be the primary pathogen in a number of disease conditions in farm animals (Table 32.1). Mixed bacterial infections are commonly implicated in foot lesions in domestic ruminants and pigs (Table 32.2). Pedal bacterial infections in farm animals, such as footrot and foot abscessation, are discussed in detail in Chapter 82. Mixed infections with non-spore-forming anaerobes are also present in aspiration pneumonias and in bovine traumatic reticuloperitonitis and pericarditis. In addition, many inflammatory conditions in domestic carnivores are caused by non-specific mixed anaerobic infections.

Calf diphtheria

This condition usually presents as necrotic pharyngitis or laryngitis in calves under 3 months of age. The aetiological agent, *F. necrophorum*, can enter through abrasions in the mucosa of the pharynx or larynx often caused by ingestion of coarse feed. Clinical signs include fever, depression, anorexia, excessive salivation, respiratory distress and a foul smell from the mouth. Untreated calves

---

Box 32.2 Gram-negative, non-spore-forming anaerobes which have been implicated in infections in domestic animals.

- *Bacteroides fragilis*
- Other *Bacteroides* species
- *Brachyspira hyodysenteriae*
- *Dichelobacter nodosus*
- *Fusobacterium necrophorum*
- *F. nucleatum*
- *F. russii*
- Other *Fusobacterium* species
- *Porphyromonas asaccharolytica*
- *Porphyromonas levii*
- *Prevotella heparinolytica*
- *P. melaninogenica*
- Spirochaetes (unclassified)

Table 32.1 Disease conditions of farm animals, not including foot conditions, in which *Fusobacterium necrophorum* plays a primary role.

Species	Disease condition	Predisposing factors
Cattle	Calf diphtheria	Rough feed producing mucosal damage
	Post-partum metritis	Dystocia
	Hepatic abscessation	Sudden dietary change leading to acidosis and rumenitis
	Black spot of teat	Trauma to region adjacent to teat sphincter
Horses	Thrush (hoof)	Poor hygiene and wet housing conditions
	Necrobacillosis of lower limbs	Poor hygiene
Pigs	Bull nose	Trauma to nasal mucosa

may develop a fatal necrotizing pneumonia. Treatment with potentiated sulphonamides or tetracyclines early in the course of the disease is usually effective.

Bovine liver abscess

Hepatic abscessation in cattle, secondary to rumenitis, is encountered most commonly in feedlot animals. The feeding of rations high in carbohydrates and the resulting rapid intraruminal fermentation can lead to the development of ulcers. *Fusobacterium necrophorum* together with other anaerobes and *Arcanobacterium pyogenes* invade the tissues, and occasional emboli which reach the liver via the portal vein initiate abscess formation. Affected cattle rarely show clinical signs and lesions are usually detected at slaughter. Management techniques in feedlots should be aimed at reducing the incidence of rumenitis. Chlortetracycline in feed during the finishing period can reduce the prevalence of liver abscess.

Necrotic rhinitis of pigs

This sporadic condition, primarily affecting young pigs, is characterised by suppuration and necrosis of the snout as a result of infection with *F. necrophorum*, often in association with other anaerobes. These organisms enter through abrasions in the nasal mucosa. Signs include swelling of the face, sneezing and a foul-smelling nasal discharge. In chronic infections, involvement of the nasal and facial bones can result in permanent facial deformity ('bull nose'). Potentiated sulphonamides administered early in the course of the infection may be beneficial.

Thrush of the hoof

This necrotic condition of the horse's hoof is associated with poor hygiene, wet conditions and lack of regular

Table 32.2 Foot conditions in farm animals associated with mixed infections including anaerobic non-spore-forming bacteria[a].

Species	Disease condition	Bacteria implicated
Sheep	Interdigital dermatitis	*Fusobacterium necrophorum* *Dichelobacter nodosus* (benign strains)
	Heel abscess and lamellar suppuration	Mixed anaerobic flora including *Arcanobacterium pyogenes*[b] *F. necrophorum*, and others
	Footrot	*Dichelobacter nodosus* *Fusobacterium necrophorum* *Arcanobacterium pyogenes*[b] Unidentified spirochaete
Cattle	Interdigital necrobacillosis (Foul-in-the-Foot)	*Fusobacterium necrophorum* *Porphyromonas levii*
	Interdigital dermatitis	*Dichelobacter nodosus* *Fusobacterium necrophorum* *Prevotella* species Spirochaetes?
Pigs	Foot abscess in young pigs and bush foot (lamellar suppuration) in older animals	Mixed anaerobes

a Bacterial and viral infections affecting the feet of cattle, sheep and pigs are reviewed in Chapter 82
b facultatively anaerobic

cleaning of the hooves. Infection with *F. necrophorum*, secondary to hoof damage, results in a localized inflammatory response. Thrush, which commonly affects the hind feet, is characterized by a foul-smelling discharge in the sulci close to the frog. The aim of therapy is to encourage regeneration of the frog by providing dry, clean stabling, regular attention to the hooves and exercise.

Black spot of bovine teats

Black spot or black pox of the teat orifice and sphincter of dairy cows presents as a localized area of necrosis with black scab formation due to invasion by *Fusobacterium necrophorum*. The condition can contribute to stenosis of the sphincter and may predispose to mastitis.

References

Emery, D.L., Dufty, J.H. and Clark, B.L. (1984). Biochemical and functional properties of a leucocidin produced by several strains of *Fusobacterium necrophorum*. *Australian Veterinary Journal*, **61**, 382–387.

Liu, D. and Yong, W.K. (1997). Improved laboratory diagnosis of ovine foot rot: an update. *Veterinary Journal*, **153**, 99–105.

Smith, G.R., Till, D., Wallace, L.J. and Noakes, D.E. (1989). Enhancement of the infectivity of *Fusobacterium necrophorum* by other bacteria. *Epidemiology and Infection*, **102**, 447–458.

Skerman, T.M. (1989). Isolation and identification of *Bacteroides nodosus*. In *Footrot and Foot abscess of Ruminants*. Eds. J.R. Egerton, W.K. Young and G.G. Riffkin, CRC Press, Boca Raton, Florida. pp. 85–104.

Stewart, D.J., Peterson, J.E., Vaughan, J.A., Clark, B.L., Emery, D.L., Caldwell, J.B. *et al.* (1986). The pathogenicity and cultural characteristics of virulent, intermediate and benign strains of *Bacteroides nodosus* causing ovine foot-rot. *Australian Veterinary Journal*, **63**, 317–326.

Further reading

Nagaraja, T.G. and Chengappa, M.M. (1998). Liver abscess in feedlot cattle: a review. *Journal of Animal Science*, **76**, 287–298.

Otter, A. (1996). *Fusobacterium necrophorum* abortion in a cow. *Veterinary Record*, **139**, 318–319.

Smith, G.R. and Thornton, E.A. (1993). Pathogenicity of *Fusobacterium necrophorum* strains from man and animals. *Epidemiology and Infection*, **110**, 499–506.

Walker, R.D., Richardson, D.C., Bryant, M.J. and Draper, C.S. (1983). Anaerobic bacteria associated with osteomyelitis in domestic animals. *Journal of the American Veterinary Medical Association*, **182**, 814–816.

Chapter 33

Mycoplasmas

The mycoplasmas are microorganisms in the class *Mollicutes*. Of the nine genera in this class, five contain species of veterinary interest (Fig. 33.1). The genus *Mycoplasma*, in which there are about 100 species, contains most of the animal pathogens. The first mycoplasma identified in 1890 was *Mycoplasma mycoides* subspecies *mycoides*, the cause of contagious bovine pleuropneumonia. Similar types of mycoplasmas which were subsequently identified were called pleuro-pneumonia-like organisms (PPLO).

Mycoplasmas, the smallest prokaryotic cells capable of self-replication, are pleomorphic organisms ranging from spherical (0.3 to 0.9 μm in diameter) to filamentous (up to 1.0 μm long). Because they cannot synthesize peptido-glycan or its precursors, they do not possess rigid cell walls but have flexible, triple-layered outer membranes. Their flexibility allows them to pass through bacterial membrane filters of pore size 0.22 to 0.45 μm. Mycoplasmas are susceptible to desiccation, heat, detergents and disinfectants. However, they are resistant to antibiotics such as penicillin which interfere with the synthesis of bacterial cell walls. Based on 5S rRNA sequence analyses, the mycoplasmas have been shown to be linked phylogenetically to Gram-positive bacteria such as *Clostridium* species which have low guanine-cytosine content in their DNA. They require enriched media for growth, characteristically forming umbonate micro-

---

Key points

- Smallest free-living prokaryotic microorganisms
- Possess triple-layered limiting membranes but lack cell walls
- Do not stain by the Gram method
- Highly pleomorphic, filterable plastic forms
- Susceptible to desiccation and disinfectants
- Microcolonies have a 'fried-egg' appearance
- Most are facultative anaerobes
- Do not replicate in the environment
- Most are host-specific
- *Mycoplasma* and *Ureaplasma* contain species of veterinary importance
- *Mycoplasma* species cause a wide range of diseases in animals, including contagious bovine pleuropneumonia

---

colonies when illuminated obliquely and microcolonies with a 'fried egg' appearance in transmitted light (Fig. 33.2). The dense central zone is due to extension of the microcolony into the agar (Fig. 33.3). Mycoplasmas, which have relatively small genomes (approximately 800 genes), are fastidious in their growth requirements.

Most mycoplasmas are facultative anaerobes and some grow optimally in an atmosphere of 5 to 10% CO_2. Non-pathogenic anaerobic mycoplasmas are found in the rumens of sheep and cattle. The genera *Mycoplasma* and *Ureaplasma* contain animal pathogens. The major diseases associated with infection by *Mycoplasma* species are summarized in Table 33.1. Other clinical conditions of lesser economic significance are listed in Table 33.2.

Usual habitat

Mycoplasmas are found on mucosal surfaces of the conjunctiva, nasal cavity, oropharynx and intestinal and genital tracts of animals and humans. Some species have tropisms for particular anatomical sites while others are found in many locations. In general, they are host-specific and survive for short periods in the environment.

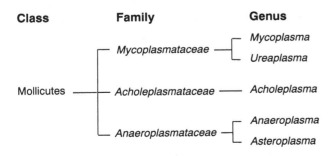

Class	Family	Genus
	Mycoplasmataceae	Mycoplasma
		Ureaplasma
Mollicutes	Acholeplasmataceae	Acholeplasma
	Anaeroplasmataceae	Anaeroplasma
		Asteroplasma

Figure 33.1 Families and genera of veterinary interest in the class *Mollicutes*, members of which may be isolated from clinical specimens. *Mycoplasma* and *Ureaplasma* are the only genera of pathogenic significance in domestic animals and humans.

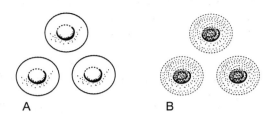

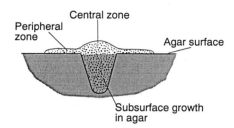

Figure 33.2 The appearance of mycoplasma microcolonies in oblique illumination (A) and in transmitted light (B). When illuminated obliquely, the microcolonies have an umbonate appearance. They have a 'fried-egg' appearance in transmitted light.

Figure 33.3 A section through a mycoplasma microcolony on agar showing surface and subsurface growth.

Differentiation of the mycoplasmas

Mycoplasmas are differentiated by their host specificity, colonial morphology, requirement for cholesterol and biochemical reactivity (Table 33.3). They can be identified by serological methods. Specific identification is usually made in specialized laboratories.

- *Mycoplasma* species and *Ureaplasma* species require enriched media containing animal protein, a sterol component and a source of DNA or adenine dinucleotide. Commercially-available mycoplasma agar or broth media (often heart-infusions) are supplemented with horse serum (20%) and yeast extract providing amino acids and vitamins. In addition, penicillin is used to inhibit Gram-positive bacteria and thallous acetate to inhibit Gram-negative bacteria and

Table 33.1 *Mycoplasma* species of veterinary significance, the disease conditions which they cause and their geographical distribution.

Mycoplasma species	Hosts	Disease conditions	Geographical distribution
M. mycoides subsp. *mycoides* (small colony type)	Cattle	Contagious bovine pleuropneumonia	Endemic in parts of Africa, Middle East, Asia; sporadic outbreaks in some European countries
M. bovis	Cattle	Mastitis, pneumonia, arthritis	Worldwide
M. agalactiae	Sheep, goats	Contagious agalactia	Parts of Europe, northern Africa, western Asia
M. capricolum subsp. *capripneumoniae* (F38)	Goats	Contagious caprine pleuropneumonia	Northern and eastern Africa, Turkey
M. capricolum subsp. *capricolum*	Sheep, goats	Septicaemia, mastitis, polyarthritis, pneumonia	Africa, Europe, Australia, USA
M. mycoides subsp. *mycoides* (large colony type)	Goats, sheep	Pleuropneumonia, mastitis, septicaemia, polyarthritis	Middle East, North America, India, parts of Europe
M. mycoides subsp. *capri*	Goats	Septicaemia, pleuropneumonia, arthritis, mastitis	Parts of Asia, Africa, Europe, Australia
M. hyopneumoniae	Pigs	Enzootic pneumonia	Worldwide
M. hyorhinis	Pigs (3-10 weeks of age)	Polyserositis	Worldwide
M. hyosynoviae	Pigs (10-30 weeks of age)	Polyarthritis	Worldwide
M. gallisepticum	Chickens Turkeys	Chronic respiratory disease Infectious sinusitis	Worldwide
M. synoviae	Poultry	Infectious synovitis	Worldwide
M. meleagridis	Turkeys	Airsacculitis, bone deformities, reduced hatchability and growth rate	Worldwide

Table 33.2 Clinical conditions of minor economic importance in animals associated with *Mycoplasma* and *Ureaplasma* species.

Hosts	Pathogen	Clinical conditions
Cattle	*Mycoplasma alkalescens*	Mastitis
	M. bovigenitalium	Seminal vesiculitis, vaginitis, mastitis
	M. bovirhinis	Mastitis
	M. bovoculi	Role in keratoconjunctivitis
	M. californicum	Mastitis
	M. canadense	Mastitis
	M. dispar	Pneumonia in calves
	Bovine mycoplasma group 7	Mastitis, polyarthritis, pneumonia
	Ureaplasma diversum	Vulvitis, infertility, abortion
Sheep, goats	*M. conjunctivae*	Keratoconjunctivitis
	M. ovipneumoniae	Pneumonia
Goats	*M. putrefaciens*	Mastitis, arthritis
Turkeys	*M. iowae*	Embryo mortality
Horses	*M. felis*	Pleuritis
	M. equigenitalium	Implicated in abortion
Cats	*M. felis*	Conjunctivitis
	M. gateae	Arthritis, tenosynovitis
Dogs	*M. cynos*	Implicated in the kennel cough complex

fungi. Media are buffered at pH 7.3 to 7.8 for *Mycoplasma* species and at pH 6.0 to 6.5 for *Ureaplasma* species. For culturing ureaplasmas, urea is added to the medium and thallium, which is toxic for these organisms, is omitted. *Acholeplasma* species occasionally grow as contaminants on mycoplasma media.

• Colonial morphology:
  — When examined microscopically at low magnification, unstained microcolonies of *Mycoplasma* species are 0.1 to 0.6 mm in diameter and have a 'fried-egg' appearance (Fig. 33.2). Some species produce colonies up to 1.5 mm in diameter which can be seen without magnification.
  — Colonies of *Ureaplasma* species are usually 0.02 to 0.06 mm in diameter and often lack a typical peripheral zone. Because their colonies are tiny, these organisms were formerly referred to as T-mycoplasmas.
  — Dienes stain facilitates recognition of microcolonies by staining the central zone dark blue and the peripheral zone a lighter blue.
  — Microcolonies of *Mycoplasma* species require differentiation from colonies of bacterial L-forms. However, L-forms often revert to normal and produce cell walls and typical bacterial colonies when subcultured on non-inhibitory media.

• *Mycoplasma* species and *Ureaplasma* species require sterols for growth, and this is reflected in their sensitivity to inhibition by digitonin. As *Acholeplasma* species are sterol-independent, they are resistant to inhibition by digitonin. In the digitonin sensitivity test, a filter paper disc impregnated with digitonin is placed on medium inoculated with the isolate. A zone of growth inhibition exceeding 5 mm around the disc indicates sensitivity to digitonin.

• Biochemical tests are carried out in liquid or solid media with the appropriate reagent added. Table 33.4 indicates the biochemical reactions of the main pathogenic mycoplasmas of sheep and goats. Unlike *Ureaplasma* species which produce urease, *Mycoplasma* species do not metabolize urea.

• Immunological tests, using specific antisera produced against each pathogenic species, are required for specific identification. Growth inhibition tests, in which filter paper discs containing specific antisera are placed on an agar surface seeded with the mycoplasma under test, are used for diagnosis. A zone of growth inhibition up 8 mm wide develops around the disc containing homologous antiserum. Fluorescent antibody staining of individual microcolonies can also be used for identification.

Pathogenesis and pathogenicity

Mycoplasmas adhere to host cells, an attribute essential for pathogenicity. This close contact facilitates toxic damage to the host cells by soluble factors produced by the pathogen. Some pathogenic species possess structures composed of unique adhesion proteins which promote

Table 33.3 Differentiating features of *Mollicutes* isolated from domestic animals.

Isolate	Effect of digitonin	Requirement for cholesterol	Urease production	Colony size
Mycoplasma species	Growth inhibition	+	−	0.1 – 0.6 mm
Ureaplasma species	Growth inhibition	+	+	0.02 – 0.06 mm
Acholeplasma species	No growth inhibition	−	−	up to 1.5 mm

Table 33.4 Biochemical tests which aid differentiation of *Mycoplasma* species pathogenic for sheep and goats.

Test	*Mycoplasma agalactiae*	*M. capricolum* subsp. *capricolum*	*M. mycoides* subsp. *mycoides* (large colony type)
Glucose fermentation	−	+	+
Arginine hydrolysis	−	+	−
Phosphatase activity	+	+	−
Casein digestion	−	+	+

attachment to mammalian cells (Krause and Stevens, 1995). Mycoplasmas can adhere to neutrophils and macrophages and can also impair phagocytic functions. In addition, individual species damage cells by active penetration.

Modulation or activation of host immune responses is critical in the pathogenesis of mycoplasmal diseases. Some pathogenic mycoplasmas, including those involved in pulmonary diseases, are mitogenic for B and T lymphocytes (Muhlradt and Schade, 1991). Activation of macrophages and monocytes leads to the release of cytokines including tumour necrosis factor and interleukins, resulting in the initiation of inflammation. Pneumonia-producing mycoplasmas, which adhere to ciliated respiratory epithelium, can induce ciliostasis, loss of cilia and cytopathic change. Inflammation can also be induced in the bovine mammary gland by a membrane-associated toxin of *M. bovis* (Geary *et al.*, 1981).

It is recognized that some mycoplasmal antigens cross-react with the antigens of host tissues. This molecular mimicry has two possible outcomes which are important in pathogenesis. The antigenic similarity to host tissues may allow mycoplasmas to establish persistent infection by avoiding recognition by the host immune system. It may also lead to the development of autoimmune disease if an immune response to mycoplasmal antigens develops and cross-reacts with host cell antigens.

Diagnostic procedures

Isolation of mycoplasmas from clinical samples does not necessarily confirm aetiological involvement because certain mycoplasmas of questionable clinical significance are widely distributed. In regions where mycoplasmal diseases are endemic, clinical findings may point to the involvement of a particular mycoplasmal pathogen.

- Specimens for laboratory examination, ideally collected early in the course of a disease, should be kept refrigerated and delivered to a laboratory within 48 hours. Suitable samples include mucosal scrapings, tracheal exudates, aspirates, pneumonic tissue, mastitic milk and fluids from joints or body cavities. Swabs from lesions or suspect material should be placed in mycoplasmal

transport media for transfer to the laboratory.
- The presence of *Mycoplasma* species or mycoplasmal antigens in samples can be demonstrated immunologically or by nucleic acid procedures:
  — Fluorescent antibody techniques
  — Peroxidase-antiperoxidase procedures on paraffin-embedded tissues
  — Polymerase chain reaction techniques
- Inoculated mycoplasmal medium is incubated, aerobically or in 10% CO_2, in a humid atmosphere at 37°C for up to 14 days.
- Fluid samples can be inoculated directly onto agar or into broth media. Tissue specimens such as lung should be freshly sampled and a cut surface moved across the surface of a solid medium. Alternatively, the tissue can be homogenized in broth and samples of the suspension used for inoculation of liquid or solid media.
- Identification criteria for isolates:
  — 'Fried-egg' microcolonies
  — Microcolony size
  — Cholesterol requirement for growth (digitonin sensitivity test)
  — Biochemical profile including urease production
  — Fluorescent antibody technique on microcolonies
  — Growth inhibition test with specific antisera
- Serological tests:
  — Complement fixation tests for the major mycoplasmal diseases of ruminants are used for certification when animals are traded internationally.
  — Tests based on ELISA are being developed for the diagnosis of economically important mycoplasmal diseases.
  — Rapid plate agglutination tests are used for screening poultry flocks and for the field diagnosis of contagious bovine pleuropneumonia.
  — Haemagglutination-inhibition tests can be used to determine the antibody levels in avian mycoplasmal diseases.

Clinical infections

Mycoplasmas are often involved in disease processes affecting mucosal surfaces. Factors such as extremes of age, stress and intercurrent infection may predispose to tissue invasion. In addition, mycoplasmas may exacerbate disease initiated by other pathogens, particularly in the respiratory tract.

Mycoplasmal infections cause respiratory diseases of major economic importance in farm animals especially in ruminants, pigs and poultry (Table 33.1). Infections associated with mastitis or conjunctivitis in cattle and with disease conditions in domestic carnivores are usually of lesser importance (Table 33.2). Several mycoplasmas have been isolated from dogs and cats but their precise role in disease has not been clearly defined. They have been implicated in respiratory and urinary tract disease in dogs (Jang *et al.*, 1984). In cats, *M. felis* can occasionally cause conjunc-tivitis and *M. gateae* is associated with arthritis (Moise *et al.*, 1983).

Contagious bovine pleuropneumonia

Contagious bovine pleuropneumonia (CBPP) is a severe contagious disease of cattle which has been recognized for more than 200 years and formerly had a worldwide distribution. It is caused by *M. mycoides* subspecies *mycoides* (small colony type), a member of the '*mycoides* cluster'. This cluster is composed of six closely related members including the *M. mycoides* and *M. capricolum* subspecies of sheep and goats (Table 33.1) and bovine mycoplasma group 7 (Table 33.2). Members of the cluster share biochemical, immunological and genetic characteristics which render individual species and subspecies difficult to differentiate (Egwu *et al.*, 1996).

Contagious bovine pleuropneumonia is endemic in central Africa, the Middle East and Asia. Sporadic outbreaks, usually of a less severe form of disease, occur in Portugal, Spain and other Mediterranean countries. The main method of transmission is by aerosols. Transmission of the disease requires close contact with clinically affected animals or asymptomatic carriers. Clinical signs become apparent three weeks after infection. The severity of the disease relates to strain virulence and the immune status of the host. Spread of infection can be relatively slow with peak morbidity (about 50%) at 7 to 8 months after introduction of infection into a herd. In severe outbreaks the mortality rate may be high.

Clinical signs and pathology

Clinical signs in the acute form of CBPP include sudden onset of high fever, anorexia, depression, drop in milk yield, accelerated respiration and coughing. Animals adopt a characteristic stance with the head and neck extended and elbows abducted. Expiratory grunting and mucopurulent nasal discharge may be present. Death can occur 1 to 3 weeks after the onset of clinical signs. Arthritis, synovitis and endocarditis may be present in affected calves.

At postmortem, the pneumonic lungs have a marbled appearance. Grey and red consolidated lobules alternate irregularly with pink emphysematous lobules and the interlobular septa are distended and oedematous. There may be abundant serofibrinous exudate in the pleural cavity. In chronic cases, fibrous encapsulation of necrotic foci is commonly found. These necrotic foci contain viable mycoplasmas and breakdown of the capsules in chronically affected animals is a major factor in the persistence and spread of CBPP in endemic areas.

Diagnosis

- In endemic regions, clinical signs and characteristic postmortem findings allow a presumptive diagnosis.
- Techniques, such as the polymerase chain reaction, based on the detection of specific DNA in tissue samples can be used to differentiate *M. mycoides* subspecies *mycoides* (small colony type) from other members of the '*mycoides* cluster'.
- The fluorescent antibody test can be used on pleural fluid to confirm the presence of the pathogen.
- Isolation and definitive identification of the pathogen from broncho-alveolar lavage, pleural fluid, lung tissue or the broncho-pulmonary lymph nodes is confirmatory. Polymerase chain reaction-based tests may be useful confirmatory tests.
- Serological tests:
  — Rapid field serum agglutination test
  — Passive haemagglutination screening test
  — Complement fixation test for determining disease status of animals crossing national boundaries
  — Dot-blot technique for confirmation (Nicholas *et al.*, 1996)
  — A competitive ELISA is presently under development.

Treatment and control

- Although treatment with antimicrobial drugs may be attempted in countries where the disease is endemic, it is generally unsatisfactory especially for chronically affected animals.
- In countries where CBPP is exotic, slaughter of affected and in-contact cattle is mandatory.
- In endemic regions, control strategies are based on prohibiting movement of suspect animals, mandatory quarantine and the elimination of carrier animals by serological testing and slaughter.
- Annual vaccination with attenuated vaccines is carried out to stimulate effective immunity in cattle in endemic areas. The virulence of attenuated vaccines varies with the strain of mycoplasma employed. Annual vaccination may be discontinued as eradication of the disease progresses.

Infections with *Mycoplasma bovis*

Strains of *M. bovis,* which is worldwide in distribution, can cause severe pneumonia in calves in the absence of other respiratory pathogens (Doherty *et al.*, 1994) and can exacerbate respiratory disease caused by *Pasteurella* and *Mannheimia* species (Gourlay *et al.*, 1989). *Mycoplasma bovis* has also been associated with mastitis and poly-arthritis. Diagnostic techniques are similar to those used for other mycoplasmas. A number of other *Mycoplasma* species cause sporadic cases of mastitis in cattle (Table 33.2). Although the mastitis may be severe, systemic involvement is uncommon. There is often a dramatic loss of milk production and the serous or purulent mastitic exudate has a high leukocyte count. Mycoplasmal mastitis should be considered when other common bacterial causal agents have been excluded. *Mycoplasma bovis* mastitis is discussed in more detail in Chapter 81.

Contagious agalactia of sheep and goats

This severe febrile disease of sheep and goats, caused by *M. agalactiae*, is prevalent in parts of Europe, northern Africa and parts of Asia. It usually becomes evident immediately after parturition and is characterized by mastitis, arthritis and conjunctivitis. Pregnant animals may abort and the disease can be fatal in young animals due to pneumonic complications. The organism is shed in milk and may remain localized in the supramammary lymph nodes between lactations. Disease due to *M. agalactiae* must be distinguished from mastitis and arthritis associated with *M. capricolum* subspecies *capricolum*, *M. mycoides* subspecies *mycoides* (large colony type) and *M. mycoides* subspecies *capri* (Gil *et al.*, 1999). Inactivated and attenuated vaccines for *M. agalactiae* are commercially available.

Contagious caprine pleuropneumonia

Contagious caprine pleuropneumonia (CCPP), caused by *M. capricolum* subspecies *capripneumoniae* (formerly *Mycoplasma* strain F38), is present in northern and eastern Africa and in Turkey. The disease is characterized by pneumonia, fibrinous pleurisy, profuse pleural exudate and a marbled appearance on the cut surface of affected lungs. Although similar in many respects to CBPP, well developed necrotic areas in the lungs in chronic CCPP are rare. The disease is highly contagious and is transmitted by aerosols. Nomadic herds often carry infection to regions free of the disease. Pleuropneumonia in goats can occasionally be caused by *M. mycoides* subspecies *capri* or *M. mycoides* subspecies *mycoides* (large colony type). However, monoclonal antibody to *M. capricolum* sub-species *capripneumoniae* is specific for this organism in a growth inhibition disc test (Belton *et al.*, 1994). Inactivated vaccines give satisfactory protection.

Enzootic pneumonia of pigs

This economically important disease, caused by

M. hyopneumoniae, occurs worldwide in intensively reared pigs. Poor ventilation, overcrowding and temperature fluctuations may precipitate an outbreak. Pigs of all ages are susceptible and the condition is characterized by coughing, poor growth rates and, in some cases, respiratory distress. At postmortem, pulmonary consolidation is confined to the apical and cardiac lobes with clear demarcation from normal lung tissue. Clinical, epidemiological and pathological findings are usually indicative of the presence of the condition. The disease can be confirmed by isolation and identification of the pathogen, by immunofluorescence using lung tissue and, on a herd basis, by the complement fixation test or by ELISA. Appropriate antimicrobial drugs such as tylosin tartrate, lincomycin or tiamulin, when incorporated into the feed, are suitable for controlling herd infections. Although inactivated and subunit vaccines are available, their efficacy is uncertain. Prevention and control are primarily based on the development of specific-pathogen-free herds.

Other mycoplasmal diseases of pigs

Mycoplasma hyorhinis causes a chronic progressive poly-serositis in pigs up to 10 weeks of age. It is characterized by fever, laboured breathing, lameness and swollen joints. At postmortem, serofibrinous pleurisy, pericarditis and peritonitis are present. The disease can be confirmed by isolation and identification of the pathogen and by serology. Tylosin or lincomycin, administered early in the course of the disease, may be of therapeutic value.

A polyarthritis caused by *M. hyosynoviae* affects pigs from 10 to 30 weeks of age. This self-limiting arthritis and synovitis produces transient lameness. Confirmation relies on isolation and identification of the pathogen.

Mycoplasmal diseases of poultry

Mycoplasma gallisepticum causes chronic respiratory disease in chickens and infectious sinusitis in turkeys. The organism is transmitted through infection of the embryo in the egg or by aerosols. Clinical signs are consistent with upper respiratory tract involvement in chickens. In turkeys, there is swelling of the paranasal sinuses. Reduced egg production may be evident. Diagnosis is based on isolation and identification of the pathogen and on flock testing using the serum plate agglutination test. Haemagglutination inhibition and ELISA tests are also used in flocks to confirm infection. Although anti-microbial medication of feed is used during outbreaks, the establishment of specific-pathogen-free flocks is the preferred method for controlling the disease. Eggs used for hatching should be dipped in a tylosin solution to eliminate the pathogen. Modified live vaccines and bacterins are available.

Mycoplasma meleagridis may be egg-transmitted and may be present in turkey semen. Aerosol transmission is less important with this pathogen than with *M. gallisepticum*. The clinical features of the infection include reduced egg hatchability, airsacculitis in young poults and joint and bone deformities in growers. Confirmation requires isolation and identification of the pathogen. The serum plate agglutination test is used for flock testing. Tylosin, administered in the water for the first 10 days of life is of therapeutic value. Eggs used for hatching should be dipped in tylosin solution. Semen should be obtained from *M. meleagridis*-free toms.

Mycoplasma synoviae, the cause of infectious synovitis in chickens and turkeys, is transmitted mainly by aerosols. Egg transmission is much less important than in *M. gallisepticum* and *M. meleagridis* infections. Synovitis, arthritis and respiratory signs are the main clinical features. Confirmation requires isolation and identification of the pathogen or positive serological tests. Tetracycline medication of the feed is used for treatment and control. Eradication is possible through the development of specific-pathogen-free flocks.

References

Belton, D., Leach, R.H., Mitchelmore, D.L. and Rurangirwa, F.R. (1994). Serological specificity of a monoclonal antibody to *Mycoplasma capricolum* strain F38, the agent of infectious caprine pleuropneumonia. *Veterinary Record*, **134**, 643–646.

Doherty, M.L., McElroy, M.C., Markey, B.K., Carter, M.E. and Ball, H.J. (1994). Isolation of *Mycoplasma bovis* from a calf imported into the Republic of Ireland. *Veterinary Record*, **135**, 259–260.

Egwu, G.O., Nicholas, R.A.J., Ameh, J.A. and Bashiruddin, J.B. (1996). Contagious bovine pleuropneumonia: an update. *Veterinary Bulletin*, **66**, 875–888.

Geary, S.J., Tourtelotte, M.E. and Cameron, J.A. (1981). Inflammatory toxin from *Mycoplasma bovis*: isolation and characterization. *Science*, **212**, 1032–1033.

Gil, M.C., Hermoso de Merdoza, M., Rey, J., Alonso, J.M., Poveda, J.B. and Hermoso de Mendoza, J. (1999). Aetiology of caprine agalactia syndrome in Extremadura, Spain. *Veterinary Record*, **144**, 24–25.

Gourlay, R.N., Thomas, L.H. and Wyld, S.G. (1989). Increased severity of calf pneumonia associated with the appearance of *Mycoplasma bovis* in a rearing shed. *Veterinary Record*, **124**, 420–422.

Jang, S.S., Ling, G.V., Yamamoto, R. and Wolf, A.M. (1984). Mycoplasmas as a cause of canine urinary tract infection. *Journal of the American Veterinary Medical Association*, **185**, 45–47.

Krause, D.C. and Stevens, M.K. (1995). Localization of antigens on mycoplasma cell surface and tip structures. In *Molecular and Diagnostic Procedures in Mycoplasmology*, Volume 1. Eds. S. Razin and J.G. Tully. Academic Press, San Diego. pp. 89-98.

Moise, N.S., Crissman, J.W., Fairbrother, J.F. and Baldwin, C. (1983). *Mycoplasma gateae* arthritis and tenosynovitis in cats: case report and experimental reproduction of the disease. *American Journal of Veterinary Research*, **44**, 16–21.

Muhlradt, P.F. and Schade, U. (1991). MDHM, a macrophage-stimulatory product of *Mycoplasma fermentans*, leads to in vitro interleukin-1 (IL-1), IL-6, tumor necrosis factor and prostaglandin production and is pyrogenic in rabbits. *Infection and Immunity*, **59**, 3969–3974.

Nicholas, R.A.J., Santini, F.G., Clark, K.M., Palmer, N.M.A., DeSantis, P. and Bashiruddin, J.B. (1996). A comparison of serological tests and gross lung pathology for detecting contagious bovine pleuropneumonia in two groups of Italian cattle. *Veterinary Record*, **139**, 89–93.

Further reading

Mohan, K., Foggin, C.M., Muvavarirwa, P. and Honeywill, J. (1997). Vaccination of farmed crocodiles (*Crocodylus niloticus*) against *Mycoplasma crocodyli* infection. *Veterinary Record*, **141**, 476.

Thiaucourt, F., Breard, A., Lefevre, P.C. and Mebratu, G.Y. (1992). Contagious caprine pleuropneumonia in Ethiopia. *Veterinary Record*, **131**, 585.

Wood, J.L.N., Chanter, N., Newton, J.R., Burrell, M.H., Dugdale, D., Windsor, H.M. *et al.* (1997). An outbreak of respiratory disease in horses associated with *Mycoplasma felis* infection. *Veterinary Record*, **140**, 388-391.

Chapter 34

Chlamydia and *Chlamydophila* species

Chlamydiae are obligate intracellular bacteria with an unusual developmental cycle during which unique infectious forms are produced. They replicate within cytoplasmic vacuoles in host cells. On account of their apparent inability to generate ATP, with resultant dependence on host cell metabolism, they have been termed 'energy parasites'. The family *Chlamydiaceae* belongs to the order *Chlamydiales*. Currently two genera, *Chlamydia* and *Chlamydophila*, and nine species are described (Fig. 34.1). Formerly a single genus and four species, *Chlamydia trachomatis*, *C. psittaci*, *C. pneumoniae* and *C. pecorum*, were recognised. This classification was based on phenotypic characteristics such as host preference, inclusion morphology, iodine staining for the presence of glycogen, and sulphonamide susceptibility. However, recent nucleic acid sequencing studies of the 16S and 23S rRNA genes confirm two distinct lineages (Everett *et al.*, 1999).

In the developmental cycle of chlamydiae, infectious and reproductive forms are morphologically distinct (Fig. 34.2). Infectious extracellular forms, called elementary bodies (EBs) are small (200 to 300 nm), metabolically inert and osmotically stable. Each EB is surrounded by a conventional bacterial cytoplasmic membrane, a periplasmic space and an outer envelope containing lipopolysaccharide. The periplasmic space does not contain a detectable peptidoglycan layer and the EB relies on disulphide cross-linked envelope proteins for osmotic stability (Hatch, 1996). Elementary bodies enter host cells by receptor-mediated endocytosis. Acidification of the

> **Key points**
> - Sperical intracellular bacteria with unique developmental cycle
> - Appropriate staining procedures include the modified Ziehl-Neelsen and Giemsa methods
> - Unable to synthesize ATP and replicate only in living cells
> - Cell walls lack peptidoglycan but contain genus-specific lipopolysaccharide
> - Species vary in virulence for particular hosts; some strains are associated with specific diseases in domestic animals
> - Produce respiratory, enteric, plural and reproductive tract diseases in animals and humans

endosome and fusion with lysosomes are prevented by mechanisms which are not fully understood. A process of structural reorganization within the pathogen, of several hours duration, results in the conversion of an EB into a reticulate body (RB). The RB, about 1 μm in diameter, is metabolically active, osmotically fragile and replicates by binary fission within the endosome. The endosome and its contents, when stained, is called an inclusion. When a number of inclusions containing RBs of *C. trachomatis*

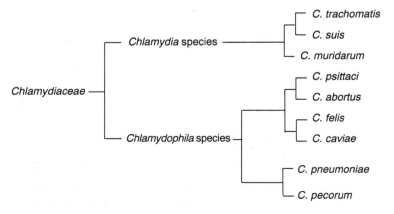

Figure 34.1 Classification of chlamydial isolates on the basis of genetic relatedness (based on Everett *et al.*, 1999)

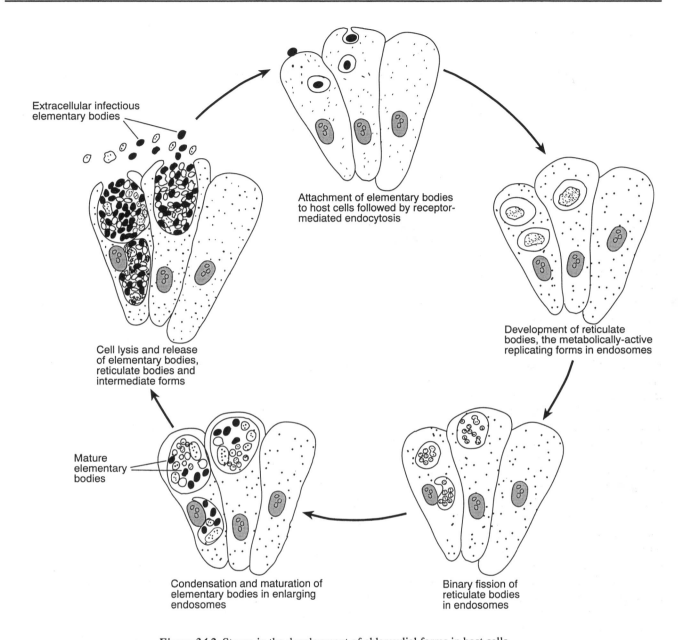

Extracellular infectious
elementary bodies

Attachment of elementary bodies
to host cells followed by receptor-
mediated endocytosis

Development of reticulate
bodies, the metabolically-active
replicating forms in endosomes

Cell lysis and release
of elementary bodies,
reticulate bodies and
intermediate forms

Mature
elementary
bodies

Condensation and maturation of
elementary bodies in enlarging
endosomes

Binary fission of
reticulate bodies
in endosomes

Figure 34.2 Stages in the development of chlamydial forms in host cells.

are formed in an infected cell, fusion of these structures may occur. About 20 hours after infection, the developmental cycle becomes asynchronous with some RBs continuing to divide while others condense and mature to form EBs. In general, replication continues for up to 72 hours after infection when the host cell lyses releasing several hundred bodies which include EBs, RBs and intermediate forms. Chlamydial replication may be delayed in the presence of gamma interferon or penicillin or when the availability of tryptophan or cysteine is limited, resulting in persistent infection. Delayed replication of this type appears to be important in the development of the immunopathological changes in humans associated with trachoma and with pelvic inflammatory reaction.

Usual habitat

The gastrointestinal tract appears to be the usual site of *Chlamydophila* species infection in animals. Intestinal infections are often subclinical and persistent. Faecal shedding of the organisms, which is typically prolonged, becomes intermittent with time. The EBs can survive in the environment for several days.

Pathogenesis and pathogenicity

Chlamydiae infect over 130 species of birds and a large number of mammalian species including man. In recent years isolations have also been made from invertebrate species. Chlamydial species are usually associated with specific diseases in particular hosts. In sheep, *C. abortus* is an important cause of abortion whereas infections with *C. pecorum* are frequently inapparent. Interspecies transmission is uncommon. When it occurs, the outcome of infection in the secondary host may be either similar, as in transmission from sheep to cattle, or severe, as in transmission from sheep to pregnant women.

Infection with *C. pecorum* is associated with conjunctivitis, arthritis and inapparent intestinal infection. The type of clinical presentation relates to the route of infection and the degree of exposure. Environmental factors and management practices can influence the prevalence of some chlamydial infections such as enzootic abortion in ewes, which tend to be more prevalent in intensively managed lowland flocks.

Many chlamydial infections are asymptomatic, particularly when they are localized in superficial epithelia. They may also persist for long periods without inducing protective immunity. However, chronic infections may repeatedly stimulate the host immune system. Chlamydiae possess a number of heat shock proteins which are partially homologous to heat shock proteins in other bacteria and to a number of human mitochondrial proteins. It is considered that repeated stimulation of the immune system with these proteins contributes significantly to the delayed-type hypersensitivity responses associated with trachoma and inflammatory pelvic disease in man. The tissue damage in these diseases is more severe than would be expected from direct infection alone. Gamma interferon has been shown to contribute to the control of primary chlamydial infections. However, there is also evidence that gamma interferon can induce latent or persistent chlamydial infections which, in turn, may be responsible for increased heat shock protein expression (Ward, 1995).

Diagnostic procedures

Consideration of the history, clinical signs and pathological changes may suggest certain chlamydial infections such as feline chlamydiosis and enzootic abortion of ewes.

- Specimens for isolation of the organism should be placed in suitable transport medium such as sucrose-phosphate-glutamate medium supplemented with foetal calf serum, aminoglycoside antibiotics and an antifungal agent (Spencer and Johnson, 1983). As chlamydiae are thermolabile, samples should be kept at 4°C. For long term storage, samples should be frozen at –70°C. However, each cycle of freezing and thawing reduces the titre of the stored organisms.
- Direct microscopy is suitable for the detection of the organisms in smears or tissue sections containing moderate numbers of organisms. Smears or histological sections of organs from aborted foetuses or from the liver and spleen in cases of avian chlamydiosis are suitable for direct examination. Placental smears from cases of chlamydial abortion typically contain large numbers of organisms. Suitable chemical staining procedures include the modified Ziehl-Neelsen, Giemsa, modified Machiavello and Castaneda methods. Methylene blue-stained smears can be examined by darkfield microscopy.
- Several commercial kit sets, employing ELISA methodology, have been developed for the detection of *C. trachomatis*. Many of these kit sets detect chlamydial lipopolysaccharide (LPS) which is common to all *Chlamydia* and *Chlamydophila* species. Consequently, they can be used to detect the LPS of species in both genera.
- Chlamydiae can be isolated either in embryonated eggs, inoculated into the yolk sac, or in a number of continuous cell lines such as McCoy, L929, baby hamster kidney and Vero. Tissue culture cells are usually grown in flat-bottomed vials or in bottles containing coverslips for ease of fixing and subsequent staining. The attachment of chlamydiae to cells is greatly enhanced by centrifugation of the sample onto the monolayer. The sensitivity of the isolation procedure is also increased by the use of non-replicating cells. This is achieved by the addition of cytotoxic chemicals such as cycloheximide, 5-iodo-2-deoxyuridine, cytochalasin B and emetine to the cell culture medium. After 2 to 3 days incubation at 37°C the monolayer is fixed, stained as described above and examined for the presence of chlamydial inclusions. Antibiotics to which chlamydiae are sensitive, such as oxytetracycline, erythromycin and penicillin, should not be used in the cell culture medium.
- Polymerase chain reaction techniques have been developed for the detection of chlamydial DNA in samples. Using these methods it is possible to distinguish different chlamydial species by employing specific primers (Sheehy *et al.*, 1996; Everett and Andersen, 1999).
- Several serological procedures are available for the detection of antibodies to chlamydiae including complement fixation, ELISA, indirect immunofluorescence and micro-immunofluorescence. Although the complement fixation test is the most widely recognised serological test, it is time-consuming and only moderately sensitive. More sensitive assays based on ELISA methodology are now available. Because chlamydial infection is widespread, an exceptionally high or a rising antibody titre must be demonstrated in order to correlate infection with clinical signs. Interpretation of results is complicated by the fact that many of the available serological procedures detect antibodies against chlamydial LPS and therefore do not allow differentiation of the chlamydial species involved in the infection. In addition, there is cross-reactivity

between the LPS of chlamydiae and that of some other Gram-negative bacteria.

Clinical infections

A wide range of animal species are susceptible to infections with chlamydiae (Vanrompay *et al.*, 1995). Both the severity and the type of disease produced by chlamydiae are highly variable, ranging from clinically inapparent infections and local infections of epithelial surfaces to severe systemic infections (Table 34.1). Diseases associated with chlamydial infections include conjunctivitis, arthritis, abortion, urethritis, enteritis, pneumonia and encephalomyelitis. Clinical signs and their severity are influenced by factors related to both host and pathogen, and one type of clinical presentation usually predominates in outbreaks of disease.

The species of *Chlamydophila* which infect humans differ in transmissibility. Although human infections can be acquired following contact with aborting ewes or cats with conjunctivitis, infected birds are considered to be more likely sources of infection. Human infections acquired from psittacine species are termed psittacosis while those from other avian species are termed ornithosis. Irrespective of the avian source of the infection, the condition typically presents as a respiratory illness.

Enzootic abortion of ewes

Enzootic abortion of ewes (EAE) caused by *C. abortus* (formerly known as ovine strains of *C. psittaci*), is primarily a disease of intensively managed flocks. The disease is economically significant in most sheep-producing countries. Although abortion associated with *C. abortus* is best documented in sheep, it has also been reported in other domestic species including cattle, pigs and goats. Chlamydial infection in cattle and goats often originates from sheep. The source of infection in pigs is less clearly defined (Schiller *et al.*, 1997).

Epidemiology

Infection is usually introduced into clean flocks when infected replacement ewes abort. Large numbers of chlamydiae are shed in placentas and uterine discharges from affected ewes. Organisms can remain viable in the environment for several days at low temperatures. Infection occurs by ingestion. The role of infected rams in venereal spread is uncertain (Appleyard *et al.*, 1985). Ewes infected late in pregnancy do not usually abort but may do so in the next pregnancy. Infection early in pregnancy can result in abortion during that pregnancy. Ewe lambs may acquire infection during the neonatal period and abort during their first pregnancy. As a result, the most dramatic outbreaks of EAE often occur in the year following the introduction of infection into a flock.

Clinical signs

Enzootic abortion of ewes is characterized by abortion during late pregnancy or by the birth of premature weak lambs. Aborted lambs are well developed and fresh. Necrosis of cotyledons and oedema of adjacent intercotyledonary tissue in affected placentas is often present along with a dirty pink uterine exudate. Aborting ewes rarely show evidence of clinical disease and their subsequent fertility is usually unimpaired. Although up to 30% of

Table 34.1 Chlamydial infections of veterinary and medical importance.

Pathogen	Hosts	Clinical conditions
Chlamydophila psittaci	Birds	Pneumonia and airsacculitis Intestinal infection and diarrhoea Conjunctivitis Pericarditis Encephalitis
	Humans (secondary hosts)	Psittacosis/ornithosis Abortion Conjunctivitis
C. abortus	Sheep	Enzootic abortion of ewes (EAE)
	Goats	Chlamydial abortion
	Cattle	Chlamydial abortion
	Pigs	Chlamydial abortion
C. felis	Cats	Conjunctivitis (feline pneumonitis)
C. caviae	Guinea-pigs	Guinea-pig inclusion conjunctivitis
C. pecorum	Sheep	Intestinal infection Conjunctivitis Polyarthritis
	Cattle	Sporadic bovine encephalomyelitis Polyarthritis Metritis
	Koalas	Conjunctivitis Urogenital infection
C. pneumoniae	Humans	Respiratory infection
	Horses	Respiratory infection
	Koalas	Conjunctivitis
Chlamydia trachomatis	Humans	Trachoma, inclusion conjunctivitis of infants Non-specific urethritis Respiratory disease of infants Proctitis Lymphogranuloma venereum Arthritis
C. suis	Pigs	Intestinal infection
C. muridarum	Mice	Respiratory infection

animals in a fully susceptible flock may abort, a rate of 5 to 10% is more usual in flocks in which the disease is endemic.

Diagnosis

- Well-preserved aborted lambs and evidence of necrotic placentitis are suggestive of EAE.
- Large numbers of EBs can be demonstrated in placental smears using suitable staining procedures.
- Commercial diagnostic kits are available for the detection of chlamydial antigen in samples.
- Isolation of chlamydiae in suitable cell lines or in the yolk sac of embryonated eggs is possible.
- Polymerase chain reaction techniques are available and can be carried out using species-specific primers to distinguish *C. abortus* and *C. pecorum*.
- A number of different serological tests can be used for the detection of chlamydial antibodies including the complement fixation test, ELISA and indirect immunofluorescence. The use of recombinant antigens specific for *C. abortus* may improve the specificity of serological tests (Rodolakis *et al.*, 1998).

Treatment and control

Control measures for EAE have been comprehensively reviewed (Aitken *et al.*, 1990).

- Chlamydiae are susceptible to a number of antibiotics which can be used during an outbreak. Administration of long-acting oxytetracycline to in-contact pregnant ewes has been shown to increase the number of live-born lambs. However, antibiotic treatment does not eliminate the infection and treated ewes may shed chlamydiae at parturition.
- Transmission of infection in an affected flock can be reduced by isolating all aborted ewes for 2 to 3 weeks, removing and destroying all placentas, thoroughly cleaning areas where abortions occurred and administering long-acting oxytetracycline to ewes which have not yet lambed.
- A decision should be made either to vaccinate or attempt to eradicate the disease by culling. A live attenuated vaccine is available which should be administered to ewes prior to breeding. An inactivated vaccine is also available which can be used in pregnant animals.
- *Chlamydophila abortus* infection is serious and potentially life-threatening for pregnant women who should avoid contact with ewes during the lambing season (Johnson *et al.*, 1985; Buxton, 1986).

Feline chlamydiosis

Chlamydophila felis (formerly known as feline strains of *C. psittaci*) is associated with conjunctivitis and less commonly rhinitis. Feline pneumonitis, the original name for feline chlamydiosis, is now considered a misnomer because of the rarity of lower respiratory tract infection caused by *C. felis* in cats.

Epidemiology

Serological surveys have revealed that up to 10% of cats become infected with *C. felis*. Infection is transmitted by direct or indirect contact with conjunctival or nasal secretions. Organisms may also be shed from the reproductive tract (TerWee *et al.*, 1998). Infection may be persistent with prolonged shedding of organisms and clinical relapses. The stress of parturition and lactation may trigger shedding of organisms by infected queens facilitating transmission to their offspring.

Clinical signs

After an incubation period of about 5 days, unilateral or bilateral conjunctival congestion, clear ocular discharge and blepharospasm become evident. If secondary infection with organisms such as *Mycoplasma felis* and *Staphylococcus* species occurs, the ocular discharge may become mucopurulent. Conjunctivitis may be accompanied by sneezing and nasal discharge. The condition usually resolves without treatment in a few weeks. However, persistent infection with recurring clinical episodes also occurs.

Diagnosis

- Stained conjunctival smears may reveal intracytoplasmic inclusions.
- The organism may be isolated in suitable cell lines or in embryonated eggs.
- Commercial diagnostic ELISA kits for detecting the genus-specific lipopolysaccharide antigen are available.
- Polymerase chain reaction protocols have been developed for samples.
- The complement fixation test or the indirect immunofluorescence test can be used to detect chlamydial antibody titres. However, the level of antibody does not necessarily correlate with active infection.

Treatment and control

- Chlamydiae are susceptible to several antibiotics. All in-contact cats should be treated at the same time.
- Modified live vaccines are available for parenteral inoculation. Vaccination reduces the clinical effects of natural infection but does not prevent infection or the shedding of organisms. Inadvertent intraocular administration of the vaccine can result in conjunctivitis (Sturgess *et al.*, 1995).
- A small number of cases of conjunctivitis in humans involving *C. felis* have been reported.

Sporadic bovine encephalomyelitis

This neurological disease, caused by *C. pecorum*, has been described in several regions of the world including the USA, Japan, Israel and central Europe. Although intestinal infection in cattle with *C. pecorum* is considered to be common, sporadic bovine encephalomyelitis occurs haphazardly and the predisposing factors are unknown. Affected animals, which are usually under 3 years of age, develop a high fever and exhibit incoordination, depression, excessive salivation and diarrhoea. Terminally, animals may become recumbent and can develop opisthotonos. The course of the disease is about 2 weeks and the mortality rate may be up to 50%. Lesions associated with vascular damage are found in the brain and other organs. Diagnosis is based on clinical signs, the presence of a serofibrinous peritonitis, histopathological changes in the brain and isolation of the organism from brain tissue. High doses of antibiotics such as tetracyclines and tylosin may be effective. No vaccines are available and there is no defined control strategy.

Avian chlamydiosis

Infections with *C. psittaci* in psittacine birds were originally designated psittacosis and ornithosis was reserved for chlamydial infection in other avian species. Avian chlamydiosis is currently the preferred designation for the condition. The disease has been recorded worldwide.

Epidemiology

A wide range of both wild and domestic avian species are susceptible to infection. Isolates can be divided into several serovars on the basis of reactivity with monoclonal antibodies. The organism is present in respiratory discharges and faeces of infected birds. Infection is usually acquired by inhalation or by ingestion. Subclinical infection is common. Clinically affected and carrier birds may shed organisms intermittently for prolonged periods. Stress arising from captivity, transportation, egg-laying, overcrowding and intercurrent infection is important in precipitating disease outbreaks.

Clinical signs

Avian chlamydiosis is a generalized infection, affecting particularly the digestive and respiratory tracts. The incubation period is up to 10 days. Clinical signs vary in nature and severity, depending on the strain of *C. psittaci* and the species and age of the affected birds. Signs include loss of condition, nasal and ocular discharges, diarrhoea and respiratory distress. The most frequent post-mortem findings are hepatosplenomegaly, airsacculitis and peritonitis.

Diagnosis

The diagnostic techniques for avian chlamydiosis have been reviewed by Andersen (1996).

- Organisms may be identified in stained impression smears of affected tissues.

- Chlamydial antigen may be detected using immuno-histochemistry or ELISA kits.
- Chlamydial DNA may be demonstrated by the polymerase chain reaction.
- Isolation of *C. psittaci* is carried out in cell culture or embryonated eggs.
- Antibodies to *C. psittaci* may be detected using suitable serological tests including the complement fixation test and ELISA. However, interpretation of antibody titres can be difficult particularly when single samples are tested. Paired serum samples or samples from several birds in a flock are more reliable for diagnosis.

Treatment and control

- Tetracyclines are the antibiotics of choice. An extended course of treatment over several weeks is required.
- No commercial vaccines are available.
- Imported birds, particularly psittacine species, should be held in quarantine and receive tetracycline-medicated feeds.
- Proper husbandry and suitable transportation minimize the occurrence of clinical disease.
- Avian chlamydial isolates are potentially zoonotic. Infection, which commonly follows aerosol inhalation, may be subclinical or result in systemic disease. Pulmonary involvement is common. Meningitis or meningoencephalitis may develop in severely affected individuals.

References

Aitken, I.D., Clarkson, M.J. and Linklater, K. (1990). Enzootic abortion of ewes. *Veterinary Record*, **126**, 136–138.

Andersen, A.A. (1996). Avian chlamydiosis. In *OIE Manual of Standards for Diagnostic Tests and Vaccines*. Third Edition. OIE, Paris, France. pp. 522–531.

Appleyard, W.T., Aitken, I.D. and Anderson, I.E. (1985). Attempted venereal transmission of *Chlamydia psittaci* in sheep. *Veterinary Record*, **116**, 535–538.

Buxton, D. (1986). Potential danger to pregnant women of *Chlamydia psittaci* from sheep. *Veterinary Record*, **118**, 510–511.

Everett, K.D.E. and Andersen, A.A. (1999). Identification of nine species of the *Chlamydiaceae* using PCR-RFLP. *International Journal of Systematic Bacteriology*, **49**, 803–813.

Everett, K.D., Bush, R.M. and Andersen, A.A. (1999). Emended description of the order *Chlamydiales*, proposal of *Parachlamydiaceae* fam. nov. and *Simkaniaceae* fam. nov., each containing one monotypic genus, revised taxonomy of the family *Chlamydiaceae*, including a new genus and five new species, and standards for the identification of organisms. *International Journal of Systematic Bacteriology*, **49**, 415–440.

Hatch, T.P. (1996). Disulfide cross-linked envelope proteins: the functional equivalent of peptidoglycan in chlamydiae?

Journal of Bacteriology, **178**, 1–5.

Johnson, F.W.A., Matheson, B.A., Williams, H. *et al.* (1985). Abortion due to infection with *Chlamydia psittaci* in a sheep farmer's wife. *British Medical Journal,* **290**, 592–594.

Rodolakis, A., Salinas, J. and Papp, J. (1998). Recent advances on ovine chlamydial abortion. *Veterinary Research,* **29**, 275–288.

Schiller, I., Koesters, R., Weilenmann, R. *et al.* (1997). Mixed infections with porcine *Chlamydia trachomatis/pecorum* and infections with ruminant *Chlamydia psittaci* serovar 1 associated with abortions in swine. *Veterinary Microbiology,* **58**, 251–260.

Sheehy, N., Markey, B., Gleeson, M. and Quinn, P.J. (1996). Differentiation of *Chlamydia psittaci* and *C. pecorum* strains by species-specific PCR. *Journal of Clinical Microbiology,* **34**, 3175–3179.

Spencer, W.N. and Johnson, F.W.A. (1983). Simple transport medium for the isolation of *Chlamydia psittaci* from clinical material. *Veterinary Record,* **113**, 535–536.

Sturgess, C.P., Gruffydd-Jones, T.J., Harbour, D.A. and Feilden, H.R. (1995). Studies on the safety of *Chlamydia psittaci* vaccination in cats. *Veterinary Record,* **137**, 668–669.

TerWee, J., Sabara, M., Kokjohn K. *et al.* (1998). Characterization of the systemic disease and ocular signs induced by experimental infection with *Chlamydia psittaci* in cats. *Veterinary Microbiology,* **59**, 259–281.

Vanrompay, D., Ducatelle, R. and Haesebrouck, F. (1995). *Chlamydia psittaci* infections: a review with emphasis on avian chlamydiosis. *Veterinary Microbiology,* **45**, 93–119.

Ward, M.E. (1995). The immunobiology and immunopathology of chlamydial infections. *APMIS,* **103**, 769–796.

Further reading

Everett, K.D.E. (2000). *Chlamydia* and *Chlamydiales*: more than meets the eye. *Veterinary Microbiology,* **75**, 109–126.

Chapter 35

Rickettsiales

Organisms in the order *Rickettsiales* form a diverse group of small (0.3 to 0.5 x 0.8 to 2.0 μm), non-motile, pleomorphic Gram-negative bacteria which replicate only in host cells. They can be cultured in the yolk sac of embryonated eggs or in selected tissue culture cell lines. Because they stain poorly with aniline dyes, these organisms should be stained by Romanowsky methods such as Giemsa or Leishman. In addition to host-cell dependence and poor affinity for basic dyes, a requirement for an invertebrate vector distinguishes them from conventional bacteria and the *Chlamydiales*.

The application of ribosomal RNA sequencing techniques and other precise analytical methods is likely to lead to a more accurate classification of the organisms in the *Rickettsiales* than at present. The family *Bartonellaceae* has been removed from the order (Brenner *et al.*, 1993) and *Coxiella burnetii*, which is genotypically and phenotypically distinct from other members of the group, may eventually be reclassified (Campbell, 1994). In addition, it has been proposed that some members of the genera *Haemobartonella* and *Eperythrozoon* should be transferred to the genus *Mycoplasma* (Neimark *et al.*, 2001). Phylogenetic investigation has shown that members of these genera are most closely related to species within the so-called pneumoniae group of *Mycoplasma*.

At present, two families, *Rickettsiaceae* and *Anaplasmataceae*, comprise the *Rickettsiales* (Fig. 35.1). Those species in the family *Rickettsiales* awaiting definitive assignment are in quotation marks in Fig. 35.1 and Table 35.1. Organisms in the family *Rickettsiaceae*, referred to as rickettsiae, generally target macrophages, leukocytes and endothelial cells. In common with conventional Gram-negative bacteria, rickettsiae have peptidoglycan in their cell walls. Species of veterinary importance in the family *Rickettsiaceae* are listed in Table 35.1. Members of the *Anaplasmataceae* parasitize erythrocytes and possess cytoplasmic membranes but lack cell walls. Species of veterinary importance in the family are listed in Table 35.2.

Epidemiology

Animal hosts and arthropod vectors are the reservoirs for most rickettsiae. A number of rickettsial organisms, including *Ehrlichia canis*, *Anaplasma marginale* and

---

Key points

- Minute, non-motile Gram-negative bacteria
- Obligate intracellular pathogens, replicating only in cells
- Demonstrated in blood smears by Romanowsky stains
- Host specificity and tropism for particular cell types evident
- Extracellular survival brief for most members apart from *Coxiella burnetii*
- Cause systemic diseases, mainly arthropod-borne, in humans and animals
- *Rickettsiaceae*
  —cell walls often contain peptidoglycan
  —cultured in specific cell lines or in fertile eggs
  —tropism for vascular endothelium or leukocytes
- *Anaplasmataceae*
  —lack cell walls, possess cell membranes
  —have not been cultured *in vitro*
  —tropism for erythrocytes

Haemobartonella felis produce latent infections. In arthropods, rickettsiae replicate in the epithelial cells of the gut before spreading to other organs, including the salivary glands and ovaries where further replication may occur. Organisms are transmitted when the arthropod feeds on the animal host. Some organisms such as *Rickettsia rickettsii* are maintained in a tick population by transovarial transmission. Trans-stadial but not transovarial transmission of *E. canis* and *E. phagocytophila* occurs in ticks. The majority of members of the *Rickettsiales* are transmitted by arthropods but the vectors of some *Ehrlichia* species have not yet been clearly defined (Table 35.1). Transmission by flukes, which has been confirmed for *Neorickettsia* species, may also occur in the life cycle of *E. risticii*. With the exception of *Coxiella burnetii*, which produces endospore-like forms and can remain viable in dust for up to 50 days, most rickettsiae are labile outside host cells. Aerosol transmission of *C. burnetii* commonly occurs in

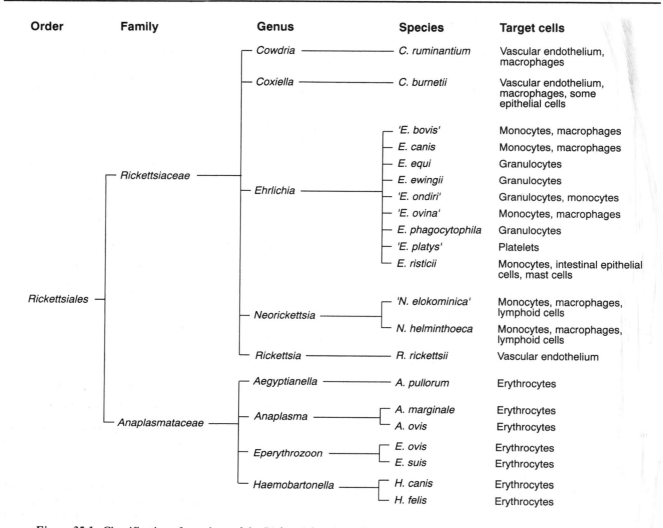

Figure 35.1 Classification of members of the *Rickettsiales* of veterinary importance and the cell types which they target.

domestic animals and humans. In addition, a silent cycle involving ticks and small wild mammals may constitute a possible source of infection for some domestic species.

Pathogenesis and pathogenicity

Many *Rickettsia* species including the causal agents of typhus (*R. prowazekii*), murine typhus (*R. typhi*) and scrub typhus (*R. tsutsugamushi*) are primarily human pathogens. Rocky Mountain spotted fever, caused by *Rickettsia rickettsii*, which is a common rickettsial disease of humans, also affects dogs. These highly pathogenic organisms have a predilection for the endothelial cells of small blood vessels. *Rickettsia* species produce phospholipase which damages the membranes of phagosomes allowing the organisms to escape into the cytoplasm. Replication in the cytoplasm induces cytotoxic effects.

Ehrlichia species, with the exception of the human pathogens *E. chaffeensis* and *E. sennetsu*, are pathogens of domestic and feral animals. They have a predilection for either leukocytes or platelets and they survive and replicate in phagosomes by inhibiting phagosome/lysosome fusion.

Cowdria ruminantium, the cause of heartwater in ruminants, probably parasitizes macrophages and other cell types in lymphoid tissues during the initial phase of infection. Organisms finally localize in membrane-bound vacuoles in endothelial cells throughout the body.

Two species in the genus *Neorickettsia* cause acute febrile disease in dogs. These organisms, which localize predominantly in lymph nodes, produce a generalized lymphadenopathy.

Coxiella burnetii grows preferentially in the acid environment of phagolysosomes and many of its metabolic activities are detectable only at pH 5 or lower (Redd and Thompson, 1995). This pathogen localizes and replicates in cells of the female reproductive tract and mammary glands of ruminants.

Members of the *Anaplasmataceae* have a predilection for erythrocytes. *Anaplasma* species and *Aegyptianella pullorum* are found within vacuoles in red blood cells, whereas *Haemobartonella* and *Eperythrozoon* species are located on erythrocyte surfaces. Although *H. felis* does

Table 35.1 Species of veterinary importance in the family *Rickettsiaceae*.

Pathogen	Hosts / Vectors	Disease	Geographical distribution
Cowdria ruminantium	Ruminants / ticks	Heartwater	Sub-Saharan Africa, Caribbean islands
Coxiella burnetii	Humans, ruminants / aerosols, ticks	Q fever in humans, sporadic abortion in ruminants	Worldwide
'*Ehrlichia bovis*'	Cattle / ticks	Bovine ehrlichiosis	Africa, Middle East, Asia, South America
E. canis	Dogs / ticks	Canine monocytic ehrlichiosis	Tropical and subtropical regions
E. equi	Horses / ticks suspected	Equine ehrlichiosis	USA, Europe, Israel
E. ewingii	Dogs / ticks	Canine granulocytic ehrlichiosis	USA
'*E. ondiri*'	Cattle / ticks suspected	Bovine petechial fever	Highlands of East Africa
'*E. ovina*'	Sheep / ticks	Ovine ehrlichiosis	Africa, Asia, Middle East
E. phagocytophila	Ruminants / ticks	Tick-borne fever	European countries
'*E. platys*'	Dogs / ticks suspected	Canine cyclic thrombocytopenia	USA, Israel
E. risticii	Horses / flukes suspected	Potomac horse fever	North America, Europe
'*Neorickettsia elokominica*'	Dogs, bears, racoons / flukes	Elokomin fluke fever	West coast of North America
N. helminthoeca	Dogs / flukes	Salmon poisoning disease	West coast of North America
Rickettsia rickettsii	Humans, dogs / ticks	Rocky Mountain spotted fever	North, Central and South America

not usually penetrate red cells, it may erode surface membranes, increasing osmotic fragility of the erythrocytes and shortening their life span. Attachment of the organism to the surface of red cells appears to alter their surface antigens, stimulating autoantibody production and immune-mediated injury to the red cells. Anaemia, due to *H. felis* infection results from a combination of haemolysis and premature removal of red cells from the circulation.

Recognition and differentiation of members of the *Rickettsiales*

Definitive classification of the members of the *Rickettsiales* is based on 16S ribosomal RNA sequencing, lipopolysaccharide content and metabolic requirements (Woldehiwet and Ristic, 1993). In diagnostic laboratories, identification of these organisms is based on the species affected, cell predilection, microscopic appearance and molecular techniques. Some of the rickettsiae can be cultured in embryonated eggs or tissue culture cells. These difficult procedures are usually performed only in laboratories engaged in research or vaccine production.

- Blood or tissue smears stained by the Giemsa technique can be used to demonstrate the morphology of many rickettsial organisms. They occur as purplish-blue, small individual organisms, sometimes in clusters, or as morulae up to 4.0 μm in diameter. *Ehrlichia* species are found in granulocytes or platelets in blood smears from animals in the early stages of disease. Those species which target monocytes are present less frequently in blood smears.
- *Coxiella burnetii* is unusual in that it stains well with aniline dyes. In MZN-stained smears from ruminant placental tissues, the organisms appears as clusters of small, red-staining coccobacilli.
- Fluorescent antibody techniques can be used to identify specific rickettsial organisms in smears.
- Some rickettsiae can be isolated in the yolk sac of embryonated eggs or in defined tissue culture cell lines. *Coxiella burnetii* and many of those *Ehrlichia* species which parasitize monocytes grow comparatively readily in the yolk sac. Neither those *Ehrlichia* species which affect granulocytes nor members of the *Anaplasmataceae* have been grown *in vitro*.
- Molecular methods, including nucleic acid probes and polymerase chain reaction techniques, have been developed to detect *Anaplasma marginale* and *Cowdria ruminantium* in host tissues.
- In outbreaks of major diseases such as bovine anaplasmosis, susceptible domestic animals can be

Table 35.2 Species of veterinary importance in the family *Anaplasmataceae*.

Pathogen	Hosts / Vectors	Disease	Geographical distribution
Aegyptianella pullorum	Poultry / ticks	Aegyptianellosis	Africa, Asia, Mediterranean region
Anaplasma marginale	Ruminants / ticks	Anaplasmosis	Tropical and subtropical regions
A. ovis	Sheep, goats / ticks	Anaplasmosis	Asia, Africa, Europe, USA
Eperythrozoon ovis	Sheep, goats / biting arthropods suspected	Eperythrozoonosis	Worldwide
E. suis	Pigs / lice, flies suspected	Swine eperythrozoonosis	USA, parts of Europe
Haemobartonella canis	Dogs / ticks suspected	Canine haemobartonellosis	Worldwide
H. felis	Cats / biting arthropods suspected	Feline infectious anaemia	Worldwide

inoculated with infected blood or tissue in order to identify an organism or confirm a diagnosis.

Clinical infections

Rickettsial organisms are relatively host-specific. Because definitive arthropod or fluke vectors are involved in the transmission of most rickettsiae, diseases associated with these organisms tend to occur in defined geographical regions (Tables 35.1 and 35.2). In many instances the clinical signs reflect the targeting of a particular cell type by the causal agent of rickettsial disease. Q fever and Rocky Mountain spotted fever are important zoonotic diseases.

Rocky Mountain spotted fever in dogs

Rocky Mountain spotted fever, caused by *Rickettsia rickettsii*, affects mainly humans and dogs. In North America, the main tick vectors are *Dermacentor variabilis* and *D. andersoni*. *Rhipicephalus sanguineus* and *Amblyomma cajennense* are the main vectors in Central and South America. Ticks acquire the pathogen while feeding on infected small wild mammals. *Rickettsia rickettsii* is maintained in the tick population by transovarial and trans-stadial transmission. An infected tick must remain attached for up to 20 hours before salivary transmission to the host occurs. The organisms, which replicate in endothelial cells of infected dogs, produce vasculitis, increased vascular permeability and haemorrhage.

Clinical signs

The incubation period of the disease is 2 to 10 days and the course is usually less than 2 weeks. Clinical signs include fever, depression, conjunctivitis, retinal haemorrhages, muscle and joint pain, coughing, dyspnoea and oedema of the extremities. Neurological disturbance, which occurs in about 80% of affected dogs, presents as stupor, ataxia, neck rigidity, seizures and coma. Dogs with mild disease and those treated early in the infection usually recover. In severe disease, death may result from cardiovascular, neurological or renal damage. At postmortem there is widespread haemorrhage, splenomegaly and generalized lymphadenopathy.

Diagnosis

- Rocky Mountain spotted fever should be considered in dogs with systemic disease which have been exposed to ticks in endemic areas.
- Indirect fluorescent antibody test or ELISA demonstrating a rising antibody titre to *R. rickettsii* are diagnostic. Antibodies are not demonstrable until at least 10 days after infection.
- A marked thrombocytopenia and leukopenia may be present during the acute phase of the disease.
- The disease must be differentiated from acute canine monocytic ehrlichiosis (Greene *et al.*, 1985).

Treatment and control

- Tetracycline therapy, which usually produces clinical improvement within 24 hours, must be continued for 2 weeks.
- Supportive therapy is necessary for severely debilitated dogs.
- Frequent removal of ticks is recommended. Because the disease is zoonotic, gloves should be worn during this procedure.

Canine monocytic ehrlichiosis

Canine monocytic ehrlichiosis, a generalized disease of *Canidae* caused by *Ehrlichia canis*, is confined to tropical and subtropical regions. *Rhipicephalus sanguineus*, the brown tick, is one of the main vectors and trans-stadial transmission occurs. After detachment from an infected host, ticks can transmit the agent to susceptible dogs for up

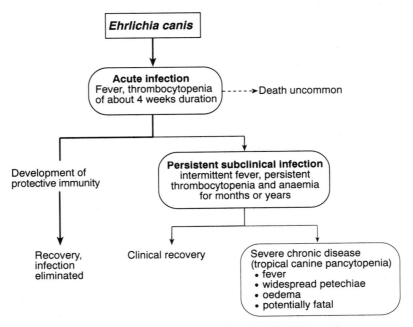

Figure 35.2 Possible consequences of infection with *Ehrlichia canis*.

to 5 months. Dogs often remain carriers for more than 2 years after recovery from acute disease. Human ehrlichiosis is caused by *E. chaffeensis* which is closely related to *E. canis*.

Clinical signs

Following an incubation period lasting up to 3 weeks, the disease can progress through acute, subclinical and chronic phases (Fig. 35.2). The acute phase, in which signs range from mild to severe, is characterized by fever, thrombocytopenia, leukopenia and anaemia. Most affected dogs recover but some progress to a subclinical phase lasting months or years during which low blood cell values persist but clinical signs are minimal. A minority of these dogs later develop a severe form of the disease known as tropical canine pancytopenia. Persistent bone marrow depression, along with haemorrhages, neurological disturbance, peripheral oedema and emaciation are characteristic of this phase of the disease. Hypotensive shock may ultimately develop, leading to death (Rikihisa, 1991). Progression to this chronic phase of the disease may be influenced by factors such as breed susceptibility, immunosuppression and the virulence of the infecting strain of *E. canis*.

Diagnosis

- Typical clinical and haematological features in dogs exposed to ticks in an endemic area may suggest canine monocytic ehrlichiosis.
- Morulae of *E. canis* may be detected in mononuclear cells in Giemsa-stained smears of the buffy-coat layer prepared from peripheral blood.

- Seroconversion can be demonstrated 3 weeks after infection using indirect immunofluorescence. Antibody titres of 1:10 or greater are considered to be indicative of infection.
- *Ehrlichia canis* can be cultured in a canine macrophage cell line.

Treatment and control

- Doxycycline therapy for 10 days is recommended. Tetracyclines and chloramphenicol are also effective.
- Fluid replacement therapy or blood transfusions may be necessary.
- Tetracyclines can be administered to susceptible dogs entering an endemic area as a short-term prophylactic measure.

Canine granulocytic ehrlichiosis

This disease, recently described in the USA, is caused by *Ehrlichia ewingii* (Anderson *et al.*, 1992). Neutrophils are the primary target cells for the pathogen. Infected dogs, which exhibit mild clinical signs, recover uneventfully.

Canine cyclic thrombocytopenia

'*Ehrlichia platys*', the cause of this condition, parasitizes platelets. Infected dogs, with thrombocytopenia recurring at intervals of about 10 days, are usually asymptomatic. Seroconversion, detected by indirect immunofluorescence, can be demonstrated about 2 weeks after infection.

Potomac horse fever

Potomac horse fever, also known as equine monocytic ehrlichiosis and equine ehrlichial colitis, is caused by *Ehrlichia risticii*. Originally described in 1970 in horses near the Potomac river in Virginia and Maryland, the disease has now been reported throughout North America and in some European countries. Potomac horse fever occurs during summer months and a fluke vector has been suggested. *Ehrlichia risticii* infects epithelial cells of the crypts in the colon and also targets monocytes, tissue macrophages and mast cells.

Clinical signs

Fever, anorexia, depression, diarrhoea, colic, leukopenia and laminitis may be evident. The case fatality rate can reach 30%. Transplacental transmission of *E. risticii* may occur and the agent may induce abortion (Holland and Ristic, 1993). Patchy hyperaemia of the large intestine may be found at postmortem (Rikihisa, 1991).

Diagnosis

- Clinical signs, although non-specific, may suggest the disease in endemic areas.
- A rising antibody titre detected by indirect immunofluorescence or ELISA tests is consistent with active infection.

Treatment and control

- Oxytetracycline intravenously for 7 days is therapeutically effective.
- Inactivated vaccines are commercially available in Northern America.

Equine granulocytic ehrlichiosis

This disease, often known as equine ehrlichiosis, is caused by *Ehrlichia equi*. It has been reported from the USA, some European countries and Israel. Clinical signs include fever, depression, ataxia, limb oedema, icterus and petechial haemorrhages on mucous membranes. The disease is relatively mild, the mortality rate is low and cases tend to occur in late autumn and in winter. The mode of transmission is not known. Diagnosis is based on the demonstration of morulae of *E. equi* in neutrophils during the acute phase of the disease. Elevated antibody titres, demonstrated by indirect immunofluorescence, and marked leukopenia are additional indicators of infection. Tetracycline therapy is effective.

Bovine petechial fever

Bovine petechial fever, also called Ondiri disease, which occurs in both wild and domestic ruminants is caused by '*Ehrlichia ondiri*'. Clinical disease is most common in cattle imported into endemic areas. The disease is limited to highland areas of Kenya and other East African countries, and the vector is considered to be a species of tick with restricted distribution. '*Ehrlichia ondiri*' is thought to replicate initially in the spleen and to spread subsequently to other organs. Clinical signs include high fluctuating fever, depressed milk yield and widespread petechiation of visible mucous membranes. Oedema and petechiation of the conjunctiva produces 'poached-egg' eye, a feature typical of severe cases. Death often results from pulmonary oedema. Recovered animals, which become carriers, are resistant to reinfection for at least 2 years. The organisms are often found in granulocytes in smears of peripheral blood stained by the Giemsa method. Tetracyclines are effective only when administered during the incubation period of the disease.

Tick-borne fever

Tick-borne fever is a rickettsial disease of domestic and wild ruminants caused by *Ehrlichia phagocytophila*. The disease tends to be endemic on certain tick-infected upland farms in some European countries. The main vector is the tick, *Ixodes ricinus*, in which trans-stadial transmission occurs. Transmission to ruminant hosts occurs through the bites of infected ticks and, less commonly, through contaminated instruments. Recovered animals remain infected for up to 2 years and act as reservoirs of infection for ticks. These carrier animals are immune to challenge with the homologous strain of *E. phagocytophila*. Since the maintenance of immunity appears to be related to repeated exposure to *E. phagocytophila*, removal of animals from tick-infected pastures results in a decline in protective immunity.

Clinical signs

Clinical signs, which develop after an incubation period of up to 13 days, include fever, inappetence and a reduced growth rate in young animals. A drop in milk production and abortions or stillbirths may occur in naive, pregnant animals after transfer to farms where the disease is endemic (Jones and Davies, 1995). Most affected animals recover within two weeks. However, *E. phagocytophila* depresses both antibody-mediated and cell-mediated immune responses, increasing the susceptibility of young lambs to tick pyaemia and louping ill, diseases which are also tick-transmitted. Haematological changes in tick-borne fever include leukopenia and transient thrombocytopenia.

Diagnosis

- The disease should be considered in sick ruminants on tick-infected pastures in endemic regions.
- In Giemsa-stained blood smears, more than 70% of neutrophils contain intracytoplasmic blue morulae during the febrile period of the disease (Fig. 35.3).

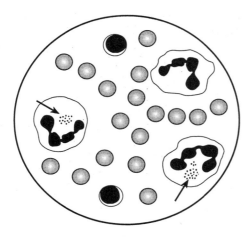

Figure 35.3 A blood smear from a sheep infected with *Ehrlichia phagocytophila*. When stained with a Romanowsky stain, groups of basophilic bodies (arrowed) are recognizable in the cytoplasm of many neutrophils.

- Indirect immunofluorescence is used to detect rising antibody titres.

Treatment and control
- Affected lactating cows should be treated with oxytetracycline.
- Tick control is an essential part of disease prevention.
- Long-acting tetracyclines, administered to lambs in the first 2 to 3 weeks of life, may protect against infection with *E. phagocytophila*.

Heartwater

Heartwater (cowdriosis), caused by *Cowdria ruminantium*, is a severe disease of ruminants limited to regions of sub-Saharan Africa and some Caribbean islands. Ticks belonging to *Amblyomma* species are the main vectors. Wild ruminants such as wildebeest become subclinically infected and the disease can be comparatively mild in indigenous breeds of domestic cattle in which a carrier state can be maintained for up to 8 months. Clinical disease develops in calves and lambs and in newly introduced breeds of *Bos taurus*.

Cowdria ruminantium replicates in reticuloendothelial cells, particularly macrophages, and in endothelial cells of capillaries, especially those of the central nervous system. Damage to vascular endothelium results in increased permeability and widespread petechial haemorrhage.

Clinical signs
Sudden onset of fever occurs following an incubation period of 1 to 4 weeks. Neurological signs are common and include chewing movements, twitching of eyelids, high-stepping gait, circling and recumbency. Death often occurs during convulsions in acute cases. In subacute disease, lesions include hydropericardium, hydrothorax and pulmonary oedema and congestion. Splenomegaly and extensive mucosal and serosal haemorrhages may be evident.

Diagnosis
- In endemic regions, nervous signs and postmortem findings provide a presumptive diagnosis.
- Squash preparations of brain tissue, stained by the Giemsa method, may disclose the organisms located close to nuclei of endothelial cells.
- Nucleic acid probes including polymerase chain reaction techniques can be used on tissues from clinically affected cattle.
- Indirect immunofluorescence, ELISA and Western blot procedures are used to demonstrate antibodies to *C. ruminantium*.

Treatment and control
- Tetracycline therapy administered early in the disease may be effective.
- Immunization by inoculating blood from infected sheep, along with tetracycline therapy, may be used.
- Tick control is expensive and often impractical. In addition, the immunity in indigenous stock may decline because challenge with the infectious agent through repeated exposure to ticks is reduced.

Salmon poisoning disease

Salmon poisoning disease, caused by *Neorickettsia helminthoeca*, is an acute and frequently fatal infection of *Canidae*. The pathogen passes through the developmental stages in a snail-fish-dog cycle of the fluke, *Nanophyetus salmincola*. Dogs become infected by ingesting raw salmon containing fluke metacercariae. *Neorickettsia helminthoeca* enters the bloodstream following attachment of the fluke to the intestinal mucosa of the canine host. Replication of the bacterium in lymphoid tissues results in generalized lymphadenopathy. The disease is limited to the northwest Pacific coast of North America and occurs close to rivers into which the salmon migrate.

Clinical signs
Signs of illness develop abruptly about 7 days after ingestion of raw fish. Fever, anorexia, weakness and depression are followed by persistent vomiting and bloody diarrhoea. Death ensues in 7-10 days in up to 90% of untreated dogs. Animals which survive are usually resistant to reinfection.

Diagnosis
- A history of access to raw fish in endemic areas and the presence of fluke eggs in the faeces of severely ill dogs are suggestive of the infection.
- Organisms can be demonstrated in macrophages in

lymph node aspirates stained by the Giemsa method.
- Infection with canine parvovirus 2 and canine distemper virus may be considered in the differential diagnosis.

Treatment and control
- Tetracyclines, sulphonamides or chloramphenicol may be effective if administered early in the course of disease.
- Supportive therapy may be necessary in dehydrated or anaemic animals.
- Raw fish should not be fed to dogs in endemic areas.
- No vaccine is available.

Elokomin fluke fever

'*Neorickettsia elokominica*', the cause of Elokomin fluke fever, is morphologically indistinguishable from *N. helminthoeca* and has the same fluke vector. The disease is milder than salmon poisoning disease and has a wider host range which includes *Canidae*, bears, racoons and ferrets. '*Neorickettsia elokominica*' infection may be concurrent with *N. helminthoeca* infection and there is no cross-protection between the two organisms.

Bovine anaplasmosis

Bovine anaplasmosis, or gall sickness, caused by *Anaplasma marginale*, affects cattle in tropical and sub-tropical regions. The disease, which is characterized by fever, anaemia and icterus, is often inapparent in animals in endemic areas. In young calves, infections are mild and result in the development of a carrier state. Carrier animals may develop mild clinical signs when stressed. Although severe clinical disease may develop in susceptible yearlings introduced into an endemic area, most recover. In contrast, the mortality rate in naive adult cattle may approach 50%. Morulae of *Anaplasma marginale* are located inside erythrocytes close to the cell membrane. The main vectors are ticks of *Boophilus* species but transmission may also occur through biting diptera. Instruments contaminated with infected blood may also be a source of infection.

Clinical signs
The incubation period ranges from 2 to 12 weeks. Clinical signs include inappetence, depression and reduced milk yield. Marked anaemia and jaundice develop in the absence of haemoglobinuria, and weight loss is pronounced. Affected cattle may die suddenly from hypoxia if they are handled roughly. Recovered animals do not develop clinical disease. Resistance is dependent on persistence of *A. marginale* in tissues.

Diagnosis
- Clinical signs and haematological findings in stressed indigenous cattle or in naive cattle introduced into an

endemic area may suggest the condition.
- Giemsa-stained blood smears may contain densely-stained bodies (0.3 to 1.0 μm in diameter) located near the periphery of erythrocytes. The organisms are most numerous about 10 days after the onset of fever, when up to 50% of erythrocytes can be affected.
- The organisms can be identified in blood smears by immunofluorescence.
- A radioactive RNA probe and a polymerase chain reaction-based method are sensitive techniques used for detecting the pathogen.
- Serological tests are of particular value in detecting latent infections. These tests include complement fixation test, card agglutination test, ELISA and dot enzyme-linked immunosorbent assay.

Treatment and control
- Long-acting oxytetracycline or imidocarb dipropionate, administered early in the disease, are effective.
- Supportive therapy is essential in severe cases.
- In endemic areas, control measures are aimed at minimizing stress in indigenously-reared cattle.
- Prior to introduction into an endemic region, animals must be vaccinated. A live *A. centrale* vaccine, which provides partial protection against *A. marginale*, is used only in calves. Attenuated and inactivated *A. marginale* vaccines are also available.

Feline infectious anaemia

Feline infectious anaemia, also referred to as feline haemobartonellosis, which is caused by *Haemobartonella felis*, occurs worldwide. The pathogen is found on the surface of erythrocytes (Fig. 35.4). The exact mode of transmission is uncertain. However, the disease is comparatively common in free-roaming tom cats between 1 and 3

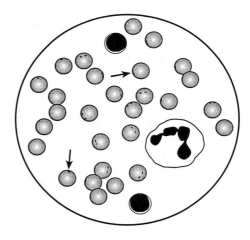

Figure 35.4 A blood smear from a cat infected with *Haemobartonella felis*. When stained with a Romanowsky stain, the organisms (arrowed) appear as dark cocci or rods which are located on the surfaces of red blood cells.

years of age, and transmission through bite-wounds or by biting arthropods has been suggested. Perinatal transmission to kittens has been recorded. Recovered cats may remain asymptomatic carriers. The prevalence of carrier cats in a population may approach 30% (Carney and England, 1993).

Clinical signs

The disease varies in clinical presentation. In peracute disease, a profound anaemia associated with immuno-suppression and an overwhelming parasitaemia rapidly results in death. The more commonly encountered acute form of the disease presents as fever, anaemia, depression, weakness and, occasionally, jaundice. A chronic form of the disease may follow, with affected animals exhibiting anaemia, lethargy and marked weight loss. In immuno-competent cats, successive waves of parasitaemia are gradually eliminated and a satisfactory regenerative bone marrow response develops. The immunosuppression resulting from infection with feline leukaemia virus is often a major factor in the development of severe feline infectious anaemia.

Diagnosis

- *Haemobartonella felis* may be demonstrated on the surface of erythrocytes in Giemsa-stained blood smears (Fig. 35.4). Because of the cyclical nature of the parasitaemia, daily blood sampling may be necessary.
- The pathogen can be demonstrated in blood smears by immunofluorescence.
- Haematological findings may include a reduced packed cell volume and evidence of regenerative anaemia.
- *Babesia felis* and *Cytauxzoon felis* should be considered in the differential diagnosis.

Treatment and control

- In acute disease, doxycycline therapy initiated early and continued for up to 21 days is effective.
- Severely affected cats may require blood transfusions.
- Control measures should include flea control and the careful selection of feline donors for blood transfusion.

Canine haemobartonellosis

Dogs infected with *Haemobartonella canis* are usually asymptomatic. Immunosuppressive drug therapy, splenectomy, splenic dysfunction or severe immuno-suppressive infections may activate latent infections resulting in the development of acute haemolytic anaemia.

Swine eperythrozoonosis

Eperythrozoon species, which appear to be host-specific, can cause sporadic, febrile disease in many mammals. *Eperythrozoon suis* infection in pigs is one of the most common of these infections. These organisms, which are

found on the surface of erythrocytes, are similar in appearance to *Haemobartonella* species. However, ring forms and chains of organisms are prominent in smears containing *Eperythrozoon* species. Most infections are subclinical and the prevalence in some pig herds can approach 20%. Transmission involves biting arthropods such as lice. It may also result from the use of instruments contaminated with infected blood. Outbreaks of disease are sporadic and may be associated with stress factors. Signs include fever, haemolytic anaemia, weakness and jaundice. Disease can be particularly severe in young pigs (Henderson *et al.*, 1997). Tetracycline therapy is effective.

Aegyptianellosis in poultry

This disease, caused by *Aegyptianella pullorum*, affects poultry and wild birds. The vector is a tick of the genus *Argus*. Infected birds have ruffled feathers, anorexia, diarrhoea, anaemia and hyperthermia. Lesions include hepatosplenomegaly and punctiform haemorrhages on serosal surfaces. Control of ticks is important and tetra-cyclines are effective for therapy.

Q fever

Q (query) fever, caused by *Coxiella burnetii*, is an influenza-like occupational disease of farmers, abattoir workers, veterinarians and others in contact with farm animals and their products. Most infections are acquired by inhalation of aerosols originating from parturient sheep, goats or cattle. *Coxiella burnetii* localizes and replicates in the female genital tract and mammary glands of ruminants with intermittent or continuous shedding of organisms in uterine discharges, foetal fluids and milk. Rare outbreaks of Q fever have been associated with exposure to part-urient cats (Langley *et al.*, 1988). Laboratory infections are common. Although several genera of ticks serve as carriers of *C. burnetii*, infection following tick bites is relatively rare. Ingestion of milk or milk products contam-inated with *C. burnetii* usually results in asymptomatic infections in humans. Most infections in domestic animals are subclinical. However, rare sporadic abortions have been described in sheep, goats, cattle and cats. In ruminants, infection may also result in infertility or the birth of weak offspring. Placentitis or endometritis may be evident. Foetal lesions include hepatitis, myocarditis and interstitial pneumonia (Campbell, 1994).

Diagnosis

To prevent human infections, specimens must be collected and handled with care, and diagnostic procedures must be carried out in a biohazard safety cabinet.

- Smears from placental tissue and uterine discharges stained by the MZN method reveal small clumps of red coccobacillary bodies.

- Immunofluorescence can be used to demonstrate the organisms in placental smears.
- Polymerase chain reaction procedures, carried out in reference laboratories, are used to detect small numbers of organisms in tissues.
- *Coxiella burnetii* can be cultured in the yolk sac of 5 to 7 day old embryonated eggs.
- Serological tests for *C. burnetii* include the complement fixation test, indirect immunofluorescence, ELISA and a competitive immunoassay (Soliman *et al.*, 1992).

Control

- Segregation of parturient ruminants and careful disposal of placentas and aborted foetuses are essential after a diagnosis has been confirmed.
- Inactivated egg-yolk vaccines are available for annual vaccination of non-pregnant ruminants.
- A vaccine suitable for laboratory and abattoir workers who are at high risk of infection, is available.

References

Anderson, B.E., Greene, C.E., Jones, D.C. and Dawson, J.E. (1992). *Ehrlichia ewingii* sp. nov., the etiologic agent of canine granulocytic ehrlichiosis. *International Journal of Systematic Bacteriology*, **42**, 299–302.

Brenner, D.J., O'Connor, S.P., Winkler, H.H. and Steigerwalt, A.G. (1993). Proposal to unify the genera *Bartonella* and *Rochalimaea*, with descriptions of *Bartonella quintana* comb. nov., *Bartonella vinsonii* comb. nov., *Bartonella henselae* comb. nov., and *Bartonella elizabethae* comb. nov., and to remove the family *Bartonellaceae* from the order *Rickettsiales*. *International Journal of Systematic Bacteriology*, **43**, 777–786.

Campbell, R.S.F. (1994). Pathogenesis and pathology of the complex rickettsial infections. *Veterinary Bulletin*, **64**, 1–24.

Carney, H.C. and England, J.J. (1993). Feline haemobartonellosis. *Veterinary Clinics of North America: Small Animal Practice*, **23**, 79–90.

Greene, C.E., Burgdorfer, W., Cavagnolo, R., Philip, R.N. and Peacock, M.G. (1985). Rocky Mountain spotted fever in dogs and its differentiation from canine ehrlichiosis. *Journal of the American Veterinary Medical Association*, **186**, 465–472.

Henderson, J.P., O'Hagan, J., Hawe, S.M. and Pratt. M.C.H. (1997). Anaemia and low viability in piglets infected with *Eperythrozoon suis*. *Veterinary Record*, **140**, 144–146.

Holland, C.J. and Ristic, M. (1993). Equine monocytic ehrlichiosis (syn. Potomac horse fever). In *Rickettsial and Chlamydial Diseases of Domestic Animals*. Eds. Z. Woldehiwet and M. Ristic. Pergamon Press, Oxford. pp. 215–232.

Jones, G.L. and Davies, I.H. (1995). An ovine abortion storm caused by infection with *Cytoecetes phagocytophila*. *Veterinary Record*, **136**, 127.

Langley, J.M., Marrie, J.J. and Covert, A. (1988). Poker players' pneumonia. An urban outbreak of Q-fever following exposure to a parturient cat. *New England Journal of Medicine*, **319**, 354–356.

Neimark, H., Johansson, K.E., Rikihisa, Y. and Tully, J.G. (2001). Proposal to transfer some members of the genera *Haemobartonella* and *Eperythrozoon* to the genus *Mycoplasma* with descriptions of 'Candidatus Mycoplasma haemofelis', 'Candidatus Mycoplasma haemomuris', 'Candidatus Mycoplasma haemosuis' and 'Candidatus Mycoplasma wenyonii'. *International Journal of Systematic and Evolutionary Microbiology*, **51**, 891–899.

Redd, T. and Thompson, H.A. (1995). Secretion of proteins by *Coxiella burnetii*. *Microbiology*, **141**, 363–369.

Rikihisa, Y. (1991). The tribe *Ehrlichieae* and ehrlichial diseases. *Clinical Microbiology Reviews*, **4**, 286–308.

Soliman, A.N., Botros, B.A. and Watts, D.M. (1992). Evaluation of a competitive immunoassay for detection of *Coxiella burnetii* antibody in animal sera. *Journal of Clinical Microbiology,* **30**, 1595–1597.

Woldehiwet, Z. and Ristic, M. (1993). The Rickettsiae. In *Rickettsial and Chlamydial Diseases of Domestic Animals*. Eds. Z. Woldehiwet and M. Ristic. Pergamon Press, Oxford. pp. 1–26.

Further reading

Bjoersdorff, A., Svendenius, L., Owens, J.H. and Massung, R.F. (1999). Feline granulocytic ehrlichiosis – a report of a new clinical entity and characterisation of the infectious agent. *Journal of Small Animal Practice*, **40**, 20–24.

Chapter 36

Bacterial species of limited pathogenic significance

This heterogeneous group contains organisms which occasionally produce disease in domestic animals (Table 36.1) and a number of bacterial species of uncertain pathogenicity which are commonly isolated from clinical specimens (Table 36.2). Most organisms in the group are Gram-negative rods except the megabacteria, which are large Gram-positive rods. *Branhamella* species and *Neisseria* species are Gram-negative cocci.

Bartonella henselae

Bartonella henselae, a thin Gram-negative slightly curved rod, is a member of the family *Bartonellaceae*, which was formerly classified in the order *Rickettsiales*. It will grow only on blood-enriched media and growth may require 3 to 4 weeks to develop. The organism is carried by healthy cats and is transmitted from cat to cat by the cat flea, *Ctenocephalides felis*. It causes no clinical signs in cats and infection is common, especially in kittens. In humans infection causes cat scratch disease with signs developing 1 to 3 weeks after the scratch or bite of a cat. In some cases, a small skin lesion which progresses to an ulcer and then heals is visible at the site of inoculation. Other signs include lymphadenitis and systemic signs such as fever, malaise and headaches. Usually the condition resolves without treatment but complications may occur. *Bartonella henselae* causes bacillary angiomatosis in immunocompromised individuals. This condition requires treatment with prolonged courses of antimicrobial therapy.

Chromobacterium violaceum

Chromobacterium violaceum is a motile Gram-negative rod which grows on MacConkey agar and on nutrient agar with the production of a non-diffusible violet pigment. This bacterium is a catalase-positive, oxidase-positive facultative anaerobe which is found in soil and water of subtropical and tropical regions. Septicaemic infections with *C. violaceum* have been recorded in humans, pigs and dogs (Gogolewski, 1983). The organism has been associated with acute pleuropneumonia in Barbary sheep (Carrasco *et al.*, 1996) and pigs (Liu *et al.*, 1989).

'Flexispira rappini'

This is the provisional name for a curved, motile, microaerophilic Gram-negative bacterium, which is closely related to *Helicobacter* species (Schauer *et al.*, 1993). It is a constituent member of the flora of the intestines of laboratory mice and has been recognized as a cause of ovine abortion in the USA and the UK (Kirkbride *et al.*, 1985; Crawshaw and Fuller, 1994). Aborted lambs have multifocal hepatic necrosis resembling the hepatic lesions caused by *Campylobacter* species.

Helicobacter species

These organisms are helical, S-shaped or curved Gram-negative rods (3.0 x 0.5 to 0.9 μm). They are related to *Campylobacter* species and *Arcobacter* species.

Table 36.1 Bacteria of limited veterinary significance.

Bacterial species	Species affected	Comments
Bartonella henselae	Cats, humans	No clinical signs in cats / cat scratch disease in humans
Chromobacterium violaceum	Pigs, dogs, sheep	Saprophyte in soil and water in tropical regions; may cause opportunistic infections
'Flexispira rappini'	Sheep	Sporadic abortion
Helicobacter species	Ferrets, dogs, cats	Chronic gastritis and gastric ulceration in ferrets; found in gastric mucosa and intestines of dogs and cats
'Megabacteria'	Budgerigars	Present in the proventriculus; implicated in megabacteriosis
Ornithobacterium rhinotracheale	Chickens, turkeys	Respiratory disease
Riemerella anatipestifer	Ducklings	Septicaemia
Streptobacillus moniliformis	Turkeys	Normal inhabitant of the upper respiratory tract of rodents; septicaemia following rat bites

Table 36.2 Bacteria of uncertain pathogenicity commonly isolated from clinical specimens.

Bacterial species	Comments
Acinetobacter species	Commonly present in soil, sewage, water, food and milk
Alcaligenes species	Saprophytes, occasionally isolated from the intestinal tract of vertebrate animals
Branhamella species	Isolated from nasopharynx and conjunctiva of clinically normal animals
Flavobacterium species	Present in soil and water
Neisseria species	Present in nasopharynx and on conjunctiva of many animal species

Helicobacter species require enriched media; some grow on Skirrow agar. They are microaerophilic, non-saccharolytic, oxidase-positive and, with the exception of *H. canis*, catalase-positive. Some helicobacters are found in the gastric mucosa and others are found in the intestine of animals and man. A strong urease reaction is characteristic of the helicobacters which colonize the gastric mucosa.

Helicobacter pylori causes gastritis and duodenal and gastric ulcers in humans and has been associated with gastric adenocarcinoma. Gastritis and gastric ulcers in ferrets have been attributed to *H. mustelae* infection. The significance of helicobacter infections in gastrointestinal disorders of domestic carnivores has not been clearly established (Hermanns *et al.*, 1995; Papasouliotis *et al.*, 1997).

'Megabacteria'

'Megabacteria' is the provisional name for a group of large (20 to 50 x 3.0 μm) Gram-positive rods which are found in the superficial mucosal glands of the lower portion of the proventriculus in budgerigars with megabacteriosis, a chronic wasting disease. They are also found in the proventriculus of clinically normal budgerigars (Baker, 1997). Large numbers of organisms are present in clinically affected birds whereas relatively few are found in asymptomatic birds. Clinical signs may include weight loss, diarrhoea and vomiting. The pH in the proventriculus changes from pH 2 to pH 7 or 8 (Simpson, 1992). The organism grows optimally on blood agar in an atmosphere of 10% CO_2 and small haemolytic colonies are detectable after incubation for 2 days. Megabacteria are catalase negative, oxidase-negative facultative anaerobes. Isolates sometimes differ in their biochemical reactions and are susceptible to a number of antibiotics *in vitro* (Scanlan and Graham, 1990). Amphotericin B has proved effective for treatment (Christensen *et al.*, 1997).

Ornithobacterium rhinotracheale

This organism has been associated with respiratory disease in chickens and turkeys (Hinz *et al.*, 1994). It is a pleomorphic Gram-negative rod which grows on blood agar producing small, grey, non-haemolytic colonies. Although *Ornithobacterium rhinotracheale* grows in an aerobic environment, growth is enhanced in 5 to 10% CO_2. The organism is oxidase-positive and catalase-negative (Charlton *et al.*, 1993). Amoxicillin administered in drinking water, on two consecutive days, at 200 ppm is usually effective.

Riemerella anatipestifer

This organism, previously designated *Pasteurella anatipestifer*, is a non-motile, asaccharolytic Gram-negative rod which grows optimally on enriched media in an atmosphere of 5 to 10% CO_2. It is non-haemolytic on blood agar and does not grow on MacConkey agar. Infection with this organism can cause septicaemia primarily affecting ducklings up to 6 weeks of age although older waterfowl, turkey poults, chickens and pheasants can also be affected (Jordan and Pattison, 1996). The disease in ducklings is usually precipitated by stress. Clinical signs include ocular and nasal discharges, head and neck tremors, and incoordination. Mortality may reach 70%. Fibrinous pericarditis and peritonitis are common postmortem findings. Meningitis and fibrinous airsacculitis may also be present. An intramuscular injection of streptomycin or dihydrostreptomycin administered in the early stages of the disease along with medication of drinking water for 3 days with sulphadimidine sodium is therapeutically effective. A bacterin and a live avirulent vaccine are available.

Streptobacillus moniliformis

Streptobacillus moniliformis, a highly pleomorphic Gram-negative rod, is a normal inhabitant of the upper respiratory tract of rodents. The organism occasionally causes outbreaks of bronchopneumonia in laboratory rats and mice and cervical lymphadenitis in guinea-pig colonies. Rare cases of synovitis and deaths are reported in turkey flocks associated with rat bites. The bacterium is responsible for Haverhill fever and rat-bite fever in humans.

References

Baker, J.R. (1997). Megabacteria in diseased and healthy budgerigars. *Veterinary Record*, **140**, 627.

Carrasco, L., Astorga, R., Méndez, A. *et al.* (1996). Acute pleuropneumonia in Barbary sheep (*Amnotragus lervia*) associated with *Chromobacterium violaceum*. *Veterinary Record*, **138**, 499–500.

Charlton, B.R., Channing-Santiago, S.E., Bickford, A.A.,

Cardona, C.J., Chin, R.P., Cooper, G.L. *et al.* (1993). Preliminary characterization of a pleomorphic Gram-negative rod associated with avian respiratory disease. *Journal of Veterinary Diagnostic Investigation*, **5**, 47–51.

Christensen, N.H., Hunter, J.E.B. and Alley, M.R. (1997). Megabacteriosis in a flock of budgerigars. *New Zealand Veterinary Journal*, **45**, 196–198.

Crawshaw, T.R. and Fuller, H.E. (1994). *Flexispira rappini* suspected in ovine abortion. *Veterinary Record*, **134**, 507.

Gogolewski, R.P. (1983). *Chromobacterium violaceum* septicaemia in a dog. *Australian Veterinary Journal*, **60**, 226.

Hermanns, W., Kregel, K., Breuer, W. and Lechner, J. (1995). *Helicobacter*-like organisms : histopathological examination of gastric biopsies from cats and dogs. *Journal of Comparative Pathology*, **112**, 307–318.

Hinz, K-H., Blome, C. and Ryll, M. (1994). Acute exudative pneumonia and airsacculitis associated with *Ornithobacterium rhinotracheale* in turkeys. *Veterinary Record*, **135**, 233–234.

Jordan, F.T.W. and Pattison, M. (1996). Anatipestifer infection. In *Poultry Diseases*. Fourth Edition. W.B. Saunders, London. pp. 49–51.

Kirkbride, C.A., Gates, C.E., Collins, J.E. and Ritchie, A.E. (1985). Ovine abortion associated with an anaerobic bacterium. *Journal of the American Veterinary Medical Association*, **186**, 789–791.

Liu, C.H., Chu, R.M., Weng, C.N., Lin, Y.L. and Chi,. C.S. (1989). An acute pleuropneumonia in a pig caused by *Chromobacterium violaceum*. *Journal of Comparative Pathology*, **100**, 459–463.

Papasouliotis, K., Gruffydd-Jones, T.J., Werrett, G. *et al.* (1997). Occurrence of gastric *Helicobacter*-like organisms in cats. *Veterinary Record*, **140**, 369–370.

Scanlan, C.M. and Graham, D.L. (1990). Characterization of a Gram-positive bacterium from the proventriculus of budgerigars (*Melopsittacus undulatus*). *Avian Diseases*, **34**, 779–786.

Schauer, D.B., Ghori, N. and Falkow, S. (1993). Isolation and characterization of '*Flexispira rappini*' from laboratory mice. *Journal of Clinical Microbiology*, **31**, 2709–2714.

Simpson, V.R. (1992). Megabacteriosis in exhibition budgerigars. *Veterinary Record*, **131**, 203.

Further reading

Barnes, A., Bell, S.C., Isherwood, D.R., Bennett, M. and Carter, S.D. (2000). Evidence of *Bartonella henselae* infection in cats and dogs in the United Kingdom. *Veterinary Record*, **147**, 673–677.

Section III

Mycology

Chapter 37

General features of fungi associated with disease in animals

Although there are more than 250,000 species in the kingdom Fungi, less than 150 are known to be pathogenic for animals and man. Fungi are eukaryotic, non-photosynthetic heterotrophs which produce exoenzymes and obtain nutrients by absorption. The three phyla in the kingdom, *Ascomycota* (ascomycetes), *Basidiomycota* (basidiomycetes) and *Zygomycota* (zygomycetes), can be distinguished by the characteristics of their sexual forms (teleomorphs). Fungi imperfecti (deuteromycetes), so-called because a sexual form has not been found, constitute a heterogeneous fourth group. Although most fungi of veterinary importance are deuteromycetes, some fungi in each of the three phyla can also produce disease in animals.

The two main morphological fungal forms are moulds and yeasts (Fig. 37.1). Moulds grow as branching filaments called hyphae (2 to 10 μm in diameter) whereas the unicellular yeasts have an oval or spherical appearance (3 to 5 μm in diameter). Dimorphic fungi occur in both mould and yeast forms. Environmental factors usually determine the form in which a dimorphic fungus occurs. Fungi such as *Candida albicans*, which produce forms additional to the two major forms, are described as polymorphic.

Fungi grow aerobically, and many are strict aerobes. Temperatures appropriate for the optimal growth of different groups of pathogenic fungi and the incubation time required for the development of distinctive colonial features are indicated in Table 37.1. Reproduction by spore formation may be either sexual or asexual. In some species both types of spore formation occur. Fungi

Key points
■ Eukaryotic, non-photosynthetic microorganisms in the kingdom Fungi
■ Widely distributed in the environment
■ Cell walls contain chitin and other polysaccharides
■ Heterotrophs; produce exoenzymes and obtain nutrients by absorption
■ Branching hyphae and unicellular yeasts are the two major forms
■ Reproduce both sexually and asexually with the production of spores
■ Grow aerobically at 25°C; some moulds are strict aerobes
■ Tolerate high osmotic pressures and low pH values; grow on Sabouraud dextrose agar, pH 5.5
■ Resistant to antimicrobial drugs which are effective against bacteria
■ Majority are saprophytes; some cause opportunistic infections
■ Dermatophytes are pathogens which cause ringworm in animals and humans

tolerate high osmotic pressures and acidic environments as low as pH 5.0.

Fungal species may be saprophytic, parasitic or mutualistic. Mutualistic fungi have obligatory associations with other microorganisms and are non-pathogenic. Saprophytic fungi, which are widespread in the environment and are involved in the decomposition of organic matter, occasionally cause sporadic opportunistic infections in animals. The parasitic dermatophytes are pathogens, causing ringworm in animals. Overgrowth of yeasts, which are often commensals on skin and mucous membranes, may cause localized lesions.

Structure

Hyphal cell walls, which impart rigidity and osmotic stability, are mainly composed of carbohydrate

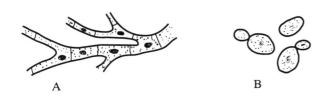

Figure 37.1 Microscopic appearance of the two main fungal forms: A. Septate branching hypha of a mould. A mass of interlacing hyphae forms a mycelium. B. Budding cells of a yeast.

Table 37.1 Incubation conditions appropriate for the aerobic culture of fungi.

Fungal group	Incubation conditions	
	Temperature (°C)	Time
Dermatophytes	25	2 to 4 weeks
Aspergillus species	37	1 to 4 days
Yeasts (pathogenic)	37	1 to 4 days
Dimorphic fungi		
mould phase	25	1 to 4 weeks
yeast phase	37	1 to 4 weeks
Zygomycetes	37	1 to 4 days

components including chitin macromolecules with cellulose cross-linkages. In yeasts, cell walls contain protein complexed with polysaccharides and, in some species, a range of lipid compounds. In the bilayered cell membrane, which lines the cell wall in the fungi, the predominant sterol is ergosterol in contrast to cholesterol, which predominates in the cell membranes of animals. Both moulds and yeasts have nuclei with well-defined nuclear membranes, mitochondria and networks of microtubules. Septa (cross-walls) are often present in hyphae.

Growth, reproduction and colonial formation

Airborne fungal spores germinate in locations where environmental conditions are favourable. Spores swell and their metabolic activity increases prior to the production of tubular projections which develop into branched hyphae (Fig. 37.2). The hyphal wall is thin and plastic at its tip and, as apical growth occurs, cross-linkage of wall constituents results in maturation of the structure. Lateral branches develop from hyphae at localized areas of plasticity which allow outgrowth from the rigid mature cell wall. Septa, formed by inward growth of the cell wall, have central pores through which nutrients and organelles

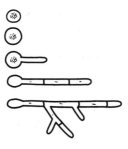

Figure 37.2 Stages in the germination of a fungal spore leading to the development of a branched hypha.

may pass. Extension of hyphae and their lateral branches results in the formation of a mycelium, an interlacing network of hyphae.

Moulds tend to form large colonies with growth and extension of hyphae at their peripheries. In some species, mature elements at the centre of colonies produce specialized aerial hyphae which support spore-bearing structures and facilitate dispersal of mature spores. In this asexual reproduction, two main types of spores, conidia and sporangiospores are recognized. Conidia are formed on conidiophores and sporangiospores are formed within a sporangium, a sac-like structure borne on an aerial hypha termed a sporangiophore (Fig. 37.3). Sporangiospores are formed only by fungi in the phylum *Zygomycota*. In dermatophytes, multicellular structures called macroconidia and single-celled microconidia are produced in cultures from lateral hyphal branches, whereas arthroconidia are formed from the disintegration of hyphae within keratinized structures. Asexual spores produced by fungi are illustrated in Fig. 37.4.

In most yeasts, asexual division is by budding. Daughter cells separate from parent cells after the formation of a cross-wall at the point of budding. The colonies of yeast-like fungi are soft, smooth and round.

Demonstration of the sexual stage of fungi, which is usually conducted in specialized laboratories, is essential for the taxonomic classification of phyla. A summary of the features of the sexual spores of the *Ascomycota*, *Basidiomycota* and *Zygomycota* is presented in Table 37.2.

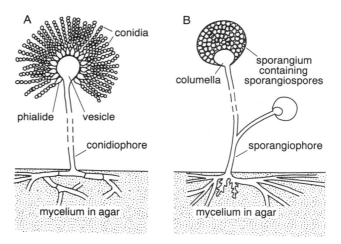

Figure 37.3 Fungal growth on agar illustrating vegetative mycelia and aerial hyphae with sporing heads. A. *Aspergillus* species. B. *Rhizopus* species.

General features of fungal disease

The pathogenetic mechanisms by which fungi produce disease are listed in Box 37.1. The fungal diseases which result from tissue invasion (mycoses) can be conveniently

Arthroconidia (arthrospores)

Spores which are formed and subsequently released during the process of hyphal fragmentation. Spores may be formed successively as in dermatophytes (A), or with intervening empty cells as in *Coccidioides immitis* (B)

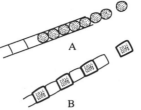

Blastoconidia (blastospores)

Conidia (arrows) which are produced by budding, as in *Candida albicans,* from a mother cell (A), from hyphae (B) or from pseudohyphae (C)

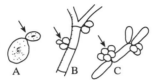

Chlamydoconidia (chlamydospores)

Thick-walled, resistant spores which contain storage products. These structures are formed by some fungi in unfavourable environmental conditions

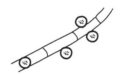

Macroconidia

Large multi-celled conidia which are produced by dermatophytes in culture

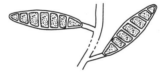

Microconidia

Small conidia which are produced by certain dermatophytes

Phialoconidia

Conidia produced from phialides. The phialides of *Aspergillus* species arise from a vesicle

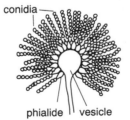

Sporangiospores

Spores (arrow), formed by zygomycetes such as *Rhizopus* species, are released when a mature sporangium ruptures

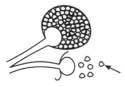

Figure 37.4 Asexual spores produced by fungi of veterinary importance.

Table 37.2 Sexual spores of fungi in the phyla *Ascomycota, Basidiomycota* and *Zygomycota*.

Spores	Comments
Ascospores	Produced by members of *Ascomycota*; develop in a sac-like structure called an ascus. Asci may be enclosed in well-defined structures termed ascocarps
Basidiospores	Produced by members of *Basidiomycota* on club-shaped structures called basidia
Zygospores	Produced by members of *Zygomycota*; develop in a thick-walled zygosporangium, formed from the fusion of side projections of two compatible hyphae

categorized according to the sites of lesions (Table 37.3). Superficial mycoses are classified either as dermatomycoses or as dermatophytoses. In the dermato-mycoses, opportunistic infections of the skin or muco-cutaneous junctions result from overgrowth of fungi such as *Candida* species or *Malassezia pachydermatis*. The dermatophytoses, which are clinically more important because of their communicability and zoonotic potential, are associated with invasion and destruction of keratinized structures by dermatophytes such as *Microsporum* species and *Trichophyton* species. Subcutaneous mycoses result from localized fungal invasion of the dermis and subcutis, often following penetration by a foreign body. When infection is caused by pigmented (dematiaceous) fungi, the condition is termed phaeohyphomycosis. Tumour-like granulomatous lesions are called mycetomas, when caused by saprophytic fungi, and pseudomycetomas, when associated with dermatophyte invasion. Systemic mycoses, which often originate in the respiratory or digestive tracts, usually follow opportunistic infection by saprophytic fungi. Factors which predispose to infection include alteration in the normal microbial flora as a result of prolonged antimicrobial therapy, immunosuppression following corticosteroid therapy or viral infection, and exposure to high infective doses of spores in confined spaces (Box 37.2).

Mycotoxicoses constitute an important group of diseases resulting from the ingestion of fungal toxins which have been pre-formed in stored food or standing crops. Although hypersensitivity reactions to fungal infections are rare in domestic animals, they can be associated with chronic pulmonary disease in cattle and horses.

Box 37.1 Mechanisms involved in fungal diseases.

- Tissue invasion (mycosis)
- Toxin production (mycotoxicosis)
- Induction of hypersensitivity

Table 37.3 Fungal diseases categorized according to sites of lesions.

Category	Sites of lesions
Superficial mycoses	Skin, other keratinized structures and mucous membranes
Subcutaneous mycoses	Dermis and subcutaneous tissues
Systemic mycoses	Respiratory and digestive tracts and other organ systems

Diagnosis of fungal diseases

Mycological cultural procedures should be performed in a biohazard cabinet because of the risk of human infection from spore aerosols. Culture of *Coccidioides immitis* should be attempted only in reference laboratories because highly infective arthrospores are produced in cultures at both 25°C and 37°C.

- Clinical signs and history may point to a presumptive diagnosis particularly in the dermatophytoses.
- Specimens for diagnosis include hair and skin scrapings from superficial mycoses and biopsy or postmortem specimens from subcutaneous and systemic mycoses.
- Direct microscopic examination of wet preparations may be confirmatory:
  — Ringworm arthrospores surrounding infected hairs or hyphae in infected tissues may be demonstrable after clearing specimens in a few drops of 10% KOH under a coverslip for some hours.
  — *Cryptococcus neoformans* can be demonstrated, in cerebrospinal fluid mixed with India ink or nigrosin, as budding cells with wide capsules.
  — Sporing heads can be examined under a coverslip after mounting a sample from a colony in a drop of lactophenol cotton blue. Other methods for direct examination include slide culture and transparent adhesive tape techniques. Yeast cells can be stained with methylene blue or by the Gram method.
- Fungi are usually isolated on Sabouraud dextrose agar (pH 5.5) which inhibits growth of most bacteria. The

---

Box 37.2 Factors which may predispose to fungal invasion of tissues.

- Immunosuppression
- Prolonged antibiotic therapy
- Immunological defects
- Immaturity, ageing and malnutrition
- Exposure to heavy challenge of fungal spores
- Traumatized tissues
- Persistent moisture on skin surface
- Some neoplastic conditions

---

addition of chloramphenicol and cycloheximide increases selectivity by inhibiting some of the fast-growing contaminating fungi such as the zygomycetes. To stimulate growth of the yeast phase of dimorphic fungi, enriched media, such as brain-heart infusion agar with 5% blood, and incubation at 37°C are required. Incubation times and temperatures for the various fungal groups are listed in Table 37.1.

- Histopathological demonstration of fungal hyphae or yeast forms is usually necessary for confirming the significance of isolates from deep mycotic infections. The periodic acid-Schiff (PAS) reaction or methenamine silver impregnation can be used to demonstrate fungal elements in tissue sections.

Differentiation of fungal species

The main morphological features used for differentiating fungi implicated in mycotic diseases are presented in Table 37.4. In addition, molecular and immunological characterization of fungal pathogens is being developed for species differentiation.

- The form of the sexual stage (teleomorph) is used for assigning a fungus to a phylum (Table 37.2).
- Examination of sporing heads for conidial arrangement and the type and morphology of spores may allow initial differentiation. The presence of a mature sporangium identifies the fungus as a zygomycete (Fig. 37.3).
- Features of vegetative hyphae which can be used for differentiation include:
  — Presence or absence of septa
  — Either hyaline (colourless) or dematiaceous (pigmented)
  — Specific hyphal structures such as racquet-shaped and spiral hyphae
- Colonial characteristics:
  — Size and appearance after specified incubation time
  — Colour of both obverse and reverse sides
  — Surface elevations or depressions

Table 37.4 Differentiating features of fungi implicated in mycotic diseases.

| Feature | Phylum | | | Fungi Imperfecti |
	Ascomycota	*Basidiomycota*	*Zygomycota*	
Sexual spores	ascospores	basidiospores	zygospores	no sexual spores
Asexual spores	conidia	conidia	sporangiospores	conidia
Septate hyphae	+	+	−	+

- Yeasts can be differentiated by colonial appearance and the size and shape of individual cells. Biochemical reactions are also used for differentiation.
- Dimorphic fungi grow as moulds when cultured on Sabouraud dextrose agar at 25°C and as yeasts when cultured on enriched media at 37°C.
- Soluble antigens produced by dimorphic fungi can be used for identification in immunological tests.
- Specific nucleic acid probes are being developed for rapid and reliable identification of dimorphic fungi.

Antifungal chemotherapy

The eukaryotic cells of fungi and animals have cell structures and metabolic pathways that are often similar. Since the plasma membranes of most fungi differ from those of animal cells in having ergosterol as a main sterol component, they are the primary target of many antifungal therapeutic agents. The polyene antifungal drugs such as nystatin and amphotericin B bind selectively to ergosterol, and anti-fungal azoles like ketoconazole inhibit ergosterol biosynthesis. Griseofulvin, which is used for the treatment of ringworm, accumulates in keratinized tissues and is absorbed by invading dermatophytes. Griseofulvin interaction with fungal microtubules and disruption of mitotic spindles inhibits dermatophyte growth.

Further reading

Ajello, L. and Hay, R.J. (1998). Medical Mycology. In *Topley and Wilson's Microbiology and Microbial Infections*. Eds. L. Collier, A. Balows and M. Sussman. Ninth Edition. Volume 4. Arnold, London.

Evans, E.G.V. and Richardson, M.D. (1989). *Medical Mycology*. IRL Press, Oxford.

Quinn, P.J., Carter, M.E., Markey, B.K. and Carter, G.R. (1994). *Clinical Veterinary Microbiology*. Mosby Year Book Europe, London. pp. 367–380.

Chapter 38

Dermatophytes

The dermatophytes, a group of septate fungi which occur worldwide, invade superficial keratinized structures such as skin, hair and claws. More than 30 species of dermatophytes are recognized. Most belong to the Fungi Imperfecti and are classified in three anamorphic genera: *Microsporum*, *Trichophyton* and *Epidermophyton*. A few species have been placed in the teleomorphic genus *Arthroderma* in the phylum *Ascomycota*. The species *Epidermophyton floccosum* is primarily a human pathogen.

Arthrospores (arthroconidia) are the infectious forms most often associated with tissue invasion by this group of fungi. They are released by fragmentation of hyphae in keratinized structures. These resistant forms can remain viable for more than 12 months in suitable environments in buildings. Dermatophytes are strict aerobes, most of which grow slowly on standard Sabouraud dextrose agar. A few require special growth factors which are supplied by the addition of yeast extract to the Sabouraud dextrose agar. Macroconidia and microconidia are produced in culture. The colonies of many dermatophytes are pigmented. Colonial morphology and the type of macroconidia produced are used for identification.

Dermatophytosis (ringworm) affects many animal species (Table 38.1). The disease is a zoonosis and most human infections are caused by *Microsporum canis* contracted from infected cats (Pepin and Oxenham, 1986).

Usual habitat

Dermatophytes can be grouped on the basis of their habitats and host preferences as geophilic, zoophilic or anthropophilic (Table 38.2). Geophilic dermatophytes inhabit and replicate in the soil in association with decomposing keratinous materials such as hairs or feathers (Weitzman and Summerbell, 1995). Animals can acquire infection with geophilic dermatophytes from soil or from contact with infected animals. Zoophilic and anthropophilic dermatophytes are obligate pathogens which are unable to replicate in soil. Their existence as pathogens of keratinized structures usually corresponds with an inability to reproduce sexually. Dermatophytes growing on keratinized structures rarely produce macroconidia and consequently rely on the production of arthrospores for transmission. Each zoophilic species tends to parasitize a particular animal species.

Key points

- Members of the Fungi Imperfecti
- Affinity for keratinized structures; colonize and invade skin, hair and nails
- Grow slowly on specially formulated laboratory media such as Sabouraud dextrose agar; some require additional growth factors
- Aerobic, tolerate cyclohexamide in media
- Colonies often pigmented
- Macroconidia formed in cultures
- Arthrospores, shed from infected animals, remain infective for many months
- Zoophilic and anthropophilic dermatophytes are obligate pathogens; geophilic dermatophytes are saprophytes in soil
- Cause characteristic circular skin lesions termed ringworm

Laboratory recognition and differentiation

Individual species are identified mainly by colonial morphology and the microscopic appearance of macroconidia, chlamydospores or other structures (Table 38.3, Figs. 38.1, 38.2).

- The colonial morphology of dermatophytes commonly isolated from animals is described in Table 38.3. The obverse and reverse of each colony should be examined.
- Macroconidial morphology is assessed under low or high dry magnification in preparations or transparent adhesive tape mounts of colony samples stained with lactophenol cotton blue (Figs. 38.1, 38.2). Other structures such as spiral hyphae, microconidia or chlamydospores can be used for differentiation.
- Special growth requirements can be determined using commercially-available trichophyton agar. Control medium, designated trichophyton agar 1 (T1), is a casein basal agar. Other media, produced by adding growth factors to the basal agar, are T3 containing

Table 38.1 Dermatophytes of animals, their main hosts and reported geographical distribution.

Dermatophyte	Hosts	Geographical distribution
Microsporum canis (var. *canis*)	Cats, dogs	Worldwide
M. canis var. *distortum*	Dogs	New Zealand, Australia, North America
M. equinum	Horses	Africa, Australasia, Europe, North and South America
M. gallinae	Chickens, turkeys	Worldwide
M. gypseum	Horses, dogs, rodents	Worldwide
M. nanum	Pigs	North and South America, Europe, Australasia
M. persicolor	Field vole	Europe, North America
Trichophyton equinum	Horses	Worldwide
T. equinum var. *autotrophicum*	Horses	Australia and New Zealand
T. mentagrophytes var. *erinacei*	European hedge-hogs, dogs	Europe, New Zealand
T. mentagrophytes var. *mentagrophytes*	Rodents, dogs, horses and many other animal species	Worldwide
T. mentagrophytes var. *quickeanum*	Mice	Australia, Canada, Eastern Europe, Italy
T. simii	Monkeys, poultry, dogs	India, Brazil, Guinea
T. verrucosum	Cattle	Worldwide

thiamine and inositol, T4 containing only thiamine and T5 containing nicotinic acid.

— *Trichophyton verrucosum*, which has a requirement for thiamine and sometimes for inositol, usually grows on T3 or T4 media.

— *Trichophyton equinum* requires nicotinic acid for growth whereas *T. equinum* var. *autotrophicum* does not. Culture on T1 and T5 media can be used to differentiate these variants.

— *Trichophyton mentagrophytes* hydrolyzes urea when grown on Christensen urea agar.

• Temperature tolerance tests are useful for differentiating *T. verrucosum* and *T. mentagrophytes*, which grow

well at 37°C, from other dermatophytes which do not tolerate this temperature.

• *In vitro* hair perforation tests are sometimes used to distinguish atypical isolates of *T. mentagrophytes* from *T. rubrum* and atypical *M. canis* from *T. equinum*. Sterilized blonde hairs from a child, placed on a culture of the dermatophyte under test, are incubated at 25°C. The hairs, stained with lactophenol cotton blue, are examined microscopically from the seventh day onwards. *Microsporum canis* and *T. mentagrophytes* penetrate the hair shafts forming wedge-shaped dark blue structures (Fig. 38.3).

• Dermatophyte test medium (DTM) has been formulated to differentiate dermatophytes from contaminating fungi. Phenol red is used as a pH indicator in this medium. Growth of dermatophytes results in alkaline metabolic products and the colour of the medium changes to red. Other fungal media should be used in conjunction with DTM because some contaminating fungi can also induce a colour change. In addition, the colour change in DTM can obscure the characteristic pigmentation required for differentiation of dermatophyte species.

Pathogenesis and pathogenicity

Dermatophytes invade keratinized structures such as the stratum corneum of the epidermis, hair follicles, hair shafts and feathers. Lesion development is influenced by the virulence of the dermatophyte and the immunological competence of the host. Young, aged, debilitated and immunosuppressed animals are particularly susceptible to infection, which occurs either directly by contact with an infected host or indirectly through infected epithelial debris in the environment. Infective arthrospores adhere to keratinized structures and germinate within 6 hours. Minor trauma such as gentle rubbing of the skin or bites from arthropods may facilitate infection. Damp skin

Table 38.2 Dermatophytes grouped according to host preference or habitat.

Zoophilic group	Geophilic group	Anthropophilic group[a]
Microsporum canis	*Microsporum cookei*	*Epidermophyton floccosum*
M. gallinae	*M. gypseum*	*M. audouinii*
Trichophyton equinum	*M. nanum*	*M. ferrugineum*
T. mentagrophytes	*M. persicolor*	*T. rubrum*
T. verrucosum	*T. simii*	*T. schoenleinii*

a Anthropophilic dermatophytes rarely infect animals

Table 38.3 Colonial appearance and growth characteristics of dermatophytes isolated from animals.

Dermatophyte	Colonial appearance on Sabouraud dextrose agar	Comments
Microsporum canis	Obverse, white to buff with bright orange periphery; reverse, yellowish-orange or yellowish-brown	Heavy sporulation occurs on rice grain media. Colony size up to 50 mm after incubation for 10 days
M. gypseum	Obverse, buff to cinnamon with white border and powdery; reverse, buff to reddish-brown	Colony size up to 50 mm after incubation for 10 days. Mouse-like odour
M. nanum	Obverse, cream to tan and powdery; reverse, reddish brown	Colony size up to 35 mm after incubation for 10 days
Trichophyton equinum	Obverse, initially white and fluffy, later buff and folded; reverse, yellow to dark reddish-brown	Nicotinic acid required for growth. Colony size up to 35 mm after incubation for 10 days
T. mentagrophytes	Obverse, cream-tan to buff and powdery; reverse, buff-tan to dark brown	Colony size up to 30 mm after incubation for 10 days. Urease-positive; grows well at 37°C
T. verrucosum	Obverse, white, heaped and velvety; reverse, white or pale buff	Growth slow, colony size up to 10 mm after incubation for 20 days. Requires thiamine and sometimes inositol for growth. Grows at 37°C

surfaces and warmth favour germination of spores. Metabolic products of hyphal growth may provoke a local inflammatory response. Hyphae grow centrifugally from the initial lesion towards normal skin, producing typical ringworm lesions. Alopecia, tissue repair and non-viable hyphae are found at the centres of lesions as they develop. Growth of hyphae can result in epidermal hyperplasia and hyperkeratosis. Secondary bacterial infection sometimes follows mycotic folliculitis.

The development of a strong cell-mediated response correlates with the onset of a delayed-type hypersensitivity which usually results in elimination of the dermatophyte, resolution of the lesion and local resistance to reinfection. Immunity to dermatophytosis is transient and reinfection may occur if the challenge dose is large (Moriello and De Boer, 1995). Other mechanisms which may be associated with the elimination of infection include an increased rate of desquamation from the stratum corneum and an increase

Microsporum canis

Spindle-shaped macroconidium (40-120 x 8-20 μm), rough, thick-walled, up to 15 septa

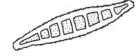

Microsporum gypseum

Boat-shaped macroconidium (25-60 x 7-15 μm), rough, thin-walled, up to 6 septa

Microsporum nanum

Pear-shaped or ovoid macroconidium (10-30 x 6-13 μm), rough, thin-walled, usually 1 septum

Figure 38.1 Morphological features of the macroconidia of some *Microsporum* species.

Trichophyton mentagrophytes

Cigar-shaped macroconidium (20-50 x 4-8 μm), smooth, thin-walled, up to 7 septa

Trichophyton verrucosum

Chlamydospores in chains; macroconidia rare

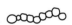

Figure 38.2 Morphological features of the macroconidia of *Trichophyton mentagrophytes* and the chlamydospores of *T. verrucosum*.

in the permeability of the epidermis allowing penetration of inflammatory fluids (Wagner and Sohnle, 1995). Animals with ringworm develop antibodies against dermatophyte glycoprotein antigens. Antibody-mediated responses do not appear to be protective. Strong humoral immune-mediated responses and weak cell-mediated responses have been demonstrated in persistently infected cats (Moriello and DeBoer, 1995).

Diagnostic procedures

Laboratory investigation of dermatophytosis is often necessary because diagnosis on clinical grounds can be difficult.

- As dermatophyte species tend to parasitize particular hosts, the animal species affected may indicate the dermatophyte most likely to be involved (Table 38.1).
- Specimens suitable for laboratory examination include plucked hair, deep skin scrapings from the edge of lesions, scrapings from affected claws and biopsy material from pseudomycetomas. Suitable material from cats can also be collected on a large sheet of paper by brushing the coat with a clean toothbrush.
- Hairs and skin scrapings treated with KOH should be

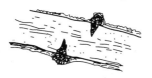

Figure 38.3 The *in vitro* hair perforation test. Wedge-shaped areas along a hair shaft stain darkly with lactophenol cotton blue. Some dermatophytes such as *M. canis* and *T. mentagrophytes* produce this hair perforation pattern.

examined microscopically for the presence of arthrospores. The arrangement of arthrospores on hair shafts is typically ectothrix (Fig. 38.4). Mites, such as *Demodex* species, may also be detected in these specimens.

- Histological sections of skin or pseudomycetomas can be stained by the PAS or methenamine silver techniques to demonstrate fungal structures.
- Specimens are cultured on Emmon's Sabouraud dextrose agar (pH 6.9) with the addition of 2 to 4% yeast extract, 0.05 g/litre chloramphenicol and 0.4 g/litre cycloheximide. Inoculated plates are incubated aerobically at 25°C to 27°C and examined twice weekly for up to 5 weeks.
- Identification criteria for isolates:
  — Colonial morphology
  — Microscopic appearance of macroconidia
  — Supplementary tests including growth on DTM medium.
- In cats and dogs with suspicious lesions, examination with Wood's lamp should always be carried out because *M. canis* infections are comparatively common in these species. A characteristic apple-green fluorescence from infected hairs is evident in more than 50% of affected dogs and cats (Sparkes *et al.*, 1993). Detection of fluorescence depends on factors such as stage of infection and the characteristics of the infecting strain. In cats with inapparent infections, fluorescing hairs should be cultured.
- Investigations for other pathogens which cause skin lesions or for mixed infections may be warranted.

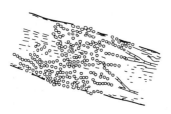

Figure 38.4 Surface (ectothrix) arthrospores on a hair shaft following clearance with 10% potassium hydroxide.

Clinical infections

Dermatophytosis is a comparatively common clinical condition in both companion and farm animals. Because of the zoonotic nature of the dermatophytoses, affected animals should be handled with care.

Dermatophytosis in cats and dogs

Most infections in cats are caused by *M. canis*. Clinical features of the disease include classical ringworm lesions, miliary dermatitis, pseudomycetomas, (Medleau and Rakich, 1994), onychomycosis and, rarely, generalized lesions in immunosuppressed animals. Inapparent infections are known to occur and cats may also carry arthrospores physically in their coats (Moriello *et al.*, 1994). The dermatophytes which commonly affect dogs are listed in Box 38.1. The disease usually presents as areas of alopecia, scaling and broken hairs surrounded by inflammatory zones. Less commonly encountered lesions include folliculitis and onychomycosis. Lesion distribution on the muzzle may relate to certain behavioural activities such as compulsive digging in soil, rat-catching and attacking and worrying hedgehogs. These activities often determine the species of dermatophyte involved in the infection, for example *T. mentagrophytes* var. *erinacei* is usually acquired from hedgehogs and *M. gypseum* from the soil. Generalized infection is uncommon in dogs and is often associated with conditions such as hyperadrenocorticism and immunosuppression.

> **Box 38.1** Dermatophytes of dogs.
>
> - *Microsporum canis*
> - *M. gypseum*
> - *Trichophyton mentagrophytes*
> - *T. mentagrophytes* var. *erinacei*

Treatment and control

Because the dermatophytoses are zoonoses, treatment and control are particularly important in domestic carnivores.

- If lesions are limited in extent, treatment with preparations such as lime sulphur or miconazole shampoo may be effective (Moriello and De Boer, 1995).
- Clipping of the haircoat is advisable, particularly if lesions are extensive. The clippings, which contain numerous infective arthrospores, must be disposed of carefully.
- Griseofulvin or itraconazole, administered orally, are the drugs of choice for systemic therapy. Because they are potentially teratogenic, they should not be given to pregnant animals. In addition, griseofulvin can induce neutropenia and should not be given to cats with feline immunodeficiency virus infection.

- Animals with suspicious lesions should be isolated.
- Early laboratory confirmation is essential.
- In-contact animals should be examined under a Wood's lamp and closely monitored for skin lesions.
- Contaminated areas should be vacuum-cleaned to remove infected skin debris and hairs.
- Contaminated bedding should be burnt and grooming equipment should be disinfected with 0.5% sodium hypochlorite.

Dermatophytosis in cattle

Trichophyton verrucosum is the usual cause of ringworm in cattle. Calves are most commonly affected and often develop characteristic lesions on the face and around the eyes. In heifers and cows lesions may be present on the neck and limbs. Oval areas of affected skin are alopecic with greyish white crusts. Infection is most common in winter months and a number of animals are usually affected. Bovine dermatophytosis is usually self-limiting. However, individual valuable animals may require treatment. Topical preparations such as 5% lime sulphur, captan (1:300) or natamycin may be effective. A vaccine containing an attenuated strain of *T. verrucosum* (LTF-130) has been used for the control of bovine dermatophytosis (Gordon and Bond, 1996). This vaccine is not available for use in the USA.

Dermatophytosis in horses

Trichophyton equinum is the main cause of ringworm in horses. *Microsporum equinum* and *T. equinum* var. *autotrophicum*, although relatively specific for the horse, are uncommon and are limited in geographical distribution. Transmission occurs by direct contact or from contaminated harness and grooming gear. The distribution of the skin lesions may indicate the likely source of the infection. Lesions may be limited to the girth strap or saddle regions or may be widely distributed if grooming gear is contaminated. Infection caused by *M. gypseum* can be acquired from rolling in soil, with lesions usually confined to the dorsum. *Microsporum canis* and *T. mentagrophytes* are occasionally isolated from horses and *T. verrucosum* infections may be acquired from contact with infected cattle. Young horses under 4 years of age are particularly susceptible to dermatophytosis. Treatment with topical preparations such as 5% lime sulphur or natamycin is usually effective. Affected animals must be isolated and contaminated harness and grooming gear should be disinfected with 0.5% sodium hypochlorite.

Dermatophytosis in pigs

Dermatophytosis in pigs is uncommon and is usually caused by *M. nanum*. The condition, which can be endemic in a herd, may not be recognized particularly in pigs with pigmented skin (Ginther, 1965). All ages are susceptible and lesions can occur anywhere on the body surface as thick brownish crusts. Ringworm in pigs is not of economic importance.

Favus in poultry

Gallinaceous birds are occasionally infected with *M. gallinae*, the cause of avian ringworm or favus. White patchy crusts develop on the comb and wattles. If the disease is severe, feather follicles may be invaded and affected birds may show signs of systemic illness.

References

Ginther, O.J. (1965). Clinical aspects of *Microsporum nanum* infection in swine. *Journal of the American Veterinary Medical Association*, **146**, 945–953.

Gordon, P.J. and Bond, R. (1996). Efficacy of a live attenuated *Trichophyton verrucosum* vaccine for control of bovine dermatophytosis. *Veterinary Record*, **139**, 395–396.

Medleau, L. and Rakich, P.M. (1994). *Microsporum canis* pseudomycetomas in a cat. *Journal of the American Animal Hospital Association*, **30**, 573–576.

Moriello, K.A. and DeBoer, D.J. (1995). Feline dermatophytosis: recent advances and recommendations for therapy. *Veterinary Clinics of North America: Small Animal Practice*, **25**, 901–921.

Moriello, K.A., Kunkle, G. and DeBoer, D.J. (1994). Isolation of dermatophytes from the haircoats of stray cats from selected animal shelters in two different geographic regions of the United States. *Veterinary Dermatology*, **5**, 57–62.

Pepin, G.A. and Oxenham, M. (1986). Zoonotic dermatophytosis (ringworm). *Veterinary Record*, **118**, 110–111.

Sparkes, A.H., Gruffydd-Jones, T.J., Shaw, S.E., Wright, A.I. and Stokes, C.R. (1993). Epidemiology and diagnostic features of canine and feline dermatophytosis in the United Kingdom from 1956 to 1991. *Veterinary Record*, **133**, 57–61.

Wagner, D.K. and Sohnle, P.G. (1995). Cutaneous defenses against dermatophytes and yeasts. *Clinical Microbiological Reviews*, **8**, 317–335.

Weitzman, I. and Summerbell, R.C. (1995). The dermatophytes. *Clinical Microbiological Reviews*, **8**, 240–259.

Further reading

DeBoer, D.J., Moriello, K. and Cairns, R. (1995). Clinical update on feline dermatophytosis - part II. *Compendium of Continuing Education*, **17**, 1471–1480.

Rosser, E.J. (1995). Infectious crusting dermatoses. *Veterinary Clinics of North America: Equine Practice*, **11**, 53–59.

Chapter 39

Aspergillus species

Among the saprophytic moulds, *Aspergillus* species are widely distributed. Although the genus contains more than 190 species, only a limited number of these have been implicated in opportunistic infections in animals and humans. *Aspergillus fumigatus* is the species most often involved in tissue invasion. Aspergillosis may also be caused by other potentially invasive species including *A. niger, A. flavus, A. terreus, A. deflectus, A. nidulans* and *A. flavipes*. Most *Aspergillus* species are grouped in the Fungi Imperfecti; some belong to the ascomycetes. The hyphae are septate, hyaline and up to 8.0 μm in diameter. Unbranched conidiophores develop at right angles from specialized hyphal foot cells. The tip of the conidiophore enlarges to form a vesicle which becomes partially or completely covered with flask-shaped phialides. The phialides produce chains of round pigmented conidia (phialoconidia) which may be smooth or rough and are up to 5.0 μm in diameter (Fig. 39.1). Aspergilli are aerobic and grow rapidly, forming distinct colonies after incubation for 2 to 3 days. The colour of the obverse side of colonies, which may be bluish-green, black, brown, yellow or reddish, varies with individual species and with cultural conditions. *Aspergillus fumigatus*, a thermotolerant species, grows at temperatures ranging from 20°C to 50°C.

> **Key points**
> - Majority are members of the Fungi Imperfecti; a few are ascomycetes
> - Ubiquitous, saprophytic moulds with septate hyaline hyphae
> - Rapidly growing pigmented colonies
> - Pigmented conidia formed from phalides borne on vesicles
> - Respiratory pathogens, acquired by inhalation of spores
> - *Aspergillus fumigatus* responsible for the majority of infections in animals
> - Toxins elaborated by *Aspergillus flavus* in stored food cause aflatoxicosis

Respiratory infections may occur following inhalation of spores. Less commonly, infection can result from ingestion of spores or following tissue trauma. Systemic infection is invariably associated with immunosuppression. Species such as *A. flavus*, which elaborate potent toxins when growing in cereals and other foods, cause mycotoxicosis (*see* Chapter 46).

Usual habitat

Aspergilli are common soil inhabitants and are also found in large numbers in decomposing organic matter. *Aspergillus fumigatus* often occurs in overheated, poor quality hay and in compost heaps. Spores of *Aspergillus* species are present in dust and air.

Recognition of *Aspergillus* species

Aspergillus species grow on standard laboratory media such as Sabouraud dextrose agar. Because the genus contains a large number of species, differentiation is difficult. A small number of the species are responsible for the majority of infections in animals and a presumptive identification may be made on the basis of colonial appearance and the conidial arrangement on sporing heads.

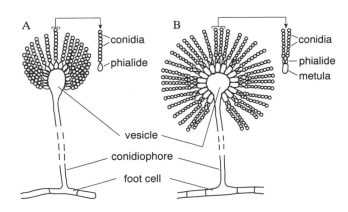

Figure 39.1 Sporing heads of two *Aspergillus* species. Differences in the shape of the vesicles and conidial arrangement is evident. The phialides of *A. fumigatus* (A) are borne directly on the vesicle (uniseriate) whereas those of *A. niger* (B) are borne on metulae (biseriate).

- Colonies can be up to 5 cm in diameter after incubation for 5 days. The colour of the reverse side is pale yellow to light tan. The colour of the obverse side is determined by the pigmentation of the conidia:
  - —*A. fumigatus* colonies rapidly become velvety or granular and bluish green with narrow white peripheries. Older colonies are slate-grey.
  - —*A. niger* colonies are black and granular, features imparted by their large pigmented sporing heads.
  - —*A. flavus* colonies are yellowish green with a fluffy texture.
  - —*A. terreus* colonies are cinnamon-brown with a granular texture.
- Sporing heads, stained with lactophenol cotton blue and examined with low and high dry magnification, have characteristic features. These include size and shape of vesicles, position of phialides and the size, shape and colour of conidia. Differentiating features of *A. fumigatus* and *A. niger* sporing heads are illustrated in Figure 39.1.
- Because their colonies can be similar in appearance, microscopic differentiation of *A. fumigatus* from some *Penicillium* species may be necessary. The conidiophores of *Penicillium* species often possess secondary branches (metulae), bearing several phialides (Fig. 39.2).
- For definitive identification, it may be necessary to induce and examine the teleomorphic form of an *Aspergillus* isolate, a procedure carried out in reference laboratories.

Pathogenesis and pathogenicity

Infection with *Aspergillus* species, mainly *A. fumigatus*, has been recorded in many species of animals. Aspergillosis, which is primarily a respiratory infection, follows spore inhalation. Because the spores of *A. fumigatus* are small, they can pass through the upper respiratory tract and may be carried to the terminal parts of the bronchial tree (Amitani *et al.*, 1995). Germination of inhaled spores and hyphal invasion of tissues depend on a number of factors. There is evidence that fragments of fibrinogen bind to the spores of *A. fumigatus* in a manner which is apparently specific for aspergilli with pathogenic potential (Annaix *et al.*, 1992). Factors which may be relevant to virulence include the production of protease and elastase. In addition, a metabolite of *A. fumigatus*, gliotoxin, inhibits both the activity of cilia and phagocytosis by macrophages.

Immune competence of the host largely determines the outcome of infection. Factors which may modify immune competence include corticosteroid therapy and long-term treatment with antimicrobial drugs. Interference with both neutrophil and monocyte function may predispose to tissue invasion. Hyphal invasion of blood vessels leads to vasculitis and thrombus formation. Mycotic granulomas may develop in the lungs and occasionally in other internal organs.

Diagnostic procedures

- Certain specific clinical conditions such as guttural pouch mycosis may suggest the involvement of *Aspergillus* species.
- Endoscopic examination can be used to detect lesions in the nasal cavity and guttural pouch.
- For confirmation of aetiological involvement, tissue invasion by fungi must be demonstrated in biopsy specimens or tissues taken at postmortem and *Aspergillus* species must be isolated from specimens.
- Tissue sections stained by methenamine silver or by the PAS method may reveal hyphal invasion.
- For isolation, small tissue specimens are applied to the scarified surface of Sabouraud dextrose agar and incubated aerobically at 37°C for 2 to 5 days. Hyphae grow from specimens to form colonies.
- Identification criteria:
  - — Colonial morphology
  - — Appearance of sporing heads including conidia (Fig. 39.1)
  - — Growth at 45°C to 50°C (thermotolerant species)
- Molecular procedures, such as the polymerase chain reaction technique, are being developed to detect *A. fumigatus* in clinical specimens (Spreadbury *et al.*, 1993).
- Serological tests are based on growth-phase or hyphal-specific antigens of *A. fumigatus*. As a consequence of constant exposure, most animals develop antibodies to conidial antigens. In dogs, the most reliable serological test is considered to be the ELISA.

Clinical infections

Clinical cases of aspergillosis are comparatively uncommon and usually sporadic. Infections often involve the respiratory tract although localized infections with *A. fumigatus* have been recorded in other organs. Mycotic mastitis occasionally results from the accidental introduction of *A. fumigatus* spores into the mammary gland on an

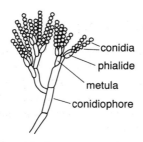

Figure 39.2 Sporing head of *Penicillium* species. Colonies can resemble those produced by *Aspergillus fumigatus*.

Table 39.1 Clinical conditions caused by *Aspergillus* species in domestic animals.

Hosts	Condition	Comments
Birds	Brooder pneumonia	Occurs in newly-hatched chickens in incubators
	Pneumonia and airsacculitis	Chickens and poults up to 6 weeks of age are most susceptible; older birds sometimes affected
	Generalized aspergillosis	Dissemination of infection usually from the respiratory tract
Horses	Guttural pouch mycosis	Confined to guttural pouch, often unilateral
	Nasal granuloma	Produces a nasal discharge and interferes with breathing. Fungi other than *Aspergillus* spp. may initiate this condition
	Keratitis	Localized infection following ocular trauma
	Intestinal aspergillosis	Enteric infection resulting in diarrhoea in foals
Cattle	Mycotic abortion	Occurs sporadically; produces thickened placenta and plaques on skin of aborted foetus
	Mycotic pneumonia	Uncommon condition of housed calves
	Mycotic mastitis	May result from the use of contaminated intramammary antibiotic tubes
	Intestinal aspergillosis	May cause acute or chronic diarrhoea in calves
Dogs	Nasal aspergillosis	Invasion of nasal mucosa and turbinate bones; occurs periodically
	Otitis externa	*Aspergillus* species may constitute part of a mixed infection
	Disseminated aspergillosis	Uncommon; may result in osteomyelitis or discospondylitis
Cats	Systemic aspergillosis	Rarely encountered; immuno-suppressed animals are at risk

intramammary tube. *Aspergillus fumigatus* is sometimes involved in mixed infections associated with otitis externa. The clinical conditions caused by *Aspergillus* species in domestic animals are summarized in Table 39.1. Rarely, other fungi such as *Penicillium* species, *Paecilomyces* species and *Scedosporium apiospermum* may cause opportunistic infections similar to those caused by *Aspergillus* species (Watt *et al.*, 1995).

Brooder pneumonia in young chickens

This disease affects newly-hatched chickens which are exposed to high numbers of *A. fumigatus* spores. Affected chickens develop somnolence and inappetence, and many die. Yellowish nodules are present in the lungs, airsacs and, occasionally, in other organs. Histopathological evidence of tissue invasion by fungi and culture of *A. fumigatus* from lesions are required for confirmation. Strict hygiene and routine fumigation of incubators are effective control measures.

Aspergillosis in mature birds

Infection in mature birds frequently follows inhalation of spore-laden dust derived from contaminated litter or feed. Poultry and captive penguins, raptors and psittacine birds may be affected. Penguins are susceptible to infection if kept at unsuitably high ambient temperatures, whereas infection in raptors has been attributed to *A. fumigatus* spores from shredded woodbark on aviary floors. Clinical signs, which are variable, include dyspnoea and emaciation. Yellowish nodules resembling lesions of avian tuberculosis can be observed in the lungs and air-sacs. Dissemination may occur to other internal organs. Diagnosis is confirmed by histopathology and culture.

Guttural pouch mycosis

This condition, which is frequently associated with *A. fumigatus* infection, is usually unilateral. Lesions, often plaque-like, develop in the mucosa of the pouch wall. When fungal hyphae penetrate to deeper tissues they cause tissue necrosis, thrombosis, erosion of blood vessel walls and neural damage. The clinical signs include epistaxis, dysphagia and laryngeal hemiplegia. Postauricular swelling and unilateral nasal discharge may follow accumulation of inflammatory exudates in the pouch. Diagnosis is based on clinical signs, radiographic evidence of fluid accumulation in the pouch and demonstration of characteristic lesions by endoscopy. Confirmation is based on demonstration of fungal hyphae in biopsy specimens and isolation of *A. fumigatus* from lesions. Therapeutic options include infusion of antifungal agents into the pouch and surgical intervention to deal with serious haemorrhage. Oral or systemic antifungal therapy is infrequently used because of potential toxicity and excessive cost.

Nasal aspergillosis in dogs

Canine nasal aspergillosis is encountered in young to middle-aged dolichocephalic breeds. Clinical signs, which are often unilateral, include persistent, profuse sanguino-purulent nasal discharge with sneezing and bouts of epistaxis. Radiography may reveal an increased radio-lucency of turbinate bones. Culture and histopathological examination of biopsy material are essential for confirmation.

Administration of enilconazole through tubes inserted

surgically in the frontal sinuses and nasal chambers may be used together with systemic treatment which should continue for 6 to 8 weeks (Sharp *et al.*, 1992).

Mycotic abortion in cows

This form of abortion occurs sporadically and its prevalence may be influenced by poor quality contaminated fodder harvested in wet seasons. *Aspergillus fumigatus* can proliferate in damp hay, in poor quality silage and in brewers grains. Infection, which reaches the uterus haematogenously, causes placentitis leading to abortion late in gestation. Affected cows usually show no signs of systemic illness. Intercotyledonary areas of the placenta are thickened and leathery and the cotyledons are necrotic. Aborted foetuses may have raised cutaneous plaques, resembling ringworm lesions. Diagnosis is based on culture of *A. fumigatus* from foetal abomasal contents and histopathological evidence of mycotic placentitis.

References

Amitani, R., Taylor, G., Elezis, E.N. *et al.*, (1995). Purification and characterization of factors produced by *Aspergillus fumigatus* which affect human ciliated epithelium. *Infection and Immunity*, **63**, 3266–3271.

Annaix, V., Bouchara, J-P., Larcher, G., Chabasse, D. and Tronchin, G. (1992). Specific binding of human fibrinogen fragment D to *Aspergillus fumigatus* conidia. *Infection and Immunity*, **60**, 1747–1755.

Sharp, N., Sullivan, M. and Harvey, C. (1992). Treatment of canine nasal aspergillosis. *In Practice*, **14**, 27–31.

Spreadbury, C., Holden, D., Aufauvre-Brown, A. *et al.* (1993). Detection of *Aspergillus fumigatus* by polymerase chain reaction. *Journal of Clinical Microbiology*, **31**, 615–621.

Watt, P.R., Robins, G.M., Galloway, A.M. and O'Boyle, D.A. (1995). Disseminated opportunistic fungal disease in dogs: 10 cases (1982–1990). *Journal of the American Veterinary Medical Association*, **207**, 67–70.

Further reading

Forbes, N.A. (1991). Aspergillosis in raptors. *Veterinary Record*, **128**, 263.

Greet, T.R.C. (1987). Outcome of treatment of 35 cases of guttural pouch mycosis. *Equine Veterinary Journal*, **19**, 483–487.

Kabay, M.J., Robinson, W.F., Huxtable, C.R.R. and McAleer, R. (1985). The pathology of disseminated *Aspergillus terreus* infection in dogs. *Veterinary Pathology*, **22**, 540–547.

Peiffer, R.L., Belkin, P.V. and Janke, B.H. (1980). Orbital cellulitis, sinusitis and pneumonitis caused by *Penicillium* species in a cat. *Journal of the American Veterinary Medical Association*, **176**, 449–451.

Thompson, K.G., diMenna, M.E., Carter, M.E. and Carman, M.G. (1978). Mycotic mastitis in two cows. *New Zealand Veterinary Journal*, **26**, 176–177.

Wolf, A.M. (1992). Fungal diseases of the nasal cavity of the dog and cat. *Veterinary Clinics of North America: Small Animal Practice*, **22**, 1119–1132.

Chapter 40

Yeasts and disease production

Yeasts are eukaryotic, unicellular, round or oval, single celled organisms. During asexual reproduction, blastoconidia, also referred to as buds or daughter cells, develop. Blastoconidia, produced linearly without separation, may elongate to form a pseudohypha. Yeasts, such as *Candida* species, can produce true septate hyphae in animal tissues or when growing deeply in agar media. Yeasts grow aerobically on Sabouraud dextrose agar and those species capable of tissue invasion grow well at 37°C. Colonies, which are usually moist and creamy in texture, resemble large bacterial colonies. Yeasts are classified as Fungi Imperfecti; if a teleomorph is demonstrated, a yeast can be assigned either to the ascomycetes or to the basidiomycetes.

Yeasts are found in the environment, often on plants or plant materials. They may also occur as commensals on the skin or mucous membranes of animals. They cause opportunistic infections which are categorized as exogenous, when derived from the environment, or endogenous, when resulting from overgrowth of commensals. Immunosuppression or factors such as antimicrobial therapy which disturb the resident flora on mucosal surfaces may facilitate yeast overgrowth leading to tissue invasion. Yeasts of importance in animal disease are *Candida* species, (particularly *C. albicans*), *Cryptococcus neoformans* and *Malassezia pachydermatis*. Other yeasts, such as *Trichosporon beigelii*, and the yeast-like mould *Geotrichum candidum* rarely cause infection.

Candida species

There are more than 200 species in the genus *Candida*. *Candida albicans*, the species most often implicated in animal disease, does not have a sexual stage. It grows aerobically at 37°C on a wide range of media including Sabouraud dextrose agar. Colonies are composed of budding oval cells approximately 5.0 x 8.0 μm. In animal tissues, *C. albicans* may exhibit polymorphism in the form of pseudohyphae or hyphae (Fig. 40.1). On certain media, it characteristically produces thick-walled resting cells, known as chlamydospores (chlamydoconidia).

Key points

- Eukaryotic, unicellular budding cells
- Asexual reproduction by blastoconidia
- Pseudohyphae or true hyphae may be formed
- Teleomorphs are either ascomycetes or basidiomycetes
- *Candida albicans:*
  —Grows at 37°C on a wide range of media
  —Chlamydospores produced on cornmeal agar
  —Germ tubes formed in serum within 2 hours at 37°C
  —Resistant to cyclohexamide
  —Commensal on mucocutaneous surfaces; uncommon in the environment
  —Opportunistic infections, related to immunosuppression, in animals and humans
- *Cryptococcus neoformans:*
  —Large mucopolysaccharide capsule produced
  —Grows at 37°C on a variety of media, producing mucoid colonies
  —Teleomorph is a basidiomycete
  —Utilizes creatinine in bird droppings
  —Opportunistic infection derived from environmental sources
  —Localized granulomas or sometimes disseminated disease in cats, dogs, horses and cattle
- *Malassezia pachydermatis:*
  —Bottle-shaped cells
  —Monopolar budding
  —Commensal on the skin of mammals and birds
  —Associated with canine seborrhoeic dermatitis and otitis externa

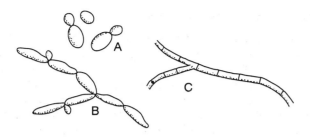

Figure 40.1 Three forms of the polymorphic yeast *Candida albicans*: budding yeast cell (A); pseudohypha (B); true septate hypha (C).

Usual habitat

Candida species occur worldwide on plant materials and, as commensals, in the digestive and urogenital tracts of animals and humans. *Candida albicans* is isolated from environmental sources less frequently than other *Candida* species, suggesting adaptation towards a parasitic rather than a saprophytic existence.

Differentiation of *Candida* species

- Most *Candida* species have a similar colonial appearance. Colonies, which are whitish, shiny and convex, are 4 to 5mm in diameter after incubation for 3 days.
- Subculturing onto an indicator medium allows presumptive identification of *C. albicans*, *C. krusei* and *C. tropicalis* on the basis of colonial appearance (Odds and Bernaerts, 1994).
- Carbohydrate assimilation and fermentation tests, which are usually performed in reference laboratories, allow definitive species identification.
- Commercially-available biochemical test kits, giving results within 24 to 48 hours, are usually used for species differentiation in diagnostic laboratories.
- Features of *C. albicans* used for presumptive identification include:
  — Growth at 37°C
  — Production of chlamydospores in submerged cultures on cornmeal agar (Fig. 40.2)
  — Production of germ tubes within 2 hours, when incubated in serum at 37°C (Fig. 40.3)
  — Growth on Sabouraud dextrose agar containing cycloheximide

Pathogenesis and pathogenicity

Candida albicans, the principal yeast involved in animal disease, possesses a number of putative virulence factors (Cutler, 1991). The organism has surface integrin-like molecules which allow adhesion to matrix proteins. In addition, surface structures can bind fibrinogen and complement components. Production of proteases and phospholipases may aid tissue invasion. Phenotypic switching, which has been demonstrated in *C. albicans*, may facilitate evasion of host defence mechanisms.

During the early stages of infection, phagocytic clearance mechanisms eliminate most of the yeast cells. Those cells which are not cleared rapidly convert to hyphal forms. Phospholipases, concentrated in hyphal tips, may enhance invasiveness. The localized mucocutaneous form of candidiasis is associated with overgrowth of resident *C. albicans* in the oral cavity or gastrointestinal and urogenital tracts. Predisposing factors include defects in cell-mediated immunity, concurrent disease, disturbance of the normal flora by prolonged use of antimicrobial drugs and damage to the mucosa from indwelling catheters. Affected mucosa is thickened and often hyperaemic.

Haematogenous spread may occur following vascular invasion by hyphae or pseudohyphae, producing systemic lesions.

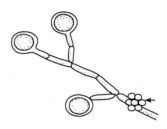

Figure 40.2 Thick-walled resting cells of *Candida albicans*, called chlamydospores (chlamydoconidia). These resting cells are formed from pseudohyphae when submerged colonies grow in cornmeal agar. The smaller cells are blastoconidia (arrow).

Diagnostic procedures

- Suitable specimens for culture and histopathology include biopsy or postmortem tissue samples and milk samples.
- Tissue sections, stained by PAS or methenamine silver methods, may reveal budding yeast cells or hyphae.
- Culture is carried out aerobically at 37°C for 2 to 5 days on Sabouraud dextrose agar, with or without cycloheximide.
- Identification criteria for isolates:
  — Characteristic colonies yielding budding yeast cells
  — Growth on media containing cycloheximide (specific for *C. albicans*)

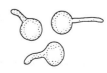

Figure 40.3 Germ tubes form within 2 hours when cells of *Candida albicans* are incubated in serum at 37°C.

— Colonial appearance on CHROMagar Candida
— Biochemical profile
— Chlamydospore and germ tube production (specific for *C. albicans*)

Clinical infections

Opportunistic infections with *Candida* species, which occur sporadically, are usually associated with immunosuppression or the prolonged use of antimicrobial drugs. The clinical conditions attributed to *Candida* species are presented in Table 40.1. Overgrowth of commensal *Candida* species may result in localized mucosal damage in parts of the digestive or urogenital tracts.

Thrush of the oesophagus or crop in young chickens may be associated with prolonged antibiotic administration. Mycotic stomatitis has been reported in pups, kittens and foals (McClure *et al.*, 1985). *Candida albicans* has been implicated in gastro-oesophageal ulceration in pigs and foals (Kadel *et al.*, 1969; Gross and Mayhew, 1985). Rarely, disseminated candidiasis may occur in pigs, calves, dogs and cats.

Bovine abortion caused by *Candida* species has been recorded (Foley and Schlafer, 1987). In addition, a number of *Candida* species have been isolated from cases of bovine mastitis (Richard *et al.*, 1980). Mycotic mastitis occurs sporadically either as a consequence of contaminated intramammary preparations or from heavy environmental contamination (Elad *et al.*, 1995). Usually one quarter is involved and spontaneous elimination of the infection frequently occurs. Rarely, yeast cells may be shed for up to 12 months.

Table 40.1 Clinical conditions associated with *Candida albicans*.

Hosts	Clinical conditions
Pups, kittens, foals	Mycotic stomatitis
Pigs, foals, calves	Gastro-oesophageal ulcers
Calves	Rumenitis
Dogs	Enteritis, cutaneous lesions
Chickens	Thrush of the oesophagus or crop
Geese, turkeys	Cloacal and vent infections
Cows	Reduced fertility, abortion, mastitis
Mares	Pyometra
Cats	Urocystitis, pyothorax
Cats, horses	Ocular lesions
Dogs, cats, pigs, calves	Disseminated disease

Cryptococcus neoformans

Although the genus *Cryptococcus* contains about 37 species, only *C. neoformans* produces opportunistic infections. The yeast cells are round to oval and 3.5 to 8.0 μm in diameter. A daughter cell is formed as a bud, on a narrow neck, from the mother cell. When recovered directly from affected animals, the yeasts have thick mucopolysaccharide capsules which can be demonstrated in India ink preparations (Fig. 40.4). The capsules can also be observed in tissue sections stained with mucicarmine. *Cryptococcus* species are aerobic, nonfermentative organisms which form mucoid colonies on a variety of media including Sabouraud dextrose agar. The ability to grow at 37°C distinguishes *C. neoformans* from other *Cryptococcus* species.

On the basis of capsular antigens, four serotypes of *C. neoformans* are recognized. Serotypes A and D are designated as *C. neoformans* var. *neoformans* while serotypes B and C have been termed *C. neoformans* var. *gattii*. *In vitro*, these serotypes produce the teleomorph *Filobasidiella neoformans*, a basidiomycete. The teleomorph has not been recognized as a free-growing form.

The clinical conditions caused by *C. neoformans* in domestic animals are presented in Table 40.2.

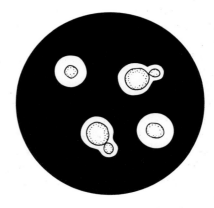

Figure 40.4 Cells of *Cryptococcus neoformans* as they appear in an India ink preparation. A narrow neck joins the mother cell and its bud. Prominent mucopolysaccharide capsules are a characteristic feature of this yeast.

Usual habitat

Cryptococcus neoformans var. *neoformans* can be isolated from the droppings of pigeons and other birds and from soil enriched by these droppings. Creatinine, present in the droppings, is utilized by this yeast. Pigeons with *C. neoformans* in their intestinal tracts can excrete the organism for several months without developing disease.

Cryptococcocus neoformans var. *gattii*, isolated from forest red gum trees (*Eucalyptus* species) in Australia, has been spread in timber products.

Table 40.2 Clinical conditions caused by *Cryptococcus neoformans* in domestic animals.

Hosts	Clinical condition
Cats	Respiratory, cutaneous, neural and ocular infections
Dogs	Disseminated disease with neural and ocular signs
Cattle	Mastitis, nasal granulomas
Horses	Nasal granulomas, sinusitis, cutaneous lesions, pneumonia, meningoencephalitis, abortion

Laboratory recognition of *C. neoformans*

- Colonies of *Cryptococcus* species, which are mucoid when first isolated due to the presence of capsular material, become dry with age. They may have a cream, tan or yellowish appearance.
- Budding yeasts with wide capsules can be demonstrated in India ink preparations (Fig. 40.4).
- Most *Cryptococcus* species produce urease, rapidly hydrolyzing urea to ammonia.
- Differentiation of species is possible using carbohydrate assimilation tests or commercially-available biochemical kits.
- Identification criteria for *C. neoformans*:
  — Ability to grow at 37°C
  — Brown colonies on birdseed agar as a result of phenol oxidase production
  — Melanin demonstrable in cell walls using the Fontana-Masson stain on tissue sections
- Variety *gattii* can utilize glycine as the sole source of nitrogen and is resistant to canavanine. In contrast, variety *neoformans* cannot utilize glycine as a sole source of nitrogen and is susceptible to canavanine.

Pathogenesis and pathogenicity

Infection occurs through inhalation of *C. neoformans* cells in contaminated dust. Some yeast cells may be trapped in the nasal cavities or sinuses while others are deposited in the lungs. Virulence factors of *C. neoformans* include the capsule, which is antiphagocytic, the ability to grow at mammalian body temperature and the production of phenol oxidase. Mutants which have lost one of these attributes are avirulent. The virulence arising from phenol oxidase activity may relate to the degradation of catecholamine which results in the accumulation of melanin in the yeast cell walls protecting against the toxic effects of free radicals (Jacobson and Emery, 1991).

    Immunocompetent animals can mount an effective cell-mediated response to *C. neoformans*. Dissemination from the respiratory tract to brain, meninges, skin and bones is usually associated with defective cell-mediated immunity.

Lesions associated with *C. neoformans* infection range from discrete granulomas to tumour-like myxomatous masses composed of yeast cells in a connective tissue matrix. Small granulomas may be present in the lungs of clinically normal animals.

Diagnostic procedures

Care must be exercised when handling material from suspect *C. neoformans* cases because of the risk of acquiring infection.

- Suitable specimens for laboratory examination include exudates, cerebrospinal fluid and biopsy or postmortem tissues.
- Budding yeasts with characteristic, thick capsules can be demonstrated in fluid samples using India ink preparations (Fig. 40.4).
- In tissue sections yeast capsules are demonstrated by Mayer's mucicarmine method. Melanin can be detected in cell walls of *C. neoformans* by the Fontana-Masson technique.
- Specimens, cultured on Sabouraud dextrose agar with chloramphenicol but without cyclohexamide, are incubated aerobically at 37°C for up to 2 weeks.
- Identification criteria for isolates:
  — Mucoid colonies
  — Presence of capsules
  — Urease activity
  — Brown colonies on birdseed agar and growth at 37°C (specific for *C. neoformans*)
- A latex agglutination test, which detects soluble capsular material of *C. neoformans* within 3 weeks of infection, can be used on samples of cerebrospinal fluid, serum and urine.

Clinical infections

Apart from sporadic cases in cats and dogs, cryptococcosis in domestic animals is relatively rare (Table 40.2). In companion animals, clinical signs of cryptococcosis usually relate to the nasal cavity or skin involvement. The disease in dogs, which is less common than in cats, is often disseminated with neurological and ocular signs (Jergens *et al.*, 1986). Cryptococcosis has been recorded infrequently in horses. Clinical signs include nasal granulomas and sinusitis (Scott *et al.*, 1974), pneumonia (Hilbert *et al.*, 1980), meningoencephalitis and abortion (Blanchard and Filkins, 1992). *Cryptococcus neoformans* is a rare cause of mastitis in dairy cattle.

Feline cryptococcosis

Nasal, cutaneous, neural and ocular forms of cryptococcosis are recognized in cats. The nasal form, which accounts for approximately 70% of cases, is characterized by flesh-coloured, polyp-like granulomas in the nasal cavity. Cutaneous lesions, often affecting the face, head and neck, are reported in about 30% of cases. Peripheral lymphadenopathy is common. Neurological signs are evident in about 25% of cases and, in some instances, chorioretinitis may be evident.

Surgical removal combined with parenteral antifungal drugs is the usual method for treating cutaneous cryptococcosis. There may be a favourable response to amphotericin B with flucytosine or to ketoconazole, itraconazole or fluconazole (Medleau *et al.*, 1990; Malik *et al.*, 1992). Therapy should continue for at least 2 months. The latex agglutination test can be used to monitor the effects of antifungal therapy and declining antigen levels indicate a favourable response to the treatment (Medleau *et al.*, 1990).

Malassezia pachydermatis

Malassezia species, commensals on the skin of animals and humans, are aerobic, non-fermentative, urease-positive yeasts which grow at 35°C to 37°C. One species, *Malassezia pachydermatis* (formerly *Pityrosporum canis*) is of veterinary importance. The cells of *M. pachydermatis*, which are bottle-shaped, thick walled and up to 6.5 μm in length, reproduce by monopolar budding on a broad base. Multiple budding may occur from the same site on a mother cell. After repeated budding, a distinct collarette forms at this site (Fig. 40.5). Pseudohyphae may be produced infrequently in tissues (Guillot *et al.*, 1998).

Usual habit

Malassezia pachydermatis can be found on the skin of mammals and birds, particularly in areas rich in sebaceous glands. The anal region, external ear canal, lips and interdigital skin of dogs are frequently colonized by this yeast (Bond *et al.*, 1995b).

Identification of *Malassezia pachydermatis*

- The unique budding pattern is demonstrable in microscopic preparations stained with methylene blue.
- *Malassezia pachydermatis* is the only member of the genus which grows on Sabouraud dextrose agar without lipid supplementation. Colonies, which are dull, opaque and cream-coloured, have a smooth surface.

Pathogenesis and pathogenicity

Malassezia pachydermatis is associated with two clinical conditions, otitis externa and dermatitis, usually in dogs. Colonization and growth of the organism in these locations may be associated with immunosuppression and other predisposing factors. When the yeast cells are present in high numbers, they apparently induce excessive sebaceous secretion, a feature of seborrhoeic dermatitis (Akerstedt and Vollset, 1996).

In otitis externa, the production of proteolytic enzymes by *M. pachydermatis* results in damage to the mucosa of the ear canal. Excessive production and retention of wax, a consequence of ceruminous gland hypersecretion, combined with the activity of *M. pachydermatis* and other microorganisms contribute to inflammatory changes. Inflammatory exudate and necrotic debris accumulate in the canal.

Diagnostic procedures

- Involvement of *M. pachydermatis* should be considered in otitis externa and in canine seborrhoeic dermatitis.
- Exudate from affected ear canals should be submitted for laboratory examination.
- In severe dermatitis, biopsy of skin may be considered.
- Characteristic yeast cells are demonstrable in exudates stained with methylene blue (Fig. 40.5).
- *Malassezia pachydermatis* can be cultured aerobically at 37°C for 3 to 4 days on Sabouraud dextrose agar containing chloramphenicol.
- Identification criteria for isolates:
  — Colonial appearance
  — Growth without lipid supplementation (consistent with *M. pachydermatis*)
  — Characteristic microscopic appearance
- In otitis externa, blood agar and MacConkey agar plates should be inoculated with exudate to isolate bacterial pathogens aetiologically associated with *M. pachydermatis*.

Clinical infections

Malassezia pachydermatis has recently been implicated in canine seborrhoeic dermatitis and also in skin infections secondary to epidermal dysplasia, a genetic disorder of West Highland terriers (Akerstedt and Vollset, 1996). This yeast is one of many organisms which may contribute

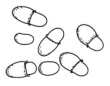

Figure 40.5 Bottle-shaped cells of the yeast, *Malassezia pachydermatis*. Monopolar budding on a broad base, with the formation of a prominent collarette, is a characteristic of this yeast.

to otitis externa in dogs. The condition occurs less frequently in cats.

Canine seborrhoeic dermatitis

Factors which predispose to canine seborrhoeic dermatitis include hypersensitivity disorders, keratinization defects, immunosuppression and persistently moist skin folds. Lesions tend to occur more frequently and with greater severity in skin folds. Pruritis and erythema are accompanied by a foul-smelling, greasy exudate with matting of hair. Concurrent bilateral otitis externa may be present (Bond *et al.*, 1995b) Treatment with miconazole-chlorhexidine shampoo (Bond *et al.*, 1995a), or a combination of topical and oral ketoconazole may be effective.

Canine otitis externa

Otitis externa is characterized by a dark pungent discharge from the ear canal and intense pruritis with head shaking, scratching and rubbing of the ears. Damage to the pinna may manifest as a haematoma. The mucosa of the ear canal is painful and swollen. The aetiology of this condition is complex. Poor ear conformation, wax retention and immunosuppression are among the factors which may predispose dogs to the disease. *Malassezia pachydermatis*, which is present in low numbers in the ear canal of clinically normal dogs, may proliferate in otitis externa. Predisposing causes should be investigated and eliminated or treated (Little, 1996). The fungal and bacterial pathogens causing the inflammatory response should be identified by microscopic examination and culture of aural exudate. Antibiotic sensitivity testing should be carried out on the bacterial isolates prior to initiating therapy. Proprietary ear drops, containing drugs effective against the bacteria and fungi usually involved, and also against *Otodectes cynotis*, may be beneficial. In chronic cases, surgical intervention may be required.

Trichosporon beigelii

Trichosporon beigelii (*T. cutaneum*), a soil saprophyte, produces yeast cells (blastoconidia), pseudohyphae, true hyphae and arthrospores (Fig. 40.6). After inoculation of Sabouraud dextrose agar, colonies appear in about one week. This yeast, which is non-fermentative and urease-positive, causes white piedra, a skin condition of humans. Rare infections in animals include skin lesions in horses and monkeys, and mastitis in cattle. Nasal granuloma, mycotic cystitis and disseminated trichosporonosis have been described in cats infected with feline leukaemia virus (Doster *et al.*, 1987).

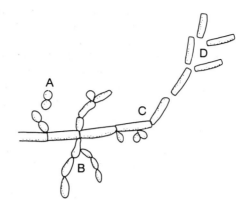

Figure 40.6 Fungal forms and structures of *Trichosporon beigelii*: yeast cells (A); pseudohyphae (B); true hyphae (C); arthrospores (D)

Geotrichum candidum

The mould, *Geotrichum candidum*, has a yeast-like colonial morphology. The hyphae fragment into chains of rectangular arthrospores (Fig. 40.7). *Geotrichum candidum* is a saprophyte in soil and decaying organic matter. It can be isolated from faeces of clinically normal animals. The fungus has been occasionally implicated in diarrhoea in dogs and apes, lymphadenitis in pigs and disseminated geotrichosis in dogs (Rhyan *et al.*, 1990).

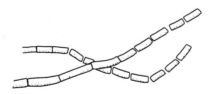

Figure 40.7 Rectangular arthrospores produced by the yeast-like mould, *Geotrichum candidum*.

References

Akerstedt, J. and Vollset, I. (1996). *Malassezia pachydermatis* with special reference to canine skin disease. *British Veterinary Journal*, **152**, 269–281.

Blanchard, P.C. and Filkins, M. (1992). Cryptococcal pneumonia and abortion in an equine fetus. *Journal of the American Veterinary Medical Association*, **201**, 1591–1592.

Bond, R., Rose, J.F., Ellis, J.W. and Lloyd, D.H. (1995a). Comparison of two shampoos for treatment of *Malassezia pachydermatis*-associated seborrhoeic dermatitis in basset hounds. *Journal of Small Animal Practice*, **36**, 99–104.

Bond, R., Saijonmaa-Koulumies, L.E.M. and Lloyd, D.H.

(1995b). Population sizes and frequency of *Malassezia pachydermatis* at skin and mucosal sites on healthy dogs. *Journal of Small Animal Practice*, **36**, 147–150.

Cutler, J.E. (1991). Putative virulence factors of *Candida albicans*. *Annual Review of Microbiology*, **45**, 187–218.

Doster, A.R., Erickson, E.D. and Chandler, F.W. (1987). Trichosporonosis in two cats. *Journal of the American Veterinary Medical Association*, **190**, 1184–1186.

Elad, D., Shipgel, N.Y., Winkler, M. *et al.* (1995). Feed contaminated with *Candida krusei* as a probable source of mycotic mastitis in dairy cows. *Journal of the American Veterinary Medical Association*, **207**, 620–622.

Foley, G.L. and Schlafer, D.H. (1987). Candida abortion in cattle. *Veterinary Pathology*, **24**, 532–536.

Gross, T.L. and Mayhew, I.G. (1985). Gastroesophageal ulceration and candidiasis in foals. *Journal of the American Veterinary Medical Association*, **186**, 1195–1197.

Guillot, J., Petit, T., Degorce-Rubiales, F., Gueho, E. and Chermette, R. (1998). Dermatitis caused by *Malassezia pachydermatis* in a Californian sea lion (*Zalophus californianus*). *Veterinary Record*, **142**, 311–312.

Hilbert, B.J., Huxtable, C.R. and Pawley, S.E. (1980). Cryptococcal pneumonia in a horse. *Australian Veterinary Journal*, **56**, 391–392.

Jacobson, E.S. and Emery, H.S. (1991). Catecholamine uptake, melaninization and oxygen toxicity in *Cryptococcus neoformans*. *Journal of Bacteriology*, **173**, 401–403.

Jergens, A.E., Wheeler, C.A. and Collier, L.L. (1986). Cryptococcosis involving the eye and nervous system of a dog. *Journal of the American Veterinary Medical Association,* **189**, 302–304.

Kadel, W.L., Kelley, D.C. and Coles, E.H. (1969). Survey of yeast-like fungi and tissue changes in esophagogastric region of stomach of swine. *American Journal of Veterinary Research*, **30**, 401–408.

Little, C. (1996). A clinician's approach to the investigation of otitis externa. *In Practice*, **18**, 9–16.

Malik, R., Wigney, D.I. and Muir, D.B. *et al.* (1992). Cryptococcosis in cats: clinical and mycological assessment of 29 cases and evaluation of treatment using orally administered fluconazole. *Journal of Medical and Veterinary Mycology*, **30**, 133–144.

Medleau, L. Greene, C.E. and Rakich, P.M. (1990). Evaluation of ketoconazole and itraconazole for treatment of disseminated cryptococcosis in cats. *American Journal of Veterinary Research*, **51**, 1454–1458.

McClure, J.J., Addison, J.D. and Miller, R.I. (1985). Immunodeficiency manifested by oral candidiasis and bacterial septicemia in foals. *Journal of the American Veterinary Medical Association*, **186**, 1195–1197.

Odds, F.C. and Bernaerts, R.I.A. (1994). CHROMagar Candida, a new differential isolation medium for presumptive identification of clinically important *Candida* species. *Journal of Clinical Microbiology*, **32**, 1923–1929.

Rhyan, J.C., Stackhouse, L.L. and Davis, E.G. (1990). Disseminated geotrichosis in two dogs. *Journal of the American Veterinary Medical Association*, **197**, 358–360.

Richard, J.L., McDonald, J.S., Fichtner, R.E. and Anderson, A.J. (1980). Identification of yeasts from infected bovine mammary glands and their experimental infectivity in cattle. *American Journal of Veterinary Research*, **41**, 1991–1994.

Scott, E.A., Duncan, J.R. and McCormack, J.E. (1974). Cryptococcosis involving the postorbital area and frontal sinus in a horse. *Journal of the American Veterinary Association,* **165**, 626–627.

Further reading

Rodriguez, F., Ferandez, A., Espinosa de los Monteros, A., Wohlsein, P. and Jensen, H.E. (1998). Acute disseminated candidiasis in a puppy associated with parvoviral infection. *Veterinary Record*, **142**, 434–436.

Chapter 41

Dimorphic fungi

Some fungi, referred to as dimorphic fungi, occur in two distinct forms, a mould form and a yeast form. They exist as moulds in the environment and when cultured on Sabouraud dextrose agar at 25°C to 30°C. In animal tissues and when cultured at 37°C on brain-heart infusion agar with the addition of 5% blood, most grow as yeasts after conversion from the more stable mould form. The dimorphic fungi most often associated with disease in domestic animals are *Blastomyces dermatitidis*, *Histoplasma capsulatum* and *Coccidioides immitis* (Table 41.1). The spores of these dimorphic fungi usually enter hosts by the respiratory route and infection may be disseminated throughout the body. A variant of *H. capsulatum*, *H. capsulatum* var. *farciminosum*, hereafter referred to as *H. farciminosum*, generally enters through skin abrasions and produces lympho-cutaneous lesions. *Sporothrix schenckii*, which can also infect dermal tissues following trauma, produces occasional opportunistic infections.

Rare asymptomatic infections, caused by *Paracoccidioides brasiliensis* (Costa *et al.*, 1995) and *Emmonsia* species, have been recorded in domestic animals.

Blastomyces dermatitidis

Blastomyces dermatitidis is a dimorphic fungus which causes blastomycosis, mainly in dogs and humans. The mould and yeast forms of this fungus are shown in Fig. 41.1. The teleomorph of *B. dermatitidis* is an ascomycete designated *Ajellomyces dermatitidis*.

Usual habitat

Although the precise natural habitat of *B. dermatitidis* is unknown, it has been isolated from acid soils rich in organic matter (Archer *et al.*, 1987).

Recognition and laboratory diagnosis

- When incubated at 25°C to 30°C on Sabouraud dextrose agar, mould colonies are white and cottony, usually becoming brown with age. Oval or pear-shaped conidia (2 to 10 μm in diameter) are borne either on

---

Key points

- Occur as moulds in the environment and as yeast forms in animal tissues
- Saprophytes in soil and in decaying vegetation
- Produce opportunistic infections in animals and humans
- *Blastomyces dermatitidis*:
  —Saprophyte in soil enriched with organic matter
  —Cells budding on a broad base in tissues
  —Causes blastomycosis in dogs and humans
- *Coccidioides immitis*:
  —Saprophyte in arid soils
  —Large spherules containing endospores demonstrable in infected tissues
  —Causes coccidioidomycosis in dogs, horses and humans; often asymptomatic in other species
- *Histoplasma capsulatum*:
  —Saprophyte in soil enriched with bird faeces
  —Small yeast cells demonstrable in macrophages
  —Causes histoplasmosis in dogs, cats and humans; uncommon in other species
- *Histoplasma farciminosum*:
  —Saprophyte in soil
  —Small yeast cells in macrophages
  —Causes epizootic lymphangitis in *Equidae*
- *Sporothrix schenckii*:
  —Saprophyte on vegetation
  —Cigar-shaped yeast cells demonstrable in infected tissues and exudates
  —Causes sporotrichosis in horses, cats, dogs, humans and other species

---

conidiophores or directly on the hyphae.

- When incubated at 37°C on brain-heart infusion agar with added cysteine and 5% blood, yeast colonies are cream to tan, wrinkled and waxy. The yeast cells (8 to

Table 41.1 Dimorphic fungi which are associated with disease in animals and humans.

Feature	*Blastomyces dermatitidis*	*Histoplasma capsulatum*	*Histoplasma farciminosum*	*Coccidioides immitis*	*Sporothrix schenckii*
Disease	Blastomycosis	Histoplasmosis	Epizootic lymphangitis	Coccidioidomycosis	Sporotrichosis
Geographical distribution	Eastern regions of North America, sporadic cases in India and the Middle East	Endemic in the Mississippi and Ohio river valleys, sporadic cases in some countries	Africa, Middle East, Asia	Semi-arid regions of southwestern USA, Mexico, Central and South America	Worldwide, most common in subtropical and tropical regions
Usual habitat	Acid soil rich in organic matter	Soil enriched with bat or bird faeces	Soil	Desert soils at low elevation	Dead vegetation, rose thorns, wooden posts, sphagnum moss
Main hosts	Dogs, humans	Dogs, cats, humans	Horses, other *Equidae*	Dogs, horses, humans	Horses, cats, dogs, humans
Site of lesions	Lungs, metastases to skin and other tissues	Lungs, metastases to other organs	Skin, lymphatic vessels, lymph nodes	Lungs, metastases to bones	Skin, lymphatic vessels

10 µm in diameter) are thick-walled and typically bud on a broad base.

- A soluble exoantigen of *B. dermatitidis* can be identified by agar gel immunodiffusion using specific antiserum (Di Salvo, 1998).
- Commercially available nucleic acid probes for use on cultures of dimorphic fungi are sensitive and specific (Stockman *et al.*, 1993).
- Yeast cells may be demonstrated in cytological and histopathological preparations from affected tissues. Exudates or aspirates for cytological examination should be stained with methylene blue or by the Giemsa method.
- Serological procedures, suitable for demonstrating rising antibody titres in affected dogs, are ELISA and counter-immunoelectrophoresis.

Mould form

Oval or pear-shaped conidia (2-10 µm in diameter) form on conidiophores or directly on septate hyphae when cultured at 25°C

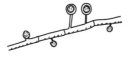

Yeast form

Thick-walled yeast cells (8-10 µm in diameter) form when cultured at 37°C. Daughter cells bud on a broad base

Figure 41.1 The mould and yeast forms of *Blastomyces dermatitidis*.

Clinical infections

Blastomycosis most commonly affects dogs and humans (Legendre *et al.*, 1981). Infection in other species is uncommon but it has been recorded in the cat (Breider *et al.*, 1988). The disease is encountered in North America, Africa, the Middle East and India.

Canine blastomycosis

Young male dogs of sporting breeds are particularly prone to infection because of frequent exposure to the fungus in the environment. Infection usually occurs by inhalation and pulmonary blastomycosis, a chronic debilitating condition, is the usual form of the disease. Presenting signs include coughing, exercise intolerance and dyspnoea. The extent of the infection, which may be limited to the lungs and associated lymph nodes, is largely determined by the immune competence of the host. Many infections are subclinical, detectable only by seroconversion. In animals with inadequate cell-mediated immunity, there may be dissemination to skin, eyes and bones. The central nervous system and, in male dogs, the urogenital tract are occasionally affected. Primary cutaneous blastomycosis is uncommon (Wolf, 1979). The clinical presentation in disseminated disease relates to the distribution and severity of the lesions which are granulomatous or pyogranulomatous. Yeast cells are numerous in these lesions.

Amphotericin B, which may be combined with ketoconazole, is effective if administered early in the course of the disease. Animals should be monitored for possible nephrotoxic effects of treatment.

Histoplasma capsulatum

Three variants of *H. capsulatum* are recognized: *Histoplasma capsulatum* var. *capsulatum* (*H. capsulatum*) which can produce systemic histoplasmosis mainly in dogs and cats; *Histoplasma capsulatum* var. *farciminosum* (*H. farciminosum*) which causes equine epizootic lymphangitis; *Histoplasma capsulatum* var. *duboisii*, a human pathogen limited to parts of equatorial Africa. The teleomorphs of these variants are ascomycetes, designated *Ajellomyces capsulatus*. The mould and yeast forms of *H. capsulatum* are shown in Fig. 41.2.

Usual habitat

Histoplasma capsulatum is found in soil, particularly when enriched with bird or bat faeces. Aerosols, following disturbance of soil beneath roosting sites, contain large numbers of infective propagules. *Histoplasma farciminosum* is a soil saprophyte.

Recognition and laboratory diagnosis

- When cultured at 25°C to 30°C on Sabouraud dextrose agar, the mould form grows as white to buff colonies with cottony aerial hyphae. Septate hyphae bear small conidia. In mature colonies, slender conidiophores produce tuberculate, sunflower-like macroconidia (9 to 15 μm in diameter).
- When cultured at 37°C on brain-heart infusion agar with added cysteine and 5% blood, yeast colonies are round, mucoid and cream-coloured. Budding yeast cells are oval to spherical (2 to 5 μm in diameter).
- A commercially available nucleic acid probe can be used for identification of isolates (Stockman *et al.*, 1993).
- Giemsa-stained smears of exudates or aspirates may be used for demonstrating yeast forms in macrophages.

Mould form

Septate hypha bearing small conidia. Later, sunflower-like macroconidia (9-15 μm in diameter) form when cultured at 25°C

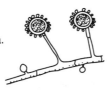

Yeast form

Small oval budding yeast cells (2-5 μm in diameter) in cultures at 37°C. Found also in tissues

Yeast cells in a macrophage

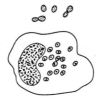

Figure 41.2 The mould and yeast forms of *Histoplasma capsulatum*.

- Histopathological examination of affected tissues reveals pyogranulomatous foci containing yeast forms.
- A positive skin test, using histoplasmin, merely indicates exposure to the fungus.
- Using histoplasmin as antigen in an agar gel immunodiffusion test, two precipitin bands H and M can be identified with serum from affected animals. The reliability of this test for the diagnosis of the disease in animals is questionable.

Clinical infections

Histoplasmosis, which occurs in many countries, is endemic in the Mississippi and Ohio river valleys and in other areas of the USA. The dog and cat are the domestic species most often affected clinically. Epizootic lymphangitis occurs in *Equidae* in Africa, the Middle East and Asia.

Canine and feline histoplasmosis

Most infections in these species are asymptomatic. Following inhalation, microconidia are ingested by pulmonary alveolar macrophages, in which the yeast forms replicate. Granulomatous lesions may be found in the lungs of both dogs and cats. Disseminated disease has been recorded in both species probably associated with impaired cell-mediated immunity. In dogs, ulcerative intestinal lesions are commonly encountered whereas intestinal involvement is rare in cats. Clinical signs in affected dogs include chronic cough, persistent diarrhoea and emaciation. Less frequently, peripheral lymphadenitis, ulcerative skin nodules, eye lesions, lameness and neurological dysfunction may be encountered. The clinical signs in cats relate mainly to pulmonary involvement and include dyspnoea, depression, fever and loss of weight. Disseminated histoplasmosis is invariably fatal. Ketoconazole and amphotericin B can be used for treatment. Animals should be monitored for signs of toxicity.

Epizootic lymphangitis

Epizootic lymphangitis, caused by *H. farciminosum*, is a contagious disease of *Equidae* which may have a high prevalence when animals are in close contact. Infection is usually acquired from environmental sources through minor skin abrasions on the limbs. However, primary ocular and pulmonary involvement have also been recorded. Characteristic lymphocutaneous lesions, which resemble those of equine farcy (*see* Chapter 19), consist of ulcerated discharging nodules usually located along the course of thickened, hard lymphatic vessels. Regional lymphadenopathy is often present. Yeast cells of *H. farciminosum* are found in large numbers in lesions mainly within macrophages (Chandler *et al.*, 1980). *Histoplasma farciminosum*, present in discharges, can be spread by biting insects and through contaminated grooming gear and harness.

In most countries where the disease is exotic, it is notifiable and a test and slaughter policy is implemented. If treatment is considered advisable, surgical excision of skin lesions may be attempted in conjunction with sodium iodide therapy.

Coccidioides immitis

The geophilic fungus *C. immitis* can infect many animal species including humans. Although grouped with the dimorphic fungi, *C. immitis* is biphasic rather than dimorphic because typical yeast forms are not produced. Large spherules containing endospores develop in tissues. The spherule and mould forms of this fungus are shown in Fig. 41.3. Respiratory infections may follow inhalation of arthroconidia (arthrospores) produced from the mould form of the fungus in soil. Systemic spread from pulmonary lesions has been described. A teleomorphic stage of *C. immitis* has not been demonstrated.

Usual habitat

Coccidioides immitis grows in the soil of arid or semi-arid low-lying areas, especially in the Americas. Dust in these areas may be heavily contaminated with arthroconidia.

Recognition and laboratory diagnosis

Because culturing of *C. immitis* is hazardous, it should be attempted only when stringent precautions are observed, including the use of a biohazard cabinet. Diagnosis is usually based on clinical findings and histopathology.

- When cultured on Sabouraud dextrose agar at 25°C to 30°C, colonies are shiny, moist and grey becoming white and cottony. Thick-walled, barrel-shaped arthroconidia, separated by empty cells which undergo degeneration, are released following hyphal fragmentation (Fig. 41.3).
- The identity of suspect cultures can be confirmed using aqueous extracts in immunodiffusion tests with specific *C. immitis* antiserum.
- A commercially available nucleic acid probe can be used on cultures for identification (Stockman *et al.*, 1993).
- The history may indicate that a suspect animal came from an endemic area.
- Spherules of *C. immitis* may be demonstrated in exudates or aspirates cleared with 10% KOH and may also be identified in stained tissue sections.
- Complement fixation and latex agglutination tests can be employed to demonstrate rising antibody titres.

- A positive skin test, using a filtrate of a mycelial culture (coccidioidin), is indicative of exposure to the fungus.
- Intraperitoneal inoculation of mice with material from cultures may be necessary to demonstrate the formation of spherules *in vivo*.

Clinical infections

Since the occurrence of *C. immitis* is limited to defined arid regions of southwestern USA, Mexico and Central and South America, most cases of coccidioidomycosis are encountered in animals from these areas. Although many animals from these regions become infected, relatively few develop clinical disease. The domestic species most often affected is the dog. Clinical coccidioidomycosis has also been described in horses.

Canine coccidioidomycosis

Dogs with mild pulmonary coccidioidomycosis, which present with non-specific signs including cough, fever and inappetence, may recover spontaneously. Animals with extensive pulmonary lesions display persistent coughing, weakness, depression, fluctuating fever and loss of weight. Dissemination from pulmonary lesions, which is frequently related to immunosuppression, often results in osteomyelitis with lameness and radiological evidence of bone destruction as the condition progresses. Other tissues, including the skin, may be affected. Ketoconazole therapy, continued for at least 6 months, may be effective.

Equine coccidioidomycosis

Clinical signs of coccidioidomycosis in horses are non-specific and include intermittent fever, abdominal pain, loss of weight and evidence of pulmonary and musculoskeletal involvement. Pulmonary disease, in which coughing may be the only presenting sign, occurs in about 60% of cases. Musculoskeletal pain, usually associated with osteomyelitis, is evident in about one third of infected

Mould form

Septate hyphae with barrel-shaped arthrospores (2-4 x 5-6 μm) separated by empty cells are formed in soil and cultures

Spherule

Mature spherules (30-100 μm) containing endospores are found in tissues

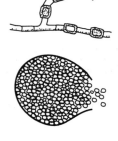

Figure 41.3 The mould form and spherule of *Coccidioides immitis*.

animals. Recurrent superficial abscessation is also a feature. Thickening of the placenta, plaque-like lesions on the umbilical cord and nodules in the lungs of the foetus were recorded in a case of abortion caused by *C. immitis* (Langham *et al.*, 1977). Treatment of disseminated coccidioidomycosis is usually unsuccessful.

Sporothrix schenckii

Sporothrix schenckii is widely distributed in the environment where it grows as a mould producing slender hyphae (1 to 2 μm in diameter) and conidiophores. The yeast and mould forms of this fungus are shown in Fig. 41.4. Infection occurs sporadically in horses, cats, dogs and humans. *Sporothrix schenckii* occurs worldwide and is particularly important in subtropical and tropical regions.

Usual habitat

The fungus is saprophytic on dead or senescent vegetation such as rose thorns, timber, hay, straw and sphagnum moss.

Recognition and laboratory diagnosis

- When cultured on Sabouraud dextrose agar at 25°C, mould colonies grow rapidly and are white, becoming black or brown, wrinkled and leathery. Pear-shaped conidia are borne in a rosette pattern on slender conidiophores. In older cultures, conidia form singly on hyphae.
- When cultured at 35°C to 37°C on brain-heart infusion agar containing 5% blood, cream to tan yeast colonies develop within 3 weeks. The yeast cells, (2 to 3 x 3 to 5 μm), are cigar-shaped.
- Direct microscopic examination of exudates from feline lesions stained with methylene blue usually reveals large numbers of yeast cells. They are sparse in exudates from other animals.

Mould form

Thin septate hyphae with tapering conidiophores bearing conidia (2x4 μm) in rosette-like clusters. Conidia occur singly along the hyphae. Both are found in cultures at 25°C

Yeast form

Cigar-shaped, pleomorphic budding yeast cell (3-5 μm) when cultured at 37°C. Found also in exudates

Figure 41.4 The mould and yeast forms of *Sporothrix schenckii*.

- Histopathological examination of tissue sections, stained by the PAS or methenamine silver techniques, may reveal yeast cells.
- Fluorescent antibody or immunoperoxidase techniques applied to tissue sections allow specific identification of the yeast cells.

Clinical infections

Sporotrichosis is a chronic cutaneous or lymphocutaneous disease which rarely becomes generalized. Dissemination usually occurs in immunocompromized individuals. Sporadic cases are recorded in horses, cats, dogs, cattle, goats, pigs and humans.

Equine sporotrichosis

Lymphocutaneous sporotrichosis is the most common form of the disease in horses (Blackford, 1984). Fungal spores usually enter through skin abrasions on the lower limbs. Nodules, which ulcerate and discharge a yellowish exudate, develop along the course of superficial lymphatic vessels. Subcutaneous oedema in the affected limb may result from lymphatic obstruction. Treatment with inorganic iodides, administered in the feed, should continue for approximately 30 days after clinical recovery. Animals undergoing treatment should be monitored for signs of iodism. Surgical excision of early lesions may be feasible.

Feline sporotrichosis

Nodular skin lesions occur most often on limb extremities, head and tail. Secondary nodules can develop along the course of lymphatics. Infection may be spread to other skin sites by grooming. Nodules ulcerate and discharge a seropurulent exudate. Following ulceration, extensive areas of underlying muscle and bone may be exposed (Dunstan *et al.*, 1986). Large numbers of yeast cells in discharges from lesions in cats may pose a health hazard to humans handling affected animals (Zamri-Saad *et al.*, 1990). Sodium iodide, administered in the food, is effective for treating the cutaneous and lymphocutaneous forms of the disease. Treatment should be continued for 30 days after clinical recovery. If signs of iodism develop, treatment should be suspended for a period. Ketoconazole may be used in conjunction with sodium iodide in intractable cases.

Canine sporotrichosis

Sporotrichosis in dogs often manifests as multiple, ulcerated and crusted, alopecic, cutaneous lesions over the head and trunk. Lymphocutaneous involvement occasionally occurs but disseminated disease is rare (Scott *et al.*, 1974). The treatment regime is similar to that for cats.

References

Archer, J.R., Trainer, D.O. and Schell, R.F. (1987). Epidemiologic study of canine blastomycosis in Wisconsin. *Journal of the American Veterinary Medical Association*, **190**, 1292–1295.

Blackford, J. (1984). Superficial and deep mycoses in horses. *Veterinary Clinics of North America: Large Animal Practice*, **6**, 47–58.

Breider, M.A., Walker, T.L., Legendre, A.M. and VanEe, R.T. (1988). Blastomycosis in cats: five cases (1979–1986). *Journal of the American Veterinary Medical Association*, **193**, 570–572.

Chandler, F.W., Kaplan, W. and Ajello, L. (1980). *Histoplasmosis farciminosi*. In *Histopathology of Mycotic Diseases*. Wolfe Medical Publications, London. pp. 70–72; 216–217.

Costa, E.O., Diniz, L.S.M. and Netto, C.F. (1995). The prevalence of positive intradermal reactions to paracoccidioidin in domestic and wild animals in Sao Paulo, Brazil. *Veterinary Research Communications*, **19**, 127–130.

Di Salvo, A.F. (1998). *Blastomyces dermatitidis*. In *Topley and Wilson's Microbiology and Microbial Infections*. Ninth Edition. Volume 4. Eds. L. Ajello and R.J. Hay. Arnold, London. pp. 337-355.

Dunstan, R.W., Reimann, K.A. and Langham, R.F. (1986). Feline sporotrichosis. *Journal of the American Veterinary Medical Association*, **189**, 880–883.

Langham, R.F., Beneke, E.S. and Whitenack, D.L. (1977). Abortion in a mare due to coccidioidomycosis. *Journal of the American Veterinary Medical Association*, **170**, 178–180.

Legendre, A.M., Walker, M., Buyukmihci, N. and Stevens, R. (1981). Canine blastomycosis: a review of 47 clinical cases. *Journal of the American Veterinary Medical Association*, **178**, 1163–1168.

Scott, D.W., Bentinck-Smith, J. and Haggerty, G.F. (1974). Sporotrichosis in three dogs. *Cornell Veterinarian*, **64**, 416–426.

Stockman, L., Clark, K.A., Hunt, J.M. and Roberts, G.D. (1993). Evaluation of commercially available acridinium ester-labelled chemiluminescent DNA probes for culture identification of *Blastomyces dermatitidis*, *Coccidioides immitis*, *Cryptococcus neoformans* and *Histoplasma capsulatum*. *Journal of Clinical Microbiology*, **31**, 845–850.

Wolf, A.M. (1979). Primary cutaneous coccidioidomycosis in a dog and cat. *Journal of the American Veterinary Medical Association*, **174**, 504–506.

Zamri-Saad, M., Salmiyah, T.S., Jasni, S., Cheng, B.Y. and Basri, K. (1990). Feline sporotrichosis: an increasingly important zoonotic disease in Malaysia. *Veterinary Record*, **127**, 480.

Further reading

Fawi, M.T. (1969). Fluorescent antibody test for the serodiagnosis of *Histoplasma farciminosum* infections in *Equidae*. *British Veterinary Journal*, **125**, 231–234.

Gabal, M.A. and Mohammed, K.A. (1985). Use of enzyme-linked immunosorbent assay for the diagnosis of equine *Histoplasma farciminosi* (epizootic lymphangitis). *Mycopathologia*, **91**, 35–37.

Kowalewich, N., Hawkins, E.C., Skowronek, A.J. and Clemo, F.A.S. (1993). Identification of *Histoplasma capsulatum* organisms in the pleural and peritoneal effusions of a dog. *Journal of the American Veterinary Medical Association*, **202**, 423–426.

Wolf, A.M. and Beldin, M.N. (1984). Feline histoplasmosis: a literature review and retrospective study of 20 new cases. *Journal of the American Animal Hospital Association*, **20**, 995–998.

Ziermer, E.L., Pappagianis, D., Madigan, J.E., Mansmann, R.A. and Hoffman, K.D. (1992). Coccidioidomycosis in horses: 15 cases (1975–1984). *Journal of the American Veterinary Medical Association*, **201**, 910–916.

Chapter 42

Zygomycetes of veterinary importance

Fungi in the phylum Zygomycota characteristically have broad (6 to 15 μm), aseptate hyphae and replicate asexually by producing sporangiospores within a sporangium. Fusion of gametangia from two different strains, resulting in the production of a thick walled zygospore, is the mode of sexual reproduction. Zygospores are seldom formed in cultures except in the case of *Basidiobolus* species. The absence of septa allows nutrients to pass along hyphae resulting in rapid growth. Septa may occasionally be observed at sites of hyphal damage and close to sporangia.

Two orders in the phylum, *Mucorales* and *Entomophthorales*, are of veterinary importance. Genera in these orders containing potentially pathogenic species are indicated in Figure 42.1. These fungi, which are widely distributed saprophytes, can cause sporadic opportunistic infections. The term zygomycosis is applied to disease caused by infection with a member of the Zygomycota. The term phycomycosis was formerly used to encompass infection by zygomycetes or by *Pythium insidiosum*, a fungal-like organism which produces opportunistic infections similar to those produced by zygomycetes (*see* Chapter 43).

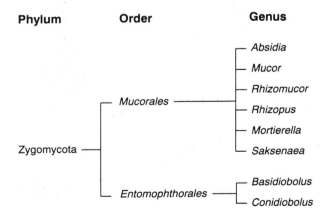

Figure 42.1 Genera of the zygomycetes which include species of veterinary importance.

Key points

- Broad aseptate hyphae (up to 15 μm diameter)
- Sporangiospores produced asexually
- Zygospores are the sexual spores
- Saprophytes, widely distributed in the environment
- Rapid growth
- Cause zygomycoses
- *Mucorales*
  —*Absidia, Mucor, Rhizomucor* and *Rhizopus* are typical zygomycetes
  —*Mortierella* and *Saksenaea* species form spores only on nutrient-deficient media
  —Immunosuppression may predispose to infection
  —Mucormycoses are often systemic diseases
  —*Mortierella wolfii* associated with abortion and pneumonia in cattle
- *Entomophthorales*
  —Sporangium functions as a single conidium
  —Hyphae, sometimes septate, produced in animal tissues (up to 20 mm diameter)
  —Characteristic aggregates around hyphae
  —Granulomas caused by *Basidiobolus* species and *Conidiobolus* species; most common in horses

Mucorales

These fungi are commonly known as 'pin' or 'bread' moulds because their dark sporangia resemble pinheads and they are often found growing on stale bread. The morphological features of some members of the *Mucorales* are illustrated in Fig. 42.2. Several genera produce root-like rhizoids which allow anchorage to surfaces. Colonies grow rapidly on culture plates.

Strains associated with animal disease, which grow well at 37°C on Sabouraud dextrose agar, are susceptible to cycloheximide. Sporulation of two species, *Mortierella*

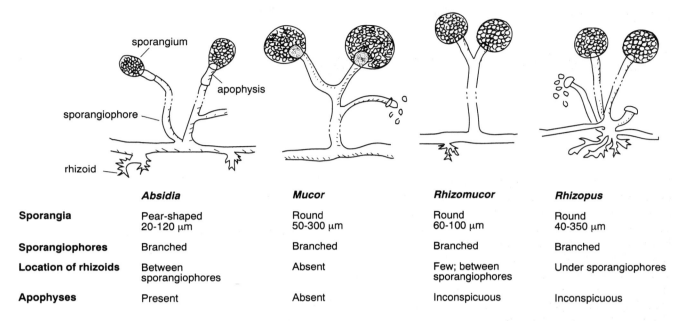

	Absidia	**Mucor**	**Rhizomucor**	**Rhizopus**
Sporangia	Pear-shaped 20-120 μm	Round 50-300 μm	Round 60-100 μm	Round 40-350 μm
Sporangiophores	Branched	Branched	Branched	Branched
Location of rhizoids	Between sporangiophores	Absent	Few; between sporangiophores	Under sporangiophores
Apophyses	Present	Absent	Inconspicuous	Inconspicuous

Figure 42.2 Morphological features of members of *Mucorales* which produce sporangia on standard fungal media.

wolfii and *Saksenaea vasiformis*, occurs only on media deficient in certain nutrients.

Mucormycoses, diseases caused by fungi belonging to the order *Mucorales*, are encountered sporadically worldwide. They often involve the gastrointestinal tract, the respiratory tract and associated lymph nodes. Dissemination to other organs may occur. Infection may be associated with immunosuppression.

Usual habitat

Members of the *Mucorales* are saprophytes present in soil and vegetation and their spores are often airborne. Although *M. wolfii* has been isolated from soil near silage and rotting hay, it is otherwise difficult to recover from environmental sources.

Differentiation of members of the *Mucorales*

- Colonial morphology:
  —Growth of *Absidia, Mucor, Rhizomucor* and *Rhizopus* species is rapid, filling the Petri dish with greyish or brownish-grey fluffy colonies within a few days.
  —*Mortierella wolfii* has characteristic white velvety colonies with lobulated outlines. Colonies are about 5 cm in diameter after incubation for 4 days.
  —*Saksenaea vasiformis* produces rapidly-growing colonies with a white downy appearance.
- Microscopic appearance:
  —Morphological features allow differentiation of the genera (Fig. 42.2).
  —Sporulation of *M. wolfii* and *S. vasiformis* can be

induced by subculturing onto nutrient-deficient media such as hay-infusion agar. These two fungi have distinctive structural features (Fig. 42.3).
- Differentiation of species in the genera *Absidia, Mucor, Rhizomucor* and *Rhizopus* is carried out in reference laboratories.

Pathogenesis and pathology

Infection with these fungi is uncommon in healthy immunocompetent individuals. Factors which may predispose to infection include immunodeficiency, corticosteroid therapy, prolonged administration of broad-spectrum

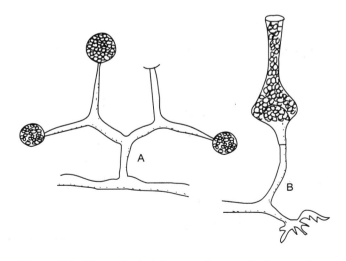

Figure 42.3 Morphological features of sporangiophores and sporangia of *Mortierella wolfii* (A) and *Saksenaea vasiformis* (B). Sporulation is induced by nutrient-deficient media.

antibiotics and viral diseases such as panleukopenia and infectious peritonitis in cats (Ossent, 1987). Infection may follow ingestion or inhalation of spores from contaminated environmental sources. Hyphae invade the mucosa, submucosa and local vessel walls producing an acute necrotizing thrombotic vasculitis. Chronic lesions are usually localized and granulomatous.

Diagnostic procedures

- Apart from *M. wolfii,* which may produce abortion followed by acute pneumonia, members of the *Mucorales* rarely cause recognizable disease syndromes in animals.
- Specimens for laboratory examination should include tissues for both histopathology and culture. Cotyledons, abomasal contents from foetuses and uterine discharges should be collected from cases of abortion. Isolation of *M. wolfii* from autolyzed tissues may be difficult.
- Staining of tissue sections by the PAS or methenamine silver techniques facilitates detection of aseptate hyphae.
- Fluorescent antibody methods have been used for identifying pathogens such as *Absidia corymbifera* (Jensen *et al.*, 1990).
- Isolation is carried out on Sabouraud dextrose agar without cycloheximide. Cultures are incubated aerobically at 37°C for up to 5 days.
- Identification criteria for isolates:
  — Colonial morphology
  — Microscopic morphological features (Fig. 42.2)
- Serological tests such as agar gel diffusion have been developed but are of uncertain diagnostic value.

Clinical infections

The zygomycoses of domestic animals are presented in Table 42.1. Laboratory procedures including isolation of the fungus and demonstration of hyphae in affected tissues are essential for the diagnosis of zygomycosis. The clinical signs, relating to the condition which predisposed to fungal invasion, may mask signs arising from the fungal infection. Irrespective of the location, mycotic lesions caused by members of the *Mucorales* are less commonly encountered than those caused by *Aspergillus* species.

Mycotic abortion

The prevalence of mycotic abortion in cattle is influenced by climatic and other environmental factors. Reports from some regions suggest that fungi may be involved in 7% of bovine abortions (Knudtson and Kirkbride, 1992).

Table 42.1 Zygomycoses of domestic animals.

Fungal disease	Hosts	Clinical conditions
Mucormycosis	Cattle	Mesenteric and mediastinal lymphadenitis Abortion Pneumonia following abortion caused by *Mortierella wolfii* Oesophagitis and enteritis in calves Rumenitis, abomasal ulcers Cranial granuloma
	Pigs	Enteritis in piglets Mesenteric and mandibular lymphadenitis Gastrointestinal ulcers
	Cats	Focal necrotizing pneumonia Necrotic enteritis
	Dogs	Enteritis
Entomophthomycosis	Horses	Cutaneous granulomas caused by *Basidiobolus* species Nasal granulomas caused by *Conidiobolus* species
	Dogs	Gastrointestinal and pulmonary granulomas caused by *Basidiobolus* species Subcutaneous granulomas caused by *Conidiobolus* species
	Sheep	Nasal granulomas caused by *Conidiobolus* species

Although *Aspergillus* species account for the majority of cases in many countries, *M. wolfii, Absidia* species, *Mucor* species and *Rhizopus* species have also been implicated and, in some regions, may predominate. Abortion, which usually occurs late in gestation, is often linked to the feeding of mouldy hay or silage. The location of lesions on cotyledons suggests haematogenous infection of the uterus, possibly from a pulmonary or enteric source. The cotyledons are enlarged and necrotic, and the intercotyledonary placental tissue is thickened and leathery. Vasculitis, associated with hyphal invasion, is demonstrable in sections of affected cotyledons. Occasionally, lesions may be observed grossly on the skin of aborted foetuses.

Abortion due to *M. wolfii*, an important cause of mycotic abortion in New Zealand, may be followed within days by an acute fibrinonecrotic fungal pneumonia (Carter *et al.*, 1973). Because of the difficulty in isolating *M. wolfii* from autolyzed tissues, abortion caused by this organism may be under-diagnosed (MacDonald and Corbel, 1981). Mycotic abortion in mares caused by *Absidia corymbifera* has been reported.

Alimentary tract infections

Mycotic rumenitis in cattle may follow mucosal damage associated with ruminal lactic acidosis. The microscopic appearance of the causal fungi in ruminal lesions suggests that, in most cases, zygomycetes are involved. In some instances, *Rhizopus* species have been isolated (Barker *et al.*, 1993). Infarction, due to thrombotic arteritis, necrosis and haemorrhage are major features of the mycotic lesions. Extension of the inflammatory process through the ruminal wall results in fibrinous peritonitis. Zygomycotic abomasitis in calves, which may follow neonatal infection, can also produce perforation and peritonitis. Acute gastrointestinal zygomycosis has been recorded in piglets (Reed *et al.*, 1987).

Mycotic pneumonia

An acute fatal pneumonia of cows, which is caused by *M. wolfii* and occasionally follows abortion due to the fungus, is a well recognized syndrome in New Zealand (Carter *et al.*, 1973). Chronic pneumonic lesions caused by other zygomycetes are encountered sporadically in cattle and other domestic species.

Entomophthorales

Two genera in the *Entomophthorales*, *Basidiobolus* and *Conidiobolus*, are sometimes associated with opportunistic infections in animals. A unique feature of these fungi is the production of a single conidium which is forcibly discharged when mature.

Usual habitat

Basidiobolus species are saprophytes in soil, decaying fruit and vegetable material, and may be present in the faeces of amphibians, reptiles, insectivorous bats and marsupials (Speare and Thomas, 1985).

  Conidiobolus species are saprophytes in soil and in decaying vegetation, particularly in rain forests.

Differentiation of the *Entomophthorales*

- Colonial morphology :
  — *Basidiobolus* species are moderately fast-growing and form flat, smooth, yellowish-grey colonies which become radially folded with a white powdery surface. They have an earthy odour similar to that of *Streptomyces* species.
  — *Conidiobolus* species grow rapidly and produce flat, smooth, cream-coloured colonies which become radially folded and brownish with a white powdery

surface. Discharged conidia adhere to the Petri dish lid.
- Microscopic appearance:
  — *Basidiobolus* species have broad (20 µm in diameter) mainly aseptate hyphae in which round, thick-walled zygospores (20 to 50 µm in diameter) form.
  — *Conidiobolus* species produce simple conidiophores which bear solitary, spherical conidia (10 to 25 µm in diameter). Germination of conidia results in the production of single or multiple hyphal tubes with secondary conidia.
- Differentiation to a specific level is carried out in mycological reference laboratories.

Pathogenesis and pathology

Although not clearly defined, the route of entry of these fungi is probably through minor abrasions in the skin or nasal mucous membranes. Hyphal invasion of blood vessels is uncommon. Spread by lymphatics sometimes occurs (Hillier *et al.*, 1994). Although disseminated disease is rare, it has been reported in a dog infected with *B. haptosporus* (Miller and Turnwald, 1984).

  Granulomatous lesions result from infection with these opportunistic pathogens. An eosinophilic deposit, around individual hyphae (Splendore-Hoeppli phenomenon) may represent an immune complex (Miller and Campbell, 1984).

Diagnostic procedures

- Specimens for laboratory examination should include biopsy or postmortem tissues for histopathology and culture.
- Fungal hyphae must be demonstrated in tissue sections. The hyphae of *Basidiobolus* species are usually up to 20 µm in diameter whereas those of *Conidiobolus* species are up to 12 µm in diameter. There may be evidence of the Splendore-Hoeppli phenomenon around hyphae.
- These fungi can be isolated on Sabouraud dextrose agar without added cyclohexamide after incubation aerobically at 37°C for up to 5 days.
- Identification criteria for isolates:
  — Colonial morphology
  — Microscopic appearance
- For identification to a specific level, specimens should be sent to a reference laboratory.

Clinical infections

The entomophthomycoses of domestic animals are indicated in Table 42.1. *Basidiobolus* species cause cutaneous lesions in the horse which resemble those associated with *Pythium insidiosum* (*see* Chapter 43). Infections with *Conidiobolus* species cause nasal granulomas in horses

(Humber *et al.*, 1989), sheep (Carrigan *et al.*, 1992) and llamas (French and Ashworth, 1994). On rare occasions, *Conidiobolus* species cause pyogranulomatous and cutaneous lesions in dogs (Hillier *et al.*, 1994).

References

Barker, I.K., van Dreumel, A.A. and Palmer, N. (1993). In: *Pathology of Domestic Animals*. Fourth Edition. Eds. K.V.F. Jubb, P.C. Kennedy and N. Palmer. Academic Press, San Diego. pp. 1–318.

Carrigan, M.J., Small, A.C. and Perry, G.H. (1992). Ovine nasal zygomycosis caused by *Conidiobolus incongruus*. *Australian Veterinary Journal*, **69**, 237–240.

Carter, M.E., Cordes, D.O., Di Menna, M.E. and Hunter, R. (1973). Fungi isolated from bovine mycotic abortion and pneumonia with special reference to *Mortierella wolfii*. *Research in Veterinary Science*, **14**, 201–206.

French, R.A. and Ashworth, C.D. (1994). Zygomycosis caused by *Conidiobolus coronatus* in a llama (*Lama glama*). *Veterinary Pathology*, **31**, 120–122.

Hillier, A., Kunkle, G.A., Ginn, P.E. and Padhye, A.A. (1994). Canine subcutaneous zygomycosis caused by *Conidiobolus* sp.: a case report and review of conidiobolus infections in other species. *Veterinary Dermatology*, **5**, 205–213.

Humber, R.A., Brown, C.C. and Kornegay, R.W. (1989). Equine zygomycosis caused by *Conidiobolus lamprauges*. *Journal of Clinical Microbiology*, **27**, 573–576.

Jensen, H.E., Schonheyder, H. and Jorgensen, J.B. (1990). Intestinal and pulmonary mycotic lymphadenitis in cattle. *Journal of Comparative Pathology*, **102**, 345–354.

Knudtson, W.U. and Kirkbride, C.A. (1992). Fungi associated with bovine abortion in the northern plain states (USA). *Journal of Veterinary Diagnostic Investigation*, **4**, 181–185.

MacDonald, S.M. and Corbel, M.J. (1981). *Mortierella wolfii* infection in cattle in Britain. *Veterinary Record*, **109**, 419–421.

Miller, R.I. and Campbell, R.S.F. (1984). The comparative pathology of equine cutaneous phycomycosis. *Veterinary Pathology*, **21**, 325–332.

Miller, R.I. and Turnwald, G.H. (1984). Disseminated basidiobolomycosis in a dog. *Veterinary Pathology*, **21**, 117–119.

Ossent, P. (1987). Systemic aspergillosis and mucormycosis in 23 cats. *Veterinary Record*, **120**, 330–333.

Reed, W.M., Hanika, C., Mehdi, N.A.Q. and Shackelford, C. (1987). Gastrointestinal zygomycosis in suckling pigs. *Journal of the American Veterinary Medical Association*, **191**, 549–550.

Speare, R. and Thomas, A.D. (1985). Kangaroos and wallabies as carriers of *Basidiobolus haptosporus*. *Australian Veterinary Journal*, **62**, 209–210.

Further reading

Hill, B.D., Black, P.F., Kelly, M., Muir, D. and McDonald, W.A.J. (1992). Bovine cranial zygomycosis caused by *Saksenaea vasiformis*. *Australian Veterinary Journal*, **69**, 173–174.

Miller, R. and Pott, B. (1980). Phycomycosis of the horse caused by *Basidiobolus haptosporus*. *Australian Veterinary Journal*, **56**, 224–227.

Chapter 43

Fungus-like organisms of veterinary importance

Three eukaryotic, fungus-like organisms *Pythium insidiosum*, *Rhinosporidium seeberi*, and *Loboa loboi* cause rare sporadic infections in animals which have contact with contaminated water. These organisms, which are found in either mycelial or unicellular forms in tissues, induce host reactions similar to those encountered in fungal infections. Pythiosis and rhinosporidiosis have been described in domestic animal species and in humans. *Loboa loboi* is mainly a human pathogen although sporadic cases have been recorded in dolphins.

Pythium insidiosum

This fungus-like organism, also known as *Hyphomyces destruens*, is classified in the kingdom Chromista and found in aquatic environments. It is an opportunistic animal pathogen whereas many other *Pythium* species are important as plant pathogens. Infection with *P. insidiosum* is rare in animals. Plant infections are essential for the propagation of the organism and the production of motile zoospores (Fig. 43.1).

Pythium insidiosum grows on a variety of laboratory media when incubated at both 25°C and 37°C. However, zoospores are produced only in water cultures. On solid media and in plant and animal tissues, the organism develops aseptate hyphae (4 to 10 μm in diameter) which are similar morphologically to those of the zygomycetes.

Pythiosis, characterized by granulomatous lesions in subcutaneous or intestinal tissues, has been reported in horses, dogs, calves and a cat.

Usual habitat

Pythium insidiosum is usually found in stagnant inland waters and occasionally in soil.

Pathogenicity

Motile zoospores, which are apparently attracted by chemotaxis to wounds and abrasions on skin or intestinal mucosa, encyst on the exposed tissues. The encysted zoospores secrete a sticky material, possibly glycoprotein,

---

Key points

- *Pythium insidiosum*
  —Member of the kingdom Chromista
  —Found mainly in bodies of stagnant water
  —Genus contains important plant pathogens
  —Grows on wide varity of media
  —Motile zoospores may invade animal tissue with mild abrasions
  —Causes cutaneous pythiosis in horses and gastrointestinal pythiosis in dogs
- *Rhinosporidium seeberi*
  —Fungal-like organism of low pathogenic potential
  —Found in stagnant water
  —Does not grow on inert media
  —Rhinosporidiosis, which occurs in horses, dogs and cattle, is characterized by nasal polyp formation
- *Loboa loboi*
  —Aquatic yeast-like organism
  —Has not been cultured *in vitro*
  —Causes cutaneous lesions in humans and dolphins

---

which allows adhesion to tissues prior to invasion. Aseptate hyphae, which develop from germ tubes produced by the zoospores at body temperature, extend into the tissues and may invade blood vessels, facilitating dissemination and producing thrombosis.

Diagnostic procedures

- The nature and distribution of lesions and a history of access to stagnant water in regions where pythiosis occurs may suggest the disease.
- Specimens, including biopsy material and samples from cutaneous lesions in horses, should be delivered immediately to the laboratory. Samples for transportation should be washed in sterile distilled water and transported at ambient temperature.

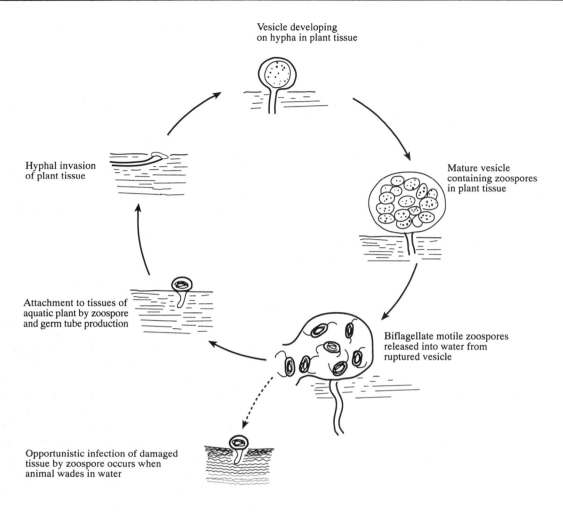

Vesicle developing
on hypha in plant tissue

Hyphal invasion
of plant tissue

Mature vesicle
containing zoospores
in plant tissue

Attachment to tissues of
aquatic plant by zoospore
and germ tube production

Biflagellate motile zoospores
released into water from
ruptured vesicle

Opportunistic infection of damaged
tissue by zoospore occurs when
animal wades in water

Figure 43.1 Stages in the life cycle of *Pythium insidiosum* in plant tissue. Sporadic invasion of animal tissue can occur at sites of minor trauma when animals are wading in water.

- Tissue sections, stained by the PAS or methenamine silver methods, are used to demonstrate hyphal forms.
- Immunofluorescence or immunoperoxidase techniques can be used to identify *P. insidiosum* in tissue sections.
- Sabouraud dextrose agar, inoculated with material from lesions, is incubated aerobically at 37°C for 24 to 48 hours. The colonies, which are flat, whitish and radiating, may be up to 20 mm in diameter after 24 hours.
- Identification criteria for isolates:
  — Colonial morphology
  — Aseptate hyphae
- Specific identification should be carried out in a reference laboratory.
- Serological tests such as agar gel diffusion and ELISA have been used for diagnosis in affected animals.

Clinical infections

Pythiosis is a rare, sporadic, non-contagious condition which occurs mainly in tropical and subtropical regions. It has been recorded in Australia, New Zealand, New Guinea, the Caribbean Islands and in South, Central and North America. Although horses and dogs are the species most commonly infected, a few cases have been reported in calves (Miller *et al.*, 1985).

Pythiosis in horses

Cutaneous pythiosis is the usual presentation in horses (Chaffin *et al.*, 1992), although intestinal pythiosis has also been reported (Morton *et al.*, 1991). Lesions usually occur on those parts of the body, particularly the limbs, which come in contact with water containing zoospores. Lesions are large, circular, granulomatous nodules which often ulcerate. Sinus tracts may develop exuding a serosanguineous discharge. Pruritis is marked. Necrotic yellowish coral-like masses ('kunkers' or 'leeches') can be removed intact from the granulomas. In addition to necrotic tissue, these masses contain eosinophils and hyphae of *P. insidiosum* (Mendoza *et al.*, 1993). Bone involvement can occur in chronic disease. Surgical excision of lesions followed by immunotherapy has been proposed (Miller, 1981). Enteric pythiosis is characterized by stenotic fibrous gastrointestinal lesions.

Pythiosis in dogs

Canine infection most commonly involves the stomach and small intestine (Miller, 1985). Subcutaneous pythiosis is less commonly encountered (Foil *et al.*, 1984). Intestinal lesions are usually extensive when an affected animal is first presented for examination. Clinical signs include vomiting, weight loss, intermittent diarrhoea and palpable abdominal masses. Extension of the infection to the pancreas, mesenteric lymph nodes and bile ducts may occur. Cutaneous lesions, which occur on limbs, face or tail, are granulomatous nodules often with discharging sinus tracts. Surgical excision of lesions and long-term treatment with itraconazole may be beneficial.

Rhinosporidium seeberi

Rhinosporidium seeberi is a fungus-like organism which has not been cultured on inert media but has been grown in monolayers of human rectal tumour cells (Levy *et al.*, 1986). Rhinosporidiosis, a non-contagious, pyogranulomatous infection of the skin or mucosa, has been recorded in horses, dogs, cattle, goats and waterfowl.

Usual habitat

It is generally considered that stagnant water and possibly soil are the natural habitats of the organism.

Pathogenicity and pathology

Rhinosporidium seeberi is of low pathogenic potential and disseminated infection is rare. The life cycle of the organism is uncertain. Rhinosporidiosis presents most commonly as a chronic polypous rhinitis characterized by the presence of large sporangia (100 to 400 μm in diameter) in affected tissues. The sporangia, which have double-contoured cell walls with an outer chitinous layer and an inner layer of cellulose, contain up to 16,000 endospores (approximately 7 μm in diameter). Mature endospores can be stained by the PAS and methenamine silver methods. Several electron-dense bodies (1.5 to 2.0 μm in diameter) containing DNA are present in the endospores.

The polyps, which may be sessile or pedunculated and up to 3 cm in diameter, are composed of soft fibromyxomatous stromal tissue covered by epithelium. Mature sporangia may be detectable grossly in the stroma as minute white spots. Cellular response to sporangia is sparse except when they rupture. The release of

endospores elicits a marked pyogranulomatous reaction (Easley *et al.*, 1986).

Diagnostic procedures

- Nasal polyposis may suggest the presence of the condition.
- Specimens for laboratory examination should include biopsy material and scrapings from lesions.
- Cytological examination demonstrates a neutrophilic response and many endospores. Neutrophils form in aggregates around endospores.
- Sporangia can be demonstrated histologically in tissue sections.

Clinical infections

Rhinosporidiosis, which is endemic in subtropical and tropical regions, has been encountered also in North America and Europe (Caniatti *et al.*, 1998). Infection occurs through minor trauma in skin or mucous membranes. The reddish-brown polyps in rhinosporidiosis may project from the nares and can occlude the nasal passages. Noisy breathing may be exacerbated by exercise. Nasal discharge is usually present and epistaxis may occur. The uncommon cutaneous lesions may be single or multiple and sessile or pedunculated. Treatment by cryosurgery or electrocauterization is suggested to avoid excessive bleeding. Diaminodiphenylsulphone (dapsone) has proved beneficial although deleterious side effects, including haemolytic anaemia and thrombocytopenia, may occur in dogs.

Loboa loboi

Loboa loboi, an unclassified yeast-like organism not yet cultured *in vitro*, causes granulomatous cutaneous disease (lobomycosis or keloidal blastomycosis) in humans and dolphins. In skin sections stained by the PAS or methenamine silver techniques, large numbers of yeast-like cells (5 to 12 μm in diameter) are present in multinucleate giant cells. They replicate by budding and some remain attached to each other by narrow bridge-like structures forming short chains (Fig. 43.2).

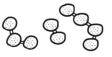

Figure 43.2 Cells of *Loboa loboi* as they appear in smears from lesions. These yeast-like cells often occur in short chains connected by short bridge-like structures.

Lobomycosis has not been reported in domestic animals. Human cases of the disease have been reported from tropical regions of South and Central America and affected dolphins have been found off the coast of Florida. Skin changes in dolphins range from white crusts to nodular or verrucose lesions which ulcerate easily and bleed (Bossart, 1984). Small lesions can be removed surgically.

References

Bossart, G.D. (1984). Suspected acquired immunodeficiency in an Atlantic bottlenosed dolphin with chronic hepatitis and lobomycosis. *Journal of the American Veterinary Medical Association*, **185**, 1413–1414.

Caniatti, M., Roccabianca, P., Scanziani, E. *et al.* (1998). Nasal rhinosporidiosis in dogs: four cases from Europe and a review of the literature. *Veterinary Record*, **142**, 334–338.

Chaffin, M.K., Schumacher, J. and Hooper, N. (1992). Multicentric cutaneous pythiosis in a foal. *Journal of the American Veterinary Medical Association,* **201**, 310–312.

Easley, J.R., Meuten, D.J., Levy, M.G. *et al.* (1986). Nasal rhinosporidiosis in the dog. *Veterinary Pathology*, **23**, 50–56.

Foil, C.S., Short, B.G., Fadok, V.A. and Kunkle, G.A. (1984). A report of subcutaneous pythiosis in five dogs and a review of the etiologic agent *Pythium* spp. *Journal of the American Animal Hospital Association*, **20**, 959–966.

Levy, M.G., Meuten, D.J. and Breitschwerdt, E.B. (1986). Cultivation of *Rhinosporidium seeberi* in vitro: Interaction with epithelial cells. *Science*, **234**, 474–476.

Mendoza, L., Hernandez, F. and Ajello, L. (1993). Life cycle of the human and animal oomycete pathogen *Pythium insidiosum*. *Journal of Clinical Microbiology,* **31**, 2967–2973.

Miller, R.I. (1981). Treatment of equine phycomycosis by immunotherapy and surgery. *Australian Veterinary Journal*, **57**, 377–382.

Miller, R.I. (1985). Gastrointestinal phycomycosis in 63 dogs. *Journal of the American Veterinary Medical Association,* **186**, 473–478.

Miller, R.I., Olcott, B.M. and Archer, M. (1985). Cutaneous pythiosis in beef calves. *Journal of the American Veterinary Medical Association*, **186**, 984–986.

Morton, L.D., Morton, D.G., Baker, G.J. and Gelberg, H.B. (1991). Chronic eosinophilic enteritis attributed to *Pythium* sp. in a horse. *Veterinary Pathology*, **28**, 542–544.

Further reading

Davidson, W.R. and Nettles, V.F. (1977). Rhinosporidiosis in a wood duck. *Journal of the American Veterinary Medical Association*, **171**, 989–990.

Meyers, D.D., Simon, J. and Case, M.T. (1964). Rhinosporidiosis in a horse. *Journal of the American Veterinary Medical Association*, **145**, 345–347.

Chapter 44

Pneumocystis carinii

Pneumocystis carinii, a unicellular organism with a life cycle resembling that of a protozoal parasite, is currently classified in the kingdom Fungi (Pixley *et al.*, 1991). Although the life cycle of *P. carinii* has not yet been fully determined, intrapulmonary infection probably involves asexual and sexual phases. In the asexual phase, a haploid trophic form (1.0 to 1.5 μm in length) replicates by binary division. In the sexual phase conjugation of haploid forms leads to the development of a cyst (5.0 to 8.0 μm in diameter) containing up to eight spores (1 to 2 μm in diameter) which are eventually released. A cell wall is present only in the cyst form of the organism. Because the main sterol in this thin cell wall is cholesterol rather than ergosterol, this form of the organism is refractory to standard anti-fungal drugs. *Pneumocystis carinii* is detected infrequently in the lungs of immunocompetent hosts. In immunocompromized individuals, infection may result in pneumonia. The organism has been found in a wide range of domestic, wild and captive mammalian species. Pneumocystosis in humans is often associated with the immunosuppression following HIV infection. Strains of *P. carinii* from different animal species have distinct molecular and antigenic profiles (Peters *et al.*, 1994). The organism is difficult to culture *in vitro*.

Usual habitat

The natural reservoir of *P. carinii* is not known but serological studies suggest that the organism may be present in young, clinically normal humans and animals.

Pathogenicity and pathology

The exact mode of transmission is uncertain but airborne spread is suspected. In the animal body, the trophic form adheres in clusters to type 1 pneumocytes. Characteristic pathological findings, which are similar in all species, include diffuse pulmonary consolidation, marked thickening of alveolar septa and proteinaceous exudate in alveoli.

Diagnostic procedures

- Specimens for laboratory examination may include lung tissue and bronchoalveolar lavage fluid.

> **Key points**
> - Member of the kingdom Fungi
> - Distinct strains appear to be associated with particular animal species
> - Difficult to culture *in vitro*
> - Trophic, cyst and spore forms may be found in lungs of affected animals
> - Pneumonia, which occurs only in immunosuppressed animals, occasionally affects horses and dogs

- Cytological and histopathological specimens are used for diagnosis. Giemsa-stained preparations can be used to demonstrate the different forms of the organism, whereas the methenamine silver method stains only the cyst form. Fluorescent-conjugated monoclonal antibody techniques are sensitive and specific.
- Immunocytochemical methods can be used for specific identification in tissue sections.
- The organism may be detected during electron microscopic examination of bronchoalveolar lavage fluid.
- The polymerase chain reaction is used in reference laboratories for DNA amplification (Peters *et al.*, 1994).
- Serological tests, employed for epidemiological surveys, are not of diagnostic value.

Clinical infections

Most cases of pneumonia caused by *P. carinii* in domestic species have been recorded in dogs and horses. Hereditary immunodeficiency has been suggested as an explanation for the frequency of the disease in miniature dachshunds (Farrow *et al.*, 1972). Arabian foals with combined immunodeficiency disorder are particularly susceptible (Perryman *et al.*, 1978). Affected animals are afebrile and present with respiratory distress. Without treatment the disease may prove fatal. Trimethoprim-sulphamethoxazole, administered orally for 2 weeks, is usually effective.

References

Farrow, B.R.H., Watson, A.D.J., Hartley, W.J. and Huxtable, C.R.R. (1972). Pneumocystis pneumonia in the dog. *Journal of Comparative Pathology*, **82**, 447–453.

Perryman, L.E., McGuire, T.C. and Crawford, T.B. (1978). Maintenance of foals with combined immunodeficiency: causes and control of secondary infections. *American Journal of Veterinary Research*, **39**, 1043–1047.

Peters, S.E., Wakefield, A.E., Whitwell, K.E. and Hopkin, J.M. (1994). *Pneumocystis carinii* pneumonia in thoroughbred foals: identification of a genetically distinct organism by DNA amplification. *Journal of Clinical Microbiology*, **32**, 213–216.

Pixley, F.J., Wakefield, A.E., Banenji, S. and Hopkin, J.M. (1991). Mitochondrial gene sequences show fungal homology for *Pneumocystis carinii*. *Molecular Microbiology*, **5**, 1347–1351.

Chapter 45

Opportunistic infections caused predominantly by phaeoid fungi

A variety of saprophytic fungi which can infect traumatized tissues produce slowly progressive inflammatory lesions. Although these lesions mainly involve the dermis or subcutis, they may be found elsewhere. In this chapter, discussion is limited to the saprophytic fungi which have been aetiologically implicated in phaeohyphomycosis and eumycetomas. Eumycetomas caused by *Sporothrix schenkii*, *Pythium insidiosum*, *Aspergillus* species and the zygomycetes are described in other chapters.

Phaeohyphomycosis is caused by species of phaeoid (dematiaceous, pigmented) fungi. Eumycetomas may be caused by phaeoid or non-phaeoid fungi. The granulomatous lesions in eumycetomas are characterized by the presence of granules, composed largely of fungal mycelia, in exudates. Granules are not present in exudates from lesions of phaeohyphomycosis. In some instances phaeohyphomycosis, especially when caused by infection with *Bipolaris specifera* or with *Exserohilum rostratum*, has been mistakenly categorized as eumycetoma (Chandler *et al.*, 1980). True eumycetomas are rare in domestic animal species (Brodey *et al.*, 1967; Lambrechts *et al.*, 1991).

The pigmentation of phaeoid fungi is due to the presence of melanin in their hyphal walls. The dark colouration of granules occasionally found in eumycetomas also derives from melanin. Some phaeoid species produce meagre amounts of melanin. In eumycetomas caused by these species, the granules are pale and their hyphae appear non-pigmented in tissue sections. Masson-Fontana silver stain can be used to demonstrate the presence of melanin.

Usual habitat

The fungi implicated in phaeohyphomycosis and eumycetoma are found in soil and in plant material. Some are distributed worldwide and others are restricted to tropical and subtropical regions.

Clinical infections

The fungal species which have been isolated from subcutaneous phaeohyphomycosis in domestic animals are presented in Table 45.1. Some of these fungal species have also been isolated from the rare eumycetomas which have been confirmed in domestic animals. The domestic

---

Key points
- Phaeoid (pigmented) fungi can infect traumatized tissue causing phaeohyphomycosis
- An uncommon manifestation of infection with both phaeoid and non-phaeoid fungi is eumycetoma formation
- The granulomatous lesions of phaeohyphomycosis and eumycetoma occur most frequently in subcutaneous tissues
- Sinus formation with serosanguineous discharges is a feature of superficial lesions
- Discharges from eumycetomas contain macroscopic granules composed of fungal elements. Granules formed by phaeoid fungi are black; those formed by other fungi lack pigmentation

---

species most often affected by phaeohyphomycosis are cats, horses and cattle. Mycetomas have been described in the horse and also in the dog (Brodey *et al.*, 1967).

Slowly enlarging subcutaneous granulomatous lesions, located mainly on the feet, limbs and head, are the most common presentations in both phaeohyphomycosis and eumycetoma. The lesions in eumycetomas are nodular. Ulceration and sinus tract formation with serosanguineous discharges are associated with both conditions. Lesions of phaeohyphomycosis in two horses presented as black denuded skin plaques (Kaplan *et al.*, 1975). The presence of distinct granules (either black or pale) in discharges, distinguishes the lesions of eumycetomas from those of phaeohyphomycosis.

Systemic lesions caused by phaeoid fungi are extremely rare. Osteolytic phaeohyphomycosis caused by *Phialemonium obovatum* (Lomax *et al.*, 1986) and *Scedosporium inflatum* (Salkin *et al.*, 1992), now termed *S. prolificans*, has been recorded in dogs. Cerebral phaeohyphomycosis caused by *Cladophialophora bantiana* has been reported in dogs and a cat (Dillehay *et al.*, 1987). A chronic granulomatous lesion in the abdominal cavity of a dog was described as a black grain eumycetoma (Lambrechts *et al.*, 1991).

Table 45.1 Dematiaceous fungi infrequently implicated in subcutaneous mycoses in domestic animals.

Fungus	Colonial appearance	Microscopic structure	Species affected
Alternaria species	Colony matures within 5 days and has a greyish woolly surface; reverse is black	Conidiophores are septate and vary in length. Conidia are formed singly or in chains	Horse (*A. alternata*) Cat (*A. infectoria*)
Bipolaris spicifera	Colony matures in about 5 days and has a greyish brown surface; reverse is black	Conidiophores are elongate and bend at the attachment point of each conidium. Conidia are cylindrical with 3 to 5 septa	Cat, dog, horse, cow
Curvularia species	Colony matures in 5 days and has a dark olive-green to brown or black surface; reverse is black	Conidiophores are simple or branched and bent at points of conidial formation. Due to the swelling of the central cell, conidia appear curved	Cow (*C. anomatum*) Dog, horse (*C. geniculata*) Cat (*C. lunata*)
Exophiala jeanselmei	Colony requires up to 15 days to mature; surface is brown and skin-like becoming velvety; reverse is black	Initially, yeast-like budding cells may be present; conidiophores bearing conidia in clusters are produced later	Cat (*E. jeanselmei, E. spinifera*)
Exserohilum rostratum	Colony matures in 5 days and has a dark grey to black cottony surface; reverse is black	Conidiophores have a uneven appearance; conidia are fusiform with 7 to 11 septa	Cow
Phialophora verrucosa	Colony matures in about 15 days. Surface is dark greenish–brown to black; reverse is black	Conidia are oval to round and accumulate at the apex of a phialide which has a cup-like colarette	Cat
Phoma glomerata	Colony matures within 5 days and is powdery or velvety and greyish-brown; reverse is brown	A pycnidium, the asexual fruiting body, is dark and round with an opening. Conidia are borne on conidiophores inside the pycnidium	Goat
Scedosporium apiospermum (*Pseudallescheria boydii*)	Colony matures in 7 days, initially white, becoming grey or brown; reverse is white becoming greyish-black	Both short and long conidiophores bear conidia which are oval with a flat base	Dog, horse

Diagnosis

- Suitable specimens for laboratory examination include fine-needle aspirates, punch biopsies and postmortem tissue samples.
- Specimens are inoculated onto Sabouraud dextrose agar and incubated aerobically at 25°C to 30°C for up to 6 weeks. Isolates should be subcultured to facilitate accurate identification by a reference laboratory.
- Isolates are identified by colonial morphology and the microscopic appearance of fruiting structures (Table 45.1).
- Both PAS and methenamine silver techniques are used for demonstrating hyphae in tissue sections.
- The Masson-Fontana silver stain is used to demonstrate melanin in the hyphae of phaeoid fungi.
- A deposit of eosinophilic material around mycelial aggregates in eumycetomas, referred to as the Splendore-Hoeppli phenomenon, may be demonstrable in tissue sections.

Treatment

- Surgical excision of lesions is effective (Beale and Pinson, 1990).
- Although antifungal therapy is usually ineffective, a combination of amphotericin B and 5-fluorocytosine may be beneficial.

References

Beale, K.M. and Pinson, D. (1990). Phaeohyphomycosis caused by two different species of *Curvularia* in two animals in the same household. *Journal of the American Animal Hospital Association*, **26**, 67–70.

Brodey, R.S., Schryver, H.S., Deubler, M.J. *et al.* (1967). Mycetoma in a dog. *Journal of the American Veterinary Medical Association*, **151**, 442–451.

Chandler, F.W., Kaplan, W. and Ajello, L. (1980). Mycetomas. In *Histopathology of Mycotic Diseases*. Wolfe Medical Publications, London. pp. 76–82 and 222–239.

Dillehay, D.L. Ribas, J.L., Newton, J.C. and Kwapien, R.P. (1987). Cerebral phaeohyphomycosis in two dogs and a cat. *Veterinary Pathology*, **24**, 192–194.

Kaplan, W., Chandler, F.W., Ajello, L., Gauthier, R., Higgins, R. and Cayouette, P. (1975). Equine phaeohyphomycosis caused by *Drechslera spicifera*. *Canadian Veterinary Journal*, **16**, 205–208.

Lambrechts, N., Collett, M.G. and Henton, M. (1991). Black grain eumycetoma in the abdominal cavity of a dog. *Journal of Medical and Veterinary Mycology*, **29**, 211–214.

Lomax, L.G., Cole, J.R., Padhye, A.A. *et al.* (1986). Osteolytic phaeohyphomycosis in a German shepherd dog caused by *Phialemonium obovatum*. *Journal of Clinical Microbiology*, **23**, 987–991.

Salkin, I.F., Cooper, C.R., Bartges, J.W., Kemna, M.E. and Rinaldi, M.G. (1992). *Scedosporium inflatum* osteomyelitis in a dog. *Journal of Clinical Microbiology*, **30**, 2797–2800.

Further reading

Kwochka, K.W., Mays, M.B.C., Ajello, L. and Padhye, A.A. (1984). Canine phaeohyphomycosis caused by *Drechslera spicifera*: a case report and literature review. *Journal of the American Animal Hospital Association*, **20**, 625–633.

Chapter 46

Mycotoxins and mycotoxicoses

Mycotoxins, secondary metabolites of certain fungal species, are produced when toxigenic strains of these organisms grow under defined conditions on crops, pasture or stored feed. The acute or chronic intoxication following ingestion of contaminated plant material is termed mycotoxicosis. More than 100 fungal species are known to elaborate mycotoxins. Many of these fungi belong to the genera *Penicillium*, *Aspergillus* and *Fusarium*.

Factors affecting mycotoxin production and the development of mycotoxicosis are presented in Fig. 46.1. For fungal growth and toxin production, a suitable substrate must be available along with moisture and optimal temperature and oxygen levels. Some mycotoxicoses have a high prevalence in particular geographical regions where agricultural practices favour their occurrence. Toxigenic strains of fungi may grow preferentially on particular parts of a plant, some favouring the carbohydrate-containing seeds or kernels and others utilizing the cellulose substrate in fibrous stems or leaves.

Mycotoxins are non-antigenic, low molecular weight compounds. Many are heat-stable, retaining toxicity following exposure to the processing temperatures used for pelleting and other procedures (Box 46.1). A particular mycotoxin may be produced by a number of fungal species. Moreover, some fungi can elaborate several mycotoxins which may differ in biological activities, producing complex clinical effects. Clinical diagnosis of the mycotoxicoses may also be complicated by the presence of a number of toxigenic species on a food source. The severity of clinical signs is influenced by the period of exposure to contaminated feed and the amount of mycotoxin ingested. Some batches of feed may be contaminated and mycotoxin may be unevenly distributed in a batch. Clinical evidence of the targeting of particular organs such as the liver or the central nervous system is a feature of some mycotoxicoses. Immunosuppression, mutagenesis, neoplasia or teratogenesis may also result from exposure. Epidemiological and clinical features of mycotoxicosis are summarized in Box 46.2.

Mycotoxicoses of defined veterinary importance are presented in Table 46.1 The role of a number of mycotoxins considered to be involved in diverse clinical conditions in domestic animals is not yet clearly defined (Griffiths and Done, 1991; Lomax *et al.*, 1984) and many diseases with suspected links to mycotoxins are poorly defined.

Key points

- Certain fungi elaborate metabolites (mycotoxins) in growing crops or stored feed under defined environmental conditions
- Mycotoxins, a diverse group of heat-stable, low molecular weight compounds, are non-antigenic
- Ingestion of contaminated plant material or contaminated crops may induce a characteristic disease process
- Susceptibility can vary with species, age and sex. The effects of mycotoxins include immunosuppression, teratogenesis or carcinogenesis
- Diseases caused by mycotoxins (mycotoxicoses) are non-contagious, tend to be sporadic, seasonal and associated with certain batches of feed
- Diagnosis is based on the presence of characteristic clinical presentation or on demonstration of significant levels of a specific mycotoxin in feed or in animal tissues

Aflatoxicosis

This disease is associated with ingestion of aflatoxins, a large group of difuranocoumarins produced by toxigenic strains of *Aspergillus flavus*, *A. parasiticus* and some other *Aspergillus* species. Maize and other cereals, groundnuts and soya beans are commonly contaminated by these saprophytic fungi. Aflatoxins B_1, B_2, G_1 and G_2 are particularly important in disease production. Aflatoxin B_1, which is the component most often encountered in disease outbreaks, appears to be the most toxic. Hydroxylated metabolites of B_1 and B_2, aflatoxins M_1 and M_2, may be detected in milk and meat. After absorption from the gastrointestinal tract, aflatoxins are metabolized by the liver to a range of toxic and non-toxic products. Toxicity relates to binding of metabolites to macromolecules, especially nucleic acid and nucleoproteins. Consequently, the toxic effects include reduced protein synthesis, carcinogenesis, teratogenesis and aplasia of the thymic cortex leading to depressed cell-mediated immunity (Osweiler, 1990).

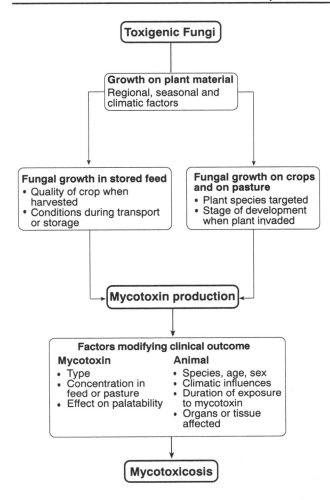

Figure 46.1 Factors affecting mycotoxin production and manifestations of clinical disease.

Clinical findings

Aflatoxicosis has been encountered worldwide in many domestic species. There is considerable variation in susceptibility between species and within age groups. Ducklings, turkey poults, calves, pigs and dogs are sensitive to toxic effects, whereas sheep and adult cattle are more resistant. Aflatoxicosis is uncommon in horses and goats. Subacute aflatoxicosis, associated with prolonged exposure to low concentrations of toxin, usually

---

Box 46.1 Characteristics of mycotoxins.

- Low molecular weight, heat-stable substances
- Unlike many bacterial toxins, non-antigenic; exposure does not induce a protective immune response
- Many are active at low dietary levels
- Specific target organs or tissues affected
- Toxic effects include immunosuppression, mutagenesis, teratogenesis and carcinogenesis
- Accumulation in tissues of food-producing animals or excretion in milk may result in human exposure

---

Box 46.2 Epidemiological and clinical features of mycotoxicoses.

- Outbreaks usually seasonal and sporadic
- No evidence of lateral spread to in-contact animals
- Certain types of pasture or stored feed may be involved
- Clinical presentation is usually ill-defined
- Severity of clinical signs is influenced by the amount of mycotoxin ingested; recovery is related to duration of exposure
- Antimicrobial medication is ineffective
- Confirmation requires demonstration of significant levels of mycotoxin in feed or in tissues from affected animals

---

presents as slowly developing ill thrift and reduced growth rate. Immunosuppression, with increasing prevalence of endemic infection and inadequate responses to routine vaccination, may also be detected in affected groups of animals. This insidious form of aflatoxicosis is often of greater economic significance than acute forms of the disease associated with high concentrations of toxin in the diet. Acute aflatoxicosis has been recorded in birds and cattle. Ataxia, opisthotonos and sudden death are features of the acute disease in ducklings. Hepatopathy is a common finding and, in birds more than 3 weeks old, subcutaneous haemorrhages may be evident. Haemorrhagic diathesis, probably related to hepatopathy, is a characteristic of acute toxicity in chickens and turkeys. In turkey X disease, the first clearly defined outbreak of acute aflatoxicosis, widespread haemorrhages may have been due to the combined effect of aflatoxins and cyclopiazonic acid, which are often produced simultaneously by *A. flavus* (Robb, 1993). Acute aflatoxicosis in cattle may rapidly result in death (Cockcroft, 1995). In affected calves, blindness, circling, tenesmus, diarrhoea and convulsions have been recorded.

Diagnosis

- Except in outbreaks of acute disease, clinical signs are vague. Epidemiological features and postmortem findings may be of diagnostic value. Aflatoxin may be demonstrated in tissues obtained at postmortem.
- Carefully selected samples of suspect feed should be stored at −20°C until analyzed.
- Procedures for aflatoxin detection in feed and tissues include:
  - Thin-layer chromatography. Chromatograms are examined under UV light for the four main toxins on the basis of position and fluorescence. The fluorescence of aflatoxins B_1 and B_2 is blue and with G_1 and G_2 it is green.
  - High performance liquid chromatography.
  - Immunoassay techniques such as ELISA and

Table 46.1 Mycotoxicoses of domestic animals.

Disease / Mycotoxins	Fungus / Crop or substrate	Species affected / Geographical distribution	Functional or structural effects / Clinical findings
Aflatoxicosis / Aflatoxins B_1, B_2, G_1, G_2	*Aspergillus flavus, A. parasiticus* / Maize, stored grain groundnuts, soybeans	Pigs, poultry, cattle, dogs, trout / Worldwide	Hepatotoxicity, immunosuppression, mutagenesis, teratogenesis, carcinogenesis / Ill-thrift, drop in milk yield, rarely death from acute toxicity
Diplodiosis / Unidentified neurotoxin	*Diplodia maydis* / Maize cobs	Sheep, cattle, goats, horses / South Africa	Neurotoxicity / Ataxia, paresis and paralysis in adults, perinatal deaths in lambs and calves
Ergotism / Ergotamine, ergometrine, ergocristine	*Claviceps purpurea* / Seedheads of ryegrass and other grasses, cereals	Cattle, sheep, deer, horses, pigs, poultry / Worldwide	Neurotoxicity and vasoconstriction / Convulsions, gangrene of extremities, agalactia, hyperthermia in hot climates
Facial eczema / Sporidesmin	*Pithomyces chartarum* / Pasture litter from ryegrass and white clover	Cattle, sheep, goats / New Zealand, Australia, South Africa, South America, occasionally USA and parts of Europe	Hepatotoxicity, biliary occlusion / Photosensitization, jaundice
Fescue toxicosis / Ergovaline	*Neophytodium coenophialum* / Tall fescue grass	Cattle, sheep, horses, / New Zealand, Australia, USA, Italy	Vasoconstriction / Dry gangrene in cold weather in cattle and sheep (fescue foot); hyperthermia and low milk yields (fescue summer toxicosis)
Leukoencephalomalacia / Fumonisins B_1, B_2, A_1, A_2	*Fusarium moniliforme*, other *Fusarium* species / Standing or stored maize	Horses, other *Equidae*, pigs / Egypt, South Africa, USA, Greece	Liquefactive necrosis in cerebrum / Neurological signs of varying severity
Mouldy sweet potato toxicosis / Derivative of 4-ipomeanol	*Fusarium solani, F. oxysporum* / Sweet potatoes	Cattle / USA, Australia, New Zealand	Cytotoxicity producing interstitial pneumonia and pulmonary oedema / Respiratory distress, sudden death may occur
Mycotoxic lupinosis / Phomopsins A, B	*Phomopsis leptostromiformis* / Growing lupins with stem blight	Sheep, occasionally cattle, horses, pigs / Worldwide	Hepatotoxicity / Inappetence, stupor, jaundice, ruminal stasis, often fatal
Ochratoxicosis / Ochratoxins A, B, C	*Aspergillus ochraceus*, other *Aspergillus* species, *Penicillium viridicatum*, other *Penicillium* species / Stored barley, maize and wheat	Pigs, poultry / Worldwide	Degenerative renal changes / Polydipsia and polyuria in pigs, fall in egg production in birds
Oestrogenism / Zearalenone	*Fusarium graminearum*, other *Fusarium* species / Stored maize and barley, pelleted cereal feeds, maize silage	Pigs, cattle, occasionally sheep / Worldwide	Oestrogenic activity / Hyperaemia and oedema of vulva and precocious mammary development in young gilts; anoestrus and reduced litter size in mature sows; reduced fertility in cattle and sheep

(continued)

radioimmunoassay procedures.
— Biological assays such as bile duct proliferation in ducklings, chick embryo bioassays, brine shrimp larvae tests and trout embryo bioassays.

Control and prevention
• The growth of fungal contaminants on stored feed should be limited by appropriate measures following harvesting and during storage.
• Batches of food for human and animal consumption may be monitored for aflatoxin contamination.
• Treatment with ammonia gas at high temperature and pressure has been used to detoxify contaminated batches of feed.
• Dilution of contaminated feed with uncontaminated supplies can be used to reduce aflatoxin concentration

Table 46.1 Mycotoxicoses of domestic animals. *(continued)*

Disease / Mycotoxins	Fungus / Crop or substrate	Species affected / Geographical distribution	Functional or structural effects / Clinical findings
Porcine pulmonary oedema / Fumonisins B$_1$, B$_2$	*Fusarium* species / Maize	Pigs / USA, South Africa	Pulmonary oedema, hydrothorax / Cyanosis, death
Slaframine toxicosis / Slaframine	*Rhizoctonia leguminicola* / Legumes, especially red clover, in pasture or hay	Sheep, cattle, horses / USA	Cholinergic activity / Salivation, lacrimation, bloating, diarrhoea, sometimes death
Tremorgen intoxications			
Perennial ryegrass staggers / Lolitrem B	*Acremonium lolii* / Perennial ryegrass	Cattle, pigs, poultry, sheep, horses, deer / USA, Australia, New Zealand, Europe	Neurotoxicity / Muscular tremors, incoordination, convulsive seizures, collapse
Paspalum staggers / Paspalinine, paspalitrems A, B	*Claviceps paspali* / Seedheads of paspalum grasses	Cattle, sheep, horses / New Zealand, Australia, USA, South America	Neurotoxicity / Muscular tremors, incoordination, convulsive seizures, collapse
Penitrem staggers / Verruculogen, paxilline, other mycotoxins	Many *Penicillium* species, some *Aspergillus* species / Stored feed and pasture	Ruminants, other domestic animals / Probably worldwide	Neurotoxicity / Muscular tremors, incoordination, convulsive seizures, collapse
Aspergillus clavatus induced tremors / Unidentified neurotoxin	*Aspergillus clavatus* / Sprouted wheat, millers' malt culms	Cattle / China, South Africa, Europe	Neurotoxicity, degeneration of neurons / Frothing from mouth and knuckling of limbs when forced to move
Trichothecene toxicoses			
Food refusal and emetic syndrome / Vomitoxin (deoxynivalenol)	*Fusarium graminearum*, other *Fusarium* species / Cereal crops	Pigs, rarely other species / Countries with temperate or cold climates	Neurotoxicity / Contaminated feed refused, vomition, poor growth
Haemorrhagic syndrome / T-2 toxin, diacetoscirpenol	*Fusarium graminearum*, *F. sporotrichoides*, other *Fusarium* species / Cereals, straw	Cattle, pigs, poultry / USA	Coagulopathy, immunosuppression / Necrotic skin lesions, necrotic lesions in alimentary tract, haemorrhages
Stachybotryotoxicosis / Satratoxin, roridin, verrucarin	*Stachybotrys atra* / Stored cereals, straw, hay	Horses, cattle, sheep, pigs / Former USSR, Europe, South Africa	Cytotoxicity, coagulopathy, immunosuppression / Stomatitis, necrotic lesions in alimentary tract, haemorrhages
Myrotheciotoxicosis / Roridins, verrucarins	*Myrothecium verrucaria*, *M. roridum* / Ryegrass, rye stubble, straw	Sheep, cattle, horses / Former USSR, New Zealand, south eastern Europe	Inflammation of many tissues, pulmonary congestion / Unthriftiness, sudden death

and minimize toxicity.

- Addition of hydrated sodium calcium aluminosilicate to feed is reported to reduce aflatoxin toxicity (Harvey *et al.*, 1989).

Diplodiosis

Diplodiosis, a neuromycotoxicosis, is associated with an unidentified toxin produced by the corncob rot fungus, *Diplodia maydis* (*D. zeae*). The condition has been recorded in southern Africa when contaminated maize cobs were fed to cattle, sheep, goats and horses. Sustained growth of the fungus on cobs over a number of weeks is necessary for toxin production. Clinical signs include salivation, lacrimation, tremors, ataxia, paresis and paralysis. Recovery usually occurs when contaminated cobs are removed from feed. Exposure of pregnant ewes and cows during the second half of pregnancy results in stillbirths and neonatal deaths. Spongiform lesions may be found in a high percentage of the brains of affected lambs and calves.

Mycotoxic leukoencephalomalacia

Ingestion of mouldy maize cobs containing the mycotoxin fumonisin B$_1$, which is produced by *Fusarium moniliforme*, is responsible for sporadic neurological disease mainly in horses, donkeys and mules. The disease has been reported from Egypt, South Africa, the USA and Greece. Neurological signs, which relate to liquefactive necrosis of the white matter in the cerebrum, include inability to swallow, weakness, staggering, circling and marked depression. Mania, described in some cases, may be due to hepatic failure. Fumonisin B_1, when fed to horses at concentrations greater than 10 μg/g of feed, is lethal (Ross *et al.*, 1991).

Ergotism

This disease, which occurs worldwide in many domestic animal species and in man, follows ingestion of toxic levels of certain ergopeptide alkaloids found in the sclerotia of *Claviceps purpurea*. This fungal species colonizes the seed heads of ryegrasses and cereals such as rye and barley. Toxicity may be retained in silage (Hogg, 1991). Ovarian tissue of the seed is destroyed and replaced by fungal mycelium which enlarges, hardens and darkens to form a sclerotium, also referred to as an ergot (Fig. 46.2). Mature sclerotia, shed from seed heads in autumn and overwintering in the soil, germinate in the following spring. They produce stromata bearing perithecia in which asci, containing ascospores, develop. Windborne ascospores, forcibly discharged from the perithecia, germinate on suitable grasses and cereal plants to form a new generation of sclerotia. The most important ergopeptide alkaloids in the sclerotia are ergotamine and ergometrine. These alkaloids, derivatives of lysergic acid, have a number of pharmacological effects including direct stimulation of the adrenergic nerves supplying arteriolar smooth muscle and inhibition of prolactin secretion.

Clinical findings

Convulsive ergotism, an uncommon acute form of the disease, is occasionally observed in cattle, sheep and horses exposed to large doses of ergotamine. Signs include staggering, convulsive episodes and drowsiness. Smaller amounts of mycotoxin absorbed over relatively long periods result in persistent arteriolar constriction and endothelial damage. The effects of these changes, most

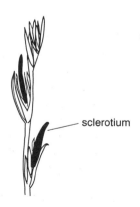

Figure 46.2 Sclerotia (ergots) of *Claviceps purpurea* in the seed head of growing ryegrass.

noticeable in body extremities, are thrombosis and ischaemia. Swelling and redness of the extremities accompanied by lameness and stiffness is followed by terminal gangrene. There is a clear line of demarcation between non-viable and viable normal tissues. Cold ambient temperatures and muddy conditions under foot may contribute to the severity of the lesions. In chickens, dry gangrene of the comb, wattles and feet may develop.

In warm climates, hyperthermia may occur in cattle ingesting ergopeptide alkaloids (Ross *et al.*, 1989). In pregnant sows, ergotism may present as poor mammary development and low litter sizes with premature births, low birth weights and high neonatal mortality due to starvation. Although ergopeptides may exert an oxytocin-like effect on the pregnant uterus, abortion is not a feature of ergotism.

Diagnosis
- Ergotism can often be diagnosed clinically. The presence of ergots in pasture grasses or in grain provides supporting evidence.
- When dealing with suspect ground grains, extraction of alkaloids and their detection by chromatography may be necessary.

Prevention
- Regular grazing or topping to prevent seed-head formation in pasture grasses reduces the possibility of sclerotia formation.
- Grain containing ergots should not be fed to animals. Removal of ergots from small batches of grain can be achieved mechanically or by flotation methods.

Facial eczema

This economically important disease of sheep and cattle occurs in Australia, New Zealand and South Africa. The skin lesions develop as a result of photosensitization following exposure to the hepatotoxin sporidesmin in the spores of the saprophytic fungus *Pithomyces chartarum*. The fungus sporulates prolifically on pasture litter during warm humid conditions in late summer or early autumn. Although most strains of *P. chartarum* isolated in New Zealand produce sporidesmin, a high proportion of non-toxigenic isolates are recovered in other countries (Collin and Towers, 1995).

Hepatobiliary lesions develop as a result of the accumulation and concentration of sporidesmin in the bile. Necrosis of biliary epithelium results in obstruction of intrahepatic ducts with cell debris and diffusion of toxin into the hepatic parenchyma producing damage to blood vessels and hepatocytes. The consequent atrophy, necrosis and fibrosis reduce the capacity of the liver to excrete phylloerythrin, a potent photodynamic compound formed from chlorophyll by enteric organisms, which is distributed to many tissues including the skin. The photodynamic activity of phylloerythrin when exposed to solar radiation produces skin lesions typical of the disease.

Clinical findings

There is a latent period of 10 to 14 days between ingestion of a toxic amount of sporidesmin and the development of photosensitization. In sheep, lesions develop in non-pigmented areas which are not covered by wool. The eyelids, muzzle and ears are inflammed and swollen. Serous exudation and scab formation may be followed by necrosis and sloughing of skin. Jaundice is usually present. In cattle, lesions are limited to areas of non-pigmented skin. Milk production may be severely reduced. Although mortality due to severe liver damage is limited, economic losses arising from debilitation may be considerable.

Diagnosis

- In ruminants, photosensitization accompanied by jaundice is suggestive of the disease.
- Environmental temperatures above 12°C along with heavy rainfall over a 48 hour period provide suitable conditions for the growth of *P. chartarum* on pasture and are likely to precipitate disease outbreaks.
- Counts of the characteristic spores of *P. chartarum* (Fig. 46.3) in pasture samples can be used for prediction of disease outbreaks. Pastures with high spore counts are toxic for grazing animals.
- Elevated serum liver enzymes such as gamma-glutamyl transferase are found in affected animals.
- Competitive ELISA techniques have been developed for field use. Sporidesmin may be detected in bile, urine, plasma or whole blood (Briggs *et al.*, 1993).

Control and prevention

- Routine monitoring of pasture spore counts can be used to evaluate their safety for grazing.
- Growth of *P. chartarum* can be controlled by spraying pastures with fungicides.
- Accumulation of pasture litter can be controlled by pasture management techniques.
- Breeding programmes which select sheep resistant to the toxic effects of sporidesmin, are employed in some countries.
- The daily administration of zinc salts reduces the toxicity of sporidesmin for liver. A zinc-containing intraruminal device for preventing the disease in sheep is available (Munday *et al.*, 1997).

Fescue toxicosis

This mycotoxicosis affects cattle and sheep in the USA, New Zealand and Australia where tall fescue (*Festuca arundinacea*) is common in pastures. An endophytic fungus, *Neophytodium coenophialum* (formerly

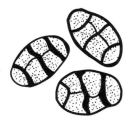

Figure 46.3 Thick-walled spores of *Pithomyces chartarum* (10-20 x 20-30 μm) with transverse and longitudinal septa.

Acremonium coenophialum), found in the foliage and seeds of tall fescue, produces the alkaloid ergovaline which has been implicated in the aetiology of fescue toxicosis (fescue foot) which resembles ergotism in herbivores. During winter months, the vasoconstrictive effects of ergovaline are exacerbated by low ambient temperatures. Dry gangrene develops on the distal extremities of hind limbs, tail and ears. During warm months, summer fescue toxicosis which occurs in cattle, sheep and horses, is characterized by hyperthermia and unthriftiness. Induced low serum prolactin leads to a drop in milk production. In addition to agalactia, prolonged gestation, weak neonates and thickened placentae are features of this toxicosis.

Mouldy sweet potato toxicity

Acute interstitial pneumonia in cattle has been attributed to eating mould-damaged sweet potatoes (*Ipomoea batatas*) in the USA, New Zealand and Australia. Phytoalexins, metabolites formed in sweet potatoes in response to structural damage, are metabolized by *Fusarium* species to lung oedema factor, 4-ipomeanol. This factor is converted by microsomal enzymes in pneumocytes to toxic products which damage the cells (Hill and Wright, 1992). Dyspnoea is the principal clinical sign. Death may occur within 10 hours of the onset of signs.

Mycotoxic lupinosis

Lupin seeds contain toxic alkaloids which can produce neurological disturbance in herbivores. This plant toxicosis is distinct from the mycotoxicosis associated with ingestion of phomopsins A and B produced by *Phomopsis leptostromiformis*, the fungal cause of stem blight in lupins. Mycotoxic lupinosis which has been reported mainly in sheep grazing lupin stubble, occurs in many countries. Acute lupinosis presents as hepatic encephalopathy with stupor, stumbling and recumbency preceding death. Surviving animals may develop jaundice and photosensitization. A skeletal myopathy associated with phomopsin toxicity has been reported in Western Australia (Allen *et al.*, 1992).

Ochratoxicosis

Ochratoxins, a group of related isocoumarin derivatives, are produced by toxigenic strains of *Aspergillus ochraceus* and *Penicillium viridicatum* when growing on stored barley, maize or wheat. Ochratoxin A is a heat stable potent nephrotoxin which is also immunosuppressive and carcinogenic. Many of the biological effects of ochratoxin A relate to interference with protein synthesis. Other mycotoxins including citrinin, which can also be produced by *A. ochraceus*, may enhance the nephrotoxic effects of ochratoxin.

Adult ruminants can detoxify ochratoxins; pigs and poultry are more likely to be affected. In pigs, inappetence, depression, loss of weight, polydipsia and polyuria are features of mycotic nephropathy. Affected poultry present with depressed growth rate, coagulopathy, reduced egg production and poor quality eggs.

Mycotoxic oestrogenism

Zearalenone is a potent non-steroidal oestrogen produced by certain *Fusarium* species particularly *F. graminearum*, when growing on stored maize and other cereals, maize stubble and silage. Pasture levels of zearalenone may be sufficient in some countries to cause reproductive problems in cattle and sheep (Towers and Sprosen, 1993).

Pigs, particularly prepubertal gilts, are commonly affected by oestrogenism. The condition, sometimes erroneously called vulvovaginitis, develops about one week after ingestion of contaminated feed. Vulval oedema and hyperaemia, hypertrophy of mammary glands and uterus and, occasionally, vaginal and rectal prolapse are features in gilts. In multiparous sows, anoestrus, pseudopregnancy, infertility and reduced litter size with small weak piglets may suggest oestrogenism (Long and Diekman, 1986).

Low conception rates have been recorded in cattle and sheep with oestrogenism. Less frequently, affected cattle may present with vaginal discharge, nymphomania and abnormal mammary development in prepubertal heifers. Zearalenone can be excreted in milk, posing a public health risk. The mycotoxin can be detected by chromatography. Oestrogen activity in feed may be assayed by injection of extracts into sexually immature mice, which develop uterine hypertrophy when extracts are positive. An ELISA technique has been developed for detecting zearalenone in pasture samples and ovine urine.

Slaframine toxicosis

Slaframine is a cholinergic mycotoxin elaborated by the phytopathogen *Rhizoctonia leguminicola*, the cause of black-patch disease of red clover, alfalfa and other leguminous pasture plants. Clinical effects in horses and cattle, consuming contaminated pasture or hay, include profuse salivation, lacrimation, bloating, diarrhoea and polyuria (Sockett *et al.*, 1982). Recovery follows removal from contaminated pasture. Mortality is uncommon.

Tremorgen intoxications

Tremorgens, a heterogeneous group of mycotoxins, produce neurological effects including muscular tremors, ataxia, incoordination and convulsive seizures following ingestion. Signs often develop after strenuous exercise or excitement. Recovery usually follows within hours of removal from contaminated pasture or withdrawal of contaminated feed. Most tremorgens produce their neurological effects without obvious morphological tissue changes. Unidentified neurotoxins of *Aspergillus clavatus* can cause neuronal degeneration and focal gliosis (Gilmour *et al.*, 1989).

Perennial ryegrass staggers

This is one of the most common mycotoxicoses of cattle, farmed deer, horses and sheep in New Zealand and, to a lesser extent, in Australia, Europe and the USA (Galey *et al.*, 1991). *Acremonium lolii*, an endophytic fungus, which affects only perennial ryegrass (*Lolium perenne*), produces lolitrems. These mycotoxins, particularly lolitrem B, are responsible for clinical signs typical of tremorgen intoxication. Strains of perennial ryegrass differ in susceptibility to colonization by the fungus. Growth of *Acremonium lolii* is largely concentrated in the older lower leaf sheaths of the grass. Consequently, clinical signs usually develop in late summer or early autumn when growth of pasture grasses declines. Signs may also develop in animals fed on contaminated hay or silage. Although morbidity in an affected flock or herd may be high, deaths are rare and recovery is rapid if animals are removed from contaminated pasture. Ryegrass staggers is seldom seen after rain or when grasses are growing rapidly, conditions which favour proliferation of *Pithomyces chartarum*. Therefore ryegrass staggers and facial eczema rarely occur concurrently.

Paspalum staggers

This disease is caused by ingestion of tremorgens present in the sclerotia of *Claviceps paspali*, which are found in the seed heads of paspalum grasses. The life cycle of *C. paspali* resembles that of *C. purpurea*. The mycotoxins, mainly paspalinine and paspalitrems A and B, produce typical tremorgen ataxia. Death is rare but may occur from respiratory failure during sustained seizures. The disease can affect many herbivorous species. Recovery is usually rapid after animals are removed from contaminated pasture. Control may be achieved by topping of pastures to prevent development of paspalum seed heads.

Penitrem staggers

Many *Penicillium* species, including *P. crustosum* and *P. verruculosum*, and some *Aspergillus* species, including *A. flavus* and *A. fumigatus*, produce tremorgens when growing on pasture plants or stored feed. The clinical signs produced by these mycotoxins, mainly the penitrems verruculogen and paxilline, are similar to those of ryegrass staggers (di Menna and Mantle, 1978). The disease, which can affect many domestic animal species, has been reported in New Zealand, Australia, the USA and South Africa.

Trichothecene toxicoses

Trichothecenes, a large group of mycotoxins which affect most cell types, often produce radiomimetic effects in tissues. Cellular protein synthesis is inhibited, and immunosuppression results from exposure to sublethal doses of trichothecenes.

Food refusal and emetic syndrome

This syndrome affects pigs exposed primarily to vomitoxin (deoxynivalenol, DON). Diacetoxyscirpenol (DAS) and T-2 toxin may also contribute to the development of clinical signs. All of these toxins are produced by *Fusarium* species, in particular *F. graminearum*, when growing in maize, barley grains or in mixed feeds containing cereals. Fungal growth can occur at relatively low temperatures and the syndrome is encountered with greater frequency in temperate regions. Intake of contaminated food is reduced even when levels of vomitoxin are relatively low. If other food sources are unavailable, pigs may continue to eat contaminated feed in sufficient quantity to induce clinical signs. The production of zearalenone by *F. graminearum* may complicate the clinical assessment of the food refusal and emetic syndrome in pigs (Côté *et al.*, 1984).

Haemorrhagic syndrome

Sporadic outbreaks of a haemorrhagic syndrome in cattle characterized by bloody diarrhoea and necrotic lesions in skin and oral cavity have been reported in the USA (Wu *et al.*, 1997). The animals were fed on oat straw contaminated with *Fusarium sporotrichioides*. The mycotoxins T-2 toxin and DAS are potent epithelial necrotizing agents which also have toxic effects on bone marrow inducing thrombocytopenia. The toxins appear to be responsible for the clinical disturbances in the haemorrhagic syndrome.

Stachybotryotoxicosis

Stachybotrys atra, when growing in harvested grain, straw or hay, produces at least 5 trichothecenes including satratoxins, roridin and verrucarin. These mycotoxins are cytotoxic and have a radiomimetic effect on tissues. Following low-level intake of the toxins over a prolonged period chronic disease can develop in horses, cattle and sheep. Horses appear to be particularly susceptible.

Necrotic stomatitis, widespread petechial haemorrhages and blood-stained diarrhoea are clinical features in all affected animals. Immunosuppression predisposes to infection; death frequently results from a combination of haemorrhage and septicaemia.

Myrotheciotoxicosis

Sudden death in sheep and cattle may be attributed to large doses of roridins, mycotoxins produced by *Myrothecium* species when growing on ryegrass or white clover plants in pasture or stored feed. Prolonged exposure to sublethal amounts of roridin may cause weight loss and unthriftiness.

References

Allen, J.G., Steele, P., Masters, H.G. and Lambe, W.J. (1992). A lupinosis-associated myopathy in sheep and the effectiveness of treatments to prevent it. *Australian Veterinary Journal*, **69**, 75–81.

Briggs, L.R., Towers, N.R. and Molan, P.C. (1993). Sporidesmin and ELISA technology. *New Zealand Veterinary Journal*, **41**, 220.

Cockcroft, P.D. (1995). Sudden death in dairy cattle with putative acute aflatoxin B poisoning. *Veterinary Record*, **136**, 248.

Collin, R.G. and Towers, N.R. (1995). Competition of a sporidesmin-producing *Pithomyces* strain with a non-toxigenic *Pithomyces* strain. *New Zealand Veterinary Journal*, **43**, 149–152.

Côté, L.M., Reynolds, J.D., Vesonder, R.F. *et al.* (1984). Survey of vomitoxin-contaminated feed grains in midwestern United States, and associated health problems in swine. *Journal of the American Veterinary Medical Association*, **184**, 189–192.

di Menna, M.E. and Mantle, P.G. (1978). The role of penicillia in ryegrass staggers. *Research in Veterinary Science*, **24**, 347–351.

Galey, F.D., Tracey, M.L., Craigmill, A.L. *et al.* (1991). Staggers induced by consumption of perennial ryegrass in cattle and sheep from northern California. *Journal of the American Veterinary Medical Association*, **199**, 466–470.

Gilmour, J.S., Inglis, D.M., Robb, J. and Maclean, M. (1989). A fodder mycotoxicosis of ruminants caused by contamination of a distillery by-product with *Aspergillus clavatus*. *Veterinary Record*, **124**, 133–135.

Griffiths, I.B. and Done, S.H. (1991). Citrinin as a possible cause of the pruritis, pyrexia, haemorrhagic syndrome in cattle. *Veterinary Record*, **129**, 113–117.

Harvey, R.B., Kubena, L.F., Phillips, T.D. *et al.* (1989). Prevention of aflatoxicosis by addition of hydrated sodium calcium aluminosilicate to the diets of growing barrows. *American Journal of Veterinary Research*, **50**, 416–420.

Hill, B.D. and Wright, H.F. (1992). Acute interstitial pneumonia in cattle associated with consumption of mould-damaged sweet potatoes (*Ipomoea batatas*). *Australian Veterinary Journal*, **69**, 36–37.

Hogg, R.A. (1991). Poisoning of cattle fed ergotised silage. *Veterinary Record*, **129**, 313–314.

Lomax, L.G., Cole, R.J. and Dorner, J.W. (1984). The toxicity of cyclopiazonic acid in weaned pigs. *Veterinary Pathology*, **21**, 418–424.

Long, G.G. and Diekman, M.A. (1986). Characterization of effects of zearalenone in swine during early pregnancy. *American Journal of Veterinary Research*, **47**, 184–187.

Munday, R., Thompson, A.M., Fowke, E.A. *et al.* (1997). A zinc-containing intraruminal device for facial eczema control in lambs. *New Zealand Veterinary Journal*, **45**, 93–98.

Osweiler, G.D. (1990). Mycotoxins and livestock: what role do fungal toxins play in illness and production losses ? *Veterinary Medicine*, **85**, 89–94.

Robb, J. (1993). Mycotoxins. *In Practice*, **15**, 278-280.

Ross, A.D., Bryden, W.L., Bakau, W. and Burgess, L.W. (1989). Induction of heat stress in beef cattle by feeding the ergots of *Claviceps purpurea*. *Australian Veterinary Journal*, **66**, 247–249.

Ross, P.F., Rice, L.G., Reagor, J.C. *et al.* (1991). Fumonisin B_1 concentrations in feeds from 45 confirmed equine leukoencephalomalacia cases. *Journal of Veterinary Diagnostic Investigation*, **3**, 328–341.

Sockett, D.C., Baker, J.C. and Stowe, C.M. (1982). Slaframine (*Rhizoctonia leguminicola*) intoxication in horses. *Journal of the American Veterinary Medical Association*, **181**, 606.

Towers, N.R. and Sprosen, J.M. (1993). Zearalenone-induced infertility in sheep and cattle in New Zealand. *New Zealand Veterinary Journal*, **41**, 223–224.

Wu, W., Cook, M.E., Chu, F.S. *et al.* (1997). Case study of bovine dermatitis caused by oat straw infected with *Fusarium sporotrichioides*. *Veterinary Record*, **140**, 399–400.

Further reading

Hollinger, K. and Ekperigin, H.E. (1999). Mycotoxicosis in food producing animals. *Veterinary Clinics of North America: Food Animal Practice*, **15**, 133–165.

Marasas, W.F.O. and Nelson, P.E. (1987). *Mycotoxicology*. The Pennsylvania State University Press, University Park, Pensylvania, USA.

Quinn, P.J., Carter, M.E., Markey, B.K. and Carter, G.R. (1994). Mycotoxins and Mycotoxicoses. In *Clinical Veterinary Microbiology*. Mosby-Year Book Europe, London. pp. 421–438.

Chapter 47

Pathogenic algae and cyanobacteria

Algae are saprophytic eukaryotic organisms which are widely distributed in the environment especially in water. Many contain chlorophyll. Infrequently, some species of algae have been implicated in disease of domestic animals (Table 47.1). The prokaryotic cyanobacteria (formerly known as blue-green algae) produce potent toxins which can affect hepatic and neurological function. Colourless eukaryotic algae belonging to the genus *Prototheca* can invade tissues causing cutaneous and disseminated disease in a number of species and mastitis in cattle. Green algae belonging to *Chlorella* species have been associated with tissue invasion in ruminants on rare occasions.

Prototheca species

Prototheca species, widely distributed, saprophytic, colourless algae, are related to green algae of the genus *Chlorella*. *Prototheca zopfii* has been associated with disseminated prototheecosis in dogs and with mastitis in cows. Cutaneous protothecosis in cats and dogs is caused by *P. wickerhamii*. Both of these *Prototheca* species grow aerobically forming yeast-like colonies on Sabouraud dextrose agar and on blood agar. During asexual reproduction 2 to 16 sporangiospores develop within a sporangium (Fig. 47.1). The sporangiospores are released through a split which develops in the sporangial wall. In cultures, the sporangiospores of *P. zopfii* are larger than those of *P. wickerhamii* (Pore, 1998).

Infections due to *Prototheca* species are opportunistic.

Table 47.1 Algae and cyanobacteria implicated infrequently in opportunistic infections or intoxications of domestic animals.

Agents	Methods of disease production	Clinical effects
Prototheca species	Tissue invasion	Skin lesions, mastitis
Chlorella species	Tissue invasion	Lymphadenopathy
Cyanobacteria	Toxin production	Hepatomegaly, photosensitization, neurological disturbance

Key points

- *Prototheca* species
  —Eukaryotic colourless algae
  —Widely distributed in sewage and organic matter
  —*P. wickerhamii* causes cutaneous infections in cats and dogs
  —*P. zopfii* causes disseminated disease in dogs and mastitis in dairy cattle
- *Chlorella* species
  —Eukaryotic green algae
  —Morphologically similar to *Prototheca* species but contain chloroplasts
  —Associated rarely with lymphadenitis in ruminants
- Cyanobacteria
  —Prokaryotic photosynthetic organisms
  —Form 'algal' blooms on fresh water surfaces
  —Produce potent hepatotoxins and neurotoxins affecting fish, birds and mammals

Organisms can enter tissues at sites of minor trauma in skin and mucous membranes or through the teat canal.

Diagnostic procedures

- Suitable specimens for laboratory examination include milk samples and biopsy or postmortem tissues.
- Methenamine silver or PAS techniques can be used to demonstrate algal cells and sporangia in histological sections of granulomatous lesions.
- Immunofluorescent techniques are used to identify *P. zopfii* and *P. wickerhamii* in tissues.
- The organisms grow on blood agar and Sabouraud dextrose agar without cyclohexamide. Organisms may be isolated from contaminated specimens on protothecha isolation medium with added phthalate and 5-fluorocytosine (Pore, 1998). Culture plates are incubated aerobically at 35°C to 37°C for 2 to 5 days.
- Carbohydrate assimilation test kits for differentiating *Prototheca* species are available commercially.

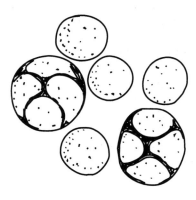

Figure 47.1 The cells and two sporangia, containing sporangiospores, of *Prototheca zopfii*.

Prototheca wickerhamii assimilates trehalose but not 1-propanol, whereas *P. zopfii* assimilates 1-propanol but not trehalose.

- Identification criteria for isolates:
  — Colonial morphology
  — Microscopic appearance of sporangiospores
  — Carbohydrate assimilation tests

Clinical infections

Although *Prototheca* species are commonly present in the environment, infections in animals are infrequent. Suppression of cell-mediated immunity may be a factor predisposing to disseminated disease (Migaki *et al.* 1981).

Cutaneous protothecosis in cats

A cutaneous form of protothecosis, caused by *P. wickerhamii,* is the only manifestation of the disease reported in cats (Dillberger *et al.*, 1988). Large, firm discrete nodules occur on limbs and feet. Similar lesions have been described on the nose, ears and at the base of the tail. Microscopically, the granulomatous lesions, located in the dermis, contain multinucleate giant cells with engulfed organisms. Surgical excision of skin lesions is the most effective method of treatment. Ketoconazole therapy is often ineffective.

Disseminated protothecosis in dogs

Infection with *P. zopfii* probably occurs through the intestinal mucosa as dissemination is often preceded by haemorrhagic colitis (Migaki *et al.*, 1981). Affected dogs may present with protracted bloody diarrhoea along with signs of neurological or ocular disturbance. There may be progressive weight loss and debility. Treatment of disseminated protothecosis is usually unsuccessful. At post-mortem, granulomatous lesions in which protothecal cells may be demonstrated, are found in skeletal muscles, brain, liver, kidneys, eyes and cochlea. In addition to disseminated protothecosis, a cutaneous form caused by *P. wickerhamii* has been recorded (Ginel *et al.*, 1997).

Protothecal mastitis in cows

Prototheca zopfii can cause chronic progressive pyogranulomatous lesions in bovine mammary glands and associated lymph nodes. Indurative mastitis may affect a number of quarters. Because protothecal cells tend to be located intracellularly they may be difficult to eliminate from the glands. Although the organisms are excreted intermittently in milk, they may not be demonstrable in samples, and some cases of the disease may be overlooked (Spalton, 1985). *Prototheca zopfii* can persist in the tissues throughout a dry period and may be excreted during the next lactation. Treatment is unsuccessful. Affected cows should be culled because they are potential sources of infection and their milk yields are permanently reduced. Disseminated protothecosis has been recorded in cattle on rare occasions (Taniyama *et al.*, 1994).

Chlorella species

Green algae cause disease in ruminants on rare occasions. *Chlorella* species are morphologically similar to *Prototheca* species. However, they are photosynthetic, possessing chloroplasts containing green pigment which imparts colour to infected tissues. The organisms have been recovered from liver and associated lymph nodes of sheep (Zakia *et al.*, 1989) and from cattle with lymphadenitis in Australia (Rogers *et al.*, 1980).

The cyanobacteria

The cyanobacteria are prokaryotic photosynthetic organisms found worldwide in fresh and marine water and in soil. Blue-green 'algal' blooms may form when conditions allow rapid replication of cyanobacteria. They may occur in water, enriched with phosphates or nitrogen, when its temperature is between 15°C and 30°C, its pH is neutral or alkaline, and wind disturbance is minimal (Carmichael, 1994). In these circumstances, domestic or wild animals drinking contaminated water are likely to be exposed to toxin released from the organisms. More than 40 species of cyanobacteria are known to produce potent hepatotoxins or neurotoxins. Selected cyanobacteria, presumed to be toxigenic, are listed in Box 47.1. *Microcystis aeruginosa* is the species most often incriminated in episodes of poisoning. Some species such as *Anabaena flos-aquae* can generate both hepatotoxin and neurotoxin.

Cyanobacterial toxicoses

Toxins of the cyanobacteria, their modes of action and their clinical effects are presented in Table 47.2. Although death may occur within a short time after ingestion of a lethal dose of toxin, the dose response curve is relatively steep and animals can ingest nearly 90% of a lethal dose without noticeable effects. The severity of intoxication depends on the degree of exposure and the toxin concentration in contaminated water. Birds and ruminants are usually more susceptible to the toxins than monogastric animals.

Clinical signs

Clinical signs, which relate to the types of toxin ingested, may be diverse. Hepatotoxic effects, which may develop within hours of exposure, include muscle tremors, dyspnoea, blood-stained diarrhoea and coma. Hepatomegaly may be detectable. Photosensitive dermatitis has been recorded in horses and ruminants. Signs of neurotoxicosis, which may develop within minutes of ingesting toxin, include hypersalivation, clonic convulsions, rigor and cyanosis (Gunn *et al.*, 1992). Death may occur rapidly after the onset of clinical signs.

Diagnosis

- There may be a history of access to contaminated water with an 'algal' bloom.
- The mouth or legs of affected animals may be stained green.
- Samples of bloom should be examined microscopically for the presence of cyanobacteria.
- Toxin must be demonstrated in the bloom or in stomach contents by chemical, biological or immunoassay techniques in a reference laboratory.
- There may be histopathological evidence of hepatotoxicosis.
- Serum concentrations of bile acids and liver enzymes may be elevated (Carbis *et al.*, 1995).
- Other possible sources of intoxication should be considered in the differential diagnosis.

Box 47.1 Toxigenic cyanobacteria.

- *Microcystis aeruginosa*
- *Anabaena flos-aquae*
- *Oscillatoria* species
- *Aphanizomenon* species
- *Nodularia* species
- *Cylindrosperum* species
- *Cylindrospermopsis* species
- *Nostoc* species
- *Lyngbya* species

Treatment

- Affected horses and ruminants, removed from the source of toxin, should be housed out of direct sunlight.
- Emetics administered to recently exposed dogs may aid recovery.
- Activated charcoal slurry or ion-exchange resins may be used for adsorbing toxins from the gastrointestinal tract.
- Although atropine reduces the anti-acetylcholinesterase activity of anatoxin-a(s), no therapeutic antagonist is effective against anatoxin-a or the saxitoxins.

Control

- Access of animals to contaminated water must be restricted.
- Companion animals should not be fed fish from contaminated waters.
- Growth of cyanobacteria can be controlled in small bodies of water by the addition of copper sulphate. However treatment of an 'algal' bloom with algicides results in the liberation of toxins from dead cells into the water.

References

Carbis, C.R., Waldron, D.L., Mitchell, G.F., Anderson, J.W. and McCauley, I. (1995). Recovery of hepatic function and latent mortalities in sheep exposed to the blue-green alga

Table 47.2 Toxins of cyanobacteria, their modes of action and clinical effects.

Toxins	Mode of action	Clinical effects
Microcystins and nodularins	Hepatotoxic; inhibition of protein phosphatases	Hepatomegaly and hepatoencephalopathy; photosensitization; raised serum liver enzyme levels; severe toxicity results in intrahepatic haemorrhage and death from hypovolaemic shock
Anatoxin–a	Neurotoxic; post-synaptic cholinergic agonist; mimics the activity of acetylcholine	Involuntary muscular contractions, convulsions; severe toxicity results in death
Anatoxin–a(s)	Neurotoxic; anti-acetylcholinesterase activity	Similar to the effects of anatoxin-a; hypersalivation
Saxitoxins and neosaxitoxins	Blockade of signal transmission in motor neurons	Flaccid paralysis; death from respiratory failure

Microcystis aeruginosa. *Veterinary Record*, **137**, 12–15.

Carmichael, W.W. (1994). The toxins of cyanobacteria. *Scientific American*, **270**, 64–72.

Dillberger, J.E., Homer, B., Daubert, D. and Altman, N.H. (1988). Protothecosis in two cats. *Journal of the American Veterinary Medical Association*, **192**, 1557–1559.

Ginel, P.J., Pérez, J., Molledo, J.M., Lucena, R. and Mozos, E. (1997). Cutaneous protothecosis in a dog. *Veterinary Record*, **140**, 651–653.

Gunn, G.J., Rafferty, A.G., Rafferty, G.C. *et al.* (1992). Fatal canine neurotoxicosis attributed to blue-green algae (cyanobacteria). *Veterinary Record*, **130**, 301–302.

Migaki, G., Font, R.L., Sauer, R.M., Kaplan, W. and Miller, R.L. (1981). Canine protothecosis: Review of the literature and report of an additional case. *Journal of the American Veterinary Medical Association*, **181**, 794–797.

Pore, R.S. (1998). *Prototheca* and *Chlorella* species. In *Topley and Wilson's Microbiology and Microbial Infections*, Volume 4. *Medical Mycology*. Eds. L. Ajello and R.J. Hay, Ninth Edition. Arnold, London. pp. 631–643.

Rogers, R.J., Connole, M.D., Thomas, J.N.A., Ladds, P.W. and

Dickson, J. (1980). Lymphadenitis of cattle due to infection with green algae. *Journal of Comparative Pathology*, **90**, 1–9.

Spalton, D.E. (1985). Bovine mastitis caused by *Prototheca zopfii*: a case study. *Veterinary Record*, **116**, 347–349.

Taniyama, H., Okamoto, F., Kurosawa, T., Furuoka, H., Kaji, Y., Okada, H. and Matsukawa, K. (1994). Disseminated protothecosis caused by *Prototheca zopfii* in a cow. *Veterinary Pathology*, **31**, 123–125.

Zakia, A.M., Osheika, A.A. and Halima, M.O. (1989). Ovine chlorellosis in the Sudan. *Veterinary Record*, **125**, 625–626.

Further reading

Anderson, K.L. and Walker, R.L. (1988). Sources of *Prototheca* spp. in a dairy cow environment. *Journal of the American Veterinary Medical Association*, **193**, 553–556.

Madigan, M.T., Martinko, J.M. and Parker, J. (1997). *Brock Biology of Microorganisms*. Eighth Edition. Prentice Hall International Inc., New Jersey. pp. 654–658.

Section IV

Introductory Virology

Chapter 48

Nature, structure and taxonomy of viruses

The term 'virus' (Latin, poison) refers to members of a unique class of infectious agents which are extremely small, contain only one type of nucleic acid and have an absolute dependence on living cells for replication (Box 48.1). The genomes of the viruses which infect animals are smaller than those of prokaryotic cells, ranging from about 2 kilobase pairs (kbp) to 200 kbp. In most viruses, the nucleic acid is present as a single molecule; in some RNA viruses the nucleic acid occurs in separate segments. Although the nucleic acid of viral genomes is usually linear, it is circular in some viruses. Genomes of DNA viruses can be single-stranded or double-stranded. Particular characteristics of DNA and RNA viruses are presented in Tables 48.1 and 48.2 and in Figs. 48.1 and 48.2.

There are two unique types of infectious agents, viroids and prions, which are structurally less complex than viruses. Viroids are composed of naked RNA and prions are proteinaceous infectious particles which are devoid of demonstrable nucleic acid.

Viruses were first recognized as unique infectious entities in the late nineteenth century. Knowledge of the nature of bacteria and fungi was well established by this time. Dmitri Ivanovsky, a Russian scientist, reported in 1892 that it was possible to transmit tobacco mosaic disease from diseased to healthy plants using filtered leaf extract as inoculum. The filters used by Ivanovsky were

---

Box 48.1 Characteristics of viruses which can infect animals.

- Small infectious agents ranging in size from 20 to 300 nm
- Composed of nucleic acid surrounded by a protein coat; in addition, some have envelopes
- Contain only one type of nucleic acid, either DNA or RNA
- Unlike bacteria and fungi, viruses cannot replicate on inert media; viable host cells are required for replication
- Some viruses have an affinity for particular cell types

Chamberland filters, porcelain filters designed to remove bacteria from drinking water. In 1898, Martinus Beijerinck, unaware of the work of Ivanovsky, also demonstrated the filterability of the agent of tobacco mosaic disease. Moreover, he realised that the disease could not be due to a toxin as the filtered sap from infected plants could be used for serial transmission of the disease without loss of potency. In the same year, Loeffler and Frosch identified the first filterable agent from animals, the virus of foot-and-mouth disease. Yellow fever virus, a filterable agent pathogenic for humans, was described by

---

Table 48.1 Characteristics of the families of DNA viruses of veterinary importance.

Family	Virion size (nm)	Capsid symmetry	Envelope	Type of genome
Adenoviridae	70–90	Icosahedral	Absent	Linear, double-stranded DNA
Asfarviridae	175–215	Icosahedral	Present	Linear, double-stranded DNA
Circoviridae	17–22	Icosahedral	Absent	Circular molecule of positive-sense or ambisense, single-stranded DNA
Herpesviridae	120–200	Icosahedral	Present	Single molecule of linear, double-stranded DNA
Papillomaviridae	55	Icosahedral	Absent	Single molecule of circular, double-stranded DNA
Parvoviridae	18–26	Icosahedral	Absent	Single molecule of linear, positive-sense or negative-sense, single-stranded DNA
Poxviridae	300 x 200	Complex	Present	Single molecule of linear, double-stranded DNA

Table 48.2 Characteristics of the families of RNA viruses of veterinary importance.

Family	Virion size (nm)	Capsid symmetry	Envelope	Type of genome
Arteriviridae	40–60	Icosahedral	Present	Linear, single molecule of positive-sense, single-stranded RNA
Astroviridae	28–30	Icosahedral	Absent	Linear, single molecule of positive-sense, single-stranded RNA
Birnaviridae	60	Icosahedral	Absent	Two segments of linear, double-stranded RNA
Bornaviridae	90	Icosahedral	Present	Linear, single molecule of negative-sense, single-stranded RNA
Bunyaviridae	80–120	Helical	Present	Three segments of linear, negative-sense or ambisense single-stranded RNA
Caliciviridae	27–40	Icosahedral	Absent	Linear, single molecule of positive-sense, single-stranded RNA
Coronaviridae	120–160	Helical	Present	Linear, single molecule of positive-sense, single-stranded RNA
Flaviviridae	40–60	Icosahedral	Present	Linear, single molecule of positive-sense, single-stranded RNA
Orthomyxoviridae	80–120	Helical	Present	Six to eight segments of linear, negative-sense, single-stranded RNA
Paramyxoviridae	150–300	Helical	Present	Linear, single molecule of negative-sense, single-stranded RNA
Picornaviridae	30	Icosahedral	Absent	Linear, single molecule of positive-sense, single-stranded RNA
Reoviridae	60–80	Icosahedral	Absent	Ten to twelve segments of linear, double-stranded RNA
Retroviridae	80–100	Icosahedral	Present	Diploid, linear, positive-sense, single-stranded RNA
Rhabdoviridae	180 x 75	Helical	Present	Linear, single molecule of negative-sense, single-stranded RNA
Togaviridae	70	Icosahedral	Present	Linear, single molecule of positive-sense, single-stranded RNA

Walter Reed and his team in 1901. Ellerman and Bang, in 1908, demonstrated the oncogenic potential of a filterable agent, the cause of avian leukosis. In 1915, Frederick Twort observed that bacteria were susceptible to a filterable agent and, two years later, Felix D'Herelle, made a similar observation. D'Herelle named these viruses 'bacteriophages' and developed a technique for establishing their concentration in active preparations. Bacteriophages have proved to be particularly useful in studies on viral replication and bacterial genetics.

Initially, the only way to recover large quantities of virus was through infecting susceptible animals. In 1913, Steinhardt and his colleagues succeeded in growing vaccinia virus in explants of guinea-pig cornea embedded in clotted plasma. Some twenty years later, Furth and Sturmia used mice as a host species for propagating viruses, while Woodruff and Goodpasture were successful in propagating fowlpox virus on the chorioallantoic membrane of embryonated eggs. A major advance was made in the early 1950s with the development of single cell cultures. Factors which were critical in this development included the availability of antibiotics to control bacterial contamination and the use of trypsin to obtain cell suspensions from embryonic or adult tissue. The separated cells could then be grown as monolayers on glass surfaces. Continuous cell lines, capable of multiplying indefinitely, provided a reliable source of cells for virus cultivation.

In 1887, Buist observed vaccinia virus using a light microscope. However, because of the limited resolving power of this type of microscopy, the structure of the virus was not discernible. In 1939, Kausche and his co-workers employed the newly developed electron microscope and a metal shadowing technique to identify tobacco mosaic virus in purified preparations. Ultrastructural studies of viruses were greatly expanded and enhanced in the 1950s by the development of negative staining and methods for cutting ultrathin sections. X-ray diffraction methods have been applied to viruses since the 1930s, when it was discovered that simple viruses could be crystallized. The first complete high resolution structure of a crystalline virus, tomato bushy stunt virus, was obtained by Harrison and his co-workers in 1978. Computer analysis of the diffraction patterns obtained by such studies has contributed to knowledge of the molecular structure of viruses.

In recent years, remarkable advances have been made in our understanding of the epidemiology, pathogenesis and

DNA viruses

dsDNA and enveloped

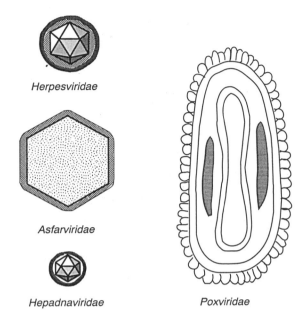

dsDNA and non-enveloped

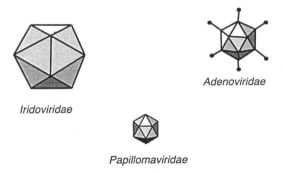

ssDNA and non-enveloped

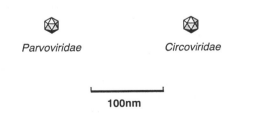

100nm

Figure 48.1 Diagrammatic representations of virions in families of DNA viruses of vertebrates. The genomes of these viruses are composed of either double-stranded (ds) or single-stranded (ss) DNA.

control of viral diseases. However, as new viral diseases are recognized in the animal and human populations, fresh challenges confront those engaged in virological research.

Origin of viruses

Viruses have evolved to a stage where they are considered to be among the most efficient and economic forms of microbial life. They can be categorized in three main groups on the basis of their nucleic acid composition: DNA viruses, RNA viruses and viruses which utilize both DNA and RNA for replication. Differences between these groups are significant and may be indicative of independent origins for each group. Although the origin of viruses is uncertain, three theories have been proposed to explain their evolution. They may have originated and evolved in parallel with primordial life forms. They may have arisen from segments of cellular nucleic acid which acquired the ability to replicate at the expense of the host cell. The third theory, the regressive theory of the origin of viruses, postulates that they arose from free-living organisms which gradually lost genetic information until they became totally dependent on the biosynthetic pathways of their host cells.

Structure of viruses

A fully assembled infective virus is termed a virion. The fundamental component of the virion is a nucleoprotein core with the ability to infect host cells and replicate in them, thus ensuring continued survival. The genome of vertebrate viruses is enclosed within a shell of proteins, called a capsid (Fig. 48.3). It is haploid except in retroviruses, in which it is diploid. The term nucleocapsid is used to describe the packaged form of the genome in the capsid. Each subunit of the capsid is composed of a folded polypeptide chain. Collections of these subunits constitute structural units or protomers which, in turn, comprise assembly units. The term capsomer or morphological unit is used to describe features such as protrusions seen on the surface of virus particles in electron micrographs. These often correspond to groups of protein subunits arranged about a local axis of symmetry. Capsids are, therefore, composed of multiples of one or more types of protein subunits. The orderly arrangement of similar protein-protein interfaces results in a symmetrical structure. Icosahedral and helical symmetries are the two types of capsid symmetry described in viruses (Fig. 48.4).

Closed-shell virions, isometric viruses, have structures based on icosahedral symmetry, a structural form which offers the maximum capacity and greatest strength for a given surface area. The icosahedron, one of the five platonic solids, has 20 equilateral triangles forming its faces, 30 edges and 12 vertices. At its simplest, a viral icosahedron has 60 identical structural units, three in each triangular face. Larger numbers of smaller units are

RNA viruses

ssRNA and enveloped

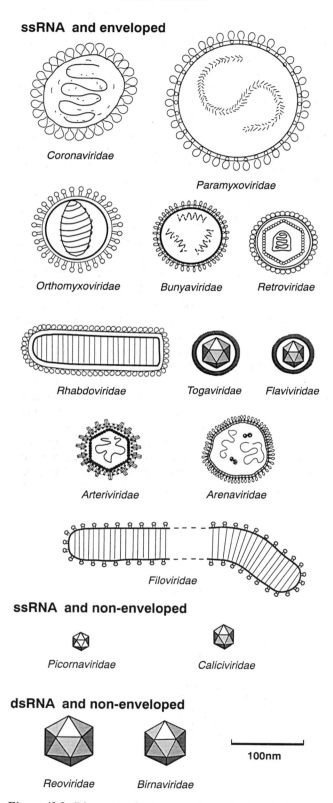

ssRNA and non-enveloped

dsRNA and non-enveloped

100nm

Figure 48.2 Diagrammatic representations of virions in families of RNA viruses of vertebrates. The genomes of these viruses are composed of either double-stranded (ds) or single-stranded (ss) RNA.

accommodated on the triangular faces only in specific multiples of 60, represented by the formula $T = h^2 + hk + k^2$ where h and k are integers having no common factors and T is the triangulation number. For caliciviruses $T = 3$ and for herpesviruses $T = 16$. The structural units at each vertex form groups of five termed pentons, while those on the faces form groups of six called hexons. There are two-fold, three-fold and five-fold axes of rotational symmetry which pass through edges, faces and vertices respectively. Viruses with icosahedral symmetry are often not seen as icosahedrons; they may appear in electron micrographs as spheres or hexagons. Icosahedral capsids are generally assembled in the host cell prior to incorporation of the viral nucleic acid. Some viral preparations may contain capsids devoid of nucleic acid. The nucleic acid of double-stranded DNA viruses is condensed into a form suitable for incorporation into capsids by the action of cellular histones and basic virus-encoded molecules. The protective capsid of many RNA viruses is formed by the insertion of protein units between each turn of the nucleic acid helix. The capsid protein helix, therefore, coincides with that of the nucleic acid and the length of the helix is determined by the length of the RNA molecule. Viral particles devoid of nucleic acid cannot be formed. In RNA viruses, each capsomere consists of a single polypeptide molecule.

In many types of viruses the nucleocapsid is covered by an envelope composed of a lipid bilayer and associated glycoproteins. The envelope is acquired when the nucleocapsid buds through a cellular membrane, usually the plasma membrane. In some viral infections, the envelope is acquired from the endoplasmic reticulum, the Golgi apparatus or the nuclear membrane. Proteins encoded by viral nucleic acid and integrated as glycoprotein into the appropriate membrane by the compartmentalization mechanisms of the host cell are an integral part of the viral envelope. These glycoproteins are associated with binding to receptors on host cells, membrane fusion, uncoating of the virion and destruction of receptors on host cells. A single envelope glycoprotein may have multiple functions. In most enveloped viruses, the envelope must be intact to maintain infectivity and, treatment with lipid solvents such as ether or chloroform, renders them non-infectious. Epitopes on envelope glycoproteins are often important for inducing protective immune responses in infected animals. Peplomers or spikes are knob-like projections from the envelope in certain viruses including coronaviruses, retroviruses, orthomyxoviruses, rhabdoviruses and paramyxoviruses. These structures are formed from oligomers of surface glycoproteins. They often bind to cell receptors and, in addition, they may have enzymatic activity. A layer of protein, termed matrix protein, is present between the nucleocapsid and the envelope in some enveloped viruses. This layer provides additional rigidity to the virion. Helical RNA viruses of animals are enveloped.

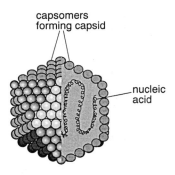

Figure 48.3 Diagrammatic representation of capsomers forming protective icosahedral capsid outside viral nucleic acid.

Taxonomy of viruses

The sole experimental indication of the minute size of viruses at the end of the nineteenth century was their ability to pass through filters which retained bacteria. Information relating to viruses derived largely from studies on the diseases which they caused. Early classification systems therefore, were based on their pathogenic effects and transmission patterns. In the 1930s, details of the structure and composition of viruses began to emerge. Subsequently, it was possible to group viruses on the basis of shared features of virions. During the 1950s and 1960s, several classification schemes were adopted. The International Committee on Nomenclature of Viruses (ICNV) was established in 1966 to develop a single universal taxonomic scheme. The successor to the ICNV, the International Committee on Taxonomy of Viruses (ICTV) established in 1973, developed and expanded the universal scheme in which virion characteristics are used to assign viruses to five main hierarchical levels namely order, family, subfamily, genus and species (Tables 48.3 to 48.8). Virus orders are designated by the suffix *-virales*. In orders, phylogenetically-related families are grouped together. Only two orders containing viruses of animals have been defined thus far. These are the *Mononegavirales* comprising the families *Paramyxoviridae*, *Rhabdoviridae*, *Bornaviridae* and *Filoviridae* and the *Nidovirales* comprising the families *Coronaviridae* and *Arteriviridae*. Families are, therefore, designated by the suffix *-viridae*. Of more than 50 families currently recognized, about 22 contain viruses of veterinary importance. The suffix *-virinae* denotes a subfamily. Viral genera are designated by the suffix *-virus*. More than 230 genera are recognized. The criteria for defining a genus differ from family to family. The species taxon is regarded as the most important level in the classification of viruses. However, its definition and application has always been difficult and controversial. In 1991, the ICTV accepted the definition of a virus species proposed by van Regenmortel (1990) which states that 'a virus species is defined as a polythetic class of viruses that constitutes a replicating lineage and occupies a particular ecological niche'. This implies that a virus species is defined by a combination of multiple properties and characteristics; no single or unique property is essential for species definition. This comprehensive type of taxonomy is the Adansonian system of classification. In the present scheme of virus taxonomy, the primary delineating criteria are the type and nature of the genome, the mode and site of viral replication and the structure of the virion. Currently, more than 1,500 virus species are recognized by the ICTV, with the

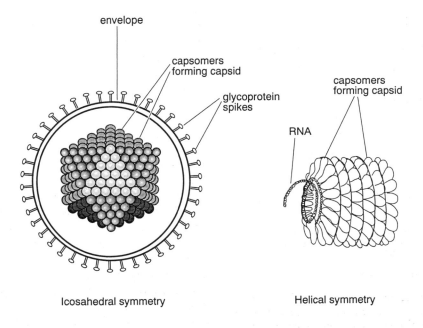

Figure 48.4 Diagrammatic representation of icosahedral and helical symmetry.

Table 48.3 The families containing the double-stranded DNA viruses of vertebrates.

Family	Subfamily	Genus	Type species
Adenoviridae		*Mastadenovirus*	Human adenovirus C
		Aviadenovirus	Fowl adenovirus A
Asfarviridae		*Asfivirus*	African swine fever virus
Herpesviridae	*Alphaherpesvirinae*	*Simplexvirus*	Human herpesvirus 1
		Varicellovirus	Human herpesvirus 3
		Marek's disease-like viruses	Gallid herpesvirus 2
		Infectious laryngotracheitis-like viruses	Gallid herpesvirus 1
	Betaherpesvirinae	*Cytomegalovirus*	Human herpesvirus 5
		Muromegalovirus	Murid herpesvirus 1
		Roseolovirus	Human herpesvirus 6
	Gammaherpesvirinae	*Lymphocryptovirus*	Human herpesvirus 4
		Rhadinovirus	Saimiriine herpesvirus 2
	Unnamed	Ictalurid herpes-like viruses	Ictalurid herpesvirus 1
Papillomaviridae		*Papillomavirus*	Cottontail rabbit papillomavirus
Poxviridae	*Chordopoxvirinae*	*Orthopoxvirus*	Vaccinia virus
		Parapoxvirus	Orf virus
		Avipoxvirus	Fowlpox virus
		Capripoxvirus	Sheeppox virus
		Leporipoxvirus	Myxoma virus
		Suipoxvirus	Swinepox virus
		Molluscipoxvirus	Molluscum contagiosum virus
		Yatapoxvirus	Yaba monkey tumour virus

Table 48.4 The families containing the single-stranded DNA viruses of vertebrates.

Family	Subfamily	Genus	Type species
Circoviridae		*Circovirus*	Porcine circovirus
		Gyrovirus	Chicken anaemia virus
Parvoviridae	*Parvovirinae*	*Parvovirus*	Mice minute virus
		Erythrovirus	B19 virus
		Dependovirus	Adeno-associated virus 2

Table 48.5 Retroviruses[a] of vertebrates

Family	Genus	Type species
Retroviridae	*Alpharetrovirus*	Avian leukosis virus
	Betaretrovirus	Mouse mammary tumour virus
	Gammaretrovirus	Murine leukaemia virus
	Deltaretrovirus	Bovine leukaemia virus
	Epsilonretrovirus	Walleye dermal sarcoma virus
	Lentivirus	Human imunodeficiency virus 1
	Spumavirus	Chimpanzee foamy virus 1

a RNA viruses with reverse transcriptase activity

Table 48.6 The families containing the double-stranded RNA viruses of vertebrates.

Family	Genus	Type species
Birnaviridae	*Avibirnavirus*	Infectious bursal disease virus
	Aquabirnavirus	Infectious pancreatic necrosis virus
Reoviridae	*Orthoreovirus*	Mammalian orthoreovirus
	Orbivirus	Bluetongue virus 1
	Rotavirus	Rotavirus A
	Coltivirus	Colarado tick fever virus
	Aquareovirus	Aquareovirus A

Table 48.7 Families containing negative-sense, single-stranded RNA viruses of vertebrates.

Family	Subfamily	Genus	Type species
Bornaviridae		*Bornavirus*	Borna disease virus
Bunyaviridae		*Bunyavirus*	Bunyamwera virus
		Hantavirus	Hantaan virus
		Nairovirus	Dugbe virus
		Phlebovirus	Rift valley fever virus
Orthomyxoviridae		*Influenzavirus A*	Influenza A virus
		Influenzavirus B	Influenza B virus
		Influenzavirus C	Influenza C virus
		Thogotovirus	Thogoto virus
Paramyxoviridae	*Paramyxovirinae*	*Respirovirus*	Sendai virus
		Morbillivirus	Measles virus
		Rubulavirus	Mumps virus
	Pneumovirinae	*Pneumovirus*	Human respiratory syncytial virus
		Metapneumovirus	Turkey rhinotracheitis virus
Rhabdoviridae		*Lyssavirus*	Rabies virus
		Vesiculovirus	Vesicular stomatitis Indiana virus
		Ephemerovirus	Bovine ephemeral fever virus
		Novirhabdovirus	Infectious haematopoietic necrosis virus

Table 48.8 Families containing the positive-sense, single-stranded RNA viruses of vertebrates.

Family	Genus	Type species
Arteriviridae	*Arterivirus*	Equine arteritis virus
Astroviridae	*Astrovirus*	Human astrovirus 1
Caliciviridae	*Vesivirus*	Swine vesicular exanthema virus
	Lagovirus	Rabbit haemorrhagic disease virus
	Norwalk-like viruses	Norwalk virus
	Sapporo-like viruses	Sapporo virus
	Hepatitis E-like viruses	Hepatitis E virus
Coronaviridae	*Coronavirus*	Infectious bronchitis virus
	Torovirus	Equine torovirus
Flaviviridae	*Flavivirus*	Yellow fever virus
	Hepacivirus	Hepatitis C virus
	Pestivirus	Bovine viral diarrhoea virus 1
Picornaviridae	*Enterovirus*	Poliovirus
	Rhinovirus	Human rhinovirus A
	Hepatovirus	Hepatitis A virus
	Cardiovirus	Encephalomyocarditis virus
	Aphthovirus	Foot-and-mouth disease virus
	Parechovirus	Human parechovirus
	Erbovirus	Equine rhinitis B virus
	Kobuvirus	Aichi virus
	Teschovirus	Porcine teschovirus
Togaviridae	*Alphavirus*	Sindbis virus
	Rubivirus	Rubella virus

periodic addition of new species. In addition, international specialist groups monitor large numbers of strains and subtypes. These latter categories have become accepted for practical reasons such as vaccine development and the diagnosis of disease. No universal definitions or formal nomenclature are recognized for strains and subtypes of virus species.

The ease with which base sequencing can be carried out on viral nucleic acids has revolutionized approaches to virus taxonomy and phylogeny. Reference genome sequences are available for all viral taxa in databases such as GenBank (http://www.ncbi.nlm.nih.gov/GenBank) which permit substantial shortcuts to specific taxonomic placements. In addition, the use of statistical methods for comparing sequence similarities has contributed to studies on the evolution of viruses. The ICTV intends to reserve the hierarchical level or order solely for the recognition of phylogenetic relationships. Recently, interest has focussed on the study of virus evolution in real time at the subspecific level. This has resulted in the development of the concept of viral quasispecies (Eigen, 1993). This concept envisages that each virus species exists as a genetically diverse, rapidly evolving population of virions with non-identical but closely related mutant and recombinant viral genomes based on a consensus sequence. The population as a whole, the quasispecies, acts as a genetic pool which is subjected to a continuous process of variation, competition and selection. The population is in dynamic equilibrium, with the expansive force of mutation balanced by the constraining force of selection. The survival of the quasispecies depends on the stability of the consensus sequence, the complexity of the information in the genome and the copying fidelity. If an advantageous mutant appears, the original quasispecies will be substituted by a new one, characterized by a new consensus sequence and a new distribution of mutants (mutant spectrum). This concept is particularly important with regard to RNA viruses with large genomes. Error rates during replication of viral RNA are much higher than those in replicating viral DNA because a cellular proof-reading mechanism for RNA is lacking. As a result, non-lethal mutations accumulate in the genome of RNA viruses.

In formal viral nomenclature, the names of families, subfamilies, genera and species are italicized. The first letter of each name is upper case. Prior to the 1998 meeting in San Diego of the ICTV, neither capital letters (with the exception of species names derived from place names) nor italics were used for species names. Lower case and plain script is always used for informal names of viruses. The informal designation is commonly used for virus species whereas formal designations tend to be reserved for taxonomic references. Confusion may arise when the same informal designation is applied both to a family and to a genus. For example, coronavirus may refer either to all members of the family *Coronaviridae* or to those of the genus *Coronavirus* only. Terms, based on virus tropisms or modes of transmission, are also used because of their convenience in categorizing viruses. Examples include enteric viruses, respiratory viruses, arboviruses and oncogenic viruses. The term arbovirus relates to the fact that the virus is 'arthropod borne'. Included in this category are viruses in the families *Togaviridae*, *Flaviviridae*, *Rhabdoviridae*, *Reoviridae*, *Asfarviridae* and *Bunyaviridae*. Oncogenic viruses, which have the potential to induce transformation of host cells, are found in the families *Retroviridae*, *Papillomaviridae*, *Adenoviridae* and *Herpesviridae*.

References

Eigen, M. (1993). Viral quasispecies. *Scientific American*, **269**, 42–49.

van Regenmortel, M.H.V. (1990). Virus species, a much overlooked but essential concept in virus classification. *Intervirology*, **31**, 241–254.

Chapter 49

Replication of viruses

Unlike bacteria, which can grow on inert media, viruses can multiply only in host cells. This requirement arises from their limited genomic composition which obliges them to utilize host cell organelles, enzymes and other macromolecules for replication. The effects of viral multiplication on host cells range from minor changes in cellular metabolism to cytolysis. Studies of viral reproduction are usually conducted in synchronously infected cell cultures. In these cultures, a single cycle of virus replication usually takes place. The duration of the cycle may range from six to 40 hours. Within hours of infection, an eclipse phase occurs when virons are difficult to detect. After this eclipse phase, virions are demonstrable both intracellularly and extracellularly. The number of viral particles increases exponentially. Fully assembled virions are released from infected cells either by budding or by cytolysis. The number of virions released is largely dependent on the species of infecting virus and may approach many thousands.

The replicative cycle of a virus can be conveniently divided into a number of stages: attachment and entry into the cell, uncoating of viral nucleic acid, synthesis of virus-specific proteins, production of new viral nucleic acid and assembly and release of newly-formed viruses from the host cell (Box 49.1). A virion must first attach to cell surface receptors in order to produce infection. Initial virus-cell interaction is a random event which relates to the number of virus particles present and the availability of appropriate receptor molecules. Virus-cell interaction determines both the host range and the tissue tropism of viral species. Viruses have evolved to the point where they can utilize a wide range of host cell surface proteins as receptors. Many of these surface molecules are highly conserved and are essential for fundamental cellular functions. Some viruses have more than one type of ligand molecule and they may bind to several cell surface receptors in sequential order during attachment. In the case of some species of virus, individual virions can detach and adsorb to another cell when infection of a particular host cell does not proceed. In the case of orthomyxoviruses and paramyxoviruses, detachment from host cells is mediated by viral neuraminidase, a receptor-destroying enzyme.

Virus uptake or penetration is an energy-dependent process which can occur in a number of ways. Receptor-mediated endocytosis occurs after virus attaches to receptors at particular sites on the plasma membrane. At these sites, which are coated internally with the protein clathrin, the virus-receptor complex is taken into the cell in specialized vesicles. The cage-like lattice formed around the vesicles by clathrin molecules breaks down after endocytosis. Acidification within the vesicles leads to degradation of viral structures. The envelopes of some viruses, such as orthomyxoviruses, rhabdoviruses and flaviviruses, fuse with the membrane of endosomes, releasing nucleocapsids directly into the cytoplasm. A second entry mechanism, which is used by some enveloped viruses including paramyxoviruses, retroviruses and herpesviruses, involves fusion of the viral envelope with the plasma membrane. This allows release of the nucleocapsid directly into the host cell cytoplasm. An additional mechanism employed by some non-enveloped viruses such as picornaviruses involves the direct introduction or translocation of viral genomes into the cytoplasm through channels in the plasma membrane.

Uncoating is the process whereby the viral genome is released in a form suitable for transcription. In the case of enveloped viruses, in which the nucleocapsid is discharged directly into the cytoplasm, transcription can usually proceed without complete uncoating. In non-enveloped viruses, uncoating is poorly understood but probably results from lysosomal proteolytic enzyme activity. In reoviruses, the genome may express all functions without complete release from the capsid. The uncoating of most other non-enveloped viruses proceeds to completion. Poxviruses are uncoated in two stages. The initial stage is mediated by host enzymes, with complete release of viral DNA from the core requiring virus-specified proteins. In some viruses, which replicate in the cell nucleus,

---

Box 49.1 Stages in virus replication.

- Attachment to a surface receptor on a susceptible host cell
- Entry into the cell
- Uncoating of viral nucleic acid
- Replication of viral nucleic acid and synthesis of virus-encoded proteins
- Assembly of newly-formed virus particles and release from host cell

uncoating may be completed at the nuclear pores.

The synthesis of viral proteins by host cells, which is the central event in replication of viruses, requires the production of viral mRNA. Those DNA viruses, which replicate in the nucleus, can avail of host cell transcriptases to synthesize viral mRNA. Other viruses utilize their own enzymes to generate mRNA. Viruses have evolved strategies which facilitate interference with the activity of cellular mRNA. Viruses direct the synthesis of either a separate mRNA for each gene or mRNA encompassing several genes. Eukaryotic cell protein-synthesizing mechanisms, however, translate only monocistronic messages. If a large precursor protein molecule is produced, cleavage into individual proteins is required and each family of viruses employs a unique strategy for this purpose.

Based on the nature of the genome and the pathways of mRNA synthesis, viruses of veterinary importance can be grouped in six classes (Baltimore, 1971). Central to this scheme is the designation of the genome of single-stranded RNA viruses as positive-sense or negative-sense nucleic acid (Fig. 49.1). In this context, the word 'sense' refers to nucleic acid polarity. The nucleic acid of positive-sense single-stranded RNA viruses is mRNA in sense and can be translated directly into virus protein.

In this chapter, specific viruses have been selected to illustrate the replicative mechanism of DNA and RNA viruses. However, individual viruses within these two groups frequently exhibit unique replicative methods. The mechanisms involved in the replication of DNA and RNA viruses, although having many similarities, are complex intracellular events which require separate discussion.

Replication of DNA viruses

Double-stranded DNA viruses, such as herpesviruses, papovaviruses and adenoviruses, which replicate in the nucleus of the cell, have a relatively direct replication strategy. The viral DNA is transcribed by cellular DNA-dependent RNA polymerase (transcriptase) to form mRNA. In contrast, the single-stranded DNA viruses, parvoviruses and circoviruses, which also replicate in cell nuclei, utilize cellular DNA polymerase to synthesize double-stranded DNA. This is then transcribed to mRNA by cellular transcriptases. Because of this transcription requirement, the replication of parvoviruses is largely confined to rapidly-dividing cells. Stages in the replication of a herpes virus, an enveloped double-stranded DNA virus are illustrated in Fig. 49.2.

A defined temporal sequence of events occurs during transcription and replication of DNA viruses. Specified genes encode for early proteins, which include the enzymes and other proteins necessary for virus replication and for suppression of the synthesis of host cell proteins. Subsequently, replication of viral nucleic acid and

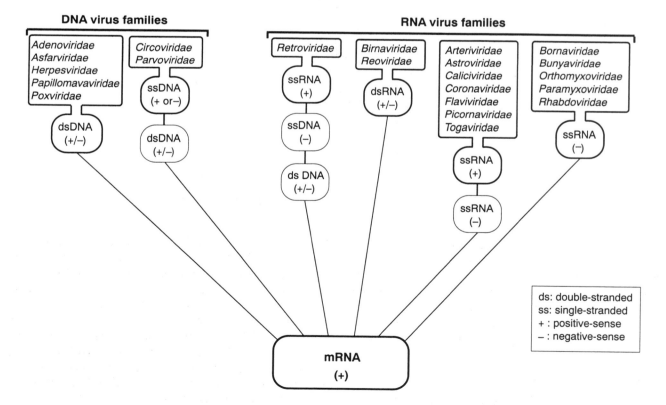

Figure 49.1 Families of DNA and RNA viruses of veterinary importance grouped according to genome types and pathways for messenger RNA synthesis (modified from Baltimore, 1971).

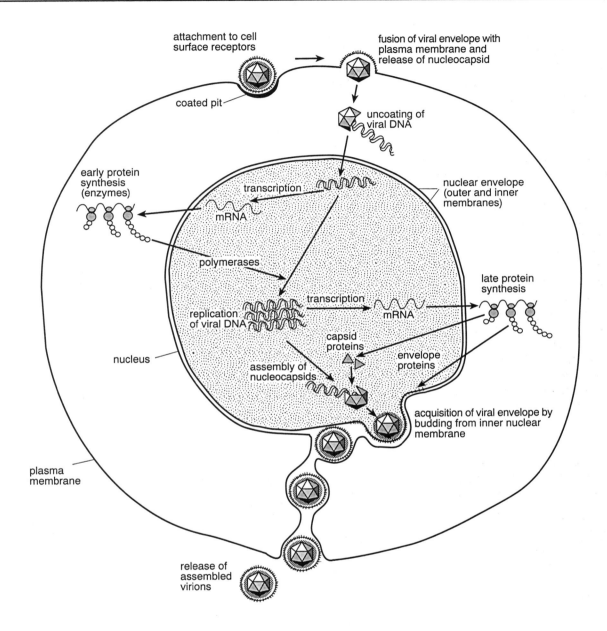

Figure 49.2 Stages in the replication of a herpes virus, an enveloped double-stranded DNA virus.

transcription of the genes which encode the late proteins occur. These late proteins, which are also often transcribed from newly-formed viral nucleic acid, are structural components synthesized late in the infection cycle. This temporal sequence is not clearly demonstrable in the replicative cycles of RNA viruses, in which most of the genetic information is expressed contemporaneously.

Replication of RNA viruses

Reoviruses and birnaviruses, double-stranded RNA viruses, have segmented genomes. Transcription occurs in the cytoplasm under the direction of a viral transcriptase.

The negative-sense strand of each segment is transcribed to produce individual mRNA molecules. In contrast, the genomes of positive-sense, single-stranded RNA viruses can act directly as mRNA after infection (Fig. 49.3). The enzymes necessary for genome replication in these viruses are produced after infection by direct translation of virion RNA. This RNA can bind directly to ribosomes and is translated to yield a single polyprotein which is then cleaved to yield both functional and structural proteins. Because direct translation can occur, naked RNA extracted from such viruses is infectious. The positive-sense, single-stranded RNA viruses utilize a number of different synthetic pathways during replication. In togaviruses, only

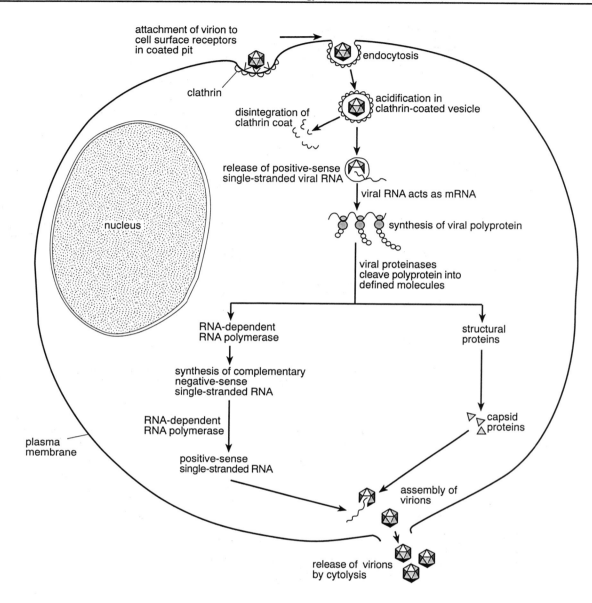

Figure 49.3 Stages in the replication of a picornavirus, a non-enveloped, positive-sense, single-stranded RNA virus.

about two-thirds of the viral RNA is directly translated during the first round of protein synthesis. Subsequently, full-length negative-sense RNA is synthesized and, from this, a full-length positive-sense RNA destined for encapsidation and a one-third length positive-sense RNA strand are formed. The genomes of caliciviruses, coronaviruses and arteriviruses also encode for mRNA which can be full length or shorter.

Negative-sense single-stranded RNA viruses possess an RNA-dependent RNA polymerase. The naked RNA of these viruses, unlike that of the positive-sense single-stranded RNA viruses, cannot initiate infection. After infection by the virion, the genomic RNA functions as a template for transcription of positive-sense mRNA and also for virus replication, utilizing the same polymerase.

The positive-sense RNA subsequently serves as the template for synthesis of negative-sense genomic RNA. Most single-stranded, negative-sense RNA viruses replicate in the cytoplasm of the cell. Notable exceptions are orthomyxoviruses and Borna disease virus which replicate in the nucleus. Part of the segmented genome of some members of the *Bunyaviridae* is ambisense, utilizing a mixed replication strategy with features characteristic of both positive-sense and negative-sense single-stranded RNA viruses. Stages in the replication of a rhabdovirus, an enveloped, negative-sense, single-stranded RNA virus are illustrated in Fig. 49.4.

The genome of retroviruses consists of positive-sense, single-stranded RNA which does not function as messenger RNA. Instead, a single-stranded DNA copy is

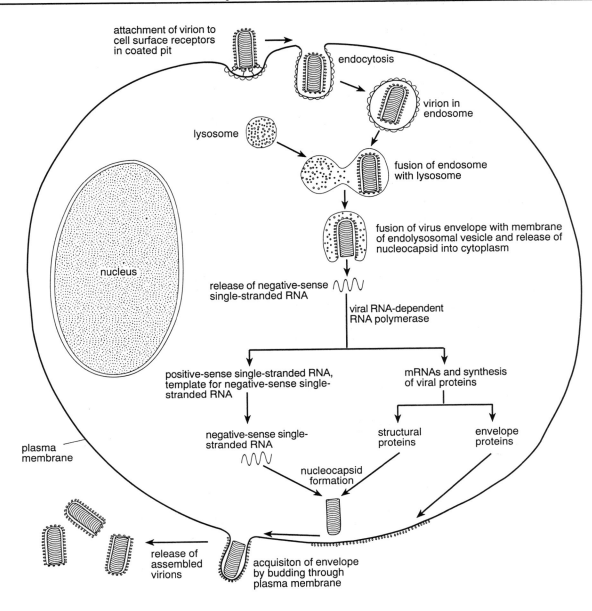

Figure 49.4 Stages in the replication of a rhabdovirus, an enveloped, negative-sense, single-stranded RNA virus.

produced by RNA-dependent DNA polymerase (reverse transcriptase) using the viral RNA as a template. As the second strand of DNA is formed, the parental RNA is removed from the RNA-DNA hybrid molecule. The double-stranded DNA is integrated into the host cell genome as a provirus (Fig. 49.5). The integrated DNA provirus, which may be incorporated into cellular chromosomes at a number of sites, can be transcribed to new viral RNA.

Protein synthesis

Within the cell, the sites at which particular proteins are synthesized relate to the type and function of the protein.

Membrane proteins and glycoproteins are synthesized on membrane-bound ribosomes while soluble proteins including enzymes are synthesized on ribosomes free in the cytoplasm. Short specific amino acid sequences, known as sorting sequences, facilitate the incorporation of proteins at various cellular locations where they are required for metabolic activity. Most viral proteins undergo post-translational modification including proteolytic cleavage, phosphorylation and glycosylation. During glycosylation, sugar side-chains are added to viral proteins in a programmed manner as the proteins are being transferred from the rough endoplasmic reticulum to the Golgi apparatus preparatory to final assembly of intact virions and their release from the cell.

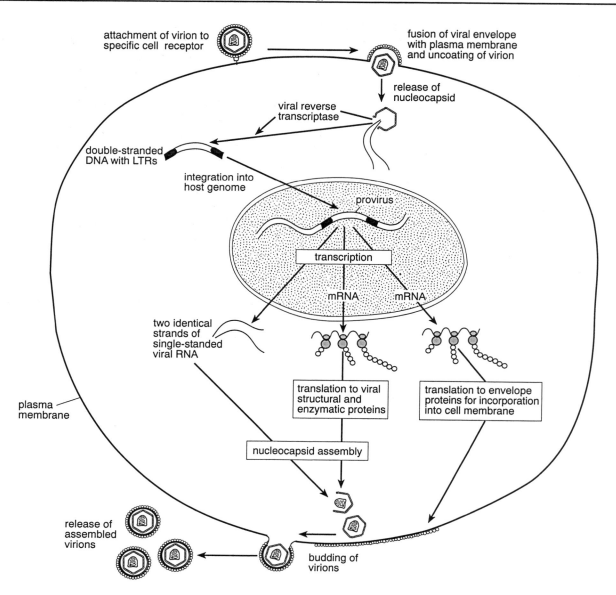

Figure 49.5 Stages in the replication of a retrovirus.
LTRs: long terminal repeats.

Assembly and release of virions

The mechanisms for the assembly and release of enveloped and non-enveloped viruses are distinct. Non-enveloped viruses of animals have an icosahedral structure. The structural proteins of these viruses associate spontaneously in a symmetrical and stepwise fashion to form procapsids. Subsequently, viral nucleic acid is incorporated into the procapsid. Proteolytic cleavage of specific procapsid polypeptides may be required for the final formation of infectious particles. Non-enveloped viruses are usually released following cellular disintegration. The assembly of picornaviruses and reoviruses occurs in the cytoplasm of the cell whereas parvoviruses, adenoviruses and papovaviruses are assembled in the nucleus.

In enveloped viruses, the final step in the process of virion assembly involves acquisition of an envelope by budding from cell membranes. Prior to budding, cell membranes are modified by the insertion of virus-specified transmembrane glycoproteins, which aggregate in patches in the plasma membrane. The presence of viral glycoproteins alters the antigenic composition of infected cells which become targets for cytotoxic T lymphocytes. Togavirus nucleocapsids bind to the hydrophilic domains of the virus-specified membrane proteins, which project slightly into the cytoplasm, and become surrounded by the altered portion of membrane. The nucleocapsids of helical viruses bind to a virus-specified matrix protein which lines the cytoplasmic side of membrane patches.

Budding of viruses through the plasma membrane does

not usually breach the integrity of the membrane and, as a result, many enveloped viruses are non-cytopathic and may be associated with persistent infections. Unlike most other enveloped viruses, togaviruses, paramyxoviruses and rhabdoviruses are cytolytic. Flaviviruses, coronaviruses, arteriviruses and bunyaviruses acquire their envelopes inside cells by budding through the membranes of the rough endoplasmic reticulum or the Golgi apparatus. These viruses are then transported in vesicles to the cell surface where the vesicle fuses with the plasma membrane releasing the virion by exocytosis. Herpesviruses, which replicate in the nucleus, are unique in that they bud through the inner lamella of the nuclear membrane and accumulate in the space between inner and outer lamellae, in the cisternae of the endoplasmic reticulum and in cytoplasmic vesicles (Fig. 49.2). Release from the cell can occur either by exocytosis or by cytolysis. The assembly and release of poxviruses is a complex process taking several hours. Although replication occurs entirely in the cytoplasm of the host cell at discrete sites, termed viroplasms or 'viral factories', nuclear factors may be involved in transcription and assembly. Maturation proceeds to the formation of infectious intracellular mature virus, which can be detected following deliberate lysis of infected host cells *in vitro*. Following assembly, virus particles move out of the assembly area and become enveloped in a double membrane derived from the trans-Golgi network. At the periphery of the cell, fusion with the plasma membrane results in loss of the outer layer of the double membrane and release of extracellular enveloped virus.

References

Baltimore, D. (1971). Expression of animal virus genomes. *Bacteriological Reviews*, **35**, 235–241.

Further reading

Fields, B.N., Knife, D.M. and Hewley, P.M. (1996). *Fundamental Virology*. Third Edition. Lippincott-Raven, Philadelphia.

Chapter 50

Genetics and evolution of viruses

Viruses exhibit enormous genetic diversity. These minute pathogens are capable of infecting not only vertebrates but also invertebrates, plants, fungi, protozoa, algae and bacteria. Viruses utilize a variety of molecular mechanisms to compensate for their limited genetic capability. They may encode genes in different reading frames. These reading frames may overlap, may be encoded in opposite directions or may be read by frameshifting. In recent years, the development of techniques in molecular biology including molecular cloning, nucleotide sequencing and the polymerase chain reaction have greatly expanded knowledge of viral genomes. Viral genetics is concerned not only with understanding the detailed structure of the viral genome and the extent to which it determines the biological and disease-producing potential of viruses but also with elucidation of the mechanisms of genetic change and virus evolution. Genomic change is responsible for alterations in antigenicity and pathogenicity which, in turn, may influence the course of viral diseases of animals and humans. Mutation is the most frequent cause of genetic change in viruses. Less commonly, genetic interactions termed recombinations, which can occur between different viruses or between a virus and its host cell, may account for alteration in virus characteristics.

Mutation

Spontaneous and random errors in the copying of viral nucleic acid, termed mutations, can occur during the replication of viruses. The rate of mutation in the genome of DNA viruses ranges from 10^{-8} to 10^{-11} per incorporated nucleotide whereas the mutation rate in the genomes of RNA viruses is much higher, ranging from 10^{-3} to 10^{-4}. When replicating in the nucleus of host cells, the genomes of DNA viruses are subjected to error-correction carried out by cellular exonucleases. The lower fidelity of genome replication in RNA viruses is attributed to poor error correction by RNA replication enzymes. In an infected cell, the genomes of the progeny of an RNA virus, such as vesicular stomatitis virus with an 11 kb genome, may differ both from the parental genome and from each other by at least one nucleotide. Exposure to X-rays, UV-irradiation or chemical mutagens increases the frequency of mutation. Point mutations, resulting from single nucleotide substitutions, are the most common type of mutation. Less common types of mutation result from the deletion or insertion of one or more nucleotides. Additive effects of point mutations occurring over several generations may account for phenotypic variations which are influenced by selection processes. Because they do not result in alteration of the amino acid composition of the coded protein, most point mutations are silent. In other instances the mutation may be lethal and virus strains containing such lethal mutations are rapidly eliminated. Occasionally, mutations conferring a selective advantage allow positive selection of the mutant virus. Non-lethal mutations may accumulate rapidly in the genomes of RNA viruses giving rise to quasispecies, genetically diverse populations of viruses centered around consensus sequences. Phenotypic expression of a mutation may be reversed by a back-mutation at the nucleotide responsible for the original mutation. Alternatively, a suppressor mutation may prevent phenotypic expression of the mutant gene. The phenotypic expression of a particular mutation may give rise to clearly distinguishable mutants including conditional-lethal, antibody-escape and defective-interfering mutants.

Conditional-lethal mutants can replicate only under defined permissive conditions. Examples of such mutants include temperature-sensitive mutants, which can multiply most efficiently at temperature ranges different from parental wild-type viruses, and host-range mutants which can infect host species different from those of parent viruses. The temperature-sensitive mutants, which replicate at temperatures slightly below core mammalian body temperature, have been particularly useful in the development of live intranasal vaccines. Such vaccines stimulate local immunity without systemic spread. When first isolated, viruses may grow poorly in cell cultures and in laboratory animals. However, adaptation can usually be achieved by serial passage, resulting in selection of rapidly growing mutants. This selection process is dependent on spontaneous mutations particularly in genes encoding surface proteins, which determine binding efficiency to host cell receptors. Host-range mutants, while often replicating more readily *in vitro*, tend to be less virulent for natural host species. This has been exploited as a method for attenuation in the production of many modified live vaccines.

Selection for antibody escape mutants can occur when viruses replicate in the presence of antibody. Because of altered antigenic surface determinants, the mutants are unaffected by neutralizing antibodies induced by the wild-type virus. Such a selection process may facilitate persistent or recurrent infections.

Defective-interfering mutants require the presence of a helper virus, usually the wild-type virus, for replication. Most defective-interfering mutants are deletion mutants. Such mutants can interfere with the replication of wild-type helper viruses and may, therefore, become progressively more numerous on serial passage. Defective-interfering mutants may play a role in disease by promoting the establishment and maintenance of persistent infections.

Viral recombination

The exchange or transfer of genetic material between different but closely related viruses infecting the same cell is termed genetic recombination. This type of genetic exchange can also occur between virus and host cells. The genomes of the recombinants contain new genetic information. The alteration of genetic information may result from intramolecular recombination, copy-choice recombination, reassortment or genetic reactivation.

Intramolecular recombination usually occurs in DNA viruses and involves dissociation and re-establishment of covalent bonds within the nucleic acid. Copy-choice recombination between positive-sense single-stranded RNA viruses occurs through a template switching mechanism. The RNA polymerase switches between template strands during synthesis of the complementary negative-sense strand. This process can occur in picornaviruses, togaviruses and coronaviruses. An exceptionally high frequency of genetic recombination has been observed in mixed infections of coronaviruses. It is suggested that western equine encephalitis virus arose through copy-choice recombination as a heterologous recombinant of the two togaviruses, eastern equine encephalitis virus and a Sindbis-like virus.

Reassortment can occur randomly in RNA viruses with segmented genomes, such as orthomyxoviruses, reoviruses and bunyaviruses. In this type of recombination, genome segments of two or more related viruses infecting the same cell are exchanged. The process is an important source of genetic variability in nature, permitting rapid adaptation of viruses to new hosts, the development of viruses with new antigenic characteristics and changes in virulence. Reassortment is generally restricted to taxonomically related viruses, either viruses of the same species, such as orthomyxoviruses, or viruses belonging to the same serogroup within a species, such as reoviruses and bunyaviruses. Genetic reassortment plays a major role in the epidemiology of human influenza A virus infections. Periodically, viruses with novel antigenic properties emerge, facilitating spread throughout the human population. There is convincing evidence that dual infection of pig populations with avian and human influenza viruses accounts for the emergence of new virulent subtypes, which can spread to the human population by close contact with pigs. In genetic reactivation, infectious progeny are produced from parental viruses, of which one or both are non-infectious, following mixed infection of a cell. When infectious progeny are produced from related viruses inactivated by lethal mutations at different loci in their genomes, the phenomenon is referred to as multiplicity reactivation. Cross-reactivation or genome rescue occurs when an inactivated virus becomes capable of replicating after acquiring genetic material from an infective virus.

Virus-host cell recombination

It is known that recombination between viral and cellular genetic material occurs. Such recombination may be important for virus evolution and virulence. Several retroviruses have become potentially oncogenic by incorporating cellular oncogenes into their genomes. Integration of the cellular DNA into the viral genome often results in a concomitant loss of viral genetic material resulting in replication-defective progeny viruses which require helper viruses for replication. The non-cytopathic biotype of bovine virus diarrhoea virus, which causes persistent infection in cattle, may become cytopathic, through mutation or recombination and cause mucosal disease. The specific change is cleavage of the non-structural fusion protein, NS2-3, and the subsequent separate expression of NS3. One mechanism which allows this change is insertion of one or more cellular ubiquitin gene sequences into a key region of the viral genome.

Other interactions involving viruses

Viruses may interact in a number of ways at the level of gene products. These types of interaction, which can result in phenotypic alteration of viral activity, include complementation and phenotypic mixing.

In cells with dual infections, complementation can occur if the defective gene product of one virus is substituted by the gene product of another virus. This results in survival or increased yields of the recipient virus. There is no lasting effect from this type of interaction because the genome remains unchanged. Complementation can occur between related and unrelated viruses; the defective viruses are termed satellite viruses. Adeno-associated viruses, which are members of the *Parvoviridae*, can replicate only in the nucleus of cells simultaneously infected with an adenovirus. Hepatitis delta virus, a satellite virus of humans, requires co-infection with hepatitis B virus for replication, especially for the provision of envelope proteins.

Structural proteins may be exchanged following infection of a cell usually by two related viruses, a process known as phenotypic mixing. One form of this type of interaction, transcapsidation, involves complete or occasionally partial exchange of capsids between non-enveloped viruses. Phenotypic mixing also occurs in enveloped viruses which acquire envelopes when budding from host cells. The progeny nucleocapsids of one virus may be released from a cell surrounded by an envelope containing glycoproteins specified by another virus. Defective oncogenic retroviruses, which are dependent on helper viruses for replication, may derive envelopes from host cell membrane which contains glycoproteins encoded by their helper viruses. As phenotypic mixing does not involve genetic change, it is a transient event.

Viral genomic sequence analysis

Cell culture techniques are no longer required for producing sufficient quantities of virus for detailed studies. It is now possible to produce large amounts of viral nucleic acid using either molecular cloning techniques or the polymerase chain reaction following extraction of viral nucleic acid from clinical samples. The nucleic acid of bovine papillomavirus and rabbit haemorrhagic disease virus has been analysed and sequenced without cultivation of these viruses *in vitro*. This has provided valuable information about both viruses, allowing alternative approaches to diagnosis and vaccination procedures. In recent years, automated methods for sequencing viral genomes have become simpler and cheaper. Sequences, both partial and complete, of a wide range of microorganisms are retrievable from international databanks such as GenBank (http://www. ncbi.nlm.nih.gov/GenBank).

Two rapid sequencing techniques are currently used, the enzymatic method of Sanger *et al.* (1977) and the chemical degradation method of Maxam and Gilbert (1977). The Sanger method is preferred for simple DNA sequencing. This method is based on the enzymatic synthesis of a strand of DNA complementary to the sample DNA which is used in single-stranded form as the template (Fig. 50.1). A primer sequence is annealed to the single-stranded DNA and the reaction mixture is divided into four aliquots. The four deoxynucleotide triphosphates (dNTPs) are added to each aliquot. These normal deoxynucleotides are radiolabelled, usually with ^{32}P or ^{35}S. A different dideoxynucleotide triphosphate (ddNTP) is then added to each of the four reaction mixtures. These deoxynucleotide analogues, ddAPT, ddCTP, ddGTP and ddTTP, contain the sugar dideoxyribose which lacks a hydroxyl group present in deoxyribose. Incorporation of a ddNTP into a growing complementary DNA strand by DNA polymerase blocks further synthesis of the chain. Incorporation of a ddNTP is random because of competition with its dNTP analogue, resulting in the production of chains of various lengths in each reaction mixture. The use of four reaction mixtures, each with a different ddNTP provides four populations of radiolabelled oligonucleotides which can be separated by polyacrylamide gel electrophoresis and identified by autoradiography in four adjacent lanes of the gel (Fig. 50.1).

The Maxam-Gilbert method involves chemical breaking of the sample DNA into fragments using four separate base-specific cleavage reactions (G, A+G, C, C+T). The fragments are radiolabelled. The four reaction mixtures contain molecules of various lengths determined by the location of a particular base along the original DNA molecule which can be determined by electrophoresis and radiography.

Viral genome sequencing has been used to great effect in the field of molecular epidemiology. The genotyping of isolates provides information on the source and epidemiology of viral diseases of veterinary importance such as foot-and-mouth disease and Venezuelan equine encephalitis. Functional genomics is concerned with the linking of phenotypic traits to specific genes. The identification of open reading frames (ORFs) is relatively easy in viruses because translatable sequences start with the methionine codon (AUG). This facilitates the identification of genes encoding viral structural and non-structural proteins. Information of this type is of considerable value in the development of diagnostic reagents and antiviral drugs, and also in the design of novel vaccines.

Restriction fragment length polymorphism

Restriction endonucleases are sequence-specific bacterial DNases that recognize a unique palindromic sequence, four to nine nucleotide pairs in length. Several hundred such enzymes, many of which are commercially available, have been identified and purified from bacteria. Restriction fragment length polymorphism, also known as DNA fingerprinting, involves cleavage of DNA into fragments. The fragments can be separated by gel electrophoresis and the pattern evaluated. The number and size of the fragments produced by the action of a specific restriction endonuclease on a particular DNA molecule are characteristic, allowing differentiation of the viral species or strain from which the nucleic acid derives.

Molecular cloning

Advances in the understanding of nucleic acid replication and the enzymatic cleavage of the molecule have paved the way for several practical applications used in genetic engineering. It is now possible to introduce foreign nucleic acid at specific sites in the genomes of viruses, bacteria, yeasts and vertebrate cells. The foreign DNA is amplified by replicating it with host DNA and, if inserted in frame with the appropriate regulatory sequences, acts as part of the host genome. Commonly, the foreign DNA is incorporated into a vector such as a plasmid or virus, especially bacteriophages. The recombinant vector can be

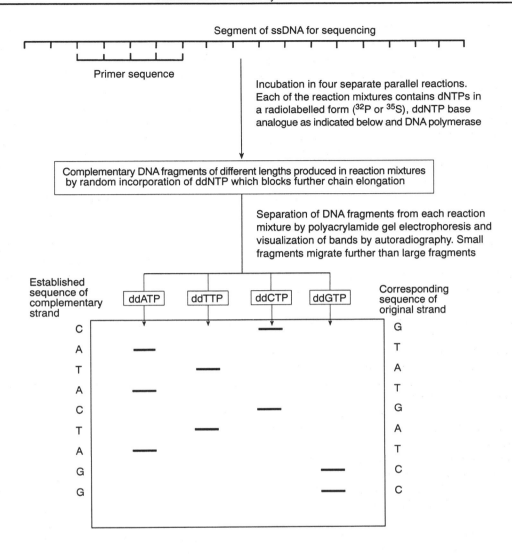

Figure 50.1 Outline of the Sanger method for DNA sequencing using dideoxynucleotide triphosphate.

ssDNA: single-stranded DNA; dNTP: deoxyribonucleotide triphosphate; ddNTP: dideoxyribonucleotide triphosphate; ddATP: dideoxyadenosine triphosphate; ddTTP: dideoxythymidine triphosphate; ddCTP: dideoxycytidine triphosphate; ddGTP: dideoxyguanosine triphosphate

delivered to bacterial, fungal, insect or mammalian cells either by infection or insertion. The vector may serve as a cloning vector, for the amplification of the foreign nucleic acid, or an expression vector, for the production of proteins encoded by the foreign DNA. Poxviruses have large DNA genomes permitting the incorporation of large amounts of foreign DNA into the non-essential areas of the genome. Vaccinia virus, in particular, has been used successfully as an expression vector. A vaccinia virus-rabies glycoprotein G recombinant has been developed and used effectively to vaccinate red foxes, the principal wildlife reservoir of rabies in Europe. This virus-vector vaccine, which is safe, relatively cheap and stable in the environment, is delivered in bait form. Other virus-vector vaccines are currently being developed.

Evolution of viruses

Genetic change, arising from mutation and recombination, occurs at different rates among families of viruses. Some genetically-controlled traits may confer a selective advantage which relates to prevailing conditions and selection pressures. Periodically, genomic change may contribute to the emergence of major outbreaks of new diseases. A point mutation in the genome of feline panleukopenia virus or a closely related virus has been proposed as the event responsible for the emergence of canine parvovirus, which causes a serious disease in dogs, first described during the late 1970s. Genomic change may also account for infection of horses with Hendra virus and of pigs with Nipah virus. Both of these paramyxoviruses have wildlife reservoirs, probably fruit bats. Subsequent transmission of these viruses to humans through contact with infected domestic animals illustrates the important unforeseen consequences of viral genomic alteration.

Influenza A virus and myxoma virus provide important insights into the evolution of viruses. Influenza A viruses can infect a wide range of animal species. Isolates of the virus from birds and humans can infect pigs and, in this species, reassortment can occur with the emergence of new subtypes. Genetic change of this type, which takes place at intervals of more than ten years, are most likely to originate in southeast Asia because of high population densities and close contact between humans and domestic pigs and ducks. Virus variants produced in this way may escape neutralization by antibodies and, by becoming the dominant circulating strain, cause pandemics. During the twentieth century, pandemics of human influenza occurred in 1900, 1918, 1957 and 1968.

Myxoma virus is a poxvirus which causes a mild infection in *Sylvilagus* species, the native American rabbit. It is transmitted mechanically by fleas and mosquitoes feeding on infected animals. The virus causes serious, often fatal, disease in European rabbits, *Oryctolagus cuniculus*. The European rabbit which had been introduced into Australia in the mid-19th century, became a major agricultural pest. Myxoma virus was released in 1950 into the Australian rabbit population in an attempt to control numbers. Case fatality rates of more than 99% during dramatic summertime epizootics were initially recorded. The disease tended to disappear during winter months due to the greatly reduced rabbit numbers and decreased mosquito activity. In such circumstances less virulent viral mutants, which caused a more prolonged disease course with a greater opportunity for transmission, were selected. Subsequently, attenuated strains of the

virus became dominant. This resulted in a recovery rate in infected rabbits exceeding 10%, with the selection of genetically more resistant rabbits. The case fatality rate for a particular strain of virus in serial infection studies on rabbits from areas where repeated outbreaks occurred declined from 90% to 50%. However, virulent strains of the virus became re-established in the genetically resistant populations ensuring further efficient transmission of the virus. In 1968, the European rabbit flea was released to improve transmission of the virus in areas where mosquitoes had not been effective vectors. In rabbit populations in which this flea flourished, the seasonal incidence of myxomatosis changed from sharp summer outbreaks to protracted winter and spring outbreaks. A dynamic equilibrium currently exists between virulence of the virus and genetic resistance of the rabbit population. However, rabbit numbers are substantially reduced when compared with the population size prior to the introduction of myxomatosis.

References

Maxam, A.M. and Gilbert, W. (1977). A new method for sequencing DNA. *Proceedings of the National Academy of Sciences*, **74**, 560–564.

Sanger, F., Nicklen, S. and Coulson, A.R. (1977). DNA sequencing with chain terminating inhibitors. *Proceedings of the National Academy of Sciences*, **74**, 5463–5467.

Further reading

Fenner, F. and Fantini, B. (1999). *Biological control of vertebrate pests. The history of myxomatosis, an experiment in evolution.* CABI Publishing, Wallingford.

Chapter 51

Propagation of viruses and virus-cell interactions

Viruses exhibit considerable diversity both in their ability to survive outside the host and in their cultural requirements. Some viruses, such as those causing enteric disease in animals, tolerate wide pH ranges and are relatively stable in the environment. In contrast, other viruses are labile and only survive for short periods outside the host. Enveloped viruses are readily inactivated by lipid solvents, such as chloroform and ether, and by various detergents such as sodium deoxycholate. Viruses are sensitive to ultraviolet and gamma irradiation. Because of their diploid genome, retroviruses are more resistant than other viruses to these forms of radiation. Enveloped viruses are more thermolabile than those without envelopes. As a rule, the rate of inactivation can be measured in seconds at 60°C, in minutes at 37°C, in hours at 20°C and in days at 4°C. Ice crystal formation during freezing damages viruses, especially enveloped viruses. The infectivity of viruses is retained for long periods when they are stored at -70°C or when they are freeze-dried. Storage at -20°C in conventional freezers is an unsatisfactory method for virus preservation. Long-term storage in liquid nitrogen at -196°C can be achieved by rapid freezing of small aliquots of high titred viral suspensions in a medium containing a high concentration of protective protein or a cryoprotective agent such as dimethyl sulphoxide. Freeze-drying involves dehydration of frozen viral suspensions under vacuum in glass ampoules which are then sealed to preserve the vacuum. Lyophilization is employed for the preservation of valuable seed stocks of viruses and for storage of modified live viral vaccines.

Propagation of viruses

As viruses replicate only in living cells, a source of viable cells is required for their propagation. Tissue culture is widely used for virus propagation; inoculation of chick embryos and experimental animals is employed for the isolation and propagation of particular viruses. Propagation is required for the isolation and identification of viruses involved in disease, for the titration of viruses for vaccine production and for the provision of stocks for research purposes.

Tissue culture
Techniques for tissue culture, the growth and maintenance

of living tissue *in vitro*, can be grouped under two headings: explant cultures and cell cultures. Originally, methods for growing cells involved using small fragments or explants of tissue. This technique is still used for isolating viruses from animals with persistent diseases such as caprine arthritis-encephalitis. In a special form of explant culture, termed organ culture, the size and type of the tissue fragment is sufficient to retain tissue architecture. Explant tracheal cultures are required for the isolation of some coronaviruses.

Digestion of tissue into individual cells is used in cell culture preparation. Dispersion of cells from tissue involves mechanical cutting or chopping of the tissue into small pieces followed by digestion using trypsin or other proteolytic enzymes. The liquid or semi-solid culture medium in which cells are grown must supply the required environmental conditions and nutrients. It must be isotonic and be maintained at physiological pH values. There must also be a supply of inorganic ions, carbohydrate (usually glucose), amino acids, vitamins, growth factors, peptides and proteins. Some cells grow in chemically defined media but usually natural products such as foetal calf serum, yeast extract or embryo extract are incorporated in the medium. Phenol red is commonly added as a pH indicator. A bicarbonate buffer is often used to maintain the correct pH. Exposure to oxygen causes the pH to rise due to loss of dissolved CO_2 and bicarbonate. Cells can be grown in sealed containers or exogenous CO_2 may be provided at a rate of 5 to 10%.

Cell cultures may be primary, semi-continuous or continuous. Primary cell cultures are derived directly from tissues and contain many cell types. Tissues from foetuses or from neonatal animals are more suitable for tissue culture preparation than those from mature animals. For the isolation of a specific virus, the most sensitive systems are primary cell lines derived from the target tissue of the virus in a susceptible animal species. The cells in these cultures retain many of the characteristics of cells in the intact organ. However, the sensitivity of a given cell culture for cultivating viruses does not appear to depend solely on the organ of origin as it is frequently possible to isolate viruses that infect one body system in cells derived from a different system. The number of cell divisions occurring in primary cultures are relatively few. Accordingly, primary cultures must be prepared at frequent intervals. Primary cultures can be passaged by dispersing the primary monolayer with trypsin, usually with added ethylenediamine tetra-acetic acid, and distributing the cells onto fresh surfaces to form secondary cell cultures. The number of further passages is finite and an end point, termed the Hayflick limit, is eventually reached. The Hayflick limit is related to the longevity of the animal species from which the cells derived. Cells which are nurtured may survive beyond the Hayflick limit, continue to grow and constitute a cell line. The cells of semi-continuous or diploid cell lines retain their characteristic diploid chromosomal constitution and can support the growth of a wide range of viruses. Such cell lines, most of which are predominantly fibroblastic, tend to die out between the 30th and 50th passage.

Continuous cell lines are derived from either normal or neoplastic tissue and can be passaged indefinitely. In these cell lines, referred to as heteroploid cell lines, the cells have an abnormal number of chromosomes. In general, they are not as sensitive as either primary or semi-continuous cell lines for virus isolation. However, viruses can usually be adapted to grow in continuous cell lines. Established cell lines facilitate large-scale growth of viruses for vaccine production or research purposes. Well characterized continuous cell lines can be obtained from commercial organizations which specialize in preserving and distributing stock. Samples can be purchased from the American Type Culture Collection and the European Collection of Cell Cultures. Continuous cell lines with recognized names include Madin Darby bovine kidney (MDBK) and Crandell feline kidney (CRFK). Following prolonged passaging, continuous cell lines may become contaminated with *Mycoplasma* species or viruses and may acquire altered characteristics such as increased or decreased susceptibility to viruses. Most virology laboratories freeze early stocks of cells and, periodically, revive cells from the frozen stock in order to ensure maintenance of characteristics. Cells can be stored in a viable state for long periods at temperatures below −130°C, typically at −196°C using liquid nitrogen. Dimethyl sulphoxide or glycerol is usually added to the medium in which cells are suspended as cryoprotective agents.

Detection of viral growth in cell cultures

Viral growth in cell culture, which results in damage to infected cells, may be detectable by light microscopy. Microscopic changes in infected cells, termed cytopathic effect (CPE), include change in shape, cell detachment, fusion leading to syncytium formation, the presence of inclusion bodies and cell death. On primary isolation, some viruses do not produce CPE. Following passage onto fresh monolayers, they may become cytopathic. The full range of the effects of viral infection on cultured cells, especially inclusion body formation, may be demonstrable only by staining. Inclusion bodies are intracellular structures which have characteristic staining features. In virus-infected cells they may be composed of viral nucleic acid, viral protein or altered cellular material. Inclusion bodies, which may be single or multiple, may be located in the cytoplasm or the nucleus. They are described as acidophilic, when stained by eosin, and basophilic, when stained by haematoxylin. Intracytoplasmic inclusions may be found in cells infected with poxviruses, reoviruses, rabies virus and paramyxoviruses while intranuclear inclusions occur in cells infected with adenoviruses, herpesviruses and parvoviruses. Infections with some viruses such as canine distemper virus may produce both intranuclear and intracytoplasmic inclusion bodies.

Non-cytopathic viruses require alternative detection methods. Enveloped viruses belonging to some families insert viral glycoproteins into the plasma membrane of infected cells. These glycoproteins may induce cell fusion, producing syncytia, or promote haemadsorption, the binding of erythrocytes to the surface of infected cells. Syncytia may be formed in cell cultures infected with lentiviruses, paramyxoviruses and some herpesviruses. Cells infected with orthomyxoviruses, paramyxoviruses and togaviruses tend to exhibit haemadsorption at sites of virion budding. Haemadsorption can be detected early in the replication cycle. The glycoproteins responsible for haemadsorption, referred to as haemagglutinins, also cause clumping of erythrocytes following mixing with free virions. Many viruses, both enveloped and non-enveloped, can cause haemagglutination with erythrocytes from particular animal species. Feline panleukopenia virus haemagglutinates porcine erythrocytes while porcine parvovirus haemagglutinates chick, guinea-pig, rat, monkey, human and cat erythrocytyes. Supernatants from infected cell cultures, lysed by freezing and thawing, can be examined for the presence of viral particles by electron microscopy. This is an insensitive technique and particle concentrations in excess of 10^6 per ml are required for detection.

Serological tests may be required for the specific identification of a viral species. A useful method for the detection and specific identification is infection of susceptible cells grown as monolayers on coverslips in Leighton tubes or in flat-bottomed vials. Following fixation of infected cells, virus can be identified employing a fluorescein-labelled antibody. Monoclonal or polyclonal conjugates may be used depending on availability and the level of specificity required. This technique is independent of any cytopathic or other property of the test virus and contributes to the speed and sensitivity of the isolation procedure. However, a separate conjugate is required for the specific detection of each virus species. Specific antibodies against viruses can also be utilized in virus neutralization tests to block cytopathic effects and in haemadsorption/haemagglutination inhibition assays to inhibit the erythrocyte-binding activity of viruses. Neutralization assays are the definitive methods for distinguishing many viruses and defining serotypes.

Although immunoelectron microscopy is more sensitive and specific than direct electron microscopy, it cannot be used as a general screening method for viruses in clinical samples.

Embryonated eggs

Formerly, embryonated eggs were used extensively for virus isolation. Decline in the use of embryonated eggs has resulted from improvements in tissue culture techniques. However, inoculation of embryonated eggs remains the preferred method for isolation of influenza A viruses and for many avian viruses. In order to exclude maternally-derived anti-viral antibodies, the source of the eggs requires careful selection, preferably eggs from specific pathogen-free flocks. Passage in embryonated eggs has proved useful for attenuating certain viruses used in the production of modified live virus vaccines.

Embryonated eggs may be inoculated using a number of defined routes (Fig. 51.1). Viruses can be inoculated into the allantoic cavity, the amniotic cavity or the yolk sac. They can also be inoculated onto the chorioallantoic membrane (CAM). In addition, well-developed chick embryos can be inoculated intravascularly. The route selected for inoculation is largely determined by the tissue affinity of each particular virus. Evidence of the effect of viral growth includes death or dwarfing of the embryo and the formation of pocks on the CAM. Haemagglutination or immunofluorescence may be used as additional tests for the detection of virus.

Experimental animals

For ethical reasons, experimental infection of animals is now used less frequently than formerly. A number of alternative methods for the growth and study of viruses is available. However, for several virus families, the use of cell culture for isolation is of limited value and animal inoculation remains the preferred procedure. Suckling mice are used for the detection of arthropod-borne viruses and for rabies virus. Inoculation of the natural host species is a requirement for the isolation of some viruses. Challenge experiments in the natural host species may be necessary to evaluate vaccines. The production of poly-clonal antisera requires inoculation of laboratory animals with virus. Investigation of the pathogenetic mechanisms relating to viral infections and the subsequent immune response of the host frequently require inoculation of either laboratory animals or natural hosts.

Determination of virus concentration

When evaluating the efficiency of vaccines, when standardizing virus neutralization or haemagglutination-inhibition assays or when producing whole virus vaccines, accurate standardization of virus concentration is essential. It is also necessary when determining the minimum dose of virus required to produce clinical disease. Titration may be used to measure the total number of virions present (employing electron microscopy) or to calculate the number of infectious virions by inoculating a susceptible

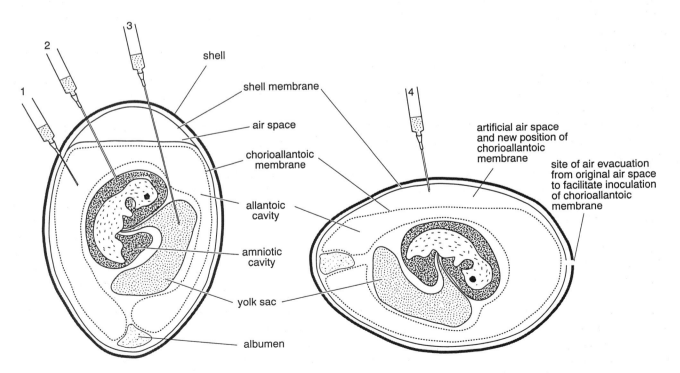

Figure 51.1 Routes for inoculation of viruses into embryonated eggs. 1: into allantoic cavity 2: into amniotic cavity 3: into yolk sac 4: onto chorioallantoic membrane

host or tissue culture system. Alternatively, a measure of a specific viral activity such as haemagglutination may be used or the concentration of viral antigen may be determined. Some titration procedures are quantal, providing an approximation of the number of virions in a preparation. Estimation of viral concentration by quantal techniques is adequate for most experimental or diagnostic purposes. Typically, these assays are carried out using serial ten-fold dilutions of a given virus preparation to inoculate several replicate host or cell culture systems per dilution. The end point in mice or embryonated eggs is usually death and the unit is expressed as the 50% lethal dose (LD_{50}). In cell culture systems, the end point is expressed as the 50% tissue culture infective dose ($TCID_{50}$). The results are usually expressed as a $\log_{10}$ value per ml of the original undiluted specimen. The statistical methods devised by Reed-Muench and by Kärber are frequently employed in these calculations.

The concentration of haemagglutinating viruses is often expressed in haemagglutinating (HA) units. The HA unit is equivalent to the highest dilution of the virus suspension causing complete haemagglutination. This simple titration method is insensitive because many thousands of virions are required to agglutinate sufficient numbers of erythrocytes for visual detection.

The plaque assay is a common and accurate method for quantifying viral infectivity. Serial ten-fold dilutions of the test virus preparation are inoculated onto monolayer cell cultures and allowed to adsorb for approximately one hour. The cell sheets are then overlaid with tissue culture medium containing agar. The solidified agar prevents spread of virus throughout the cell culture while permitting cell-to-cell transfer. As a result, cytopathic viruses produce foci of cell death around the replication sites, which then appear as clear areas called plaques. Based on the number of plaques and the dilution and size of the inoculum, the titration end point is calculated and expressed as plaque forming units (pfu) per ml. Although it is possible for a single virion to produce one plaque, in practice the virion:pfu ratio for most animal viruses is seldom less than 10:1. Even within a single virus preparation, there appears to be substantial microheterogeneity as not all virus particles in a preparation can form plaques.

Virus-host cell interactions

Virus infections may produce effects ranging from latency to cell death (Table 51.1). Infections may be productive or non-productive, consequences influenced by the ability of the virus to replicate effectively in a given cell type. When a host cell allows virus replication to proceed, it is said to be permissive. This state may not be static as occurs when latent infections are reactivated following a period of quiescence or non-productive interaction. Reactivation tends to occur when latently-infected animals are subjected to stressful environmental conditions.

Mechanisms of cell injury

Cytopathic viruses kill cells which they infect. Frequently, cell necrosis is the result of the cumulative effects of a number of biochemical changes induced by viral replication, resulting in the production of ultrastructural lesions. Cell death due to necrosis tends to occur late in the viral replication cycle after progeny virus production is complete and cytolysis may in fact facilitate the release of virions. Reoviruses, poxviruses, picornaviruses, paramyxoviruses and rhabdoviruses can inhibit the transcription of host cell RNA to permit synthesis of viral mRNA. This alteration of host cell metabolism may relate to interference with protein synthesis due to the production of virus-encoded factors. Herpesviruses, influenza viruses and vesicular stomatitis virus inhibit processing of host cell mRNA by interfering with the splicing of the primary cellular mRNA transcripts. Rapid and pronounced shut down of protein synthesis occurs in cells infected with picornaviruses, poxviruses and herpesviruses. Other viruses such as adenoviruses cause a gradual shut down of cellular activity at a late stage in the viral replicative cycle. The viral mechanisms which block protein synthesis include competition for ribosomes from large amounts of viral mRNA, degradation of cellular mRNA by viral enzymes, interference with cellular mRNA translation and the alteration of the intracellular ionic environment in favour of viral mRNA translation. Viral proteins of lentiviruses and adenoviruses inhibit the processing of cellular proteins and their transport from the endoplasmic reticulum. Accumulations of viral structural proteins occurring late in infection may be directly toxic for host cells. *In vivo* humoral and cellular immune responses directed against viral proteins incorporated into the plasma membrane of the host cell, may be cytotoxic.

Programmed cell death, apoptosis, can be induced by viral infection. In apoptosis, activation of cellular endonuclease leads to fragmentation of cellular DNA. The resulting DNA fragments produce a characteristic pattern of evenly spaced bands when electrophoresed in agarose gel. Apoptosis may be triggered by certain viruses in the early stages of infection, resulting in the death of individual cells prior to virus replication. This event could

Table 51.1 Virus-host cell interactions.

Virus	Production of progeny virus	Outcome
Cytopathic	Productive	Necrosis
	Non-productive	Apoptosis
Non-cytopathic	Productive	Persistence Transformation
	Non-productive	Latency Transformation

be an important host defence mechanism. Some viruses produce substances which block apoptosis, thus prolonging cell survival.

Non-cytopathic viral infections

Viruses such as retroviruses, which are usually non-cytopathic, do not interfere with protein synthesis in host cells. These viruses frequently produce persistent infections with progressive changes which eventually lead to cell death. Members of the sub-family *Alphaherpesvirinae* typically produce productive lytic infections, usually in epithelial cells. At the sites of productive infection, progeny virus enters sensory nerve fibres and is transported in the axoplasm to sensory nerve ganglia. Latent infection develops within the neuronal perikarya. Viral replication is restricted because stimuli for replication are not produced in the non-dividing neurons. The intracellular viral DNA is present in a circular episomal form in association with nucleosomes and transcription is limited to a few latency-associated transcripts (LATs). The function of LATs is not known. They do not appear to be translated into proteins and they are not essential for the maintenance of the latent state. The lack of viral protein expression allows infected neurons to remain undetected by the immune system. Multiple copies of the viral DNA may be demonstrable in latently infected host cells. Episodes of reactivation with production of infectious progeny virus can occur periodically. The newly produced virions are transported in the sensory nerve fibres to the superficial sites of the primary infection where they may again induce lytic lesions. The mechanism of reactivation is not fully understood. Certain stimuli or stress factors, such as trauma, immunosuppression, hormonal changes and intercurrent disease, can trigger reactivation. This frequently coincides with circumstances in which transmission of virus to susceptible animals may readily occur.

Retroviruses integrate a DNA copy of their RNA genome, termed provirus, into the host chromosome. This allows propagation of the provirus along with host chromosomes. Integration of provirus, while not destroying the cell, may alter the host genotype and the expression of host genes. The genomes of DNA viruses such as papillomaviruses are maintained in cells as circular episomal molecules. Viral replication, which is promoted by viral proteins, is synchronized with host cell division.

Viral oncogenesis

A number of DNA and RNA viruses cause neoplastic transformation of cells (Table 51.2). Transformation results from interference with growth signals in cells. Central to the understanding of the mechanisms involved in tumour production by viruses was the discovery of oncogenes. Originally recognized in retroviruses, more

Table 51.2 Some oncogenic viruses of veterinary importance.

Virus classification	Family	Virus
DNA	*Herpesviridae*	Marek's disease virus
	Papillomaviridae	Bovine papillomavirus Equine papillomavirus Canine oral papillomavirus
RNA	*Retroviridae*	Avian leukosis virus Feline leukaemia virus Jaagsiekte sheep retrovirus

than 60 oncogenes, termed v-*onc* genes, have been identified. Cellular genes, c-*onc* genes or proto-oncogenes, corresponding to most v-*onc* genes, are present in normal cells in which they regulate cell division and differentiation. Cellular oncogenes encode proteins which function as growth factors, growth factor receptors, transcription factors and intracellular signal transducers. It is generally accepted that v-*onc* genes of retroviruses were acquired during the evolution of these viruses following virus-host cell interaction. Central to this process is the possession of a unique enzyme, reverse transcriptase, and the incorporation of a DNA copy of viral RNA into the host genome. Retroviruses may exert an oncogenic effect by carrying v-*onc* genes or alternatively by causing over-expression or inappropriate expression of c-*onc* genes. The v-*onc* genes carried by rapidly transforming retroviruses differ in certain respects from the c-*onc* genes from which they were derived. They are under the control of strong viral promoters known as long terminal repeats (LTRs), carry mutations as a result of the high error rate of reverse transcriptase and may be joined to other viral genes in a way that modifies their function. As a result they are outside of the control of normal cellular gene regulation and oncogene proteins may be over-produced or may function in an abnormal way leading to uncontrolled cell division. In contrast, slowly transforming retroviruses lack a v-*onc* gene and give rise to tumours in a random manner. Insertion of provirus (insertional mutagenesis) with its strong LTR promoter sequences close to a c-*onc* gene may greatly increase the production of the normal c-*onc* gene protein.

The oncogenes of DNA viruses are not usually derived from cellular genes. The DNA viruses are generally present in cells as circular episomal nucleic acid and their oncogenes encode proteins necessary for viral replication. If the replication cycle of the virus is curtailed, over-expression of the gene products may occur, inducing uncontrolled replication of the host cell. The genome of the herpesvirus, Marek's disease virus, appears to contain a number of v-*onc* genes similar to those of retroviruses.

pathogens of the GIT, which damage intestinal cells, are usually unaffected by gastric acid, are tolerant to bile salts and are resistant to inactivation by proteolytic enzymes. Remarkably, the infectivity of some viruses such as coronaviruses and rotaviruses is enhanced by exposure to proteolytic enzymes. With the notable exception of coronaviruses, enteric viral pathogens are non-enveloped. Bile salts generally have an adverse effect on viral envelopes. The basis for the resistance of the envelopes of coronaviruses to bile salts is unknown.

Arboviruses

Arboviruses are defined as viruses maintained in nature through biological transmission between vertebrate hosts by haematophagous arthropods. The viruses multiply in the tissues of the arthropod vector. The most important arthropod vectors are mosquitoes, ticks, sandflies and midges. The vector remains infected for life. The term 'arbovirus' has no taxonomic status. It is applied to viruses belonging to several viral families including *Togaviridae, Flaviviridae, Reoviridae, Rhabdoviridae, Arenaviridae* and *Bunyaviridae*. Most arboviruses are maintained in complex sylvatic life cycles involving a primary vertebrate host and a primary arthropod host. Such cycles usually remain undetected unless domestic animals and man encroach. Alternatively the virus may escape its primary cycle by means of a secondary vector or vertebrate host due to ecological change. As a result the virus is brought into the peridomestic environment. Domestic animals and man are generally 'dead-end' hosts as they do not develop sufficient viraemia to contribute to the transmission of the virus. The majority of arbovirus infections are zoonoses and are found in tropical developing countries and have a distinct geographical distribution. Ecological factors limiting the distribution of particular arboviruses include temperature, rainfall and distribution of both vertebrate reservoir host and arthropod vector.

Dissemination in the host

Following infection, local spread from cell to cell frequently occurs. When viruses bud from cells dissemination may be influenced by the manner and site of budding. Release of viral progeny from the apical surface of mucosal cells favours localized infection in tubular structures such as the air passages and the intestine. In contrast, release of virus from the basal surface into subepithelial tissues facilitates systemic infection. Factors which may limit the ability of some viruses to spread systemically include the absence of suitable cell receptors and lack of permissive cells. In addition, optimal viral replication may occur only in dividing cells or at a temperature lower than core body temperature. These virus and host factors may play an important role in determining the tropism of a virus, and account for the selective infection of certain cells in particular organs. In subepithelial

tissues, viruses often enter the lymphatic network and may be transported to the regional lymph nodes either as free virions or in infected macrophages. From the nodes, virus may pass to the efferent lymphatics and the thoracic duct, eventually entering the blood stream, the most important route of dissemination. Some viruses are transported along peripheral nerves. The preferential use of one route of spread does not necessarily exclude spread by other routes.

Haematogenous spread

Primary replication at the site of entry is frequently followed by transitory low-titred primary viraemia which results in infection of various organs including those of the reticuloendothelial system and the vascular endothelium. Further multiplication at these locations is followed by a sustained, high-titred secondary viraemia. In the blood-stream, virus may be free in the plasma or associated with cellular elements.

The body employs a number of mechanisms for clearing virus from the circulation. These include complement and antibody, and the phagocytic cells of the reticuloendothedial system in the liver, spleen, lung and lymph nodes. The magnitude and duration of a viraemia are determined by the amount of virus entering the blood-stream and the effectiveness of the clearance mechanisms. Large viruses are cleared more rapidly from the circulation than small viruses. There is rapid removal of viruses opsonized by antibody or by complement. Viraemias in which virus remains free in the plasma, such as those associated with parvoviruses, flaviviruses, togaviruses and picornaviruses, are usually of short duration, with clearance usually coinciding with the appearance of neutralizing antibodies in the serum. Prolonged viraemias are features of infections with viruses such as canine distemper virus, feline leukaemia virus and Marek's disease virus, which are associated with circulating cells. These viruses are often unaffected by the action of antibodies and complement. Some viruses like lentiviruses can replicate in monocytes or lymphocytes and, in many instances, produce persistent viraemias.

Invasion of tissues and organs from the blood can occur in a number of ways, which may relate to virus interaction with macrophages or vascular endothelial cells. Viruses such as picornaviruses, retroviruses, togaviruses and parvoviruses can infect endothelial cells and, following replication, are released into the tissues of target organs. In other instances, after endocytosis by endothelial cells, viruses may be translocated to the basal surface and released into tissues by exocytosis. In some anatomical locations such as the choroid plexuses, virions may pass from the bloodstream into surrounding tissues through fenestrated endothelium. Viruses can be transported into tissue spaces inside lymphocytes or monocytes as these cells migrate from the circulation. Engulfment and destruction of viruses by the phagocytic cells of the reticuloendothelial system is an important defence mechanism which limits viraemia. In some instances, phagocytosis of viruses by these cells may result in transfer of virions to adjoining tissues.

Neural spread

Neurotropic viruses such as rabies virus, Aujeszky's disease virus and Borna disease virus can invade the CNS through peripheral nerves. Enveloped viruses are usually transported as naked nucleocapsids by axoplasmic flow. Within the CNS, dissemination often involves spread across synaptic junctions. In addition, spread within peripheral nerves from the CNS to other locations may occur. Alphaherpesviruses can spread in peripheral nerves from the site of infection to ganglia, causing latent infections. Reactivation of infection may result in recrudescence of superficial lesions following transport of virus from the ganglia along nerve fibres.

Clinical signs

The signs of viral infections reflect both virus replication in tissues and host responses. Some viruses kill the cells in which they replicate, producing clinical signs which relate to the anatomical locations of the affected cells. Because of the considerable reserve and regenerative capacity of the liver, the loss of large numbers of hepatocytes may not result in significant clinical disturbance. In contrast, loss of relatively few neurons may have severe clinical consequences. In some viral infections, loss of specialized functions or reduction in functional efficiency in infected cells may induce clinical signs. Viral infections of the respiratory and intestinal tracts are frequently complicated by secondary bacterial infections, which may contribute to the development of clinical signs. Bacterial species present in the normal flora may contribute to these opportunistic infections. Denuded epithelial surfaces, impaired clearance mechanisms or increased availability of bacterial nutrients may promote secondary infections.

A number of viruses, including infectious bursal disease virus of poultry and feline immunodeficiency virus, target cells of the immune system. Progressive depletion of lymphocytes can lend to an immunodeficient state. As a consequence, affected animals may present with a variety of clinical signs due to secondary bacterial infection. In most viral infections, the immune system has an important protective role. However, there are viral infections in which the principal lesions result from hypersensitivity reactions and subsequent immunopathological changes. Immune complexes formed in persistent viral infections such as feline infectious peritonitis and equine infectious anaemia are responsible for vasculitis and glomerulo-nephritis.

Abortion following viral infection is usually indicative of substantial damage to the tissues of the placenta or foetus. The effect on the foetus is often influenced by the stage of gestation and by the virulence of the virus. Infection with virulent virus early in gestation generally results in foetal death with resorption or abortion. Infection of pregnant cattle with bovine viral diarrhoea virus (BVDV) before 100 days gestation may result in abortion, congenital defects or immunotolerance. If infection occurs at a later stage during pregnancy calves may be born with congenital defects whereas infection towards the end of pregnancy induces a protective immune response.

When viral epidemics occur in susceptible populations, the outcome in individual animals ranges from asymptomatic infection to fatal infection. Host factors which may influence the outcome include age, immune status, inheritance and nutrition. Young animals are generally more susceptible to viral infections than older animals whose increased resistance can usually be attributed to maturation of the immune system and to immunological memory. Reverse age resistance, although uncommon, is well documented in rabbit haemorrhagic disease. In this condition, rabbits less than 5 weeks of age do not develop disease because the target organ, the liver, does not appear to be susceptible early in life. Severe malnutrition may exacerbate certain viral diseases; a possible consequence of which may be depressed cell-mediated immunity. Success in the breeding of birds with enhanced resistance to avian leukosis and Marek's disease illustrates the influence of genetic factors on disease susceptibility.

Virus shedding and patterns of infection

The shedding of infectious virions from surfaces or orifices allows transfer to other susceptible hosts. Although shedding usually coincides with the onset of clinical signs, it may begin earlier in some viral infections. Respiratory viruses are usually transmitted in aerosols generated by coughing and sneezing. Enteric viruses are frequently shed in enormous quantities in faeces and can generally survive in harsh environments. Viruses which produce generalized infections may be shed by a number of routes. Body fluids such as saliva, semen, urine and milk may contain particular viruses. Arboviruses usually produce high titred viraemias of short duration and they rely on appropriate haematophagous vectors for transmission. Surgical procedures or blood sampling may facilitate spread of blood-borne viruses. Some viruses can be transmitted vertically by the transplacental route. Endogenous retroviruses are transmitted in the DNA of germ cells.

The maintenance of infection in a population requires continuous infection of susceptible animals. Two main strategies have been adopted by viruses for this purpose, namely acute infection and long-term persistence.

Acute infection is characterized by a short clinical course with rapid elimination of virus from the tissues. In these infections, there may be shedding of large amounts of virus over a short period. To maintain infection in a susceptible population viruses which cause acute infections must either be highly contagious, such as influenzaviruses, or be capable of surviving for long periods in the environment, such as parvoviruses.

Persistent viral infections are characterized by a prolonged course with constant or intermittent shedding. These infections, which may be acute initially, can persist either in latent or chronic forms. Latent infections are characterized by persistence of the virus in a non-productive form. Periodic reactivation of productive infection with shedding of infectious virus may occur. This type of infection is best exemplified by alpha-herpesviruses, which produce productive infections in epithelial cells and latent infections in sensory neurons. In chronic infections, virus is constantly present and may be shed intermittently or continuously. This type of infection can occur when the immune response of the host fails to eliminate virus from the tissues.

Infections characterized by long incubation periods of months or years are referred to as slow infections. Infections of this type, produced by lentiviruses, jaagsiekte sheep retrovirus and prions, have a progressive clinical course usually resulting in death.

Mechanisms of persistence

Viruses which persist in the body usually employ a number of strategies to ensure prolonged infections. For a virus to persist in host tissues, some infected cells must survive. Viruses have evolved a number of different strategies to reduce pathogenic effects on host cells. Viruses which produce non-lytic infections are likely to cause chronic infections. A number of viruses that are normally lytic have been shown to be capable of establishing persistent infections. Alphaherpesviruses, by exploiting the fact that sensory neurons are only partly permissive, have the ability to set up latent infections in such cells. In these non-dividing cells, the viruses persist as circular episomal DNA until adverse environmental factors induce immunosuppression which permits virus replication. Adenoviruses may persist in the body by producing low-grade, cycling infection with small numbers of cells infected at any given time. The evolution of defective-interfering or less cytolytic variants

may permit this type of infection to occur.

Viruses have evolved several strategies to evade the immune response and so avoid elimination from an immunocompetent host. Certain tissues in the body, referred to as immunologically privileged sites, are exempt from immune surveillance. The blood-brain barrier restricts contact between lymphocytes and CNS tissues. In addition, neurons do not express the major histocompatibility complex (MHC) class I or class II molecules which are required for T cell recognition of virus-infected cells. During latent infection of host cells by herpesviruses, viral gene expression is diminished and viral proteins are not expressed on the cell surface. Such infected cells are not easily recognized by the immune system. Viruses, particularly RNA viruses, undergo frequent mutation. Variants with altered epitopes at sites important for antibody neutralization or T cell recognition can emerge. These variants may evade immune detection and become the predominant infecting strain. This type of antigenic variation has been described in influenzavirus infections as a consequence of alterations in the surface glycoproteins, haemagglutinin and neuraminidase. Although these viruses do not persist in individual infected animals, they may persist in animal populations. Lentiviruses, such as equine infectious anaemia (EIA) virus, exhibit significant antigenic variation during replication in infected animals. Recurrent episodes of clinical disease can occur in EIA, in association with the emergence of antibody-escape variants and subsequent viraemia. It has been shown that some viruses can down-regulate expression of host cell surface markers such as MHC class I and class II molecules. Some viral proteins appear to act defensively by interfering with the function of anti-viral cytokines. Immune tolerance of the type associated with congenital BVDV infection permits persistent infection in calves. Affected calves have a lifelong viraemia and are the principal source of infection for other cattle.

Further reading

Tyler, K.L., Fields, B.N. (1996). Pathogenesis of viral diseases. In *Fields Virology*. Volume 1. Third Edition. Eds. B.N. Fields, D.M. Knipe and P.M. Howley. Lippincott-Raven, Philadelphia. pp. 173–218.

Chapter 53

Laboratory diagnosis of viral infections

Many viral diseases of animals can be diagnosed on the basis of clinical signs together with postmortem findings and histopathological changes. However, confirmation of the involvement of specific viral pathogens often requires special laboratory procedures. Surveillance for particular viruses is an important aspect of the management of valuable animals such as bulls used for artificial insemination and stallions, which have the potential to spread infection to many other animals. As part of international trade regulations, certification of freedom from certain viral diseases must accompany animals exported to countries in which the diseases are exotic. Moreover, rapid and accurate laboratory confirmation of exotic viral diseases, including those with zoonotic potential, is essential for the successful implementation of eradication policies and for the protection of human health. Surveillance of animal populations for new or emerging viral diseases is an important responsibility of national veterinary services.

More than 200 major viral diseases affect animal species of veterinary importance. Because of the considerable resources required for the provision of comprehensive diagnostic services in virology, national diagnostic services are usually concentrated on those diseases prevalent in a country. Moreover, laboratories often provide a diagnostic service for particular animal species. Special laboratory containment facilities are mandatory for some viruses which cause highly contagious diseases such as foot-and-mouth disease. The Office International des Épizooties (OIE) in Paris monitors and publishes details of significant animal disease outbreaks worldwide. This work is possible only through international cooperation and a network of laboratories dealing with viral diseases of international importance.

Collection, preservation and transportation of samples

Ideally, specimens for laboratory examination should be collected as early as possible from affected animals before secondary bacterial or fungal infections become established. It is advisable to collect samples from apparently normal in-contact animals because some of these animals may be actively shedding virus. The specimens selected for laboratory examination should relate to the clinical signs or to lesion distribution postmortem. Swabs from the oropharynx or nasopharyngeal aspirates are suitable specimens for investigation of respiratory diseases. In enteric viral diseases, large numbers of virus particles are shed in faeces. In those diseases characterized by viraemia, virus may be demonstrable in cells of the buffy coat.

Preservation of the infectivity or antigenicity of viruses may be required for particular tests. As many viruses are labile, specimens for virus isolation should be collected into transport medium, refrigerated and transmitted to the laboratory without delay. Samples should be frozen at -70°C if delay in delivery is anticipated. Freezing in a domestic freezer at -20°C decreases the infectivity of most viruses. Transport medium consists of buffered isotonic saline containing a high concentration of protein, such as bovine albumin or foetal calf serum, which prolongs virus survival. Antibiotics and antifungal drugs are added in order to inhibit the growth of contaminants. Samples for electron microscopy, in which demonstration of virion morphology is the primary objective, require less exacting conditions for storage and transportation. Air-dried smears for fluorescent antibody (FA) staining should be fixed in either acetone or methanol for up to 10 minutes in order to preserve viral antigens. This fixation process allows penetration of FA conjugates into cells. A similar fixation procedure is required for cryostat sections of frozen tissues prior to FA staining. Formalin-fixed tissue samples embedded in paraffin wax can be stored for many years and used to demonstrate the presence of viral antigen by immunohistochemical techniques.

Guidance from clinicians regarding the possible aetiology of the disease under investigation is essential for deriving maximum benefit from laboratory tests. This requires an accurate assessment of the history and clinical signs together with a tentative clinical diagnosis. In some instances, postmortem and histopathological examination of tissues may be sufficient for diagnostic purposes, particularly if specific inclusion bodies are found in infected tissues.

Detection of virus, viral antigens or nucleic acid

The presence of virus in tissues can be confirmed by

isolation of live virus, by demonstration of virus particles or viral antigen and by detecting viral nucleic acid.

Isolation of live virus

Virus isolation using cell culture, fertile eggs or experimental animals is the standard against which other diagnostic methods are usually compared. A monolayer composed of a particular cell type cannot be expected to support the growth of the many viruses which cause animal diseases. Laboratories usually have a limited range of cell lines most often used for virus isolation and appropriate to the range of samples received. Embryonated eggs are widely used for the isolation of influenza A virus and avian viruses. Because of ethical considerations and cost, virus isolation in experimental animals is now seldom employed.

Virus isolation is a sensitive procedure when cultural conditions are optimal for a particular virus and also generates a supply of virus for further studies. However, it is labour-intensive, slow and expensive. A number of blind passages may be required before a virus becomes adapted to a particular cell line and, as a consequence, a test result may not be available for some weeks. Because some viruses do not produce a cytopathic effect, additional detection procedures such as haemadsorption and FA staining may be needed to demonstrate their presence in cell cultures. Even when a virus produces a pronounced cytopathic effect, additional tests are often required for definitive identification.

Electron microscopy

Viruses can be demonstrated in diagnostic specimens by electron microscopy. This method can be used not only to recognize mixed viral infections but also to detect viruses which cannot be grown *in vitro*. Although this technique is particularly useful for identifying enteric viruses, it has serious limitations. Large numbers of viral particles (usually greater than 10^7 per ml) must be present in clinical samples. Sufficient concentrations of virus may be found in samples of faeces, scabs, vesicular fluids and wart tissues to allow detection. Moreover, viruses with similar morphology may be difficult to distinguish by electron microscopy. Members of a viral family usually have identical morphology and cannot be distinguished on this basis alone. In a few viral families, such as *Poxviridae* and *Reoviridae*, morphological differences do exist at the generic level.

A number of methods are used for the preparation of samples for examination. When preparing fluid samples, low speed centrifugation to remove large particulate debris is followed by ultracentrifugation to sediment virus particles. Negative staining with heavy metal compounds such as phosphotungstic acid or uranyl acetate increases contrast so that the brighter virions stand out against a dark background. The addition of antiserum to the specimen in immmunoelectron microscopy enhances the sensitivity of the procedure by clumping virus particles and facilitating their recovery by centrifugation. Alternatively, antiserum, when applied to the copper grid used for examining the specimen, can aggregate virions in the specimen.

Immunofluorescence and immunohistochemistry

Antiviral antibodies labelled with fluorochromes can be used to detect viral antigens in clinical specimens. Enzyme-labelled antiviral antibodies can also be used for this purpose. When using procedures involving immuno-fluorescence, a microscope with a special light source is required in order to visualize fluorescing material. Specific antibodies labelled with fluorochromes, usually fluorescein isothiocyanate or rhodamine isothiocyanate, are employed to detect virus-infected cells in specimens. The fluorochrome, exposed to light of a particular wavelength, emits light at a slightly longer wavelength allowing demonstration of the labelled antibody bound to virus particles. The technique is used to detect virus-infected cells in fixed smears, cryostat sections or monolayers.

Direct and indirect immunofluorescent techniques can be used to demonstrate virus or viral antigen in specimens (Fig. 53.1). In direct immunofluoresence, conjugated antibody specific for the particular virus is applied to the fixed specimen. After incubation, the specimen is washed to remove unbound antibody before microscopic examination. The indirect method employs unlabelled antiviral antiserum and a labelled antiglobulin specific for the species of animal from which the unlabelled antiserum was derived. Immunofluorescence techniques are rapid and sensitive but require careful interpretation as non-specific fluorescence can occur in certain specimens.

Enzyme-labelled antibodies can also be used to identify

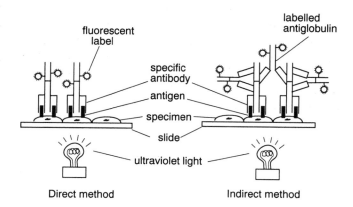

Figure 53.1 Direct and indirect immunofluorescent techniques for demonstrating viral antigen in cryostat (frozen tissue) sections, cell smears or monolayers. In the direct method, specific antibody is labelled with fluorescein isothiocyanate whereas in the indirect method, specific antibody bound to the viral antigen is demonstrated by the addition of labelled anti-globulin for the species of origin of the antibody.

viruses or viral antigen in clinical specimens. Horseradish peroxidase is the most common enzyme employed for conjugation with specific antiserum. After binding to viral antigen, antibody is identified by the addition of hydrogen peroxide and a benzidine derivative to the preparation. During the ensuing reaction, the colourless soluble benzidine derivative is converted to a coloured insoluble precipitate. For this technique, paraffin-embedded and resin-embedded tissues can be used and stained preparations do not fade when stored for long periods. Moreover, the stained preparations can be examined by conventional light microscopy. Endogenous tissue peroxidases, however, may produce misleading reactions unless suitable controls are included.

An avidin-biotin system can be used for enhancing immunohistochemical reactions. Biotin can be covalently linked to antibody without interfering with its antigen-binding capacity. Avidin bound either to a fluorochrome or an enzyme has a high affinity for the biotin molecules linked to the antibody.

Solid-phase immunoassays

In these assays, either antigen or antibody is immobilized on a surface. Suitable surfaces include polystyrene or synthetic membranes for enzyme immunoassays and radioimmunoassays; latex beads are often employed for agglutination tests. These assays are sensitive and relatively uncomplicated. Commercial tests based on these methods have been developed for particular viruses.

Radioimmunoassays employ antibodies labelled with radioisotopes and the bound antibody is measured using a gamma counter. These types of assays have been largely superseded by safer immunoassay procedures. Enzyme immunoassays, usually termed enzyme-linked immunosorbent assays (ELISA), are currently widely used for the immunodiagnosis of viral infections. In these assays, antibodies are labelled with enzymes which produce a colour change when they react with appropriate substrates. This colour change can be assessed visually or spectrophotometrically. For the detection of virus, wells in polystyrene plates are coated with specific anti-viral antibody and test material is added (Fig. 53.2). If present in the test material, viral antigen binds to the antibody during incubation and is not removed by washing. Enzyme-labelled antibody specific for the viral antigen is then added. Following incubation and washing, substrate for the enzyme is added; a colour change indicates a positive reaction.

Large numbers of samples can be processed quickly using ELISA. Rapid one-step assays suitable for use in veterinary practices are commercially available. Many of these kits utilize a membrane as the solid phase in order to increase the surface area on which antigen-antibody reactions can occur, thereby reducing incubation and washing times.

Latex particles, coated with anti-viral antibodies, agglutinate in the presence of viral antigen. No special equipment is required for these tests, which are simple and inexpensive. However, factors which decrease the reliability of these tests include non-specific reactions and prozone effects due to high antigen concentrations.

Immunodiffusion

This procedure is carried out in agar. The technique involves placing a fluid sample containing the virus under test in a well in the agar opposite a well containing antiserum. As the fluids diffuse out of the wells, a line of precipitate forms if the sample under test contains viral antigen. Although this test is easy to perform and inexpensive, it is relatively insensitive.

Complement fixation test for antigen detection

When antigen binds to antibody to form immune complexes, complement becomes activated and fixes to the complexes. In the complement-fixation test, the test sample is added to a known antiserum which has been heat-inactivated to destroy complement. Following incubation, a precise amount of guinea-pig complement is added. If viral antigen is present in the test sample, immune complexes formed during incubation fix the guinea-pig complement. Sheep red cells treated with specific rabbit antibody are added as an indicator to detect residual complement activity. If the guinea-pig complement is not bound, indicating the absence of viral antigen

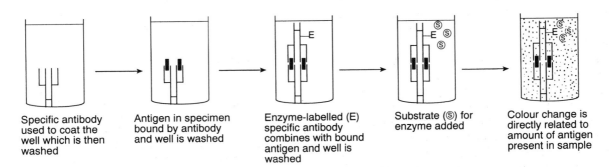

Specific antibody used to coat the well which is then washed

Antigen in specimen bound by antibody and well is washed

Enzyme-labelled (E) specific antibody combines with bound antigen and well is washed

Substrate (S) for enzyme added

Colour change is directly related to amount of antigen present in sample

Figure 53.2 Steps in ELISA for detecting antigen in a test sample (antigen capture method).

from the test sample, red cell lysis occurs. If viral antigen is present in the test sample, red cell lysis does not occur. The CFT requires rigorous standardization of reagents and careful interpretation.

Haemagglutination and haemadsorption

Viruses belonging to several families including *Orthomyxoviridae*, *Paramyxoviridae*, *Adenoviridae*, *Parvoviridae* and *Togaviridae* can interact with erythrocytes of many animal species causing haemagglutination. This unique ability derives from viral glycoproteins (haemagglutinins) which attach to receptors on erythrocytes resulting in the formation of aggregates which settle out of suspension. The haemagglutinins of orthomyxoviruses and paramyxoviruses allow these viruses to bind to neuraminic acid-containing receptors on erythrocytes. These viruses also possess neuraminidases which can destroy the erythrocyte receptors, causing dissociation. The surface structures (spikes) of influenza viruses which contain haemagglutinin and neuraminidase activity can be used to type influenza virus A isolates using specific antibody. As large numbers of virus particles are required to produce visible haemagglutination, this test is relatively insensitive.

The term haemadsorption is used to describe binding of erythrocytes to cells infected with haemagglutinating viruses. The haemagglutinating glycoproteins of these viruses are incorporated into cell membranes during viral replication.

Nucleic acid detection

The sensitivity and versatility of methods for the detection of viral nucleic acids has greatly improved in recent years and they are now becoming the method of choice for viral identification. These methods are particularly valuable when dealing with viruses which are either difficult to grow or cannot be grown *in vitro*. They are useful for latent infections in which infectious virus is absent and also for specimens containing inactivated virus. Cloned viral DNA is available for probing of samples and tissues by nucleic acid hybridization. This technique, however, has been largely replaced in recent years by the polymerase chain reaction which has the advantage of amplifying the target gene sequences.

Hybridization methods

Single-stranded DNA can hybridize to a complementary single strand of DNA or RNA by hydrogen-bonded base pairing. Under defined conditions of ionic concentration and elevated temperature, the strands of a target nucleic acid molecule can be dissociated and, on cooling, can hybridize with labelled DNA or RNA oligonucleotide probes when these are present in excess in the reaction mixture (Fig. 53.3). The temperature and ionic concentration employed largely determine the degree of discrimination of the test. Under stringent conditions, a

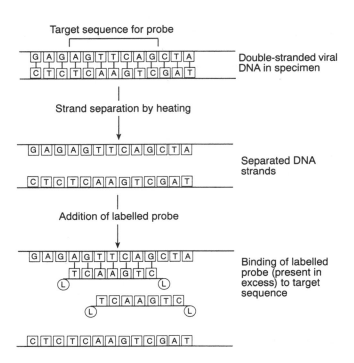

Figure 53.3 Outline of method for detecting viral DNA in clinical specimens using a labelled DNA probe specific for a target sequence. Suitable labels (L) include enzymes or radioactive isotopes. Detection of labelled probe by appropriate methods confirms the presence of viral nucleic acid.

high degree of specificity is achieved. Under conditions of low stringency, a probe containing mismatched base pairs can anneal to the dissociated nucleic acid strand. The length of the probe and the target region of the genome influence both the specificity of the test and the interpretation of the result. The oligonucleotide probes are synthesized or produced by cloning. Radioactive isotopes, which were extensively used as labels for probes, have been largely replaced by non-radioactive labels including alkaline phosphatase and horseradish peroxidase. Affinity labelling with biotin or digoxigenin and chemoluminescent labelling with acridinium esters are also employed.

Hybridization can be detected in a liquid phase or solid phase. Reactions in solution allow the target nucleic acid and the probe to interact freely. A modification of this hybridization procedure is the hybridization protection assay which employs a chemoluminescent probe. In this method, the chemoluminescent ester of the probe is protected from alkaline hydrolysis if the probe forms a stable molecular hybrid with the target molecule; unbound esterified probes are degraded giving negative results. A useful solid phase assay, termed dot-blot hybridization employs charged nylon or nitrocellulose membranes. Nucleic acid extracted from a sample, spotted directly onto the membrane, binds firmly after baking. The labelled probe is added, allowed to hybridize and unbound material is washed off. Another method based on solid phase assay is Southern blotting. In this method, extracted DNA is digested with restriction endonucleases and the resulting fragments are separated by gel electrophoresis. The separated fragments are then transferred by blotting onto a membrane for evaluation by hybridization.

Hybridization procedures can also be applied to intact cells or tissue sections. This *in situ* hybridization method is based on liberation of target nucleic acid while retaining cellular integrity and allows identification of the exact site of virus location.

Polymerase chain reaction

This *in vitro* method is based on the amplification of a particular nucleic acid sequence using a thermostable DNA polymerase and two oligonucleotide primers (Fig. 53.4). The polymerase was originally isolated from the thermophilic bacterium *Thermus aquaticus* and is known as *Taq* polymerase. In order to amplify the nucleic acid sequence of interest, primers complementary to sequences at each end of that particular portion of nucleic acid must be synthesized. Reactions, involving target DNA, primers, DNA polymerase and a mixture of individual nucleotides, are carried out under carefully controlled conditions in a programmable thermocycler. In most polymerase chain reaction (PCR) procedures, 30 to 50 thermal cycles take place. Each thermal cycle consists of a step in which the double-stranded DNA is separated at high temperature, an annealing step which allows primers to hybridize with complementary target sequences during a cooling phase, and an extension step, at an intermediate temperature, during which primer products are extended by DNA polymerase. These primer products act as new templates for the production of nucleic acid in each subsequent cycle. The number of target DNA copies approximately doubles with every cycle. The amplified DNA fragments can be separated by agarose gel electrophoresis and stained with ethidium bromide. Exact information on the DNA fragments requires the use of restriction endonuclease analysis, direct sequencing or probe analysis. An important modification of the PCR is the reverse transcriptase polymerase chain reaction (RT-PCR) which has extended the application of the technique to RNA viruses.

Quantitative PCR methods, which can be used to measure the amount of target DNA or RNA in a sample, have been developed. In addition, retrospective PCR analyses are now possible with the development of *in situ* PCR which can be applied to paraffin-embedded tissues and museum specimens. Multiplex PCR involves the use of multiple primer pairs in the same amplification reaction to increase the number of detectable target sequences. This has allowed the development of assays capable of detecting multiple pathogens or virulence-associated genes in a single sample. Nested PCR is a popular modification of PCR involving two sets of primers. The second pair of primers is designed to amplify an internal region of the sequence amplified by the first pair. It is possible to design the first primer set to be less specific, capable of detecting a range of related pathogens, while the second primers set is species- or strain-specific. Because of their exquisite sensitivity, PCR techniques require rigorous standardization to exclude cross-contamination and ensure reproducibility and reliability. When collecting clinical specimens, contamination from the environment or from other sources must be avoided. The possible presence of viral 'passengers' and degraded viral genomes becomes an important issue as the sensitivity of detection tests increases.

Diagnostic serology

Serological procedures can be used for the retrospective diagnosis of viral diseases and for epidemiological surveys. These procedures can be automated and diagnostic reagents for many viral pathogens are commercially available. Single blood samples from animals in susceptible populations suffice for establishing the prevalence of a disease. When using serological procedures for the diagnosis of endemic disease in flocks or herds, paired serum samples taken at an interval of at least three weeks, are required to demonstrate rising antibody titres. Initial samples should be collected when clinical signs are first evident and the second samples during convalescence. A single blood sample may be adequate for diagnosis if reagents are available for demonstrating IgM antibodies, which are indicative of a primary immune response. Difficulties with the interpretation of serological tests may arise due to cross-reactions with antigenically related viruses. In young animals, passively acquired maternal antibodies which may persist for several months, can lead to misinterpretation of results.

Enzyme-linked immunosorbent assay

The procedure used for carrying out ELISA to detect antibodies is different from that already described for the demonstration of virus in specimens. The essential difference is that viral antigen is bound to the solid phase (polystyrene wells or membranes). Dilutions of test serum are added and allowed to react with the antigen. After washing, enzyme-conjugated antiglobulin is added and, following further incubation and washing, appropriate substrate is added. The intensity of the colour change is proportional to the amount of antibody in the test serum (Fig. 53.5). Either polyclonal or monoclonal labelled conjugates may be used; the choice depends on whether or not the immunoglobulin isotype is required for estimating the duration of the infection.

Immunofluorescence for antibody detection

Using indirect immunofluorescence, test serum is added to known viral antigen fixed on a microscope slide

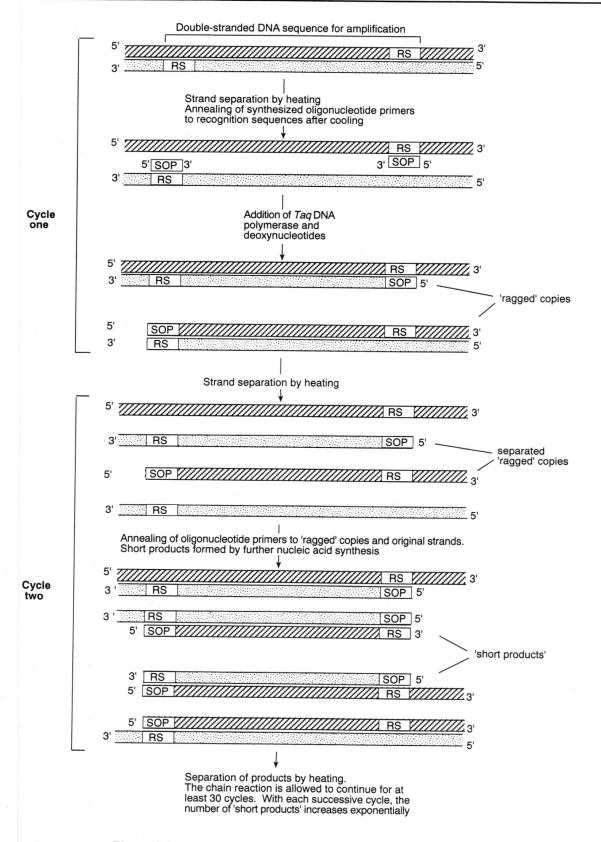

Figure 53.4 Outline of the steps involved in the polymerase chain reaction.

RS, recognition sequence; SOP, synthesized oligonucleotide primer;
Taq DNA polymerase, heat-stable enzyme derived from the bacterium *Thermus aquaticus*.

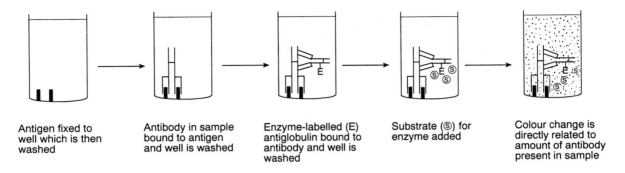

Figure 53.5 Steps in ELISA for detecting antibody in a test sample (indirect method).

(Fig. 53.6). Following incubation, the slide is washed and, after the addition of fluorescein isothiocyanate-conjugated antiglobulin, incubated for a further period. The slide is again washed before examination under UV light. The test is both sensitive and rapid but requires careful interpretation. Antibody production by plasma cells can be demonstrated in cryostat sections by the sandwich method (Fig. 53.7).

Serum neutralization test

This test is highly specific and sensitive for viruses which produce cytopathic effects (CPE). It is considered to be the definitive standard against which other serological tests are compared. Neutralizing antibodies usually correlate closely with immune protection. In this test, which is typically carried out in microtitre plates, a constant amount of stock virus is added to doubling dilutions of a test serum. Cells susceptible to the virus are added to the wells. The presence of neutralizing antibodies in the serum prevents infection of the cells and CPE. The titre of the serum is the highest dilution at which the virus is neutralized. The neutralizing effect of test serum can also be evaluated in susceptible experimental animals and in chick embryos. Neutralizing antibodies tend to persist in recovered animals for long periods, often for many years.

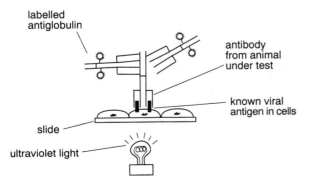

Figure 53.6 Indirect immunofluorescence technique for demonstrating antibodies in serum.

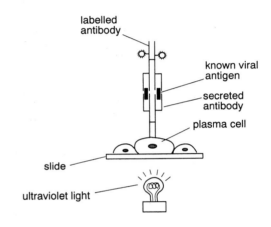

Figure 53.7 Sandwich method for demonstrating antibody production in tissue specimen.

Haemagglutination inhibition test

Because viruses in certain families have the ability to haemagglutinate, the inhibitory effect of antibodies on haemagglutination can be used for the diagnosis of infection with these viruses. The haemagglutination inhibition (HAI) test is specific, reliable and easily performed. The test, usually carried out in microtitre plates, involves serial twofold dilutions of serum to which a known concentration (four haemagglutinating units) of virus is added. The highest dilution which inhibits erythrocyte agglutination is the HAI titre of the test serum. Non-specific inhibitors of haemagglutination, sometimes present in sera, can be inactivated by heating or by treatment with kaolin, trypsin, periodate or bacterial neuraminidase.

Complement fixation tests

Due to difficulties with standardization, complement fixation tests have been superseded by more convenient diagnostic tests such as ELISA. Complement-fixing antibodies tend to appear before neutralizing antibodies but do not persist. Sera from some species are difficult to titrate by this method due to the presence of anti-complementary activity.

Western blotting (immunoblotting) technique

This test, which was primarily developed as a research procedure for the identification of antigenic proteins, can also be used for the diagnosis of viral disease. Purified virus, solubilized with an anionic detergent such as sodium dodecyl sulphate, is electrophoresed in a polyacrylamide gel. Separated proteins are transferred electrophoretically onto a nitrocellulose membrane, which is then washed, dried and cut into longitudinal strips. Following incubation in test sera, the strips are washed and incubated with enzyme-labelled antiglobulin. Addition of substrate produces an insoluble coloured product where test antibody is bound to the separated viral proteins.

Interpretation of test results

Because false-positive and false-negative results can occur in many test procedures, inclusion of positive and negative controls is essential. The sensitivity and specificity of a particular diagnostic test should be established. The sensitivity of a diagnostic test, expressed as a percentage, is the number of animals identified as positive out of the total number of animals with the disease. The specificity of a test is the percentage of uninfected animals in which the result is negative. In order to detect all animals with an important viral infection, a test with high sensitivity is required. For laboratory confirmation of a viral infection in an individual animal, a test with high specificity is essential.

The isolation of virus or the demonstration of antibody to a specific virus does not necessarily confirm an aetiological link with a disease state. For the conclusive confirmation of test results, it may be necessary to demonstrate a correlation between the site of virus recovery and the nature and extent of lesions. Circumstantial evidence for the aetiological involvement of a virus in a clinically affected animal is supported by the recovery of the same virus from susceptible in-contact animals. Moreover, a rising antibody titre to the putative causal virus, demonstrated by the use of paired serum samples, is of diagnostic importance. Published reports on the potential importance of a similar disease syndrome and its aetiology may point to the requirement for particular laboratory investigations.

Further reading

Mullis, K.B. (1990). The unusual origin of the polymerase chain reaction. *Scientific American*, **262**, 56–65.

Saiki, R.K., Scharf, S., Faloona, F. *et al.* (1985). Enzymatic amplification of β-globulin genomic sequences and restriction site analysis for the diagnosis of sickle-cell anaemia. *Science*, **230**, 1350–1354.

Section V

Viruses and Prions

Chapter 54

Herpesviridae

The family *Herpesviridae* contains more than 100 viruses. Fish, amphibians, reptiles, birds and mammals including humans are susceptible to herpesvirus infection. These viruses are of special importance because of their widespread occurrence, their evolutionary diversity and their involvement in many important diseases of domestic animals and humans. The name, herpesvirus (Greek *herpein*, to creep), refers to the sequential appearance and local extension of lesions in human infection. Herpesviruses are enveloped and range from 120 nm to 200 nm in diameter. They contain double-stranded DNA within an icosahedral capsid (Fig. 54.1). A layer of amorphous material, the tegument, lies between the envelope and the capsid. Herpesviruses enter cells by fusing with the plasma membrane. Replication occurs in the cell nucleus. The envelope, which derives from the nuclear membrane of the host cell, incorporates at least eight viral encoded glycoproteins. Enveloped virions accumulate in the endoplasmic reticulum prior to final processing of the glycoproteins in the Golgi apparatus and release by exocytosis. Active infection results in cell

<table>
<tr><td>

Key points

- Enveloped DNA viruses with icosahedral symmetry
- Replicate in the nucleus
- Labile in the environment
- Three subfamilies of veterinary importance: *Alphaherpesvirinae, Betaherpesvirinae, Gammaherpesvirinae*
- Cause diseases of the respiratory, reproductive and nervous systems; may cause cell transformation in some species
- Latency is a common outcome of infection with these viruses

</td></tr>
</table>

death. Intranuclear inclusions are characteristic of herpesvirus infections. Extension of viral infection occurs through points of cell contact without exposure of virus to neutralizing antibodies in blood or interstitial fluids. Protective antibody responses are usually directed against the envelope glycoproteins. Herpesvirus virions, which are fragile and sensitive to detergents and lipid solvents, are unstable in the environment.

The family is divided into three subfamilies (Fig. 54.2), *Alphaherpesvirinae, Betaherpesvirinae* and *Gammaherpesvirinae*. The subfamilies comprise nine genera. A tenth unnamed genus Ictalurid herpes-like viruses contains herpesviruses of fish and is currently unassigned to a subfamily. Alphaherpesviruses replicate and spread rapidly, destroying host cells and often establishing latent infections in sensory ganglia. Betaherpesviruses, which replicate and spread slowly, cause infected cells to enlarge, hence their common name cytomegaloviruses. They may become latent in secretory glands and lymphoreticular cells. Gammaherpesviruses, which infect T or B lymphocytes, can produce latent infections in these cells. When lymphocytes become infected, there is minimal expression of viral antigen. Some gammaherpesvirus species also replicate in epithelial and fibroblastic cells causing cytolysis. A number of gammaherpesviruses are implicated in neoplastic transformation of lymphocytes.

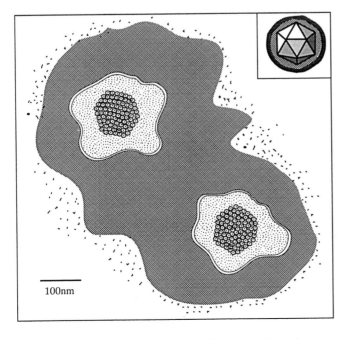

Figure 54.1 Herpesvirus particles as they appear in an electron micrograph and a diagrammatic representation (inset).

| Family | Subfamily | Virus |

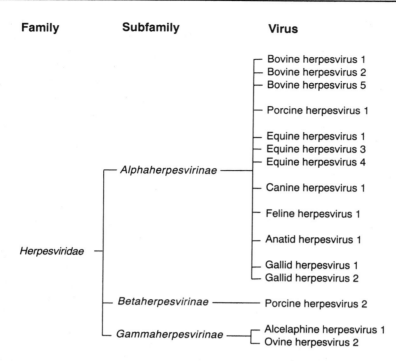

Figure 54.2 Classification of herpesviruses of domestic animals.

Clinical infections

Herpesviruses establish life-long infections with periodic reactivation resulting in bouts of clinical disease. Shedding of virus may be periodic or continuous. During latency, the episomal viral genome becomes circular and gene expression is limited. Reactivation of infection is associated with various stress factors including transportation, adverse weather conditions, overcrowding and intercurrent infection. Natural infections with particular herpesviruses are usually restricted to defined host species. Because these viruses are highly adapted to their natural hosts, infections may be inapparent or mild. However, in very young or immunosuppressed animals, infection can be life-threatening. Some herpesviruses such as Marek's disease virus and Epstein-Barr virus are implicated in neoplastic transformation of cells.

Herpesviruses can cause respiratory, genital, mammary and CNS diseases in cattle (Table 54.1). Aujeszky's disease, which affects pigs and other domestic species, is the major porcine herpesvirus infection (Table 54.2). In horses, herpesviruses can cause respiratory, neurological and venereal diseases, and abortion along with neonatal infection (Table 54.3). The herpesviruses of domestic carnivores are presented in Table 54.4 and those of birds in Table 54.5.

Infectious bovine rhinotracheitis and pustular vulvovaginitis

Bovine herpesvirus 1 (BHV-1), which infects domestic and range cattle, is associated with several clinical conditions including infectious bovine rhinotracheitis, infectious pustular vulvovaginitis, balanoposthitis, conjunctivitis and generalized disease in newborn calves. Infection with BHV-1 is an important cause of losses in livestock worldwide. A single antigenic type of BHV-1 which contains subtypes 1.1, 1.2a and 1.2b, has been

Table 54.1 Herpesvirus infections of ruminants.

Virus	Genus	Comments
Bovine herpesvirus 1	*Varicellovirus*	Causes respiratory (infectious bovine rhinotracheitis) and genital (infectious pustular vulvovaginitis, balanoposthitis) infections. Occurs worldwide
Bovine herpesvirus 2	*Simplexvirus*	Causes ulcerative mammillitis in temperate regions and pseudo-lumpy-skin disease in tropical and subtropical regions
Bovine herpesvirus 5	*Varicellovirus*	Causes encephalitis in calves; described in several countries
Ovine herpesvirus 2	*Rhadinovirus*	Causes subclinical infection in sheep and goats worldwide. Causes malignant catarrhal fever in cattle and in some wild ruminants
Alcelaphine herpesvirus 1	*Rhadinovirus*	Causes subclinical infection in wildebeest in Africa and in zoos. Causes malignant catarrhal fever in cattle, deer and in other susceptible ruminants

Table 54.2 Herpesvirus infections of pigs.

Virus	Genus	Comments
Porcine herpesvirus 1 (Aujeszky's disease virus)	*Varicellovirus*	Causes Aujeszky's disease (pseudorabies) primarily in pigs. Encephalitis, pneumonia and abortion are features of the disease. In many species other than pigs, pseudorabies manifests as a neurological disease with marked pruritis. Occurs worldwide
Porcine herpesvirus 2	Unassigned	Causes disease of the upper respiratory tract in young pigs (inclusion body rhinitis)

recognized using restriction enzyme analysis. Subtype 1.1, implicated in respiratory disease, is included in most vaccines. Subtypes 1.2a and 1.2b cause mild respiratory disease and are implicated in the infectious balanoposthitis/infectious pustular vulvovaginitis (IBP/IPV) syndrome. Subtypes 1.1 and 1.2a rarely cause abortion; the less virulent subtype 1.2b has not been associated with abortion.

Pathogenesis and pathology
The virus which causes infectious bovine rhinotracheitis is usually acquired through aerosols. Replication occurs in the mucous membranes of the upper respiratory tract and large amounts of virus are shed in nasal secretions. Virus also enters local nerve cell endings and is transported intra-axonally to the trigeminal ganglion where it remains latent. In most instances, infection is contained within two weeks by a strong immune response. However, tissue necrosis may facilitate secondary bacterial infection with severe systemic effects and, possibly, death. Rarely, a lymphocyte-associated viraemia in pregnant cows may produce foetal infection and abortion. Necrotic foci may be present in various organs of aborted foetuses, particularly in the liver.

Table 54.3 Herpesvirus infections of horses.

Virus	Genus	Comments
Equine herpesvirus 1	*Varicellovirus*	Causes abortion, respiratory disease, neonatal infection and neurological disease. Occurs worldwide
Equine herpesvirus 3	*Varicellovirus*	Causes mild venereal infection in both mares and stallions
Equine herpesvirus 4	*Varicellovirus*	Causes rhinopneumonitis in young horses and sporadic abortion. Occurs worldwide

Following genital infection with subtypes 1.2a and 1.2b, virus replicates in the mucosa of the vagina or prepuce, and latent infection may become established in the sacral ganglia. Focal necrotic lesions on genital mucosae may eventually coalesce to form large ulcers. An intense inflammatory reaction can develop in the reproductive tract with secondary bacterial infection leading to endometritis. Viraemia is not a feature of genital infection with BHV-1 subtypes and infected pregnant cows rarely abort.

Clinical signs
In outbreaks of disease, either the respiratory or the genital form usually predominates. The incubation period is up to four days. The severity of the clinical signs in the respiratory form of the disease are largely determined by the extent of secondary bacterial infection. Affected animals develop a high temperature and nasal discharge accompanied by anorexia. The nares are inflamed ('red nose'), and conjunctivitis, lacrimal discharge and corneal opacity are often present. In uncomplicated infections, animals recover after about a week. If bacterial infection becomes established, animals develop dyspnoea, coughing and open-mouth breathing. Death may ensue. In severe outbreaks in feedlot cattle, morbidity may approach 100% and mortality may be as high as 10%. Cows with infectious pustular vulvovaginitis exhibit vaginal discharge and frequent urination. Animals usually recover within two weeks. However, secondary bacterial infection may result in metritis, temporary infertility and purulent vaginal discharge persisting for several weeks. Infected bulls have lesions on penile and preputial mucosae.

A fatal generalized disease with fever, oculonasal discharge, respiratory distress, diarrhoea, incoordination and convulsions has been described in young calves.

Diagnosis
- Swabs collected from the nares and genitalia of several affected animals during the early acute phase of the disease are suitable for virus isolation. Because the virus is fragile, specimens for transport to the laboratory should be placed in viral transport medium and kept refrigerated. The virus produces a rapid cytopathic effect in bovine cell lines.
- Smears from nasal or genital swabs and frozen sections of tissues from aborted foetuses can be used for the rapid demonstration of viral antigen using immunofluorescence. Viral antigen can also be detected using ELISA.
- The presence of characteristic gross and microscopic lesions in aborted foetuses is suggestive of infection with BHV-1.
- The polymerase chain reaction has been adapted for detection of BHV-1 DNA in appropriate samples.
- The evidence of a rising antibody titre in paired serum samples using virus neutralization or ELISA is

Table 54.4 Herpesvirus infections of domestic carnivores.

Virus	Genus	Comments
Canine herpesvirus 1	*Varicellovirus*	Causes a fatal generalized infection in neonatal pups
Feline herpesvirus 1	*Varicellovirus*	Causes feline viral rhinotracheitis in young cats

indicative of active infection.
* As part of a surveillance programme, bulk milk samples can be tested for antibodies using ELISA.

Control

Inactivated, subunit and modified live vaccines are available for the control of BHV-1 (van Oirschot *et al.*, 1996). Vaccination reduces the severity of clinical signs but may not prevent infection. Modified live vaccines may cause abortion and should not be administered to pregnant animals. Vaccine strains, which are temperature-sensitive, do not replicate at temperatures above 37°C and should be administered by the intranasal route. Appropriate serological tests permit differentiation of vaccinated animals from those infected with field virus. Marker vaccines, based either on genetically engineered viruses lacking one or more genes encoding surface glycoproteins or on subunit preparations containing one or more glycoproteins, are available. A serological test, usually a blocking ELISA, is used to detect antibodies against a glycoprotein not present in the marker vaccine. The availability of marker vaccines enables either eradication or reduction of infection in national herds to proceed economically. Successful eradication programmes based on test and slaughter policies have been carried out in Denmark and Switzerland.

Table 54.5 Herpesvirus infections of birds.

Virus	Genus	Comments
Gallid herpesvirus 1	Infectious laryngotracheitis-like viruses	Causes infectious laryngotracheitis. Present in many countries
Gallid herpesvirus 2 (Marek's disease virus)	Marek's disease-like viruses	Causes Marek's disease, a lymphoproliferative condition in 12 to 24 week old chickens. Occurs worldwide
Anatid herpesvirus 1	Unassigned	Causes acute disease in ducks, geese and swans characterized by oculonasal discharge, diarrhoea and high mortality. Occurs worldwide

Bovine herpes mammillitis and pseudo-lumpy-skin disease

Infection with bovine herpesvirus 2 (BHV-2) is associated with outbreaks of a severe ulcerative condition of the teats of dairy cows. The condition has been reported in many countries around the world. Bovine herpesvirus 2 infection resulting in a generalized mild skin infection, termed pseudo-lumpy-skin disease to distinguish it from the more serious lumpy skin disease caused by a poxvirus, has been reported in tropical and subtropical regions.

Epidemiology

In temperate regions, outbreaks of herpes mammillitis are sporadic and usually occur in autumn or early winter. Latent infection and subsequent reactivation are important factors in the spread and perpetuation of infection within herds. In cows calving for the first time, lesions appear a few days after parturition Serous exudate from lesions contains large quantities of virus and transmission to other cows in the herd occurs through direct and indirect contact during milking. Infection occurs through small abrasions in the skin. Insects may transmit the virus from animal to animal mechanically. Calves suckling affected cows can become infected and may transmit the virus. In Africa, a wide range of wild animal species appear to act as subclinical reservoirs of infection. Insect transmission is considered to be important in warm climates and may account for the occurrence of the generalized skin form of the disease in those regions.

Pathogenesis

The virus replicates optimally at a temperature lower than normal body temperature. Following intradermal or subcutaneous inoculation, BHV-2 replicates without dissemination to other sites. In contrast, generalized infection with widespread skin nodules develops in experimental animals following intravenous inoculation of BHV-2.

Clinical signs

The number of animals displaying clinical signs during outbreaks is variable and subclinical infection is common. First-lactation cows which have recently calved, particularly animals with udder oedema, are most severely affected. The incubation period is up to eight days. Lesions appear as thickened plaques on one or more teats. Ulceration of the skin leads to scar formation. The lesions are painful and there is a reduction in milk yield due to difficulty with milking. In severe cases, lesions may also appear on the skin of the udder. Circular ulcers may be present on the lips, nostrils or muzzle of calves suckling affected cows. In pseudo-lumpy-skin disease, a variable number of nodules appear on the skin over the neck, shoulders, back and perineum. The nodules, which are circular and hard, have depressed centres. They heal without scar formation within a couple of weeks.

Diagnosis

Diagnosis is based on demonstration of virus in scrapings or in vesicular fluid by direct electron microscopy or by virus isolation in tissue culture. The optimal incubation temperature for inoculated cell cultures is 32°C.

Control

Commercial vaccines are not available. Affected animals should be isolated and milked separately. Teat dipping and disinfection of milking machine clusters between cows is advisable. The most susceptible animals, first-lactation cows, should be milked first. Insect control measures may help to limit the spread of disease within a herd.

Malignant catarrhal fever

This severe, sporadic disease of cattle, deer and other ruminants is frequently fatal. Malignant catarrhal fever (MCF) is caused by two related but distinct viruses, alcelaphine herpesvirus 1 (ALV-1) and ovine herpesvirus 2 (OHV-2). As the wildebeest is the natural host of ALV-1, infection with this virus is confined to Africa. Sheep are the natural hosts of OHV-2 and infection occurs worldwide in sheep and goats. In these species infection is common and subclinical.

Epidemiology

Alcelaphine herpesvirus 1 is transmitted vertically and horizontally in wildebeest populations. There is evidence that latency occurs in lymphoid cells. Some wildebeest calves are infected transplacentally but most acquire infection shortly after birth through nasal secretions from their mothers or from other calves. Viraemia persists in young wildebeest for the first few months of life. This facilitates shedding of large quantities of virus in nasal and ocular secretions. In-contact cattle may become infected. The pattern of virus shedding is thought to be similar in sheep especially at lambing, when transmission to cattle and farmed deer is most likely to occur. Infection in cattle and deer is thought to be acquired through contact with young lambs. Some studies suggest that most lambs do not become infected before seven months of age (Li *et al.*, 1998). Cattle and deer are considered to be 'end-hosts' because they do not appear to transmit virus.

Pathogenesis

The pathogenesis of MCF is poorly understood. It is presumed that virus enters the body through the upper respiratory tract. A cell-associated viraemia occurs. However, virus is virtually absent from the sites of lesions and it is thought that tissue changes in MCF have an immunopathological basis. Cell-mediated reactions have been implicated in lesion development. It has been proposed that stimulation of T lymphocytes through overproduction of IL-2 by deregulated natural killer (NK) cells contributes to lesion development.

Clinical signs

The incubation period, although variable, generally lasts three to four weeks. The most common clinical presentation is characterized by sudden onset of fever, oculonasal discharge, enlarged lymph nodes, conjunctivitis, corneal opacity and erosive mucosal lesions in the upper respiratory tract. Profuse mucopurulent nasal discharge leads to encrustation of the muzzle. Some animals display neurological signs including muscle tremors, incoordination and head pressing. An intestinal form of the disease presents with diarrhoea or dysentery.

The course of this usually fatal disease is up to seven days. Some animals may linger for weeks or months and may recover (O'Toole *et al.*, 1997). In peracute disease, particularly in deer, death may occur without premonitory signs.

Diagnosis

Diagnosis is based on clinical presentation along with extensive vasculitis characterized histologically by fibrinoid degeneration and marked lymphoid infiltration. Ulceration of surface epithelia is a prominent feature of MCF. Viral DNA can be detected in circulating leukocytes using PCR (Muller-Doblies *et al.*, 1998). Although a competitive inhibition ELISA has been developed for the detection of serum antibodies to ALV-1 and OHV-2 (Li *et al.*, 1994), it is not as reliable as PCR or histopathological examination. This ELISA test can be used to determine the prevalence of antibodies in sheep populations. Although ALV-1 can be isolated from the buffy coat of animals with wildebeest-associated MCF, ovine herpesvirus 2 has not yet been isolated.

Control

As no vaccine is available, control depends on the separation of susceptible species from reservoir hosts. Identification and elimination of sheep harbouring OHV-2 using the PCR assay in order to establish a virus-free flock may be worthwhile in defined circumstances.

Aujeszky's disease

This disease, also called pseudorabies, is caused by Aujeszky's disease virus (ADV). A single serotype of the virus is recognized. The pig, in which subclinical and latent infections can occur, is the natural host of the virus. Other domestic animals are susceptible and infection in these incidental hosts is usually fatal.

Epidemiology

Infection is endemic in the pig populations of most countries. The disease has been eradicated from Denmark and the United Kingdom. Outbreaks of disease in naive herds can be devastating with rapid spread to pigs of all ages. The virus is shed in oronasal secretions, milk and semen. Transmission usually occurs by nose-to-nose contact or by aerosols. Transplacental transmission occurs and aborted foetuses are a source of virus. Although the virus is not stable in the environment, it may remain infectious for a few days under suitable conditions. Wind-borne transmission over distances of a few kilometres has been recorded. Sheep, which are highly susceptible, may acquire infection following direct contact with pigs or when sharing the same airspace. Scavenging carnivores may become infected after eating pig meat; cats are particularly susceptible to infection. Because the incubation period and clinical course in these incidental hosts are short, the opportunity for transmission of virus from these animals is limited.

Pathogenesis

Following infection, the virus replicates in the epithelium of the nasopharynx and tonsils. Virus spreads from these primary sites to regional lymph nodes and to the CNS along axons of the cranial nerves. Virulent strains of ADV produce a brief viraemia and become widely distributed around the body, particularly in the respiratory tract. Virus replication which occurs in alveolar macrophages interferes with their phagocytic function. Transplacental transfer results in generalized infection of foetuses. Infected animals excrete virus for up to three weeks following infection. Latency occurs in a high percentage of infected animals with virus localized in the trigeminal ganglia and tonsils.

Clinical signs

The age and susceptibility of infected pigs and the virulence of the infecting strain influence the severity of the clinical signs. Young pigs are most severely affected; mortality may approach 100% in suckling piglets. In neonatal piglets, the incubation period may be as short as 36 hours compared with five days in older pigs. Neurological signs including incoordination, tremors, paddling and convulsions predominate in young pigs. Affected animals usually die within two days. Mortality is much lower in weaned pigs although neurological and respiratory signs are often present. Fever, weight loss, sneezing, coughing, nasal discharge and dyspnoea may be evident in fatteners. Neurological signs are uncommon in these older animals and they usually recover within a week. Infection in sows early in pregnancy usually results in resorption of foetuses and return to oestrus. Later in pregnancy, infection frequently produces abortion; full-term piglets may be still-born, or weak. In herds with endemic ADV infection, neonatal animals are protected by maternally-derived antibody.

Disease in other domestic animals occurs sporadically and is characterized by neurological signs resembling those of rabies. Intense pruritis ('mad itch') leading to self-mutilation is a feature of the disease, particularly in ruminants. The clinical course is short with most affected animals dying within a few days.

Diagnosis

The history, clinical signs and lesions may suggest ADV infection. Laboratory confirmation is based on virus isolation, detection of viral antigen, serology and histopathological findings.

- Specimens of brain, spleen and lung from acutely affected animals are suitable for virus isolation. Nasal swabs, collected from live animals, may also be used. In the event of a delay between collection and tissue culture inoculation, samples should be refrigerated.
- Cryostat sections of tonsil or brain are suitable for detection of viral antigen by immunofluorescence.
- Serological tests, including virus neutralization, ELISA and latex agglutination, are available for detecting ADV antibodies. In young pigs, maternally-derived antibodies may be present up to the age of four months. Differential ELISA methods have been introduced for the detection of antibodies to the surface glycoproteins gC, gE and gG. These assays are designed to differentiate animals infected with field virus from those vaccinated with a gene-deleted mutant lacking a surface glycoprotein.

Control

If used strategically, vaccination can prevent the development of clinical disease. Modified live, inactivated and gene-deleted vaccines are available. Vaccines have been produced in which the thymidine kinase (TK) gene has been deleted together with a gene encoding one of the non-essential surface glycoproteins. Because endogenous levels of TK are low in neurons, this gene-deleted virus cannot replicate in neurons and as a consequence is significantly reduced in virulence. However, such vaccinal strains may fail to prevent latent infection caused by field virus in the trigeminal ganglia. In addition, the possibility of recombination of field virus with a gene-deleted virus and the subsequent generation of a virulent ADV has been suggested (Maes *et al.*, 1997). Eradication of Aujeszky's disease can be achieved by depopulation, by test and removal, or by segregation of litters. The availability of effective marker vaccines makes eradication feasible and economically worthwhile.

Equine rhinopneumonitis and equine herpesvirus abortion

Equine herpesvirus 1 (EHV-1) and equine herpesvirus 4 (EHV-4), which are endemic in horse populations world-wide, are responsible for outbreaks of respiratory disease in young horses and for abortion. Before 1981, it was considered that a single virus, EHV-1 composed of two subtypes, was responsible for both clinical syndromes. However, restriction endonuclease analysis showed that the subtypes were two distinct viruses. Infection with EHV-1 is associated with respiratory disease, abortion, fatal generalized disease in neonatal foals and encephalomyelitis. Although infection with EHV-4 is primarily associated with respiratory disease, sporadic abortions have also been attributed to this virus.

Epidemiology

Close contact facilitates transmission of these fragile viruses. Transmission usually occurs by the respiratory route following contact with infected nasal secretions, aborted foetuses, placentae or uterine fluids. Both EHV-1 and EHV-4 can occur as latent infections. Serological studies using a type-specific ELISA have shown that there is a high prevalence of antibody to EHV-4 approaching 100% in some surveys (Gilkerson et al., 1999b). It is thought that episodes of reactivation of latent EHV-4 infection without coincident clinical disease occur in adult horses, resulting in transmission to foals. The prevalence of antibody to EHV-1 is about 30% in adult horses; it is lower in foals (Gilkerson et al., 1999b). It appears that foals become infected with EHV-1 from their dams or from other lactating mares in the group. Foal-to-foal spread may occur both before and after weaning (Gilkerson et al., 1999a). Mares infected with EHV-1 are potential sources of infection even without aborting. When reactivation of infection in a latent carrier mare occurs in a stud farm, exposure of non-immune, in-contact pregnant mares may lead to an abortion storm.

Pathogenesis

These viruses replicate initially in the upper respiratory tract and regional lymph nodes with spread, in some cases, to the lower respiratory tract and lungs. Latent infection of the trigeminal ganglia with both EHV-1 and EHV-4 may occur. Infections with EHV-4 appear to be restricted to the respiratory tract and viraemia is uncommon. In contrast, local replication of EHV-1 may be followed by a cell-associated viraemia which can result in abortion or neurological disease. The virus can spread directly from infected leukocytes to contiguous cells, thus avoiding neutralization by circulating antibody. Equine herpesvirus 1 has a predilection for vascular endothelium. Vasculitis and thrombosis in the placenta along with transplacental infection of the foetus result in abortion. Vasculitis and thrombosis, associated with EHV-1 infection, may be present in the CNS especially in the spinal cord. Neurological changes appear to be related to infection with particular strains of EHV-1.

Clinical signs

Respiratory disease caused by EHV-4 occurs in foals over two months of age, in weanlings and in yearlings. Following an incubation period of two to ten days, there are signs of fever, pharyngitis and serous nasal discharge. Secondary bacterial infection is common, giving rise to mucopurulent nasal discharge, coughing and, in some cases, bronchopneumonia. In the absence of serious secondary infection, recovery usually occurs within two weeks. Respiratory disease associated with EHV-1 is clinically indistinguishable from that caused by EHV-4. Outbreaks of disease caused by EHV-1 are less common. Immunity, following primary respiratory tract infection, lasts only a few months and is restricted to infection with antigenically similar viruses. Multiple infections result in significant cross-protection against the heterologous herpesvirus. Mares which abort following infection with EHV-1 rarely show premonitory signs. Abortion occurs several weeks or months after exposure, usually during the last four months of gestation. Such infected mares rarely abort during subsequent pregnancies and their fertility is unaffected. Infection close to term may result in the birth of an infected foal which usually dies due to interstitial pneumonia and viral damage in other tissues, sometimes complicated by secondary bacterial infection. Although neurological signs associated with EHV-1 infection are relatively uncommon, they may present in several horses during an outbreak of abortion or respiratory disease on a farm. The signs range from slight incoordination to paralysis, recumbency and death.

Diagnosis

- Virus isolation and identification are used routinely for the laboratory confirmation of herpesvirus infection in horses. Nasopharyngeal swabs should be collected during the early stages of respiratory infections and dispatched in suitable transport medium to the laboratory. Viral antigen may be demonstrated in cryostat sections of lung, liver and spleen from aborted foetuses using immunofluorescence.
- The characteristic gross and microscopic lesions, particularly intranuclear inclusions, may be sufficient for confirmation of herpesvirus abortion. Vasculitis is commonly found in the myeloencephalopathy caused by herpesvirus.
- The polymerase chain reaction has been adapted for the detection of viral DNA in clinical specimens.
- Demonstration of a fourfold rise in antibody titre in paired serum samples is useful for confirmation of a recent outbreak. Most serological tests do not distinguish infection with EHV-1 from infection with EHV-4 because of antigenic cross-reactivity. Recent ELISA-type assays employing monoclonal antibody or recombinant glycoprotein G antigens can discriminate between the two viruses.

Control

Effective management practices and vaccination are essential for control. Animals returning from sales, races or other events should be segregated for up to four weeks. On large stud farms, horses should be kept in small, physically-separated groups. It is essential that pregnant mares be segregated in a stress-free environment. Following an outbreak of disease, affected animals should be isolated. Premises should be disinfected and movement should be restricted until animals on the premises have been clear of the disease for at least one month.

Modified live and inactivated virus vaccines are commercially available. Vaccination with live vaccines is not permitted in some countries. Many vaccine preparations contain both EHV-1 and EHV-4. As vaccination is not considered to be fully protective, frequent boosters are recommended. Vaccination appears to reduce the severity of clinical signs and to decrease the likelihood of abortion.

Equine coital exanthema

This benign venereal disease of horses, caused by equine herpesvirus 3 (EHV-3), is thought to occur worldwide.

Epidemiology
Serological surveys indicate that the prevalence of infection in breeding animals is about 50%. The reported incidence of the disease is much lower, presumably because many infections are subclinical. The principal mode of transmission is venereal but transfer of EHV-3 may also occur through contaminated instruments.

Pathogenesis
Although latent infection with EHV-3 has not been conclusively demonstrated, it is thought that it probably occurs in sacral ganglia and that outbreaks of disease are initiated by reactivation of latent infection. The virus has a tropism for keratinized epithelium and is temperature sensitive with replication restricted at core body temperature. Viraemia and abortion are not associated with EHV-3 infection.

Clinical signs
The incubation period is up to ten days. Lesions on external genitalia appear initially as red papules which develop into vesicles and pustules. The pustules rupture leaving ulcers that may coalesce. Lesions are occasionally encountered on the teats, lips and nares. Secondary bacterial infection is common. In uncomplicated cases, lesions heal within two weeks. On pigmented skin, sites of healed lesions appear as white spots. Infection can affect the fertility of stallions as they may refuse to serve mares when penile lesions are severe.

Diagnosis
Clinical diagnosis is based on the distribution and appearance of the lesions. Electron microscopy of lesion scrapings or virus isolation in tissue culture at 33°C to 35°C can be used to confirm infection. Virus neutralization and ELISA are suitable assays for demonstrating a rising antibody titre in paired serum samples.

Control
Affected horses should be isolated and should not be used for breeding until lesions have completely healed. Disposable gloves should be used for genital examination and equipment should be thoroughly disinfected after use. An effective vaccine is not available.

Canine herpesvirus infection

Infection in domestic and wild *Canidae* caused by canine herpesvirus 1 (CHV-1) is common worldwide. Clinical disease caused by the virus, which is characterized by high mortality following generalized infection in neonatal pups, is uncommon.

Epidemiology
Prevalence rates, based on serological surveys of dogs are 88% in England and 42% in the Netherlands (Reading and Field, 1998; Rijsewijk *et al.*, 1999). Infection usually occurs by the oronasal route following direct contact between infected and susceptible animals. During periods of stress latent infections may be reactivated with shedding of virus. The sites of latency include sensory ganglia (Burr *et al.*, 1996; Miyoshi *et al.*, 1999). Virus is shed in oronasal and vaginal secretions. Newborn pups, which can acquire infection either during parturition or *in utero*, may transmit infection to littermates.

Pathogenesis
Following infection, CHV-1 replicates in the nasal mucosa, pharynx and tonsils. The virus replicates most effectively at temperatures below normal adult body temperature with the result that infection in adults is usually confined to the upper respiratory tract or to the external genitalia. Because the hypothalamic regulatory centre is not fully operational in pups under four weeks of age, they are particularly dependent on ambient temperature and maternal contact for maintenance of normal body temperature. A cell-associated viraemia and widespread viral replication in visceral organs can occur in infected neonatal animals with subnormal body temperatures.

Clinical signs
In adult dogs and pups over four weeks of age, infection is usually asymptomatic. Occasionally, vesicular lesions on external genitalia and mild vaginitis or balanoposthitis may be observed. Primary infection of pregnant bitches may result in abortion, stillbirths and infertility. Pups infected during parturition or shortly after birth develop clinical signs within days. Affected pups stop suckling, show signs of abdominal pain, whine incessantly and die within days. Morbidity and mortality rates in affected litters are high. Bitches whose pups are affected tend to produce healthy litters subsequently. Pups which receive colostral antibodies may become infected without developing clinical signs.

Diagnosis

Diagnostically significant postmortem findings include focal areas of necrosis and haemorrhage particularly, in the kidneys. Intranuclear inclusions are usually present. Virus isolation can be carried out in canine cell lines from fresh specimens of liver, kidney, lung and spleen.

Control

No commercial vaccine is available although administration of inactivated virus to pregnant bitches has been shown to be protective (Poulet et al., 2001). Affected bitches and their litters should be isolated to prevent infection of other whelping bitches. Heating lamps and pads, which raise the body temperature of pups to 39°C, may help to reduce the severity of infection if initiated prior to or at the time of exposure to the virus.

Feline viral rhinotracheitis

This acute upper respiratory tract infection of young cats is caused by feline herpesvirus 1 (FHV-1). The virus, which is distributed worldwide, accounts for about 40% of respiratory infections in cats. Both domestic and wild species of Felidae are susceptible.

Epidemiology

Close contact is required for transmission. The prevalence of infection is higher in cats in colonies than in cats reared individually. Virus is shed in oral and oculonasal secretions. Due to its relative lability, the virus survives for short periods in the environment. Most recovered cats are latently infected. Reactivation with virus replication and shedding is particularly associated with periods of stress such as parturition, lactation or change of housing. Several days elapse between exposure to stress and shedding of virus. The kittens of carrier queens may become infected subclinically while protected by maternally-derived antibody. These kittens may become carriers and, as adults, perpetuate the infection. In common with many herpesvirus infections in other species, the trigeminal ganglia are important sites of latency.

Pathogenesis

Initially, FHV-1 replicates in oronasal or conjunctival tissues before infecting the epithelium of the upper respiratory tract. Viraemia and generalized infection does not appear to occur except in animals at the extremes of age and in immunocompromized cats. Secondary bacterial infections, which commonly occur, exacerbate the clinical signs.

Clinical signs

The incubation period is usually short, about 2 days, but may be up to six days. Young cats display signs of acute upper respiratory tract infection including fever, sneezing, inappetence, hypersalivation, conjunctivitis and oculonasal discharge. Crusts form around the eyes, sometimes causing the eyelids to stick together. In more severe disease, pneumonia or ulcerative keratitis may be evident. The mortality rate is low except in young or immunosuppressed animals. Rarely, cats may present with facial and nasal dermatitis, which has been linked to reactivation of latent infection (Hargis and Ginn, 1999).

Diagnosis

Clinical differentiation of feline viral rhinotracheitis from feline calicivirus infection is difficult.

- Virus can be isolated in feline cell lines from oropharyngeal or conjunctival swabs.
- Specific viral antigen can be demonstrated in acetone-fixed nasal and conjunctival smears using immunofluorescence.
- The virus neutralization test on paired serum samples can be used to demonstrate a rising titre for confirmation of diagnosis.

Treatment and control

Treatment is non-specific and supportive. Antibiotics are used to control secondary bacterial infections. The protection provided by vaccination is incomplete as vaccinated cats can become infected but clinical signs tend to be much reduced. Inactivated vaccines are suitable for use in pregnant queens and help to boost levels of maternal antibody available for kittens. Intranasal vaccines may give rise to mild upper respiratory signs. When cats are at low risk of exposure to infection, booster vaccinations at three year intervals may be sufficient (Elston et al., 1998; Scott and Geissinger, 1999). Commercial vaccine preparations also contain feline calicivirus. Recent developments in vaccine production include the use of avirulent deletion mutant virus strains and, in addition, the insertion of the feline calicivirus capsid gene into the modified FHV-1 genome (Gaskell and Willoughby, 1999). Good husbandry practices and disease control procedures should be implemented in catteries in conjunction with regular vaccination schedules to minimize the impact of clinical disease.

Infectious laryngotracheitis

This highly contagious respiratory disease of chickens and sometimes pheasants is caused by gallid herpesvirus 1 (GaHV-1). Infectious laryngotracheitis (ILT) occurs in many countries. Although strains of GaHV-1 vary in virulence, they are antigenically homogeneous. In areas of intensive poultry production, the disease is usually well-controlled by a combination of vaccination and biosecurity. However, the virus tends to persist in small enterprises and specialized chicken flocks as an endemic infection.

Epidemiology

Infection is acquired through aerosols, especially in intensively reared birds. Latency occurs in the trigeminal ganglia and carrier birds may shed virus intermittently after periods of stress such as the onset of laying or when groups of birds are mixed. Indirect transmission from one production unit to another may occur through contaminated fomites.

Pathogenesis

Following inhalation, virus replicates locally in the upper respiratory tract. Spread along sensory nerves results in localization in the trigeminal ganglia.

Clinical signs

The incubation period is up to 12 days. The epidemic form of the disease, caused by virulent strains of GaHV-1, is characterized by coughing, gasping, moist rales, oculonasal discharge, expectoration of bloodstained mucus and head shaking. Mortality may reach 70%. Death is often due to severe obstructive haemorrhagic laryngotracheitis. Mild respiratory signs, conjunctivitis and decreased egg production are features of infection with strains of low virulence.

Diagnosis

In severe outbreaks of ILT, the clinical signs and postmortem findings may be sufficiently characteristic for diagnosis. In outbreaks of the mild form of the disease, laboratory confirmation is necessary. Virus isolation can be carried out on the chorioallantoic membrane of embryonated eggs or in avian cell cultures. Rapid methods of diagnosis include demonstration of herpesvirus particles in tracheal samples by electron microscopy and detection of viral antigen in smears or frozen sections by immunofluorescence. Viral antigen can be detected in tracheal samples by ELISA or AGID. Antibodies to GaHV-1 can be demonstrated by virus neutralization, ELISA or AGID.

Control

Flock management systems and vaccination protocols form the basis of control methods. In broiler flocks, short production cycles and all-in all-out management systems ensure that they remain free of the disease. In layer flocks, vaccination is usually carried out using live vaccines administered by aerosols or in drinking water. Vaccination protects against clinical disease but is ineffective against infection by field virus and the establishment of latency. Genetically engineered vaccines are currently being evaluated.

Marek's disease

This contagious lymphoproliferative disease of chickens is caused by gallid herpesvirus 2 (Marek's disease virus), which is cell-associated and oncogenic. The disease, which is of major economic significance in the poultry industry, occurs worldwide. Herpesviruses of chickens and turkeys in the genus Marek's disease-like viruses can be divided into three serotypes or species. Serotype 1 (Gallid herpesvirus 2) includes all pathogenic strains and the attenuated variants derived from these strains; serotype 2 (Gallid herpesvirus 3) contains avirulent and non-oncogenic strains; the third serotype, meleagrid herpesvirus 1, is an avirulent herpesvirus of turkeys. Serotype 1 strains can be categorized as mildly virulent, virulent and highly virulent.

Epidemiology

Productive replication with release of infective virus occurs only in the epithelium of the feather follicle. Cell-free virus is released from the follicles along with desquamated cells. This dander can remain infective for several months in dust and litter in poultry houses. Infected birds remain carriers for life and their chicks, which are protected initially by maternally-derived antibody, acquire infection within a few weeks, usually by the respiratory route. In addition to the virulence of the infecting strain of herpesvirus, host factors which contribute to the severity of the disease include the sex, age at the time of infection and genotype. Two relevant genetic loci have been identified. One, associated with the major histocompatibility complex allele, influences the immune response to Marek's disease, and the other influences the susceptibility of T lymphocytes to transformation. Female birds are more susceptible to the disease than male birds; the reason for this difference is unknown. Resistance to the development of disease increases with age. Transportation, vaccination, handling and beak trimming are stress factors which increase susceptibility to disease.

Pathogenesis and pathology

Following inhalation, virus replicates locally before transfer, probably within macrophages, to the major lymphoid organs where it causes cytolysis, primarily of B cells. Latent infection occurs in T cells activated by the cytolytic process involving B cells. A persistent cell-associated viraemia results in dissemination of the virus throughout the body. Infection of epithelial cells in feather follicles occurs about two weeks after infection. Cytolysis of these epithelial cells results in shedding of virus particles into the environment. Genetically susceptible chickens are prone to tumour development and immunosuppression, associated with apoptosis of T cells and thymocytes along with downregulation of CD8 molecule expression. Lymphomatous lesions may become evident in these birds from two weeks to several months after infection. Transformation of T cells probably relates to oncogenes in certain serotype 1 strains. Multiple copies of the virus genome are found in transformed cells, both as episomal DNA and as a form integrated into host cell

DNA. Several genomic regions with potential roles in transformation have been identified (Venugopal, 2001) including *meq* (which resembles the *Jun/Fos* family of oncogenic transcription factor proteins), a basic-leucine zipper gene (Calnek, 1998). Defective immune surveillance mechanisms can allow transformed cells to form lymphoid tumours. The peripheral nerves are often affected, exhibiting proliferative (type A), inflammatory (type B) or minor infiltrative (type C) changes. Demyelination, which is found in type A and type B lesions, causes paralysis. The acute form of Marek's disease is characterized by diffuse infiltration of many internal organs with neoplastic lymphoid cells. A surface antigen, expressed on transformed lymphocytes, formerly called Marek's disease tumour-associated antigen (MATSA) is now considered to be merely a marker for activated T cells.

Clinical signs

Birds between 12 and 24 weeks of age are most commonly affected. Clinically, Marek's disease presents as partial or complete paralysis of the legs and wings. The mortality rate rarely exceeds 15% with deaths occurring over a number of weeks or months. In the acute form of the disease, birds are severely depressed before death or may die without clinical evidence of disease. The mortality rate in the acute form of the disease is usually between 10% and 30%; outbreaks with mortality as high as 70% have been reported.

Diagnosis

The diagnosis of Marek's disease is based on clinical signs and pathological findings.

- Paralysis of legs and wings in conjunction with thickening of the peripheral nerves is typical of Marek's disease.
- Nerve involvement is not always evident in adult birds. In these circumstances, differentiation from lymphoid leukosis is particularly important.
- Differentiation from lymphoid leukosis is based on the age of affected birds, the incidence of clinical cases and the histopathological findings.
- Virus can be isolated from the buffy coat of blood samples from infected birds. Chicken kidney cells or duck embryo fibroblasts can be used for isolation of the virus.
- Viral antigen can be detected in preparations of skin or feather tips, using a radial precipitin test.
- Serum antibodies to GaHV-2 may be demonstrated using AGID, ELISA, immunofluorescence or virus neutralization.
- Primers, which can distinguish attenuated and wild-type strains, have been developed for PCR assays.
- In the absence of characteristic clinical signs, infection with gallid herpesvirus 2 is not indicative of Marek's disease in a flock.

Control

The use of appropriate management strategies, genetically resistant stock and vaccination have reduced losses from Marek's disease. Disinfection, all-in all-out policies, and rearing young chicks away from older birds for the first two or three months of life reduce exposure to infection, decreasing the likelihood of serious disease. A range of modified live vaccines containing the three avian herpesvirus serotypes are commercially available. Although a single dose of virus injected into day-old chicks provides good lifelong protection, it does not prevent superinfection with virulent field viruses. A synergistic protective effect is obtained by using two or three strains in a vaccine. Consequently meleagrid herpesvirus 1 is commonly incorporated into bivalent or trivalent vaccines. Novel vaccines, based on recombinant DNA technology are being developed because of a reduction in the efficacy of conventional vaccines due to emergence of virulent mutants (Witter, 1998). Relatively recently the introduction of automated *in ovo* vaccination at the eighteenth day of incubation has replaced conventional vaccination methods in large commercial units (Ricks *et al.*, 1999).

References

Burr P.D., Campbell, M.E.M., Nicolson, L. and Onions, D.E. (1996). Detection of canine herpesvirus 1 in a wide range of tissues using the polymerase chain reaction. *Veterinary Microbiology*, **53**, 227–237.

Calnek, B.W. (1998). Lymphomagenesis in Marek's disease. *Avian Pathology*, **27**, S54–S64.

Elston, T., Rodan, I., Flemming, D., Ford, R.B. *et al.* (1998). Feline vaccine guidelines: from the Advisory Panel on Feline Vaccines. *Feline Practice*, **26**, 14–16.

Gaskell, R. and Willoughby, K. (1999). Herpesviruses of carnivores. *Veterinary Microbiology*, **69**, 73–88.

Gilkerson, J.R., Whalley, J.M., Drummer, H.E. *et al.* (1999a). Epidemiological studies of equine herpesvirus 1 (EHV-1) in thoroughbred foals: a review of studies conducted in the Hunter Valley of New South Wales between 1995 and 1997. *Veterinary Microbiology*, **68**, 15–25.

Gilkerson, J.R., Whalley, J.M., Drummer, H.E. *et al.* (1999b). Epidemiology of EHV-1 and EHV-4 in the mare and foal populations on a Hunter Valley study farm: are mares the source of EHV-1 for unweaned foals. *Veterinary Microbiology*, **68**, 27–34.

Hargis, A.M. and Ginn, P.E. (1999). Feline herpesvirus 1-associated facial and nasal dermatitis and stomatitis in domestic cats. *Veterinary Clinics of North America: Small Animal Practice*, **29**, 1281–1290.

Li, H., Shen, D.T., Knowles, D.P. *et al.* (1994). Competitive inhibition enzyme-linked immunosorbent assay for antibody in sheep and other ruminants to a conserved epitope of malignant catarrhal fever virus. *Journal of Clinical Microbiology*, **32**, 1674–1679.

Li, H., Snowder, G., O'Toole, D. and Crawford, T.B. (1998). Transmission of ovine herpesvirus 2 in lambs. *Journal of Clinical Microbiology*, **36**, 223–226.

Maes, R.K., Sussman, M.B., Vilnis, A. and Thacker, B.J. (1997). Recent developments in latency and recombination of Aujeszky's disease (pseudorabies) virus. *Veterinary Microbiology*, **55**, 13–27.

Miyoshi, M., Ishii, Y., Takiguchi, M. *et al.* (1999). Detection of canine herpesvirus DNA in the ganglionic neurons and the lymph node lymphocytes of latently infected dogs. *Journal of Veterinary Medical Science*, **61**, 375–379.

Muller-Doblies, U.U., Li, H., Hauser, B. *et al.* (1998). Field validation of laboratory tests for clinical diagnosis of sheep-associated malignant catarrhal fever. *Journal of Clinical Microbiology*, **36**, 2970–2972.

O'Toole, D., Li, H., Miller, D. *et al.* (1997). Chronic and recovered cases of sheep-associated malignant catarrhal fever in cattle. *Veterinary Record*, **140**, 519–524.

Poulet, H., Guigal, P.M., Soulier, M. *et al.* (2001). Protection of puppies against canine herpesvirus by vaccination of the dams. *Veterinary Record*, **148**, 691–695.

Reading, M.J. and Field H.J. (1998). A serological survey of canine herpesvirus 1 infection in the English dog population. *Archives of Virology*, **143**, 1377–1488.

Ricks, C.A., Avakian, A., Bryan, T. *et al.* (1999). *In ovo* vaccination technology. In *Advances in Veterinary Medicine*. Volume **41**. Ed. R.D. Schultz. pp. 495–515.

Rijsewijk, F.A.M., Luiten, E.J., Daus, F.J. *et al.* (1999). Prevalence of antibodies against canine herpesvirus 1 in dogs in The Netherlands in 1997–1998. *Veterinary Microbiology*, **65**, 1–7.

Scott, F.W. and Geissinger, C.M. (1999). Long-term immunity in cats vaccinated with an inactivated trivalent vaccine. *American Journal of Veterinary Research*, **60**, 652–658.

van Oirschot, J.T., Kaashoek, M.J. and Rijsewijk, F.A.M. (1996). Advances in the development and evaluation of bovine herpesvirus 1 vaccines. *Veterinary Microbiology*, **53**, 43–54.

Venugopal, K. (2001). Marek's disease: an update on oncogenic mechanism and control. *Research in Veterinary Science*, **69**, 17–23.

Witter, R.L. (1998). Control strategies for Marek's disease: a perspective for the future. *Poultry Science*, **77**, 1197–1203.

Chapter 55

Papillomaviridae

Viruses in the family *Papillomaviridae* are non-enveloped with icosahedral capsids which contain a single molecule of circular double-stranded DNA. The family contains a single genus, *Papillomavirus*. Papillomaviruses are 55 nm in diameter (Fig. 55.1). Replication takes place in the nucleus and release of new virions occurs by lysis of the infected cell. Members of the genus are resistant to lipid solvents, acid, and heating at 60°C for 30 minutes. Infections are often persistent and usually established early in life.

Formerly papillomaviruses were grouped with polyomaviruses in the family *Papovaviridae*. The name *Papovaviridae* is derived from the first letters of the names of important members of the family: **pa**pillomaviruses, **po**lyomaviruses and **va**cuolating agent (originally designated simian virus 40). Infections with polyomaviruses are of minor veterinary significance. Although they produce no clinical effects in natural hosts, most polyomaviruses (*polyoma*, many tumours) are oncogenic when inoculated into newborn rodents. Budgerigar fledgling

---

Key points

- Non-enveloped, double-stranded DNA viruses
- Icosahedral symmetry
- Contains one genus, *Papillomavirus:*
  —Have not been cultured *in vitro*
  —Cause papillomas and fibropapillomas in domestic animals
  —Malignant transformation of alimentary and urinary tract papillomas may occur in cattle ingesting bracken fern
  —Bovine papillomas type 1 and 2 are aetiologically involved in equine sarcoids

---

disease, caused by an avian polyomavirus, is characterized by outbreaks of acute generalized infection with high mortality in young budgerigars.

Clinical infections

The epitheliotropic, host-specific papillomaviruses (Latin *papilloma*, nipple) cause proliferative lesions (warts) in many mammalian and avian species. Although they have not been grown in cell culture, the DNA sequences of several papillomaviruses have been elucidated, allowing specific detection in lesions. In infected cells, the viral DNA is usually episomal. Papillomaviruses are used experimentally for inserting foreign DNA into cultured cells.

The clinical conditions associated with papillomavirus infections in domestic animals are presented in Table 55.1. Each papillomavirus tends to be host-specific and to produce proliferative lesions in specific anatomical sites. Although infections with papillomaviruses occur in many animal species, only those which affect cattle, horses and dogs are of clinical significance. Lesions are most commonly observed in young animals and usually regress spontaneously after weeks or months. Regression is attributed to the development of cell-mediated immunity. Typical papillomas are composed of finger-like projections of proliferating epithelium supported by a thin core of

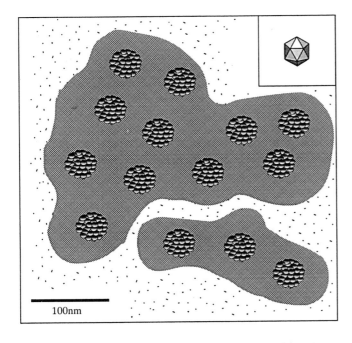

Figure 55.1 Papillomavirus particles as they appear in an electron micrograph and a diagrammatic representation (inset).

mature fibrous tissue. In fibropapillomas, the fibrous tissue component predominates. In some host species, several types of papillomaviruses can cause neoplastic change. More than 80 types have been identified in humans, while in cattle six types are recognized. Individual types of virus share less than 50% sequence homology and exhibit differences in reciprocal serological assays. The six types of bovine papillomavirus (BPV), types 1, 2 and 5 (group A) and types 3, 4 and 6 (group B), are categorized on the basis of size of genome and the type and location of associated lesions. Progression of papillomas to malignant tumours has been documented in humans, cattle and rabbits.

Pathogenesis

Papillomaviruses usually infect the basal cells of squamous epithelium as a result of minute abrasions. They may also gain entry at vulnerable sites such as junctions between different types of epithelia. Infected cells proliferate and differentiation is delayed. Viral gene expression is restricted during this proliferative phase. Full gene expression results in the production of viral capsids only after cellular differentiation begins in the upper layers of the epithelium. New virions can be visualized by electron microscopy in the nuclei of differentiated keratinized cells. The release of virus occurs during desquamation of infected cells from the surface of lesions.

Diagnosis

- The clinical appearance of papillomas (warts) is distinctive. Laboratory confirmation is not usually required for papillomatous lesions.
- Histopathological examination may be required to determine the nature of some lesions, especially equine sarcoids.
- Electron microscopic examination of specimens from the epidermis may reveal characteristic virus particles.
- Hybridization assays and PCR methods are available for the detection of papillomavirus DNA, but are not used routinely. Isolates can be typed by extraction of DNA and restriction endonuclease analysis or by Southern blotting.

Bovine cutaneous papillomatosis

Bovine cutaneous papillomatosis is caused by several types of bovine papillomavirus. Cutaneous fibro-papillomas are generally associated with BPV types 1, 2 or 5, whereas BPV types 3 or 6 are commonly linked to papillomas in which the fibrous tissue component is minimal. The different gross appearances of the two types of proliferative response are exemplified by lesions produced by types of papillomavirus on teats of cows. Teat fibropapillomas, associated with BPV-5 infection,

Table 55.1 Papillomaviruses of domestic animals and associated clinical conditions.

Virus	Clinical conditions
Bovine papillomavirus	
Types 1 and 2	Fibropapillomas in young cattle; occur mainly on the head and neck and occasionally on the penis. Implicated in the pathogenesis of equine sarcoids. Type 2 is implicated in bladder neoplasia and enzootic haematuria
Type 3	Cutaneous papillomas with a tendency to persist
Type 4	Papillomas in the alimentary tract; malignant transformation may result from ingestion of bracken fern
Type 5	Fibropapillomas on the teats ('rice grain' type)
Type 6	Papillomas on the teats ('frond' type)
Equine papillomavirus	Papillomas in young horses; occur mainly around lips and on nose
Canine oral papillomavirus	Irregularly-shaped papillomas in the oral cavity of young dogs
Ovine papillomavirus	Papillomas and fibropapillomas (rare)

have smooth surfaces and are described as 'rice grain' type. In contrast, 'frond' type teat papillomas arise from infection with BPV-6. The localization of the proliferative lesions caused by these two bovine papillomaviruses on the teats demonstrates the predilection of viruses in this group for particular anatomical sites.

Fibropapillomas arising from infection with BPV types 1 or 2 are often found on the head and neck of cattle under two years of age. Spontaneous regression of the lesions generally occurs within 1 year. Cutaneous papillomas caused by BPV-3 tend to persist. Because infection with BPV is usually self-limiting, treatment is seldom required. Surgical removal of large lesions on teats may be necessary because of interference with milking. Although inactivated autogenous vaccines are used therapeutically, their efficacy is unproven. Inactivated vaccines can be used prophylactically.

Bovine alimentary papilloma-carcinoma complex

Papillomas of the oesophagus, rumen and reticulum are associated with BPV-4 infection. The lesions, which are often solitary and relatively small, are found incidentally at postmortem examination. Epidemiological and experimental studies have demonstrated that there is an increased frequency in the occurrence of malignant transformation of virus-induced alimentary papillomas to squamous cell carcinomas when animals are ingesting bracken fern (Jarrett *et al.*, 1978; Campo *et al.*, 1994). Such malignant lesions, which are found in anatomical sites identical to those of the papillomas, may cause difficulty in swallowing, ruminal tympany and loss of condition. Nodular fibropapillomas caused by BPV-2, which are occasionally found in similar upper alimentary tract locations, do not appear to become malignant.

Enzootic haematuria

Enzootic haematuria is encountered worldwide in cattle on poor pastures with abundant bracken fern growth. The haemorrhage originates from tumours in the bladder wall. Individual neoplastic lesions derive from either epithelial or mesenchymal tissues. Experimental studies suggest that BPV-2 and toxic compounds from bracken contribute to oncogenesis (Campo *et al.*, 1992). It is probable that immunosuppression following ingestion of bracken may allow activation of latent BPV-2 in bladder tissues and this effect, together with the action of carcinogens also present in bracken, is responsible for the induction and progression of neoplastic lesions.

Equine papillomatosis

Papillomas are commonly encountered in horses between 1 and 3 years of age. Two types of equine papillomavirus have been identified based on DNA studies. Type 1 is associated with papillomas on the muzzle and legs while type 2 is associated with papillomas of the genital tract. Spread may occur by direct or indirect contact. The lesions usually regress spontaneously after several months and recovered animals are immune to reinfection.

Equine sarcoid

The equine sarcoid, a locally invasive fibroblastic skin tumour, is the most common neoplasm of horses, donkeys and mules (Marti *et al.*, 1993). Bovine papillomavirus types 1 and 2 or closely related viruses are implicated in sarcoid development. Experimental inoculation with these viruses results in fibromatous lesions which resemble sarcoids but which regress spontaneously. Viral DNA with a high degree of homology to BPV has been identified in tissue from sarcoids using both *in situ* hybridization (Lory *et al.*, 1993) and PCR (Otten *et al.*, 1993).

Lesions usually develop in horses between three and six years of age. Multiple cases can occur in families or groups of horses in close proximity. However, the incidence of equine sarcoid (estimated at 0.5 to 2%) is comparatively low for a viral disease. This may indicate that the horse is a non-permissive host (Marti *et al.*, 1993).

Sarcoids can occur on any part of the body, either singly or in clusters. The most commonly affected sites are the head, ventral abdomen and limbs. They are highly variable in appearance but can be arbitrarily categorized as verrucous or fibroblastic. Clinical diagnosis should be confirmed histologically. Surgical removal is the usual form of treatment. Recurrence is common following conventional surgery and cryosurgery is more successful. Radiation therapy, CO_2 laser surgery and chemotherapy have also been used with varying degrees of success (Knottenbelt *et al.*, 1995). Immunotherapy, aimed at stimulating cell-mediated immunity, may be effective in some cases. This involves intralesional injection of BCG or cell wall extract of *Mycobacterium bovis* into horses previously sensitized to tuberculoprotein.

Canine oral papillomatosis

Multiple transmissible papillomas in the oropharyngeal region of dogs are often encountered. The disease, which is caused by canine oral papillomavirus, is common in young dogs and is readily transmitted. While the aetiology of this oral condition is well established, the cause of papillomas occurring at other sites in the dog is uncertain (Narama *et al.*, 1992).

Canine oral papillomavirus is transmitted by direct and indirect contact. The incubation period is up to 8 weeks. Lesions are usually multiple and although generally confined to the oral mucosa, are sometimes found on the conjunctiva, eyelids and muzzle. The papillomas initially appear as smooth, white, raised lesions but later they become rough and cauliflower-like. Spread may occur inside the oral cavity. There is spontaneous regression within months. Surgical removal is generally unnecessary unless the papillomas persist or cause physical discomfort. Inactivated vaccines have been used but do not appear to be effective. Live, unattenuated vaccines, which are effective, may produce neoplastic lesions at the injection site (Bregman *et al.*, 1987).

References

Bregman, C.L., Hirth, R.S., Sundberg, J.P. and Christensen, E.F. (1987). Cutaneous neoplasms in dogs associated with canine oral papillomavirus vaccine. *Veterinary Pathology*, **24**, 477–487.

Campo, M.S., Jarrett, W.F.H., Farron, R., O'Neill, B.W. and Smith, K.T. (1992). Association of bovine papillomavirus type 2 and bracken fern with bladder cancer in cattle. *Cancer Research*, **52**, 6898–6904.

Campo, M.S., O'Neill, B.W., Barron, R.J. and Jarrett, W.F.H. (1994). Experimental reproduction of the papilloma-carcinoma complex of the alimentary canal in cattle. *Carcinogenesis*, **15**, 1597–1601.

Jarrett, W.F.H., McNeill, P.E., Grimshaw, W.T.R., *et al.* (1978). High incidence area of cattle cancer with a possible interaction between an environmental carcinogen and a papilloma virus. *Nature*, **274**, 215–217.

Knottenbelt, D., Edwards, S. and Daniel, E. (1995). Diagnosis and treatment of the equine sarcoid. *In Practice*, **17**, 123–129.

Lory, S., von Tscharner, C., Marti, E. *et al.* (1993). *In situ* hybridization of equine sarcoids with bovine papilloma virus. *Veterinary Record*, **132**, 132–133.

Marti, E., Lazary, S., Antczak, D.F. and Gerber, H. (1993). Report of the first international workshop on equine sarcoid.

Equine Veterinary Journal, **25**, 397–407.

Narama, I., Ozaki, K., Maeda, H. and Ohta, A. (1992). Cutaneous papilloma with viral replication in an old dog. *Journal of Veterinary Medical Science*, **54**, 387–389.

Otten, N., von Tscharner, C., Lazary, S. *et al.* (1993). DNA of bovine papillomavirus Type 1 and 2 in equine sarcoids: PCR detection and direct sequencing. *Archives of Virology*, **132**, 121-131.

Chapter 56

Adenoviridae

Adenoviruses (Greek *adenos*, gland), first isolated from explant cultures of human adenoids, are icosahedral (70 to 90 nm in diameter) and contain a single linear molecule of double-stranded DNA. Fibres project from each of the twelve vertices of the capsid (Fig. 56.1). Agglutination of rat or monkey erythrocytes, a property of many adenoviruses, is dependent on the fibre proteins which possess type-specific immunodeterminants. The family *Adenoviridae* is composed of two genera, *Mastadenovirus* and *Aviadenovirus*, and a group of unassigned viruses. Mammalian adenoviruses, assigned to the genus *Mastadenovirus*, infect mammals only, share a common antigen and are serologically distinct from those that infect birds. Serogroups and serotypes are defined on the basis of neutralization assays. Haemagglutination inhibition is used to confirm serospecificity. Adenoviruses are moderately stable in the environment in which they can survive for many weeks. They can withstand freezing, mild acid and lipid solvents. Infectivity is abolished by heating at 56°C for more than 10 minutes.

> **Key points**
> - Non-enveloped, double-stranded DNA viruses,
> - Icosahedral symmetry
> - Replicate in nuclei, forming intranuclear inclusion bodies
> - Moderately stable in the environment
> - Two genera:
>   —*Aviadenovirus*, avian adenoviruses
>   —*Mastadenovirus*, mammalian adenoviruses
> - Systemic and respiratory diseases in dogs
> - Systemic diseases in poultry

Adenoviruses replicate in cell nuclei. Newly assembled virions form crystalline aggregates, demonstrable as intranuclear basophilic inclusions in stained tissue sections. Adenoviruses have a natural host range generally confined to a single species or to closely related species. Infection is common in animals and man. Fifty one human serotypes have been recognized, grouped into six species (human adenovirus A to F). Most human infections appear to be subclinical or mild although immunodeficient individuals may develop severe clinical disease. In contrast to human infections, certain animal infections result in severe illness. Genera and species belonging to the *Adenoviridae* are listed in Fig. 56.2 (adapted from van Regenmortel *et al.*, 2000). Adenoviruses of veterinary importance are presented in Table 56.1.

Clinical infections

Adenovirus infections can be particularly severe in dogs and domestic fowl. Two serotypes of canine adenovirus are recognised. Infection with canine adenovirus type 1 (CAV-1) causes infectious canine hepatitis, a severe generalized disease, whereas infection with canine adenovirus type 2 (CAV-2) is commonly linked to localized respiratory disease. In other domestic mammals, adenovirus infections are associated occasionally with enteric or respiratory problems. Pulmonary infection with equine adenovirus A is invariably fatal in Arabian foals with combined immunodeficiency disease.

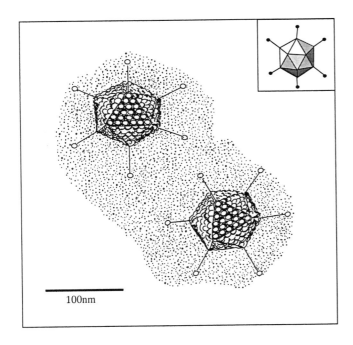

100nm

Figure 56.1 Adenovirus particles as they appear in an electron micrograph and a diagrammatic representation (inset).

weeks and at 12 to 14 weeks of age. Booster injections, either annually or at intervals of two years, are recommended. Inactivated CAV-1 vaccines, which do not induce obvious side effects, require boosters at more frequent intervals in order to maintain adequate antibody levels.

Infection with canine adenovirus type 2

Canine adenovirus type 2, which is readily transmitted by aerosols, replicates in both upper and lower respiratory tract. Clinical signs are generally mild or inapparent. Affected dogs may present with clinical signs similar to those of canine infectious tracheobronchitis (kennel cough). Most dogs recover and are immune to subsequent challenge. Occasional cases of bronchopneumonia may develop due to secondary bacterial infection. Virus shedding continues for about 9 days after infection.

Inclusion body hepatitis

Although inclusion body hepatitis (IBH) mainly affects broilers, it sometimes occurs in pullets. There is uncertainty about the cause of IBH and a number of fowl adenovirus serotypes have been aetiologically implicated. In affected flocks, a sudden increase in mortality is a feature of the disease and it may reach 30% if there is immunosuppression due to infectious bursal disease or chicken anaemia virus infection. Lesions include an enlarged liver with scattered haemorrhages and necrosis, intramuscular haemorrhage and anaemia. Intranuclear inclusions in hepatocytes are prominent. Diagnosis is based on characteristic hepatic lesions. Because apparently healthy birds excrete adenoviruses and may be serologically positive, the significance of positive serological tests is questionable. As vaccines are not readily available and the aetiology of IBH is uncertain, specific control measures cannot be recommended.

Egg drop syndrome

Egg drop syndrome caused by an adenovirus prevalent in ducks and probably introduced into chickens through a contaminated vaccine, was first described in 1976. In flocks the disease is characterized by a drop in egg production or by failure to reach peak production. Infected hens may lay abnormal eggs. Laying hens up to 36 weeks of age are those most commonly affected. Inflammatory lesions are found in the oviduct, particularly the pouch shell gland. Intranuclear inclusions may be present in the epithelial cells of this gland. Samples of oviduct, including material from the pouch shell gland, are suitable specimens for virus isolation in avian cell lines, especially duck kidney or fibroblast cell lines. As the virus agglutinates avian red cells, haemagglutination inhibition is the preferred method for serological screening of flocks. Control of egg drop syndrome relies on the use of inactivated vaccines before laying begins. Appropriate hygiene combined with disinfection can be used to limit the spread of infection. Because of the high risk of cross-infection, chickens and ducks should be housed separately.

References

Kiss, I., Matiz, K., Bajmoci, E., Rusvai, M. and Harrach, B. (1996). Infectious canine hepatitis: detection of canine adenovirus type 1 by polymerase chain reaction. *Acta Veterinaria Hungarica*, **44**, 253–258.

Morrison, M.D, Onions, D.E. and Nicolson, L. (1997). Complete DNA sequence of canine adenovirus type 1. *Journal of General Virology*, **78**, 873–878.

van Regenmortel, M.H.V., Fauquet, C.M., Bishop, D.H.L., *et al.*, (2000). *Virus Taxonony, Seventh Report of the International Committee on Taxonomy of Viruses*. Academic Press, San Diego.

Further reading

McCracken, R.M. and Adair, B.M. (1993). Avian adenoviruses. In *Virus Infections of Birds*. Eds. J.B. McFerran and M.S. McNulty. Elsevier Science Publishers, Amsterdam. pp. 121–144.

Chapter 57

Poxviridae

The family *Poxviridae* contains the largest viruses which cause disease in domestic animals. Poxvirus symmetry is complex. The virions in this family are either brick-shaped (220 to 450 nm x 140 to 260 nm) with a surface membrane composed of tubular or globular proteins or ovoid (250 to 300 nm x 160 to 190 nm) with a surface membrane composed of a regular spiral filament (Figs. 57.1 and 57.2). They contain more than 100 proteins including several virus-encoded enzymes. A biconcave core or nucleoid contains linear double-stranded DNA and one or two lateral bodies within a surface membrane (Fig. 57.3). A cell-derived envelope encloses some of the mature extracellular virions.

The family is divided into two subfamilies, *Chordopoxvirinae*, the poxviruses of vertebrates, and *Entomopoxvirinae*, the poxviruses of insects (Fig. 57.4). The subfamily *Chordopoxvirinae* is comprised of eight genera, namely *Orthopoxvirus, Parapoxvirus, Avipoxvirus, Capripoxvirus, Leporipoxvirus, Suipoxvirus, Molluscipoxvirus* and *Yatapoxvirus*. Genetic recombination within genera results in extensive serological

> **Key points**
> - Enveloped DNA viruses
> - Complex symmetry
> - Replicate in cytoplasm
> - Stable in the environment
> - Skin lesions a prominent feature
> - Individual poxviruses tend to infect particular host species; some poxviruses are not species-specific

cross-reactions and cross-protection. Replication in the cytoplasm of host cells takes place within defined areas (viral factories). Virus envelopes, derived from host cell membranes, contain host cell lipids and virus-encoded proteins such as the haemagglutinin protein of the orthopoxviruses. Both enveloped and non-enveloped forms of the virus are infectious. Virions are stable at room temperature under dry conditions but sensitive to heat, detergents, formaldehyde and oxidizing agents. The genera differ in ether sensitivity.

Infections with poxviruses, which can affect many vertebrate and invertebrate hosts, usually result in vesicular skin lesions (Table 57.1). Smallpox, caused by variola virus, was formerly a human disease of major international significance. The use of vaccinia virus for the prevention of smallpox, first introduced by Jenner in the late 18th century, eventually led to the eradication of this highly contagious disease at the close of the twentieth century.

Clinical infections

Transmission of poxviruses can occur by aerosols, by direct contact, by mechanical transmission through arthropods and through fomites. Skin lesions are the principal feature of these infections. Several virus-encoded proteins are released from infected cells including a homologue of epidermal growth factor which stimulates cell proliferation. Typically, pox lesions begin as macules and progress through papules, vesicles and pustules to scabs which detach leaving a scar. In generalized infections there is a cell-associated viraemia and recovered

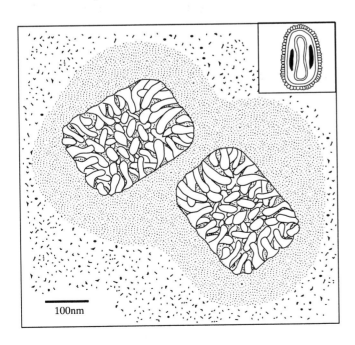

Figure 57.1 Orthopoxvirus particles as they appear in an electron micrograph and a diagrammatic representation (inset).

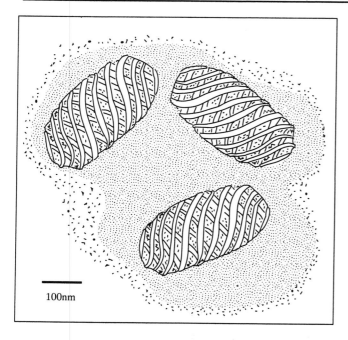

Figure 57.2 Parapoxvirus particles as they appear in an electron micrograph.

animals have solid immunity. Some localized pox infections may induce transient immunity and reinfection can occur.

Three closely related parapoxviruses, namely pseudo-cowpox virus, bovine papular stomatitis virus and orf virus, infect ruminants. These viruses are transmissible to humans producing lesions which are clinically similar. Moreover, the three viruses are morphologically indistinguishable and identification of the causal agent relies on nucleic acid analysis.

Capripoxviruses are economically important viruses producing generalized infections with significant mortality in domestic ruminants. Sheeppox virus, goatpox virus and lumpy skin disease virus are closely related and share a group-specific structural protein (p32), which allows the same vaccine to be used against each virus.

Many avian species are susceptible to infection with members of the genus *Avipoxvirus*. Although antigenic relationships exist among avian poxviruses, this relatedness is variable. Virus species within the genus, named in accordance with their affinity for particular host species, include fowlpox virus, canarypox virus, pigeonpox virus and turkeypox virus. The type species of the genus is fowlpox virus.

Infections caused by vaccinia virus

Although the natural host species of vaccinia virus is unknown, mild infections have been described in a wide range of species including sheep, cattle, horses and humans. Formerly, the virus was used to vaccinate against smallpox. Buffalopox virus and rabbitpox virus are considered to be subspecies of vaccinia virus. Spread of vaccinia virus among cattle and transmission to humans occurs at milking. The lesions on the teats of cows resemble those caused by cowpox virus. A clinical condition similar to horsepox or equine papular dermatitis can be produced experimentally using vaccinia virus (Studdert, 1989). In recent years, vaccinia virus has been used as a recombinant virus vector for vaccination against several diseases including rabies, canine distemper and measles.

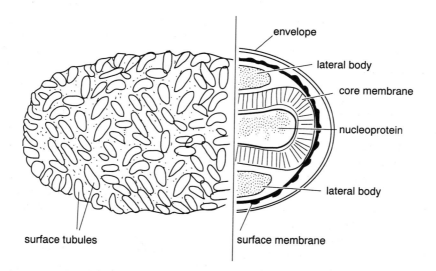

Figure 57.3 Diagrammatic representation of an orthopoxvirus displaying the surface structure of an unenveloped virion (left) and a cross-section of an enveloped virion (right).

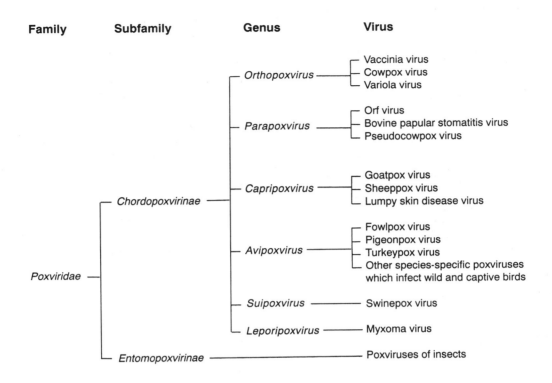

Figure 57.4 Classification of poxviruses with emphasis on those which affect domestic animals.

Infections caused by cowpox virus

Cowpox is endemic in parts of Europe. Although infection and disease have been described in cattle, cats, humans and a range of mammals in zoos, these species are considered to be incidental hosts. The reservoir hosts are probably wild rodents. There is evidence that voles and woodmice are the principal reservoir hosts in western Europe (Bennett *et al.*, 1997). In milking cows, lesions are usually confined to the teats. The domestic species in which the disease is most often recognized is the cat. Affected cats usually come from rural areas and are described as good hunters. Moreover, infections in cats tend to peak in the autumn when small rodent populations are high, suggesting rodent-derived infections. Although cat-to-cat transfer occurs, this mode of transmission is rare. Small papules on the head or forelimbs, the first recognizable signs of the infection, eventually ulcerate. Scab formation is usually followed by complete resolution in about six weeks. Secondary skin lesions develop in some cats and a few animals may show signs of coryza or conjunctivitis. Rarely, pneumonia and pleural exudation have been described. Diagnosis can be confirmed by histopathology, electronmicroscopy or virus isolation. No specific control measures are warranted. Human infections, which are usually contracted from infected cats, are uncommon.

Infections caused by pseudocowpox virus

Pseudocowpox, also known as milker's nodule, is caused by pseudocowpox virus, a parapoxvirus with worldwide distribution. It is a common mild condition affecting the teats of lactating cows. Infection spreads slowly through milking herds with variation in the number of affected animals at any particular time. Transmission is by direct or indirect contact. Transfer of infection can occur through teat cups and on milkers' hands. Transmission can also occur mechanically by flies or when calves are being suckled. Small red papules on teats or udder develop into ulcers with overlying scab formation. Healing at the centre of the lesions produces characteristic ring- or horseshoe-shaped scabs. Typical parapoxvirus particles can be demonstrated in scab material using electron microscopy. Control is based on appropriate hygienic measures at milking including the use of effective teat dips. In human infections, lesions are usually confined to the hand, forearm or face.

Bovine papular stomatitis

This mild viral disease of young cattle occurs worldwide. It is caused by a parapoxvirus, bovine papular stomatitis virus, which is transmitted by direct or indirect contact.

Table 57.1 Members of the *Poxviridae* of veterinary significance.

Virus	Genus	Host species	Significance of infection
Vaccinia virus	*Orthopoxvirus*	Wide host range	Infections in sheep, water buffaloes, rabbits, cattle, horses and humans. Used as a recombinant virus vector for rabies vaccine
Cowpox virus	*Orthopoxvirus*	Rodents, cats, cattle	Small species of rodents are the likely reservoir hosts. Cats are the principal incidental hosts; infection results in skin lesions. Rare cause of teat lesions in cattle. Transmissible to humans
Uasin gishu virus	*Orthopoxvirus*	Unknown wildlife reservoir, horses	Rare disease, reported in Kenya and neighbouring African countries. Causes papilloma-like skin lesions in horses
Camelpox virus	*Orthopoxvirus*	Camel	Widely distributed in Asia and Africa. Causes systemic infection with typical pox lesions; severe infection in young camels
Pseudocowpox virus	*Parapoxvirus*	Cattle	Common cause of teat lesions in milking cows; causes milker's nodule in humans
Bovine papular stomatitis virus	*Parapoxvirus*	Cattle	Produces mild papular lesions on the muzzle and in the oral cavity of young cattle. Transmissible to humans
Orf virus	*Parapoxvirus*	Sheep, goats	Primarily affects young lambs; causes proliferative lesions on the muzzle and lips. Transmissible to humans
Sheeppox / Goatpox virus	*Capripoxvirus*	Sheep, goats	Endemic in Africa, Middle East and India. Causes generalized infection with characteristic skin lesions and variable mortality
Lumpy skin disease virus	*Capripoxvirus*	Cattle	Endemic in Africa. Causes generalized infection with severe lesions and variable mortality
Swinepox virus	*Suipoxvirus*	Pigs	Causes mild, skin disease. Occurs worldwide. Transmitted by the pig louse (*Haematopinus suis*)
Fowlpox virus	*Avipoxvirus*	Chickens, turkeys	Causes lesions on the head and on the oral mucous membrane. Occurs worldwide. Transmitted by biting arthropods
Myxoma virus	*Leporipoxvirus*	Rabbits	Causes mild disease in cottontail rabbits, the natural host, and severe disease in European rabbits. Introduced into Europe, Australia and Chile as a biological control measure

Infection is common and usually subclinical. Mature cattle are considered to be reservoirs of infection.

Affected calves commonly develop lesions in the buccal cavity and on the muzzle. These lesions are characterized by hyperaemic foci that develop into papules with concentric zones of inflammation. Affected animals usually recover within three weeks. A more severe chronic form of the disease, which may be associated with concurrent infections or immunosuppression, has been described (Yeruham *et al.*, 1994). Virions can be demonstrated in skin scrapings by electron microscopy. The virus is transmissible to humans.

Orf

This important disease of sheep, also known as contagious pustular dermatitis or contagious ecthyma, occurs worldwide and is caused by a parapoxvirus. Goats, camels and humans are also susceptible to infection.

Epidemiology

The virus is transmitted through direct or indirect contact. Under dry environmental conditions, it is stable and can survive in scab material for months. Infectivity is substantially reduced after exposure to adverse climatic conditions. In most flocks, infection is maintained by sheep with chronic lesions (McKeever and Reid, 1986).

Pathogenesis

The virus, which is epitheliotropic, produces proliferative wart-like lesions following entry through skin abrasions. The virus replicates in epidermal keratinocytes and infected cells release an endothelial growth factor which is implicated in epithelial cell proliferation (Haig and Mercer, 1998). Papular lesions progress to vesicles, pustules and eventually to scab formation. Proliferation of cells underlying scabs produces verrucose masses. In the absence of secondary bacterial infection, lesions usually heal within four weeks.

Clinical signs

The disease primarily affects young sheep. The incubation period is up to seven days. Although lesions most often occur on the commissures of the lips and on the muzzle, they may also develop in the mouth and on the feet, genitalia and teats. Mild lesions may go unnoticed. Severely affected lambs with lesions in the buccal cavity often fail to eat, lose condition and may die. Outbreaks last for some months and vary in severity from farm to farm and from year to year. The disease does not usually recur until the birth of new susceptible lambs in the flock. Although isolates from individual flocks can differ in genotype, there is no evidence that the severity of the disease correlates with the strain of the virus involved (Gilray *et al.*, 1998). Environmental management factors may influence the outcome of infection (Gumbrell and McGregor, 1997).

Immunity following natural infection may not confer complete protection. However, lesions in animals previously affected are usually less severe and heal more rapidly than those developing after first exposure. In chronically infected sheep, lesions may be either mild or proliferative. Neonatal lambs are susceptible to infection despite receipt of colostrum from previously infected ewes.

Diagnosis

Lesions of orf are readily recognized by their characteristic appearance and distribution. Virus present in lesion material can be identified by electron microscopy.

Treatment and control

There is no specific treatment for infection with orf virus. Antibiotic therapy reduces the effect of secondary bacterial infection in young lambs.

In endemically infected flocks, control is based on the use of a fully virulent live vaccine derived from scab material or cell culture. Ewes should be vaccinated by scarification in the axilla at least eight weeks before lambing. When close to lambing, they must be moved to a new grazing area in order to minimize exposure of lambs to infectious vaccinal scab material. Lambs should be vaccinated only if an outbreak occurs in a flock. If carried out effectively, thorough cleaning and disinfection of surfaces and equipment between periods of housing may reduce the amount of virus in the buildings.

Humans are susceptible to infection with orf virus. Typically, a single lesion occurs on hands, forearm or face. Care should be exercised when handling affected sheep and when using live vaccines.

Sheeppox and goatpox

Both of these diseases are endemic diseases in south eastern Europe, the Middle East, Africa and Asia. The viruses of sheeppox and goatpox are members of the genus *Capripoxvirus*. A range of capripoxvirus strains have been isolated from sheep and goats and there is evidence of recombination between strains (Gershon *et al.*, 1989). Although some strains are extremely pathogenic in both sheep and goats, other strains produce severe disease in only one of these species.

Epidemiology

Virus particles are shed from skin lesions and in ocular and nasal discharges during the acute stages of the disease. Infection occurs through skin abrasions or by aerosol. Biting insects may also transmit the virus mechanically. Housing or stockading animals facilitates transmission of the virus. Following infection, capripoxvirus strains induce immunity. In endemic areas, where indigenous animals frequently have a high level of naturally acquired immunity, generalized disease and mortality are rare. In isolated flocks, outbreaks of severe disease may occur.

Pathogenesis and pathology

The virus replicates locally either in the skin or in the lungs. Spread to the regional lymph nodes is followed by viraemia and replication in various internal organs. Skin lesions, typical of poxvirus infection, appear about seven days post infection. Lung lesions often present as areas of consolidation and haemorrhage.

Clinical signs

Following an incubation period of about one week, infected animals develop fever, oedema of the eyelids, conjunctivitis and nasal discharge. Within a few days, macules which rapidly develop into papules appear on the skin and external mucous membranes. Scabs form over necrotic papules. The severity of the clinical signs depends on the breed of host animal and the strain of capripoxvirus. Lesions in mild afebrile disease may be minimal and confined to the skin beneath the tail.

Mortality rates with infections from some strains of capripoxvirus may be up to 50% even in indigenous breeds. The disease is most severe in young animals and in imported breeds. Some European breeds are extremely susceptible and mortality rates may approach 100%. Secondary bacterial infection or dissemination of the virus to other sites may result in a more severe form of the disease.

Diagnosis

Diagnosis can often be made solely on clinical grounds. Skin biopsies or postmortem specimens may be used for laboratory confirmation.

- Eosinophilic intracytoplasmic inclusions may be demonstrable histologically in epidermal cells.
- Electron microscopy can be used for the rapid identification of poxvirus particles in material from

lesions. Capripoxviruses can be readily distinguished from parapoxviruses.

- Virus may be isolated in lamb testis or kidney cell monolayers.
- An antigen-trapping ELISA has been developed for the detection of capripoxvirus antigen (Carn, 1995).
- Several serological methods including virus neutralization, Western blot analysis and the indirect fluorescent antibody test are available.

Control

In endemic areas, control is based on annual vaccination. Modified live and inactivated vaccines are available. A subunit vaccine has also been developed (Carn *et al.*, 1994). Inactivated vaccines are less effective than modified live vaccines because cell-mediated immunity is the predominant protective response.

Capripoxviruses are being employed as vectors for important ruminant viral vaccines (Romero *et al.*, 1993). These vector vaccines may provide protection against diseases caused by capripoxviruses as well as diseases such as rinderpest and peste des petits ruminants.

Lumpy skin disease

This acute disease, which is endemic in sub-Saharan Africa, the Malagasy Republic and Egypt, is caused by lumpy skin disease virus (Neethling virus), a capripoxvirus.

Epidemiology

Although virus is present in the saliva of infected animals and transmission may occur through environmental contamination, lumpy skin disease is not particularly contagious (Carn and Kitching, 1995). The principal method of transmission is by mechanical transfer through biting insects. As a consequence, disease outbreaks usually occur during the rainy season when insect activity is high and epidemics are often associated with heavy rains. New outbreaks may appear in areas far removed from an initial outbreak. It is unclear how the virus persists between epidemics but subclinically infected cattle are probably important. There is some evidence for a wildlife reservoir, possibly the African Cape buffalo.

Pathogenesis and pathology

Virus, which is transmitted mechanically by biting insects, rapidly disseminates through a leukocyte-associated viraemia. Many cell types including keratinocytes, myocytes, fibrocytes and endothelial cells become infected. Damage to endothelial cells, which results in vasculitis, thrombosis, infarction, oedema and inflammatory cell infiltration, accounts for the nodular skin lesions.

Clinical signs

The incubation period is up to 14 days. There is a persistent fever accompanied by lacrimation, nasal discharge and a drop in milk yield. Superficial lymph nodes become enlarged and there is oedema of the limbs and dependent tissues. Circumscribed skin nodules develop particularly on the head, neck, udder and perineum. Nodules also develop on the mucous membranes of the mouth and nares. Some skin lesions may develop into 'sit-fasts'. These are composed of a central plug of necrotic tissue which sloughs producing a deep ulcer. Secondary bacterial infection or myiasis can exacerbate the condition. Recovery may take several months. Affected animals are often debilitated and pregnant cows may abort. The severity of the disease relates to the strain of virus and the breed of cattle. Domestic breeds (*Bos taurus*) are more susceptible than zebu (*Bos indicus*). Some animals have few skin lesions and no systemic reaction while others display the full spectrum of clinical signs. Although the mortality rate is usually less than 5%, the economic impact of the disease can be considerable.

Diagnosis

- Generalized skin nodules in cattle in an endemic area are highly suggestive of lumpy skin disease.
- Intracytoplasmic inclusions may be demonstrable histologically in recently developed lesions.
- Capripoxvirus particles in biopsy material or desiccated crusts can be identified using electron microscopy.
- The virus can be isolated in lamb testis cell monolayers.
- An antigen trapping ELISA is available for the detection of capripoxvirus antigen (Carn, 1995).
- Serological assay methods include virus neutralization, Western blot analysis and the indirect fluorescent antibody test.

Control

In endemic regions vaccination is the method of control. Two modified live vaccines, one based on a South African strain of lumpy skin disease virus and the other on a Kenyan strain of sheeppox virus, are available. A recombinant vaccine providing protection against lumpy skin disease and rinderpest has been developed (Romero *et al.*, 1993). Imported cattle should be vaccinated before introduction into high risk areas. Surveillance and eradication policies are appropriate control measures in countries bordering on endemic regions (Yeruham *et al.*, 1995).

Swinepox

This disease, which occurs worldwide, is mild and often goes unrecognized. Swinepox virus is the sole member of the genus *Suipoxvirus*. The virus is transmitted mechanically by the pig louse, *Haematopinus suis*. Following an incubation period of about one week, infected animals display a slight fever and rash. Papules and pustules with scab formation resolve within three to four weeks. These skin lesions are similar to those which occur in pigs infected with vaccinia virus. Virus particles can be demonstrated in material from the lesions by electron microscopy. No vaccine is available. Control within a herd can be achieved by improved hygiene together with louse eradication.

Fowlpox

This disease, affecting domestic poultry, including chickens and turkeys, is caused by infection with fowlpox virus. The infection is slow-spreading and characterized by proliferative skin lesions and diphtheritic lesions in the upper digestive and respiratory tracts. Fowl pox has a worldwide distribution.

Epidemiology

Fowlpox, pigeonpox and turkeypox viruses are closely related and are not strictly host-specific. Several avian species are susceptible to infection with fowlpox virus. Transmission occurs by contact and by mechanical transfer on the mouthparts of biting arthropods, particularly mosquitoes. Virus enters the body through abrasions on unfeathered skin, on oral mucosa or on respiratory mucosa. Aerosols generated from scab material may result in transmission by inhalation. There is some evidence that persistence as latent infection and reactivation by stress may occur in a few birds.

Pathogenesis

Virus multiplication occurs at the site of introduction and may be confined to that site when the strain of infecting virus is of low virulence. Infections caused by virulent strains result in viraemia with replication in internal organs. The route of introduction influences the distribution and severity of lesions. Factors such as malnutrition, debilitation and stress may contribute to the severity of the disease.

Clinical signs

The incubation period is up to 14 days. Two forms of fowlpox have been described, a cutaneous form (dry pox) and a diphtheritic form (wet pox). In the cutaneous form, nodular lesions develop on the comb, wattles and other unfeathered areas of skin. Progression to vesicle formation is followed by ulceration and scab formation. Healing occurs within two weeks. In severely affected birds, lesions may involve both feathered and unfeathered areas of skin, and involvement of the eyelids may lead to complete closure. In the diphtheritic form of the disease, yellowish necrotic lesions (cankers) develop on the mucous membranes of the mouth, oesophagus and trachea.

Oral lesions may interfere with eating. Tracheal involvement may lead to laboured breathing and rales.

The mortality rate, which is higher in birds with the diphtheritic form, may approach 50% in severe outbreaks, particularly when accompanied by secondary bacterial or fungal infection. Economic losses are largely due to a transient drop in egg production in laying birds and reduced growth in young birds.

Diagnosis

- Large intracytoplasmic inclusions (Bollinger bodies) containing small elementary bodies (Borrel bodies) may be demonstrable in epithelial cells. Immuno-fluorescence and immunoperoxidase techniques can be used to identify viral antigen in intracytoplasmic inclusions.
- Typical poxvirus particles can be demonstrated by electron microscopy in material from lesions.
- Virus may be isolated on the chorioallantoic membrane of nine to 12 day old embryonated eggs.
- Nucleic acid probes can be used for diagnosis.
- Suitable serological tests include ELISA, virus neutralization, agar gel precipitation and passive haemagglutination.

Treatment and control

There is no specific treatment. Control of secondary bacterial infection is desirable. In endemic areas, improved management and hygiene along with regular vaccination have reduced the effect of the disease on commercial poultry production. Modified live fowlpox or pigeonpox virus vaccines, produced in tissue culture or chick embryo, are available commercially. Chickens are usually vaccinated at about one month of age. Recombinant vaccines employing fowlpox and canarypox viruses are being developed.

Myxomatosis

This severe generalized disease of European rabbits is caused by myxoma virus, the type species of the genus *Leporipoxvirus*.

Epidemiology

The natural hosts of myxoma virus are New World species of rabbits, *Sylvilagus brasiliensis* in South America and *S. bachmani* in California. Infection has long been endemic in South America and western North America. In natural hosts, myxoma virus infection causes a benign cutaneous fibroma. In contrast, infection in the European rabbit (*Oryctolagus cuniculus*) is lethal. South American isolates of myxoma virus were introduced during the 1950s into populations of *O. cuniculus* in Europe, Chile and Australia as a method for controlling rabbit numbers. More than 99% of infected rabbits died and the disease is now endemic in these regions. Both attenuated virus strains and resistant rabbit populations have emerged. Virus is transmitted mechanically on the mouthparts of mosquitoes and fleas. Epidemics, which may occur annually, relate to the presence of arthropod vectors and large numbers of young susceptible rabbits.

Pathogenesis and pathology

Virus replicates at the site of inoculation and in regional lymph nodes and the subsequent viraemia is mainly cell-associated, with most virus particles in lymphocytes. Gelatinous, myxoma-like swellings are evident in the skin about one week after infection.

Clinical signs

Subcutaneous gelatinous swellings are particularly prominent in the head and anogenital areas. Blepharo-conjunctivitis, accompanied by an opalescent ocular discharge, develops. Affected animals are febrile and listless, and some may die within 48 hours. Activation of *Pasteurella multocida* infection can result in nasal discharge. The mortality rate, which ranges from 25% to 90%, is influenced by the genetic resistance of the rabbit population and the virulence of the virus strain. Low ambient temperatures increase the severity of the disease.

Diagnosis

The clinical signs are characteristic. Isolation of virus or detection of poxvirus particles in exudate or in material from lesions by electron microscopy is confirmatory.

Control

Commercial and laboratory rabbit stocks can be protected by vaccination with modified live myxoma virus or with rabbit fibroma virus, a related *Leporipoxvirus*. Control of flea infestation in colonies, and insect proofing of accommodation to reduce transmission of infection by other arthropods, may be necessary in endemic areas.

References

Bennett M., Crouch, A.J., Begon, M., *et al.* (1997). Cowpox in British voles and mice. *Journal of Comparative Pathology*, **116**, 35–44.

Carn, V.M. (1995). An antigen trapping ELISA for the detection of capripoxvirus in tissue culture supernatant and biopsy samples. *Journal of Virological Methods,* **51**, 95–102.

Carn, V.M. and Kitching R.P. (1995). An investigation of possible routes of transmission of lumpy skin disease virus (Neethling). *Epidemiology and Infection*, **114**, 219–226.

Carn, V.M., Timms, C.P., Chand, P. *et al.* (1994). Protection of goats against capripox using a subunit vaccine. *Veterinary Record*, **135**, 434–436.

Gershon, P.D., Kitching, R.P. Hammond, J.M. and Black, D.N. (1989). Poxvirus genetic recombination during natural virus transmission. *Journal of General Virology*, **70**, 485–489.

Gilray, J.A., Nettleton, P.F., Pow, I., *et al.* (1998). Restriction endonuclease profiles of orf virus isolates from the British Isles. *Veterinary Record*, **143**, 237–240.

Gumbrell R.C. and McGregor, D.A. (1997). Outbreak of severe fatal orf in lambs. *Veterinary Record*, **141**, 150–151.

Haig, D.M. and Mercer, A.A. (1998). Orf. *Veterinary Research*, **29**, 311–326.

McKeever, D.J. and Reid, H.W. (1986). Survival of orf virus under British winter conditions. *Veterinary Record*, **118**, 613–614.

Romero, C.H., Barrett, T., Evans, S.A., *et al.* (1993). Single capripoxvirus recombinant vaccine for the protection of cattle against rinderpest and lumpy skin disease. *Vaccine*, **11**, 737–742.

Studdert, M.J. (1989). Experimental vaccinia virus infection of horses. *Australian Veterinary Journal*, **66**, 157–159.

Yeruham, I., Abraham, A. and Nyska, A. (1994). Clinical and pathological description of a chronic form of bovine papular stomatitis. *Journal of Comparative Pathology*, **111**, 279–286.

Yeruham, I., Nir, O., Braverman, Y., *et al.* (1995). Spread of lumpy skin disease in Israeli dairy herds. *Veterinary Record*, **137**, 91–93.

Chapter 58

Asfarviridae

African swine fever virus (ASFV), formerly assigned to the family *Iridoviridae*, has recently been reassigned to a newly created family, *Asfarviridae*, containing the single genus *Asfivirus*. African swine fever virus is the type species of this genus. The virus has similarities in genome structure and method of replication to poxviruses but is different in other respects. Virions are 175 to 215 nm in diameter and consist of a membrane-bound nucleoprotein core inside an icosahedral capsid surrounded by an outer lipid-containing envelope (Fig. 58.1). This complex virus contains more than 50 proteins, including a large number of structural proteins and several virus-encoded enzymes required for transcription and post-translational modification of mRNA. The genome consists of a single molecule of linear double-stranded DNA. Following replication in the cytoplasm of host cells, virus is released either by budding through the plasma membrane or following cellular disintegration. African swine fever virus is stable in the environment over a wide range of temperature (4°C to 20°C) and pH values. The virus may persist for months

in meat. Infectivity can be destroyed by heating and by treating with lipid solvents and some disinfectants such as orthophenylphenol.

African swine fever

African swine fever (ASF) is an economically important viral disease of pigs, characterized by fever, haemorrhages in many tissues and a high mortality rate. It is endemic in sub-Saharan Africa and Sardinia. Outbreaks have occurred in Belgium, Italy, Malta, Brazil, Cuba, Haiti and the Dominican Republic. The Iberian Peninsula was declared free of the disease in 1995, almost 30 years after initial introduction into the region, but ASFV reappeared in 1999 in Portugal.

Epidemiology

Domestic and wild pigs are the only species susceptible to infection. In Africa, ASFV is maintained in a sylvatic cycle involving soft ticks of the genus *Ornithodorus* and inapparent infection of warthogs and bushpigs (Fig. 58.2). Adult warthogs with persistent inapparent infection rarely develop viraemia. In contrast, young warthogs develop viraemia and are a major source of virus for soft ticks. Replication of virus occurs in the ticks and both trans-ovarial and trans-stadial transmission have been described. Soft ticks feed for short periods on hosts before dropping off and sheltering in crevices in walls or cracks in the ground. The presence of ticks in a particular region makes the eradication of ASF difficult. The principal tick species involved in transmission are *O. moubata* in Africa and *O. erraticus* in Spain and Portugal. Experimentally, several other *Ornithodorus* species support virus replication. Virulent strains of ASFV, producing high mortality in infected animals, are widely distributed in

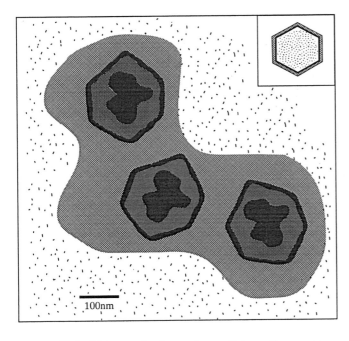

Figure 58.1 African swine fever virus particles as they appear in an electron micrograph and a diagrammatic representation (inset).

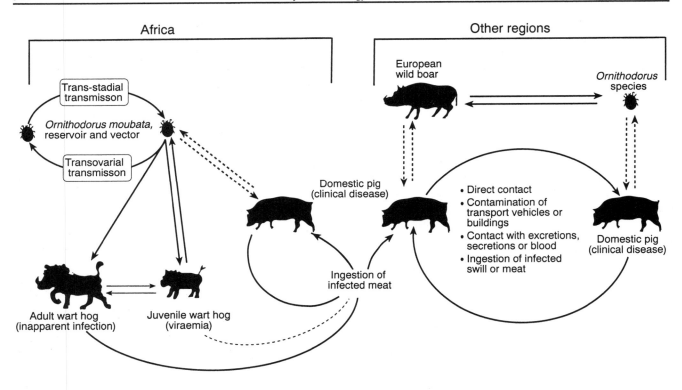

Figure 58.2 The maintenance and transmission of African swine fever virus in wild and domestic pig populations and in tick vectors.

Africa. Many isolates from other parts of the world are less virulent and mortality rates are usually below 50%.

Following infection of domestic pigs with virulent virus, body fluids and tissues contain large quantities of virus until death or recovery occurs. Ingestion of uncooked meat from infected warthogs or domestic pigs is a major method of transmission. Spread can also occur by direct contact usually through oral or nasal secretions. Occasionally, animals become infected by contact with blood shed as a result of fighting. Indirect transmission can occur through contaminated transport vehicles, fomites and footwear. Feeding uncooked swill is an important mechanism of spread of ASF internationally, with outbreaks often starting in herds close to airports and harbours.

Pigs which have recovered from clinical disease may remain infected for long periods. Carrier pigs are considered to be important sources of virus dissemination. Although recovered pigs are clinically unaffected by challenge with genotypically related ASFV, the challenge virus may replicate and spread to other pigs.

Pathogenesis and pathology

Infection in domestic pigs is usually acquired via the oronasal route. The virus replicates initially in pharyngeal mucosa, tonsils and the regional lymph nodes. Infection then spreads by the bloodstream to other lymph nodes, bone marrow, spleen, lung, liver and kidneys. Secondary replication in these sites results in prolonged viraemia.

Although the virus replicates primarily in cells of the lymphoreticular system, it can also infect megakaryocytes, endothelial cells, renal epithelial cells and hepatocytes. Lesions include splenic enlargement, swollen haemorrhagic gastrohepatic and renal lymph nodes, subcapsular petechiation in the kidneys, petechial and ecchymotic haemorrhages on serosal surfaces, oedema of the lungs and hydrothorax. The widespread haemorrhages result from disseminated intravascular coagulation, endothelial damage and destruction of megakaryocytes (Rodriguez *et al.*, 1996). Leukopenia is marked. Because the virus does not appear to replicate in T and B lymphocytes, it has been suggested that the lymphopenia follows apoptosis of lymphocytes and necrosis of lymphoid organs (Carrasco *et al.*, 1996). Lesions in chronic disease include pneumonia, fibrinous pleuritis and pericarditis, pleural adhesions and hyperplasia of lymphoreticular tissues.

Clinical signs

The clinical signs of ASF, which range from inapparent to peracute, relate to the challenge dose and virulence of the virus and to the route of infection. The incubation period, which may extend from four to 19 days, is typically five to seven days in acute cases. Animals with peracute disease die suddenly without premonitory clinical signs. Fever, inappetence, depression and recumbency are features of acute disease. Cutaneous hyperaemia and, in some cases, haemorrhages may be evident. Other signs include dyspnoea, conjunctivitis, diarrhoea, bleeding from the nose and rectum, and abortion. The mortality rate is high. Subacute disease has a course of three to four weeks. Clinical signs include pneumonia, swollen joints, emaciation, depression and inappetence. Mortality rates, which are variable, depend on the age and general health of infected pigs. Animals may recover clinically or may develop a chronic form of the disease, which usually occurs in regions where ASFV is endemic. The immune mechanisms responsible for recovery and protection from ASFV are poorly understood. Neutralizing antibodies are not demonstrable in the sera of recovered animals. Cell-mediated immunity is considered to be an important component of the immune response.

Diagnosis

Laboratory confirmation of ASF is mandatory because the clinical signs and lesions, which occur in some other important pig diseases such as classical swine fever, erysipelas and septicaemic salmonellosis, are similar.

- Suitable samples for laboratory examination include blood, serum, tonsil, spleen and lymph nodes.
- The most convenient and frequently used tests for detection of ASFV are direct immunofluorescence and haemadsorption (Sanchez-Vizcaino, 1999). Direct immunofluorescence, which is fast and economical, can be carried out on impression smears or cryostat sections. However, the sensitivity of the test is only 40% in pigs with subacute or chronic ASF because of the blocking action of bound antibody in antigen- antibody complexes. Most field strains of ASFV induce haemadsorption. Pig erythrocytes adhere to the surface of infected monocytes and macrophages, forming a characteristic rosette. The haemadsorption test can be carried out by employing leukocytes from blood samples of pigs under investigation or by inoculating primary blood leukocyte cultures with blood or homogenized tissue from suspect pigs.
- A challenge experiment, involving the inoculation of suspect material into pigs vaccinated against classical swine fever and into unvaccinated pigs, may be used to differentiate the two diseases.
- The polymerase chain reaction can be used to detect DNA from ASFV in tissues unsuitable for virus isolation or antigen detection.
- Antibodies persist for long periods in recovered animals. Serological testing may be the only means of detecting animals infected with strains of low virulence. Techniques for detecting antibodies to ASF include ELISA, immunoblotting, indirect immunofluorescence, complement fixation and radioimmunoassay.

Control

A successful vaccine is not yet available. Inactivated vaccines do not induce protection. Although live attenuated vaccines induce protection against challenge with homologous virus strains in some pigs, a proportion of these animals become carriers and may develop chronic lesions.

Countries maintain disease-free status by prohibiting importation of pigs and pig products. Waste food scraps from aircraft and ships must be boiled before inclusion in pig feed. In the face of an outbreak of ASF in countries free of infection, an eradication policy is implemented. The occurrence of low virulence strains renders eradication difficult.

Restriction of pig movement, serological monitoring of carrier pigs and prevention of contact between domestic pigs and warthogs or ticks are important control measures in countries where the disease is endemic. Eradication of tick species which act as vectors of ASFV is an essential part of a control programme.

References

Carrasco. L., Chacon, M-L., Martin de las Mulas, J. *et al.* (1996). Apoptosis in lymph nodes in acute African swine fever. *Journal of Comparative Pathology*, **115**, 415–428.

Rodriguez, F., Fernandez, A., Perez, J. *et al.* (1996). African swine fever: morphopathology of a viral haemorrhagic disease. *Veterinary Record*, **139**, 249–254

Sanchez-Vizcaino, J.M. (1999). African swine fever. In *Diseases of Swine*. Eighth Edition. Eds. B.E. Straw, S. D'Allaire, W.L. Mengeling, and D.J. Taylor. Blackwell Science, Oxford. pp. 93–102.

Chapter 59

Parvoviridae

Viruses belonging to the family *Parvoviridae*, referred to as parvoviruses, are small (Latin *parvus*, small) and range in size from 18 to 26 nm in diameter (Fig. 59.1). These non-enveloped, icosahedral viruses possess a linear genome of single-stranded DNA. There are two sub-families: *Parvovirinae* which includes viruses of vertebrates and *Densovirinae*, members of which infect arthropods. Of the three genera within the subfamily *Parvovirinae* (Fig. 59.2) only the genus *Parvovirus* contains viruses of veterinary importance.

Parvoviruses replicate only in the nuclei of dividing host cells, a feature which determines the tissues targeted. After entering a cell, the virion is uncoated and its single-stranded DNA genome is converted to double-stranded DNA by DNA polymerases in the nucleus. Following viral replication, cell lysis occurs as virions are released.

Parvoviruses are stable in the environment. They are resistant to many factors including lipid solvents, a wide range of pH values (pH 3 to 9) and heating at 56°C for more than 60 minutes. They are inactivated by formalin, β-propiolactone, sodium hypochlorite and oxidizing

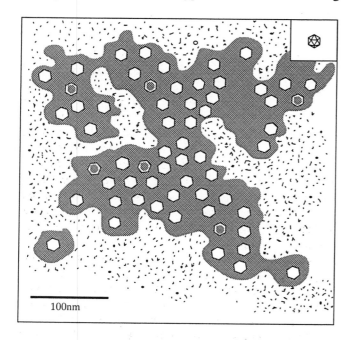

Figure 59.1 Parvovirus particles as they appear in an electron micrograph and a diagrammatic representation (inset).

> **Key points**
> - Small, non-enveloped, single-stranded DNA viruses
> - Icosahedral symmetry
> - Replicate in the nucleus, form intranuclear inclusion bodies
> - Require rapidly-dividing cells for replication
> - Stable in the environment
> - Resistant to heat, solvents, disinfectants and pH changes
> - Genus *Parvovirus:*
>   —Many have haemagglutinating activity
>   —Shed in large numbers in faeces
>   —Enteric and systemic diseases in dogs and cats
>   —Reproductive failure, SMEDI syndrome, in pigs

agents. With the exception of Aleutian mink disease virus and goose parvovirus, parvoviruses of vertebrates agglutinate erythrocytes. Haemagglutination inhibition (HAI) by specific antisera is widely used for their identification. Mink enteritis virus, canine parvovirus and racoon parvovirus are considered to be host-range mutants of feline panleukopenia virus.

Clinical infections

Parvoviruses can infect many domestic and wild animals (Table 59.1). Although most members of the group produce acute systemic diseases, some such as canine minute virus and bovine parvovirus are of uncertain pathogenic significance. Two distinct parvoviral diseases of mink, Aleutian mink disease and mink enteritis, are recognized. Mink enteritis, first described in the 1940s, affects kits and clinically resembles feline panleukopenia. Aleutian mink disease is a persistent infection, primarily affecting animals which are homozygous for pale coat colour. The disease is characterized by B lymphocyte stimulation leading to plasmacytosis, hypergammaglobulinaemia and immune complex-related lesions in the kidneys and other organs. Aleutian mink disease can also

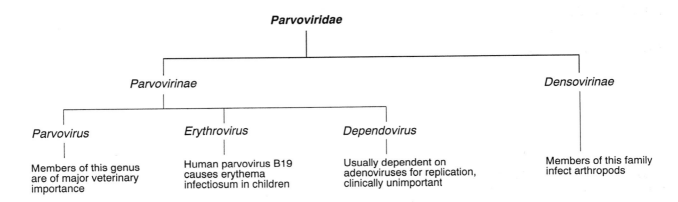

Figure 59.2 The family *Parvoviridae*, subfamilies *Parvovirinae* and *Densovirinae* and the genera of *Parvovirinae* which can infect mammalian species.

Table 59.1 *Parvoviruses of veterinary significance.*

Virus	Hosts	Consequences of infection
Feline pan-leukopenia virus	Domestic and wild cats	Highly contagious systemic and enteric disease most common in weaned kittens, manifested as depression, vomiting, diarrhoea. Intrauterine infection : abortion or cerebellar ataxia in neonatal kittens
Canine parvovirus (Canine parvovirus 2)	Dogs	Highly contagious enteric disease with depression, vomiting, dysentery and immunosuppression. Intrauterine or perinatal infection: myocarditis in pups (now rare)
Porcine parvovirus	Pigs	Major cause of stillbirths, mummified foetuses, embryonic deaths and infertility (SMEDI syndrome)
Mink enteritis virus	Mink	Generalised disease of mink kits, analagous to feline panleukopenia
Aleutian mink disease virus	Mink, ferrets	Chronic, progressive disease of mink homozygous for pale coat colour. Persistent viraemia, plasmacytosis, hypergamma-globulinaemia and immune complex-related lesions
Goose par-vovirus (goose plague virus)	Geese	Highly contagious, fatal disease of 8-30 day old goslings (Derzsy's disease): hepatitis, myositis, including myocarditis
Canine minute virus (Canine parvovirus 1)	Dogs	Role of virus in disease is uncertain; serological surveys suggest the virus is widespread
Bovine parvovirus	Cattle	Associated with sporadic outbreaks of diarrhoea in calves

occur in domestic ferrets (Welchman *et al.*, 1993). Goose parvovirus infection, which causes hepatitis and myositis in goslings, is highly contagious and often fatal. The most important parvoviral diseases of domestic animals are feline panleukopenia, canine parvovirus infection and porcine parvovirus infection.

Feline panleukopenia

Feline panleukopenia, also known as feline infectious enteritis or feline distemper, is a highly contagious generalized disease of domestic and wild cats caused by feline panleukopenia virus. Only one serotype of this virus has been identified. The disease, which is worldwide in distribution, is one of the most common feline viral infections.

Epidemiology

Most species of *Felidae* are highly susceptible to infection which is generally endemic in unvaccinated cat populations. Some species of *Mustelidae*, *Procyonidae* and *Viverridae* can also become infected but they seldom develop clinical disease. Although cats of all ages are susceptible to infection, disease occurs predominantly in young recently-weaned kittens, as maternally-derived antibody levels wane. Many infections are subclinical, particularly in older cats and in kittens partially protected by maternally-derived immunity. The disease may have a cyclical or seasonal pattern which is related to the births of kittens. Transplacental infection occurs in fully susceptible queens.

High rates of virus excretion occur during the acute stage of the disease, mainly in faeces but also in saliva, urine, vomitus and blood. Faecal shedding usually continues for some weeks following clinical recovery. Although long-term, low-grade shedding of virus by some subclinical carriers may occur, the stability of the virus in the environment is of greater significance in its persistence and spread. In cool, moist, dark environments, infectivity may last for more than a year. Fleas and humans may act as mechanical vectors.

Pathogenesis and pathology

Following ingestion or inhalation, replication occurs in the mitotically active lymphoid tissues of the oropharynx and associated lymph nodes. Viraemia develops within 24 hours, producing infection of mitotically active cells in other tissues, particularly the cells of the intestinal crypts and the lymphopoietic cells of the bone marrow, thymus, lymph nodes and spleen. Destruction of these target tissues results in panleukopenia and villous atrophy. The crypts of Lieberkühn are dilated and contain necrotic epithelial cells. Intranuclear inclusions are sometimes evident in crypt cells. Intestinal villi become blunted and may fuse. The effects of transplacental infection on foetuses generally relate to the stage of gestation at the time of viral invasion and range from cerebellar hypoplasia and retinal dysplasia to foetal death.

Clinical signs

The incubation period of feline panleukopenia ranges from two to ten days but is typically four to five days. Subclinical infection is common and results in a mild fever and leukopenia, usually followed by life-long immunity. Subacute disease presents as depression, fever and diarrhoea lasting one to three days, followed by rapid recovery. The disease is most severe in young, unvaccinated kittens between 6 and 24 weeks of age and is characterized by sudden onset of pronounced depression, anorexia and fever. Vomiting, sometimes accompanied by diarrhoea or dysentery, follows within two days and can result in severe dehydration and electrolyte imbalance. Abdominal pain may be evident. The mortality rate ranges from 25 to 90% with most deaths occurring within three to five days of the onset of illness. Animals which survive require several weeks for full recovery. Immunity is strong and long-lasting. Subnormal temperatures are followed by death within 24 hours. Although intrauterine infection of the developing foetuses often occurs, infected pregnant queens usually show no signs of illness. Foetal infections early in gestation may result in resorption or abortion. Because of developing foetal immune competence, infections after mid-gestation are usually less severe. However, stillbirths, early neonatal death and teratological changes such as cerebellar hypoplasia and retinal dysplasia may occur in the litters of queens infected during late pregnancy. Kittens with cerebellar hypoplasia exhibit cerebellar ataxia manifested as hypermetria, incoordination and, frequently, intention tremors. These signs persist for life.

Diagnosis

- Feline panleukopenia should be considered when unvaccinated cats present with diarrhoea.
- A white cell count of less than 7 x 10^9/L is often

encountered in acutely affected animals. Neutropenia is more common than lymphopenia. Cell counts return to normal after a few days in those cats which survive.

- Specimens for virus isolation in primary feline cell lines include oropharyngeal swabs, faeces, spleen, mesenteric lymph nodes and ileum.
- Large numbers of virus particles may be demonstrated by electron microscopy in faecal samples from cats with acute disease.
- Typical histopathological changes may be present in sections of the ileum and jejunum. Intranuclear inclusion bodies may be detected in crypt cells.
- Viral antigen can be detected in faeces using ELISA or haemagglutination employing pig or Rhesus monkey red cells. Commercially available canine parvovirus kit sets can be used for the detection of feline panleukopenia virus antigen (Addie *et al.*, 1998).
- A rising antibody titre may be detected in serum samples by a number of tests including the haemagglutination-inhibition (HAI) or virus neutralization (VN) tests.

Treatment

No specific treatment is available.

- Intensive supportive therapy is usually necessary:
  — Appropriate fluid therapy for dehydration should be given.
  — Whole blood or plasma from immune donors may be beneficial in cats with anaemia or hypoproteinaemia.
  — Parenterally administered broad-spectrum antibiotics can be used to combat secondary bacterial infections.
- Affected animals should be housed in a clean, warm environment and maintained on an optimal diet supplemented with B complex vitamins.

Control

Vaccination is the principal control measure. There is only one serotype of feline panleukopenia virus and immunity following natural infection is strong and long-lasting.

- Modified live and inactivated vaccines are commercially available:
  — Inactivated vaccines are less effective than modified live vaccines and require booster inoculations. They are safe for pregnant queens and might be considered for vaccination of Siamese and Burmese kittens which can have adverse reactions to modified live vaccines (Carwardine, 1990).
  — Modified live vaccines can be used to immunize kittens at 8 to 10 weeks of age, with a booster dose at 12 to 14 weeks of age. Annual booster vaccinations are recommended by vaccine manufacturers. These vaccines should not be used in pregnant queens because replicating virus may cause cerebellar hypoplasia in developing foetuses.
  — Cats should have completed a vaccination schedule

or should be given a booster injection at least two weeks before introduction to premises where feline panleukopenia has recently occurred.

- Clinical infections cause heavy environmental contamination. Premises should be thoroughly disinfected with 1% sodium hypochlorite or 2% formalin (Scott, 1980). Cats on such premises should be vaccinated without delay.

Canine parvovirus infection

Infection with canine parvovirus (CPV) emerged in the late 1970s as a worldwide disease in dogs with high morbidity and mortality. Acute or subacute heart failure in pups infected *in utero* or during the perinatal period, was a common manifestation of the disease. With the gradual development of immunity in the adult dog population, as a consequence of both natural exposure and vaccination, the clinical pattern of the disease changed. The most common clinical presentation now encountered is acute enteric disease in young dogs between weaning and 6 months of age. Since the appearance of CPV in 1978, further mutations affecting the genome and antigenicity of the virus have occurred. Three subtypes of the virus are currently recognized. Infection or vaccination with one subtype confers immunity against the other subtypes (Greenwood *et al.*, 1995). Canine parvovirus is now considered to be a host-range mutant of feline panleukopenia virus or a closely related parvovirus.

Epidemiology
Many canine species are susceptible to infection and transmission is predominantly by the faecal-oral route. Infected dogs shed large numbers of viruses in their faeces. The number of viruses in faeces may be 10^9/g from the fifth or sixth day after infection. Persistent shedding is uncommon and the continued presence of the disease in dog populations depends mainly on the stability of the virus in the environment. The low dose of virus required to establish infection and the ease with which mechanical transfer can take place are important additional factors contributing to the spread of infection.

Pathogenesis and pathology
The virus replicates initially in pharyngeal lymphoid tissues and Peyer's patches. Viraemia develops and the main target tissues are those with rapidly multiplying cell populations. During the first two weeks of life there is active cardiac myocyte division allowing viral replication with resultant necrosis and myocarditis. In older pups, the virus invades the actively dividing epithelial cells of the crypts in the small intestine. Loss of cells from the intestinal crypts leads to blunting of villi, with resultant reduced absorptive and digestive capacity leading to diarrhoea. There may be extensive haemorrhage into the intestinal lumen in severely affected pups. Destruction of lymphoid tissues of the intestinal mucosa and mesenteric lymph nodes contributes to immunosuppression which allows proliferation of Gram-negative bacteria with secondary invasion of damaged intestinal tissues. Endotoxaemia, leading to endotoxic shock, may follow.

Clinical signs

The age and the immune status of the animal largely determine the form and severity of the disease. After a short incubation period of four to seven days, animals with enteric disease show sudden onset of vomiting and anorexia. Depression and fever may also be observed. Diarrhoea, often blood-stained, develops within 48 hours and in severe cases, there may be frank haemorrhage. The faeces have a foetid smell. Concurrent intestinal parasitism and viral or bacterial infections may exacerbate the condition. Affected dogs deteriorate rapidly due to dehydration and weight loss. Prolonged illness is uncommon; severely affected animals die within three days. Animals which survive the disease develop a long-lasting immunity.

In the myocardial form of the disease, which is now rare, affected pups usually show signs of acute heart failure before eight weeks of age. Some pups may develop congestive heart failure months after the initial infection, as a result of extensive fibrosis following myocardial necrosis.

Diagnosis
- Samples for laboratory examination should include faeces, blood and other tissues, particularly affected portions of intestines and myocardium.
- The nature and distribution of the gross and microscopic enteric lesions may point to a parvoviral infection. Immunocytochemical staining can confirm the presence of viral antigen in tissue sections.
- The presence of basophilic intranuclear inclusions in cardiac myocytes is confirmatory.
- A leukopenia may be detected, particularly in severely affected animals.
- Definitive diagnosis in clinically affected animals early in the course of the disease relies on the demonstration of virus or viral antigen in faeces:
  — Numerous virus particles can be demonstrated by electron microscopy.
  — ELISA or HA may be used to demonstrate viral antigen.
- Virus can be isolated in a number of suitable canine and feline cell lines.
- Serological tests, including HAI, VN and indirect immunofluorescence, may confirm the diagnosis.

Treatment
No specific treatment is available.

- Intensive supportive therapy including anti-emetics and fluid administration is required for the treatment of parvoviral enteritis.
- Broad-spectrum antibiotics, administered parenterally, reduce the risk of secondary bacterial infections.
- Dogs with subacute or chronic heart failure may improve with rest and diuretic therapy.

Control

Vaccination alone usually cannot control the cycle of endemic parvovirus infection in kennels and therefore it is important to minimize exposure of pups to the virus until they reach 20 weeks of age (Pollock and Coyne, 1993). Non-protective, low levels of maternal antibody can interfere with the efficacy of some modified live vaccines. In many pups these critical levels last until eight to twelve weeks of age, but in some instances interference with vaccination continues until 18 weeks of age (O'Brien, 1994).

- Inactivated and modified live vaccines are commercially available:
  — Inactivated vaccines usually provide protection for up to one year and are safe to use in pregnant bitches.
  — Although modified live vaccines generally give good, long-lasting protection, annual boosters may be required. These vaccines should not be used for pregnant bitches. Modified live vaccines vary in their degree of viral attenuation. The less attenuated strains of vaccinal viruses can replicate in pups despite the presence of residual maternal antibodies (Churchill, 1987; Burtonboy *et al.*, 1991) and vaccination of pups at 12 weeks of age is often claimed by vaccine manufacturers to be protective.
- Thorough disinfection of premises must be carried out following a disease outbreak:
  — Effective disinfectants include 1% sodium hypochlorite and 2% formalin.
  — Fumigation with formaldehyde gas, where feasible, is the most efficient disinfection procedure.

Porcine parvovirus infection

Porcine parvovirus is an important cause of reproductive failure in pigs. The virus, which occurs as a single serotype, is found worldwide and infection is endemic in many conventional pig herds.

Epidemiology

On farms where the disease is endemic, many sows are immune. They remain seropositive for up to four years and transmit passive protection through colostrum to their piglets. Maternally-derived immunity usually persists for about four months, but it can persist in some pigs until they are six to nine months of age. During this period, the maternally-derived antibodies may interfere with the development of active immunity and consequently some gilts can be seronegative and susceptible to infection at mating. Infected pigs shed virus in their faeces and other secretions, including semen, for only a few weeks. However, pens may remain contaminated for several months because of the exceptional stability of the virus.

Pathogenesis

After infection by the oronasal route and occasionally through semen, local replication of virus is followed by viraemia. The virus has a predilection for the mitotically active cells of foetal tissues. Transplacental infection in pregnant sows occurs 10 to 14 days after exposure to the virus. The major damage to foetuses arises before onset of immunocompetence, at about 60 to 70 days of gestation (Huysman *et al.*, 1992). Infection of embryos in the first weeks of life results in death and resorption. When infection occurs later in gestation, but before day 70, foetuses die and become mummified. Infection after 70 days of gestation usually results in the birth of healthy seropositive piglets.

Clinical signs

Porcine parvovirus infection is a major cause of SMEDI, an acronym used to describe porcine reproductive failure in which **s**tillbirths, **m**ummified foetuses, **e**arly **e**mbryonic **d**eath and **i**nfertility occur. Abortion and neonatal deaths have been reported occasionally. Generally, small litters with mummified piglets of different sizes are produced following transplacental infection and subsequent sequential exposure of foetuses by intrauterine spread. If the number of viable embryos is reduced below four, the entire litter is usually lost. Infection with porcine parvovirus does not appear to damage the male reproductive tract.

Diagnosis

- When reproductive failure is detected in young or recently introduced sows, particularly if associated with mummified foetuses, infection with porcine parvovirus must be considered.
- Several foetuses should be submitted for laboratory examination.
- Demonstration of viral antigen in cryostat sections of foetal tissues, particularly in the lungs, by immunofluorescence is reliable and sensitive.
- Agglutination of guinea-pig erythrocytes by homogenates of foetal tissue indicates the presence of viral haemagglutinin.
- Swine kidney cell lines may be used for virus isolation. However, viral infectivity is gradually lost following death of the foetus and isolation from mummified tissues may be unsuccessful.
- Serological techniques include HAI and VN tests. Antibodies may be detected in sera or body fluids of

older foetuses or aborted piglets. However, serological testing is usually of little diagnostic value in endemically infected herds.

Control

Control in herds in which the disease is endemic is based on exposure of gilts and susceptible sows to porcine parvovirus prior to mating, thereby inducing immunity. Vaccination can be used to enhance immunity in herds with endemic disease. It can also be used for male or female breeding stock introduced into these herds.

- Natural exposure can be achieved by increasing the contact between susceptible gilts and older seropositive sows. Methods of stimulating immunity include exposing animals to contaminated faeces or to placental or foetal tissue from infected sows.
- Modified live and inactivated vaccines against the single serotype of porcine parvovirus have been developed experimentally, but only inactivated vaccines are available commercially. Gilts and susceptible seronegative sows and boars should be vaccinated two to four weeks before mating. Vaccination prevents intrauterine infection for a limited period. Most vaccination strategies rely on subsequent natural exposure to the virus to reinforce immunity (Huysman et al., 1992).

References

Addie, D.D., Toth, S., Thompson, H. *et al.* (1998). Detection of feline parvovirus in dying pedigree kittens. *Veterinary Record*, **142**, 353–356.

Burtonboy, S., Charlier, P., Hertoghs, J., *et al.* (1991). Performance of high titre attenuated canine parvovirus vaccine in pups with maternally derived antibody. *Veterinary Record*, **128**, 377–381.

Carwardine P. (1990). Adverse reactions to vaccine. *Veterinary Record*, **127**, 243.

Churchill, A.E. (1987). Preliminary development of a live attenuated canine parvovirus vaccine from an isolate of British origin. *Veterinary Record*, **120**, 334–339.

Greenwood, N.M., Chalmers, W.S.K., Baxendale, W. and Thompson, H. (1995). Comparison of isolates of canine parvovirus by restriction enzyme analysis, and vaccine efficacy against field strains. *Veterinary Record,* **136**, 63–67.

Huysman, C.N., van Leengoed, L.A.M.G., de Jong, M.C.M. and van Osta, A.L.M. (1992). Reproductive failure associated with porcine parvovirus in an enzootically infected pig herd. *Veterinary Record*, **131**, 503–506.

O'Brien, S.E. (1994). Serologic response of pups to the low-passage modified live canine parvovirus-2 component in a combination vaccine. *Journal of the American Veterinary Medical Association*, **204**, 1207–1209.

Pollock, R.V.H. and Coyne, M.J. (1993). Canine parvovirus. *Veterinary Clinics of North America: Small Animal Practice*, **23**, 555-568.

Scott, F.W. (1980). Virucidal disinfectants and feline viruses. *American Journal of Veterinary Research*, **41**, 410–414.

Welchman, D. de B., Oxenham, M. and Done, S.H. (1993). Aleutian disease in domestic ferrets: diagnostic findings and survey results. *Veterinary Record*, **132**, 479–484.

Further reading

Tijssen, P. (1990). *CRC Handbook of Parvoviruses*, Volumes. 1 and 2. CRC Press, Florida.

Chapter 60

Circoviridae

Viruses in the recently established family *Circoviridae* cause disease in vertebrate animals and plants. Circoviruses (17 to 22 nm in diameter), are non-enveloped with icosahedral symmetry (Fig. 60.1). They are stable in the environment at pH 3 to pH 9 and are resistant to heating at 60°C for 30 minutes.

The genome consists of a molecule of circular single-stranded DNA. Replication occurs in the nuclei of dividing cells. Recent genetic sequencing studies suggest that circoviruses fall into three groups (Niagro *et al.*, 1998) and this is reflected in recent classification changes. Chicken anaemia virus (22 nm in diameter), the type species, has been assigned to the newly created genus, *Gyrovirus*. The animal circoviruses (17 nm in diameter), porcine circovirus and beak and feather disease virus have been assigned to the genus *Circovirus*. The third grouping contains plant viruses which have now been removed from the family and placed in the unassigned genus *Nanovirus*.

Key points

- Small, non-enveloped single-stranded DNA viruses with icosahedral symmetry
- Replicate in the nucleus of dividing cells
- Stable in the environment
- Circoviruses cause infections in chickens, pigs and plants

Clinical infections

Circoviruses, which are host-specific and have a world-wide distribution, infect cells of the haemolymphatic system. Infections with chicken anaemia virus and with porcine circovirus are of veterinary interest. Beak and feather disease virus is associated with a debilitating, immunosuppressive disease of young pscittacine birds, particularly cockatoos.

Chicken anaemia virus infection

Young birds infected with chicken anaemia virus (CAV) develop aplastic anaemia and generalized lymphoid atrophy. This virus, which infects only chickens, is present in poultry flocks worldwide. All of the field isolates of the virus appear to be equally pathogenic and belong to a single serotype.

Epidemiology
Both horizontal and vertical transmission occur. Infection is by the faecal-oral route. Vertical transmission through the egg occurs during the one to three week viraemic period following infection in laying hens. Once infection is established in a breeder flock, most birds develop antibody before laying begins. Maternally-derived antibodies do not prevent chicks from becoming infected and shedding the virus. However, they prevent the development of clinical disease. An age resistance to disease but not to infection develops in chicks at about two weeks of age. In breeding flocks containing many serologically-positive adult birds, subclinical infection is common in chickens. However, age resistance and the

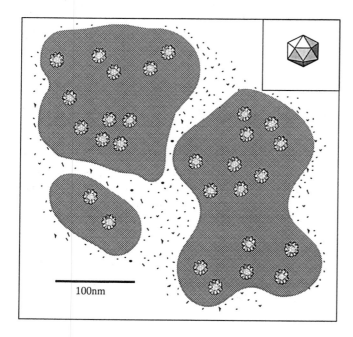

Figure 60.1 Circovirus particles as they appear in an electron micrograph and a diagrammatic representation (inset).

100nm

protective effect of maternally-derived antibodies can be overcome if infections with other immunosuppressive viruses, such as infectious bursal disease virus or gallid herpesvirus 2, are present.

Pathogenesis and pathology

Viraemia develops following infection of susceptible day old chicks and virus can be recovered from most organs and from faeces for about three or four weeks. The principal target cells are precursor T cells in the thymus and haemocytoblasts in the bone marrow. Destruction of these cells results in immunosuppression and anaemia. Gross postmortem findings include atrophy of the thymus tissues and bursa, pale bone marrow and haemorrhages under the skin and in skeletal muscle.

Clinical signs

Chickens develop clinical signs at about two weeks of age. Affected birds are depressed, anorexic and pale. The mortality rate, which is usually about 10%, may be up to 50%. Birds which survive the acute phase of the disease recover slowly. Subclinical infection in broilers from breeder flocks can adversely affect weight gains.

Diagnosis

A presumptive diagnosis is based on the clinical signs and gross lesions at postmortem. Laboratory confirmation relies on detection of viral antigen by immunocytochemical techniques. Viral DNA can be demonstrated in bone marrow and thymus by *in situ* hybridization, by dot-blot hybridization or by PCR. Virus isolation, although possible, is exacting and expensive. Serum antibodies can be detected using virus neutralization, indirect immunofluorescence and ELISA. A commercial ELISA is available and can be used to identify seronegative breeder flocks before laying begins.

Control

Because infection with CAV is common, it is difficult to maintain breeder flocks free of infection. Breeding birds should be exposed to infection before laying commences. Seronegative flocks can be deliberately exposed to virus by transfer of old litter from CAV-positive farms or by the addition of crude tissue homogenates from affected birds to drinking water but such exposure is unreliable and inherently unsafe.

A live vaccine is available in some European countries. Vaccination does not prevent economic losses in broilers due to subclinical infection. Control of other immunosuppressive viruses in CAV-positive flocks is essential due to the additive effects of these infections.

Pig circovirus infection

Porcine circovirus was first described as a picornavirus-like contaminant of the continuous pig kidney cell line PK/15. Experimental challenge suggests that this virus, termed porcine circovirus 1, is of doubtful pathogenicity. Recently, an antigenically and genomically distinct circovirus, porcine circovirus 2 (PCV 2) was isolated from piglets with wasting disease. Sero-epidemiological studies indicate that infection with PCV 2 is widespread in pig populations worldwide. Post-weaning multisystemic wasting syndrome (PMWS), a progressive wasting condition with lesions in several organ systems, was first described in Canada in 1991 in specific pathogen-free herds (Allan and Ellis, 2000). This syndrome is believed to be caused by infection with PCV 2. Affected animals, which are usually about six weeks of age, present with weight loss, dyspnoea and enlarged lymph nodes. The mortality rate may reach 10% in severe outbreaks. Adverse environmental factors or concurrent infections with other agents appear to be essential for the development of clinical disease. The diagnosis of PMWS is based on clinical signs and pathological findings. Antibodies to PCV 2 may be detected using indirect immunofluorescence or ELISA. Virus isolation in pig cell lines is also indicative of infection. A definitive diagnosis requires demonstration of PCV 2 antigen or viral nucleic acid in association with lesions. No vaccine is currently available. The resistance of the virus to detergents makes decontamination of infected premises difficult. Control is based on good husbandry, rapid removal of affected animals and the elimination of other infectious agents. It has been suggested that PCV 2 may be aetiologically involved in the porcine dermatitis and nephropathy syndrome.

References

Allan, G.M. and Ellis, J.A. (2000). Porcine circoviruses: a review. *Journal of Veterinary Diagnostic Investigation*, **12**, 3–14.

Niagro, F.D., Forsthoefel, A.N., Lawther, R.P. *et al.* (1998). Beak and feather disease virus and porcine circovirus genomes: intermediates between the geminviruses and plant circoviruses. *Archives of Virology*, **143**, 1723–1744.

Further reading

Done, S., Gresham, A., Potter, R. and Chennells, D. (2001). PMWS and PDNS – two recently recognised diseases of pigs in the UK. *In Practice*, **23**, 14–21.

Chapter 61

Retroviridae

Retroviruses (Latin *retro*, backwards) are labile enveloped RNA viruses, 80 to 100 nm in diameter. Seven genera are currently assigned to the family: *Alpharetrovirus*, *Betaretrovirus*, *Gammaretrovirus*, *Deltaretrovirus*, *Epsilonretrovirus*, *Lentivirus* and *Spumavirus* (Fig 61.1). The family name refers to the presence, in the virion, of a reverse transcriptase which is encoded in the viral genome.

The envelope, which is acquired from the plasma membrane of the host cell, surrounds an icosahedral capsid containing two linear, positive-sense, single strands of RNA and core proteins including the enzymes reverse transcriptase and integrase (Fig. 61.2). Historically, based on electron microscopy, retroviruses were categorized as A-type, B-type, C-type and D-type particles.

Reverse transcriptase acts as an RNA-dependent DNA polymerase, which transcribes from RNA to DNA. Four major genes, contained in the RNA genome of members of the *Retroviridae*, are *gag*, *pro*, *pol* and *env*. The *gag* (group specific antigen) gene encodes internal structural proteins. The *pro* (protease) gene encodes the enzyme protease while the *pol* (polymerase) gene encodes the enzymes reverse transcriptase and integrase. The *env* (envelope) gene encodes surface (SU) and transmembrane (TM) envelope glycoproteins. Cell entry follows attachment of an envelope glycoprotein to specific cell receptors. Under the influence of the reverse transcriptase, double-stranded DNA copies of the viral genome are synthesized in the cytoplasm of the host cell. During this process, repeat base sequences, containing several hundred base-pairs and called long terminal repeats (LTR), are added to the ends of the DNA transcripts. Transcripts are integrated into the chromosomal DNA, as provirus, at random sites through the action of viral integrase. The sites of proviral integration determine the extent and nature of cellular changes. The LTR contain important promoter and enhancer sequences, which are involved in the transcription of mRNA and virion RNA from provirus. Release of mature virions often occurs by budding from cell membranes (Figs. 61.3 and 61.4). If the provirus of certain retroviruses is inserted close to the host genes which regulate cell division, the proviral LTR may increase the rate of mitosis resulting in neoplasia (insertional mutagenesis).

A high mutation rate is a feature of retroviral replication because errors are relatively frequent during reverse transcription. In addition, recombination between retroviral genomes in doubly-infected cells can occur because reverse transcriptase can transfer from the RNA template of one virus to that of another. Consequently, antigenically different retroviruses frequently emerge and classification of species and subtypes often proves difficult.

Retroviruses can be categorized as endogenous or exogenous. Endogenous retroviruses occur widely among vertebrates. They resulted at some time from infection of germline cells and are transmitted only as provirus in germ cell DNA from parent to offspring. They are regulated by cellular genes and are usually silent. Endogenous retroviral genomes may contribute *env* genes to produce recombinant feline leukaemia viruses and avian leukosis viruses. Occasionally, they can be activated by irradiation, mutagens or carcinogens with the production of new virions. Endogenous retroviruses of pigs may be potentially dangerous in humans receiving xenotransplants.

Key points

- Enveloped, spherical labile viruses
- Diploid, containing two linear positive-sense single strands of RNA
- Icosahedral capsid surrounds helical nucleocapsid
- Members of this family are unique in possessing a reverse transcriptase which transcribes viral RNA to double-stranded DNA
- Double-stranded DNA is inserted as a provirus into the host genome
- Mutation and recombination occur with high frequency
- The family is composed of seven genera:
  —*Lentivirus* contains viruses which usually cause immunodeficiency diseases
  —*Spumavirus* contains viruses which cause cell vacuolation *in vitro* but do not produce disease
  —Viruses in the remaining five genera can induce neoplastic change in specific cell types

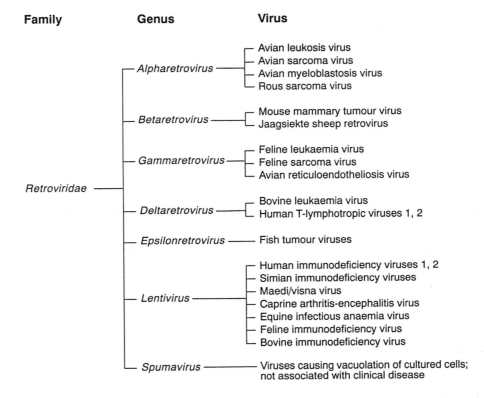

Figure 61.1 Classification of retroviruses with emphasis on those which produce disease or induce cellular changes *in vitro*.

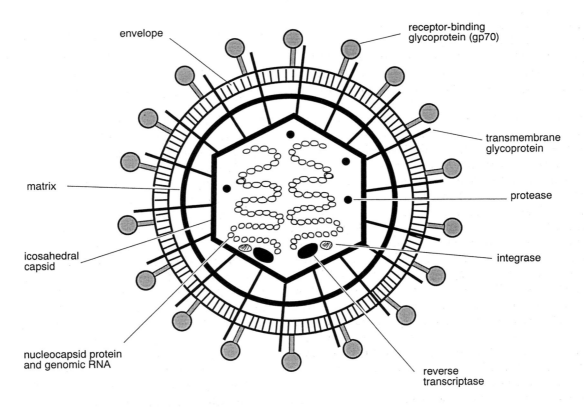

Figure 61.2 Schematic representation of the structures and components of a retrovirus virion.

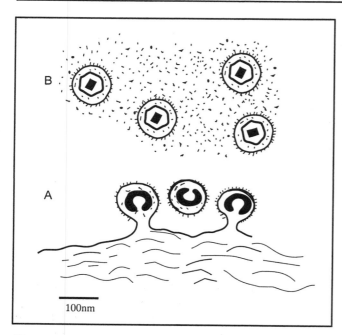

Figure 61.3 A. Budding of a typical type C retrovirus, with crescent-shaped nucleocapsid, from a cell membrane; B. Mature, extracellular type C retrovirus virions.

Retroviruses are sensitive to heat, lipid solvents and detergents. Because of their diploid genomes, they are relatively resistant to UV light.

Clinical infections

Retroviruses in the genera *Alpharetrovirus*, *Betaretrovirus*, *Gammaretrovirus*, *Deltaretrovirus* and *Epsilonretrovirus* are frequently referred to as oncogenic retroviruses because they can induce neoplastic transformation in cells which they infect.

On the basis of the interval between exposure to the virus and tumour development, exogenous oncogenic retroviruses are designated either as slowly transforming (*cis*-activating) viruses or as rapidly transforming (transducing) viruses. Slowly transforming retroviruses induce B cell, T cell or myeloid tumours after long incubation periods. For malignant transformation to occur, the provirus must be integrated into the host cell DNA close to a cellular oncogene (c-*onc*, proto-oncogene), resulting in interference with the regulation of cell division. Rapidly transforming retroviruses, which can induce tumour formation after short incubation periods, contain viral oncogenes (v-*onc*). Viral oncogenes are considered to be cellular oncogenes acquired by recombination during virus evolution. If the oncogene is integrated into the viral genome without loss of replicative virus genes, as in Rous sarcoma virus, the retrovirus is described as replication-competent. Frequently, as a consequence of cellular oncogene integration, existing viral sequences necessary for replication are deleted. Such replication-defective retroviruses, which cannot multiply without helper viruses, are rarely transmitted under normal field conditions. Occasionally, they may cause rapidly-developing neoplastic disease. A third method of tumour induction is exemplified by bovine leukaemia virus which depends on the *tax* gene encoding for a protein capable of up-regulating both viral LTR and cellular promoter sequences, even when the provirus is integrated into a different chromosome (*trans*-activation). A schematic representation of the important genes in various categories of oncogenic viruses is presented in Fig. 61.5.

The newly-established *Epsilonretrovirus* genus contains viruses associated with neoplasia in fish. The oncogenic retroviruses of poultry are presented in Table 61.1 and those of domestic mammals in Table 61.2.

Lentiviruses (Latin *lentus*, slow) cause diseases with long incubation periods and insidious protracted courses. Important animal and human diseases caused by lentiviruses include acquired immunodeficiency syndrome (AIDS), feline immunodeficiency, equine infectious anaemia and maedi/visna. Lentiviruses of domestic animals are presented in Table 61.3. Although spumaviruses (Latin *spuma*, foam) cause vacuolation of cultured cells, they are not associated with clinical disease. Spumaviruses have been identified in humans, cats and cattle.

Avian leukosis

The avian leukosis virus (ALV) group includes both replication-competent and replication-defective retroviruses. Neoplastic conditions in chickens including the

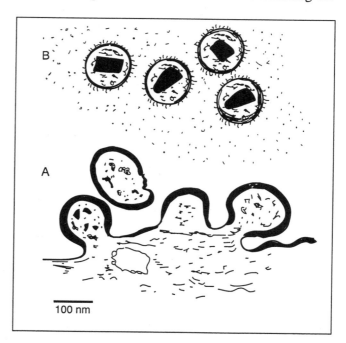

Figure 61.4 A. Budding of lentivirus particles from a cell membrane; B. Mature, extracellular lentivirus virions.

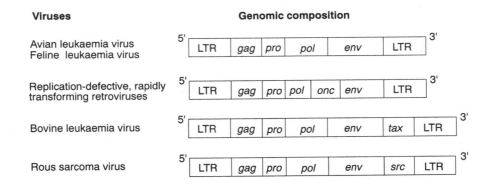

Viruses **Genomic composition**

Avian leukaemia virus
Feline leukaemia virus
5' LTR | gag | pro | pol | env | LTR 3'

Replication-defective, rapidly
transforming retroviruses
5' LTR | gag | pro | pol | onc | env | LTR 3'

Bovine leukaemia virus
5' LTR | gag | pro | pol | env | tax | LTR 3'

Rous sarcoma virus
5' LTR | gag | pro | pol | env | src | LTR 3'

Figure 61.5 Schematic representation of the important genes present in oncogenic retroviruses.

LTR: long terminal repeat sequences; *gag*: gene encoding group-specific antigen (core and capsid proteins); *pro*: gene encoding protease; *pol*: gene encoding polymerase (reverse transcriptase); *env*: gene encoding envelope glycoproteins; *onc*: oncogene; *tax*: transactivating gene; *src*: sarcoma gene

lymphoid, erythroid and myeloid leukoses, fibrosarcoma, haemangiosarcoma, and nephroblastoma are caused by viruses in the group. Lymphoid leukosis, a B cell lymphoma, is the most common of these neoplastic conditions and is economically the most important.

Avian leukosis viruses are divided into ten subgroups (A to J) on the basis of differences in viral envelope glycoproteins. Isolates from chickens belong to subgroups A, B, C, D, E and J; viruses in the other subgroups infect other avian species. Most isolates from outbreaks of disease in chickens belong to subgroup A. Endogenous avian leukosis viruses, which are commonly present in chickens and are transmitted vertically in the germ line cells, usually belong to subgroup E. Members of subgroup J, a group recently recognized in broilers, are associated with myeloid leukosis and have arisen from recombination of a novel family of endogenous viruses (ev/J) and exogenous avian leukosis viruses (Benson *et al.*, 1998).

There is usually an incubation period of months to years between natural infection with ALV and the development of neoplasia, because of the time required for the genetic events to occur that lead to transformation of cells to malignancy. Neoplastic conditions associated with ALV include lymphoid leukosis, myeloid leukosis, sarcomas and renal tumours. Avian leukosis virus is also associated with osteopetrosis. One of the final steps in oncogenesis can be the generation of recombinant, rapidly transforming viruses, which have incorporated a cellular oncogene into their genome. Viruses isolated from such tumours include avian erythroblastosis virus, avian myeloblastosis virus and Rous sarcoma virus, all of which rapidly cause tumours when inoculated experimentally into susceptible chickens. These viruses are usually defective and require a helper ALV for replication. Rous sarcoma virus is exceptional in that it has an oncogene (*src*) in addition to a complete ALV genome, and consequently is replication competent as well as capable of rapid cell transformation *in vivo* and *in vitro*. This type of acutely transforming virus is very seldom, if ever, transmitted under natural conditions. The endogenous ALVs carried by chickens in most flocks do not directly cause tumours.

Epidemiology
Exogenous ALV is transmitted both vertically, through virus present in egg albumen, and horizontally, by close contact. Chicks which hatch from infected eggs are usually immunotolerant and exhibit persistent viraemia. They are the principal source of virus in a flock. Virus is transmitted in saliva and faeces to in-contact birds. Viral shedding into oviducts results in transmission to chick embryos. Chicks infected after hatching develop a transient viraemia before they produce neutralizing

Table 61.1 Oncogenic retroviruses of poultry.

Genus	Virus	Hosts	Comments
Alpharetrovirus	Avian leukosis virus	Chickens, pheasants, partridge, quail	Endemic in commercial flocks. Exogenous and endogenous transmission of virus can occur. Causes lymphoid leukosis in birds between 5 and 9 months of age
Gammaretrovirus	Reticuloendotheliosis virus	Turkeys, ducks, chickens, quail, pheasants	Infection usually subclinical. Sporadic disease may present with anaemia, feathering defects, impaired growth or neoplasia. Disease outbreaks have occurred following use of vaccine contaminated with reticuloendotheliosis virus

Table 61.2 Oncogenic retroviruses of domestic mammals.

Genus	Virus	Hosts	Comments
Betaretrovirus	Jaagsiekte sheep retrovirus (ovine pulmonary adenocarcinoma virus)	Sheep	Causes jaagsiekte, a slowly progressive neoplastic lung disease of adult sheep which is invariably fatal. Occurs worldwide except in Australasia
	Enzootic nasal tumour virus	Sheep	Closely related to Jaagsiekte sheep retrovirus. Causes adenocarcinoma of low grade malignancy which affects the nares
Gammaretrovirus	Feline leukaemia virus	Cats	Important cause of chronic illness and death in young adult cats. Causes immunosuppression, enteritis, reproductive failure, anaemia and neoplasia. Worldwide in distribution
Deltaretrovirus	Bovine leukaemia virus	Cattle	Causes enzootic bovine leukosis in adult cattle. A small percentage of infected cattle develop lymphosarcoma

antibodies. These birds often become carriers, shed virus intermittently and may produce infected chicks. Natural exposure of adult birds to infection does not usually result in virus shedding. Neoplasms develop most often in persistently-viraemic birds. Virus-neutralizing antibodies are passed from antibody-positive hens in the yolk sac to their chicks, providing passive immunity to infection for the first few weeks of life.

Pathogenesis

Following infection, virus spreads throughout the body, replicating in most tissues. Avian leukosis virus transforms B cells after integration of provirus close to the c-*myc* gene which induces cellular replication under the influence of the viral LTR promoter. Less commonly, ALV has been associated with erythroblastosis when the c-*erb*B gene in an erythroid cell is activated. Subgroup J isolates are associated with late onset myeloid leukosis in broilers (Benson *et al.*, 1998). Rapidly-transforming viruses are formed rarely in individual birds by transfer of a c-*onc* (proto-oncogene) into the ALV provirus during its integration. Multiple insertions of the provirus into the host cell genome results in exaggerated gene expression and over-production of a transformation-associated protein. More than a dozen different oncogenes have been identified in transforming avian retroviruses. The protein products of oncogenes may act as hormone or growth factor receptors, transcription control factors and kinases in signal transduction pathways. Although a particular virus strain may be capable of producing neoplasia of more than one cell type, usually one cell type predominates in an affected animal.

Table 61.3 Lentiviruses of domestic animals.

Genus	Virus	Hosts	Comments
Lentivirus	Feline immunodeficiency virus	Cats	Causes life-long infection with persistent viraemia and immunosuppression in cats over 5 years of age. Worldwide distribution
	Equine infectious anaemia virus	Horses, mules, donkeys	Causes life-long infection with recurring febrile episodes. Anaemia is a prominent clinical sign
	Maedi/visna virus	Sheep	Causes life-long infection with progressive respiratory disease and indurative mastitis in older sheep. Clinical signs develop in a small percentage of infected animals. Some infected sheep develop progressive neurological disease
	Caprine arthritis-encephalitis virus	Goats	Causes life-long infection. Associated with polyarthritis and indurative mastitis in adults and progressive nervous disease in kids. Common in dairy goat herds. Worldwide distribution
	Bovine immunodeficiency virus	Cattle	Widely distributed; pathogenicity currently uncertain
	Jembrana disease virus	Cattle	Closely related to bovine immunodeficiency virus but disease described only in Bali cattle in Indonesia. Acute disease which occurs within days of infection is characterized by fever, anorexia, enlarged lymph nodes and, in some instances, death. Animals which recover remain viraemic

Clinical signs

The incubation period for lymphoid leukosis is usually more than four months. Disease is generally sporadic in infected flocks but occasional epidemics have been described. Affected birds become inappetent, weak and emaciated. They have pale wattles and the liver and bursa of Fabricius may be enlarged. Osteopetrosis, in which the long bones of the legs become visibly thickened, sometimes accompanies lymphoid leukosis. Subclinical infections with ALV are associated with depressed egg production and fertility, decreased hatchability and growth rate, and increased death rates. Economic loss from lymphoid leukosis is mainly due to deaths in egg-laying and breeding birds between five and nine months of age.

Diagnosis

- Postmortem findings and histopathological determination of tumour type are usually diagnostic.
- Differentiation from Marek's disease is important and is based on the age of affected birds, the presence of bursal tumours, absence of thickening of peripheral nerves and histological assessment of neoplastic cell types.
- Virus isolation is difficult and not usually attempted.
- Commercial ELISA kits for the detection of ALV group-specific antigen are available. The presence of flock infection can be demonstrated by detecting antibodies in serum or egg yolk. Suitable assays include virus neutralization, ELISA and indirect immunofluorescence.
- The polymerase chain reaction has been adapted for the detection of ALV nucleic acid.

Control

The eradication of exogenous subgroup A ALV infection has been successfully achieved in most commercial chicken flocks. The cycle of vertical transmission is interrupted by hatching and rearing infection-free chicks in isolation. Ongoing monitoring for the presence of infection is essential. Because autosomal genes encode subgroup-specific cell surface receptors through which ALV gains entry to the cell, genetically resistant birds can be bred with decreased numbers of specific cell surface receptors. Attention has focussed largely on resistance to subgroup A viruses. Selection for genetic resistance is an ongoing process because mutant viruses capable of overcoming host resistance frequently arise. Control of ALV infection in commercial flocks is based on high standards of hygiene and effective management aimed at reducing levels of infection. Birds from disease-free or genetically-resistant stock should be used for breeding. Because the virus is labile, all-in all-out management systems along with thorough washing and disinfection programmes between batches of birds are effective. Chicks of uncertain status should not be mixed with disease-free chicks. Chick rearing should take place remote from older birds.

Vaccination with inactivated or modified live ALV vaccines has not been successful. Recombinant avian leukosis and fowlpox viruses expressing subgroup A envelope glycoproteins have been shown to have potential as effective vaccines.

Feline leukaemia and associated clinical conditions

Infection with feline leukaemia virus (FeLV) not only results in feline leukaemia but is also associated with a variety of other clinical conditions. Isolates of FeLV, a gammaretrovirus, are assigned to three subgroups (A, B and C) on the basis of differences in the gp70 envelope glycoprotein. Feline leukaemia virus A (FeLV-A), the predominant subgroup, is isolated from all FeLV-infected cats. Viruses of subgroup B, which arise through recombination between the *env* genes of FeLV-A and endogenous FeLV-related proviral DNA, are present in about 50% of isolates. FeLV-B is only transmitted together with FeLV-A. In a proportion of cats exposed to a mixture of FeLV-A and FeLV-B, the FeLV-B component is lost. Therefore, the continuing survival of FeLV-B depends upon the generation of new recombinants in cats persistently infected with FeLV-A. Cats that are infected with both FeLV-A and FeLV-B have a higher risk of developing tumours than those infected with FeLV-A alone. Each FeLV-C isolate is unique, arising *de novo* in a FeLV-A infected cat through mutations in the receptor-binding region of the FeLV-A *env* gene. Once generated, FeLV-C viruses rapidly cause a fatal anaemia and consequently are not transmitted to other cats.

Like the ALVs, FeLV causes tumours by several means, including insertional mutagenesis and recombination with a variety of cellular proto-oncogenes to produce acutely transforming, replication-defective viruses. Examples of the latter are FeLVs isolated from thymic lymphomas, and feline sarcoma viruses (FeSV) that are isolated from rare multicentric fibrosarcomas in young cats. These viruses are not transmitted under natural conditions.

Epidemiology

Infection with feline leukaemia virus, which occurs in domestic cats worldwide, is an important cause of mortality. Close contact is required for transmission of this labile virus and the incidence of infection is related to population density. Highest infection rates are found in catteries and multicat households. Large amounts of virus are shed in saliva with smaller quantities present in tears, urine, milk and faeces. Infection is usually acquired by licking, grooming and through bite wounds. Young kittens are more susceptible to infection than adults. Although maternally-derived antibody is protective in kittens up to six weeks of age, a significant proportion of those exposed before 14 weeks of age become persistently infected. Such animals constitute the main reservoir of FeLV and they are prone to develop an FeLV-related disease. Most cats, which are exposed after four months of age, develop immunity and eliminate the virus. Kittens born to persistently-infected queens develop persistent infection, acquired either transplacentally or through ingestion of milk.

Pathogenesis

Following oronasal exposure, virus replicates in the lymphoid tissues of the oropharyngeal region. The virus spreads in infected mononuclear leukocytes to other lymphoreticular tissues and bone marrow. In most cats, cell mediated immunity and neutralizing antibodies to the gp70 envelope glycoprotein are produced at this stage, usually resulting in virus elimination. However, a latent bone marrow infection, which is eliminated after several months, is present in about 50% of cats. Failure to contain the infection results in extensive virus production in the bone marrow and persistent viraemia. The virus, present in both leukocytes and the plasma, is disseminated to glandular and mucosal epithelia. Large quantities of virus are shed from the salivary glands and the upper respiratory tract. Because the production of virus particles requires cellular DNA synthesis, tissues with high mitotic activity such as bone marrow and epithelia are targeted. Prolonged periods of viral replication in haemolymphatic tissues can lead to depletion of lymphoid and myeloid cells producing immunosuppression and anaemia. Severe immunosuppression is caused by infection with certain strains of FeLV-A. Isolates of FeLV-C are associated with severe non-regenerative anaemia.

Neoplastic changes in lymphoid or myeloid cells follow insertion of provirus close to a cellular oncogene with activation or deregulation of the gene, or generation of acutely transforming viruses.

Clinical signs

The incubation period ranges from months to years. The majority of persistently-infected cats die within three years of infection. About 80% of these cats die from non-neoplastic FeLV-associated disease; the remaining 20% of infected cats succumb to neoplasia, particularly lymphosarcoma. During the early phase of infection, cats may develop fever, malaise and lymphadenopathy, which may not be detected clinically. A variable period as asymptomatic carriers follows. Clinical signs, which are often non-specific and chronic, are usually seen in young adult cats between two and four years of age. Anaemia, reduction in reproductive performance, enteritis and a variety of secondary infections due to the immunosuppressive effects of the virus are important features of the disease. Immune complex formation initiated by circulating antigen may give rise to glomerulonephritis.

Lymphosarcoma, the most commonly occurring feline tumour, is usually linked to infection with FeLV. Thymic, alimentary, multicentric and leukaemic forms of lymphosarcoma are described and clinical signs relate to the anatomical sites involved. Fibrosarcoma and myeloid tumours, which have also been associated with FeLV infection, occur less frequently than lymphosarcoma.

Diagnosis

Detection of viral antigen in blood or saliva is the method commonly used for the laboratory diagnosis of feline leukaemia. Virus isolation, which is expensive and time-consuming, is used as a confirmatory test.

- Commercial ELISA and rapid immunomigration tests, designed to detect the major capsid protein (p27), are available.
- The immunofluorescent antibody test can be used to detect viral antigen in the cytoplasm of leukocytes in blood smears. It is commonly employed as a confirmatory test because it is more sensitive and specific than ELISA.
- Serological testing for antibodies is not used for diagnosis since viraemic cats are immunotolerant and do not have anti-FeLV antibodies. However, the demonstration of virus neutralizing antibodies indicates that a cat is immune and resistant to infection.
- An antigen termed feline oncovirus-associated cell membrane antigen (FOCMA) is expressed in all FeLV- and FeSV-transformed cells. The development of antibodies to FOCMA provides protection against FeLV-associated neoplasia.

Control

A test and removal policy has been shown to be effective in eradicating infection from catteries. The status of individual cats should be confirmed by retesting after 12 weeks. Infected cats, which must be separated from susceptible animals, should be excluded from breeding programmes. Serological testing at intervals of six months is recommended and cats about to be introduced into a cattery should be isolated until test results are known. Several commercial vaccines, including killed whole virus, recombinant canarypox virus, subunit and recombinant subunit types, are available. Vaccination does not alter the course of infection in persistently-infected cats. Accordingly, cats should be tested prior to vaccination. Vaccination does not provide complete protection and other appropriate control measures should be implemented.

Enzootic bovine leukosis

This retroviral disease of adult cattle is characterized by persistent lymphocytosis, the presence of circulating antibody to the causal agent bovine leukaemia virus (BLV) and the development of B cell lymphosarcoma in a number of infected animals. Enzootic bovine leukosis (EBL) has a worldwide distribution. Some countries have eradicated the disease; other countries are embarking on eradication programmes.

Epidemiology

Transmission, which can occur by direct contact or transplacentally, usually takes place through transfer of blood or secretions such as colostrum and milk containing infected lymphocytes. Infection with BLV is lifelong. The labile virus is intimately cell-associated.

Less than 10% of calves born to infected dams are infected at birth. Calves are protected from contact infection for several months by maternally-derived antibody. Animals are usually infected between six months and three years of age (Hopkins and DiGiacomo, 1997). Iatrogenic transmission is important and has been linked to reuse of needles, multidose injectors, contaminated surgical instruments and rectal examination procedures. While biting flies may transmit the virus mechanically, their importance as vectors is uncertain. The prevalence of infection is higher in dairy cattle than in beef cattle. Susceptibility to infection is influenced by genotype and related to the bovine major histocompatability antigen type.

Pathogenesis

The primary target cell is the B lymphocyte. Bovine leukaemia virus does not possess an oncogene. Nucleic acid sequences at the 3' end of the *env* gene termed the X region, encode for the regulatory proteins Tax and Rex which are central to neoplastic transformation. The Tax protein interacts with cellular transcription factors resulting in transactivation of the promoter in the LTR of integrated BLV provirus. Upregulation of some cellular genes including those coding for IL-2 and its receptor may also occur.

Clinical signs

Although infections are lifelong, most animals remain subclinically infected. About 30% of infected animals develop persistent lymphocytosis, an increase in lymphocyte numbers in the blood without clinical signs of disease. A small percentage of BLV-seropositive cattle eventually develop lymphosarcoma. Clinical disease usually occurs in adult animals between four and eight years of age. The presenting signs, which relate to the sites of tumour formation, include enlargement of superficial lymph nodes, digestive disturbance, inappetence, weight loss and general debility.

Diagnosis

Enzootic bovine leukosis (EBL) must be differentiated from sporadic bovine leukosis which usually affects calves and young adult cattle. Formerly, blood lymphocyte counts were employed for laboratory diagnosis of infected animals and for the eradication of EBL. However,

all infected cattle do not develop lymphocytosis. Serological testing for virus-specific antibody is now used for diagnosis and eradication.

- Several serological tests including AGID, ELISA and radioimmune assay are suitable for the detection of antibodies to BLV. Antibodies detected in calves less than six months of age may be of colostral origin.
- Although virus can be isolated by cultivation of peripheral blood lymphocytes, this technique is not performed routinely.
- The polymerase chain reaction has been developed as a sensitive research tool for the detection of provirus in peripheral blood lymphocytes.

Control

No commercial vaccine is currently available. Test and removal strategies have been successfully used for both national and individual herd eradication programmes. Serological testing at six month intervals is recommended (Brunner *et al.*, 1997). In countries in which the prevalence of BLV infection is too high to permit removal of all seropositive animals from herds, management practices aimed at reducing the spread of infection should be adopted. Such practices include separating infected and susceptible animals, rearing calves on milk from non-infected cows and serological testing of replacement animals.

Jaagsiekte

This lentiviral disease, also called ovine pulmonary adenomatosis, is a slowly-progressing neoplastic disease of adult sheep. It is caused by jaagsiekte sheep retrovirus (JSRV), also known as ovine pulmonary adenocarcinoma virus. Jaagsiekte is an Afrikaaner word meaning 'panting sickness'. With the exception of Australasia, jaagsiekte has a wide geographical distribution. The infection occurs rarely in goats. Multiple copies of endogenous retroviruses related to JSRV have been found in the genomes of both sheep and goats. Jaagsiekte sheep retrovirus is not considered to be endogenous.

Epidemiology

Respiratory exudates from affected sheep are infectious and transmission occurs by the respiratory route. Close contact facilitates spread of infection with the incidence of disease highest in housed animals. Within an infected flock, disease incidence may be up to 20%; it is influenced by breed and type of flock management.

Pathogenesis

The virus replicates in two types of pulmonary cells, type II alveolar cells and non-ciliated bronchial cells. Tumours arising from these cell types progressively replace normal lung tissue leading to death from asphyxia. About 10% of the tumours metastasize to regional lymph nodes. Metastasis to heart or skeletal muscle occurs rarely. As the presence of an oncogene has not been demonstrated in the viral genome, the mechanism of neoplastic transformation is unclear. Recent studies indicate that the envelope protein has transformation potential (Maeda *et al.*, 2001).

Clinical signs

The incubation period may range from several months up to two years. Tumour nodules have been detected in lambs as early as ten days after experimental inoculation. Affected animals are usually three to four years of age and in poor bodily condition. They display respiratory embarrassment and mouth breathing, particularly after exercise. By raising the hindlegs and lowering the head (wheelbarrow test), a clear fluid flows from the nostrils. Moist rales may be heard. Often, only a single animal in a flock may be clinically affected. The course of the disease may extend over weeks or months. Secondary pasteurellosis is a frequent complication.

Diagnosis

The characteristic clinical signs may be masked in individual cases by secondary infection. Histopathological confirmation is desirable. Attempts to culture the virus in monolayers have been unsuccessful. It is possible to detect virus in lung exudates or washings by ELISA and viral nucleic acid may be detected by PCR. As infected animals do not appear to develop a specific humoral immune response (Ortin *et al.*, 1998), it is not possible currently to confirm infection by serology.

Control

Jaagsiekte was successfully eradicated from Iceland in 1952 after drastic depopulation procedures. The incidence of disease in a flock can be reduced by strict isolation and elimination of suspect animals immediately after clinical or laboratory confirmation.

Feline immunodeficiency virus infection

This condition was first reported in 1987 and infection with feline immunodeficiency virus (FIV), a lentivirus, is now recognised worldwide as an important cause of disease in cats. The infection in cats is sometimes referred to as 'feline AIDS' on account of similarities to acquired immunodeficiency syndrome (AIDS) caused by human immunodeficiency virus. Five subtypes of FIV have been identified based on diversity in the envelope gene amino acid sequences. This diversity may account for differences in the pathogenesis and clinical progression of the disease associated with different isolates.

Epidemiology

Infection with FIV occurs in domestic cats. Related lentiviruses have been isolated from a number of wild *Felidae*, including pumas and lions. Animals remain infected for life. Virus is shed mainly in the saliva and transmission usually occurs through bites. Accordingly, infection rates are highest in free-roaming, adult male cats. Non-aggressive intimate contact may also be important in transmission under natural conditions. Queens may transmit infection to kittens *in utero*, during parturition or in milk, particularly during the acute phase of infection.

Pathogenesis

The virus replicates principally in CD4$^+$ (helper) T lymphocytes. Replication also occurs in macrophages, astrocytes and microglial cells. Infected cats remain persistently viraemic. Viraemia, the level of which increases rapidly after infection, peaks at seven to eight weeks before gradually declining and increasing again during the terminal stage of the disease. Humoral responses are normal, or occasionally enhanced, with antibodies appearing two weeks after infection. However, there is progressive deterioration in cell-mediated immunity due to depletion of CD4$^+$ T lymphocytes. Lymphocyte depletion is attributed to the cytopathic effect of virus in addition to decreased production of lymphocytes and apoptosis. Other immunological abnormalities associated with the infection include reduced interleukin-2 responsiveness and production, impaired lymphocyte blastogenesis in response to mitogens and reduced antibody response to T cell-dependent antigens. Reduction in CD4$^+$ lymphocyte numbers, increased production of virus, the emergence of variants with increased virulence and infection with opportunistic pathogens contribute to the development of clinical immunodeficiency.

Clinical signs

The prevalence of clinical disease is highest in cats over six years of age. The course of the disease may be divided into an acute phase, an asymptomatic phase, a phase characterized by vague clinical signs and a terminal phase with marked immunodeficiency (Hartmann, 1998). The acute phase which may last several weeks or months is manifested by pyrexia, generalized lymphadenopathy and neutropenia. A prolonged period during which infected cats appear clinically normal follows. The third phase is marked by recurrent fever, leukopenia, anaemia, weight loss, lymphadenitis, chronic gingivitis and behavioural changes. Opportunistic infections are frequent in the terminal phase of the disease. Chronic stomatitis and gingivitis are common findings. Other manifestations include chronic respiratory, enteric and skin infections. Many cats present with weight loss, anaemia and leukopenia. Neurological signs, usually due to direct viral damage, develop in a small number of infected cats. Concurrent FeLV infection may exacerbate the immunodeficiency and accelerate the appearance of clinical signs. An increased incidence of neoplasia, particularly B cell lymphomas, is recorded in FIV-infected cats. Not all infected cats develop disease.

Diagnosis
- Serological testing for antibodies to FIV is the principal method for confirming infection. Commercial ELISA and immunoconcentration kit-sets are available. Alternative tests include immunoblotting and indirect immunofluorescence. Some cats fail to produce antibodies for several months following infection; antibody levels may become undetectable in terminally-ill cats. The kittens of infected queens may remain seropositive for up to five months due to ingestion of colostral antibodies.
- Although virus isolation from blood or saliva is possible, it is not considered realistic for routine diagnostic purposes.
- Proviral DNA can be detected using the polymerase chain reaction.

Treatment and control
Treatment is primarily aimed at the control of secondary infections. A number of antiviral drugs, such as azidothymidine, directed against viral reverse transcriptase have a beneficial effect in clinically ill cats but do not eliminate infection. A commercial vaccine is not currently available. Development of an effective vaccine is complicated by several factors including the existence of multiple virus subtypes (Torres *et al.*, 1997). Control is based on prevention of exposure by separating infected and non-infected cats in multicat households, by preventing cats from roaming freely, by using seronegative queens for breeding and by screening all cats before introduction into seronegative populations.

Equine infectious anaemia

This disease, also called swamp fever, affects horses, mules and donkeys in many countries. It is caused by a lentivirus, equine infectious anaemia virus (EIAV). Infected *Equidae* remain viraemic for life.

Epidemiology
Virus is transmitted mechanically by haematophagous insects particularly *Tabanus* species and *Stomoxys* species. The virus survives for only short periods on the mouthparts of biting flies. These haematophagous insects usually obtain a complete blood meal from a single host. If interrupted during feeding, they may transfer virus to another host when they resume feeding. Transmission occurs most often in the summer, during periods of high insect activity, in low-lying swampy areas close to woodlands, the preferred habitat of tabanids. Iatrogenic transmission can occur through contaminated needles or surgical instruments. Although *in utero* transmission occurs, it is uncommon.

Pathogenesis
Virus replicates in macrophages, monocytes and Kupffer cells. A cell-associated viraemia develops with dissemination throughout the body (Oaks *et al.*, 1998). Infected horses fail to eliminate the virus despite mounting a strong immune response. They become persistently-infected following insertion of provirus into the genome of host cells. With the continuous production of virus particles, many target cells become infected. In the course of further provirus production by reverse transcription in infected cells, mutations frequently arise due to errors during the transcription process. This can result in the emergence of new virus strains exhibiting antigenic variation in envelope glycoproteins (antigenic drift). Febrile episodes and marked immune stimulation signal the emergence of these new strains. Non-neutralizing antibodies produced against virus early in the course of infection lead to the formation of immune complexes. Such immune complexes activate complement contributing to fever, anaemia and thrombocytopenia, and initiating glomerulonephritis. Haemolysis, enhanced erythrophagocytosis and depressed erythropoiesis are responsible for the anaemia in chronically affected horses. In most animals, clinical episodes eventually cease, probably as a consequence of a broad based neutralizing response against a wide range of viral epitopes.

Clinical signs
The majority of infected horses display mild signs which may go undetected. Most of the clinical signs are attributed to the host's immune response rather than to direct viral damage. Following an incubation period of up to three weeks, infected animals may present with fever, depression and petechiae on mucous membranes and conjunctivae. Rarely, severe epistaxis and ventral oedema may be followed by death. However, most horses recover from this phase and remain clinically normal for several weeks when recrudescence of signs may recur. The number and severity of recurring disease episodes varies widely. Most occur during the first year after infection and decline in number thereafter. Many horses which appear clinically normal remain carriers. Some exhibit a chronic form of the disease characterized by weight loss, anaemia, ventral oedema and debilitation, leading eventually to death.

Diagnosis
Laboratory confirmation of infection is based on the demonstration of serum antibodies to the core virus protein p26.

- The serological test recognized for international trade is the AGID test (Coggins test). Although the ELISA is a suitably sensitive assay, positive results should be confirmed by the more specific AGID test. Results can also be confirmed by immunoblotting.

Further reading

Caney, S. (2000). Feline immunodeficiency virus: an update. *In Practice*, **22**, 397–401.

Murphy, F.A., Gibbs, E.P.J., Horzinek, M.C. and Studdert, M.J. (1999). *Veterinary Virology*. Third Edition. Academic Press, San Diego.

Sparkes, A.H. (1997). Feline leukaemia virus: a review of immunity and vaccination. *Journal of Small Animal Practice*, **38**, 187–194.

Chapter 62

Reoviridae

Viruses in the family *Reoviridae* were originally isolated from respiratory and enteric sources without any associated disease, namely orphan. These icosahedral viruses, 60 to 80 nm in diameter, are non-enveloped and possess a layered capsid which is composed of concentric protein shells (Fig. 62.1). The genome of the virion is composed of ten to twelve segments of double-stranded RNA. Genetic reassortment readily takes place in cells co-infected with viruses of the same species. Replication occurs in the cytoplasm of host cells often with the formation of intracytoplasmic inclusions. The family contains nine genera. Members of the genera *Orthoreovirus*, *Rotavirus* and *Orbivirus* infect animals and man (Fig. 62.2). Members of the genus *Coltivirus*, which primarily infect rodents and humans, occasionally cause clinical disease in domestic animals. The genera *Fijivirus*, *Phytoreovirus* and *Oryzavirus* contain viruses of plants. The genus *Cypovirus* contains viruses of arthropods while members of the genus *Aquareovirus* infect fish. Viruses in the family are moderately resistant

---

Key points

- Non-enveloped viruses with double or triple layered capsid and icosahedral structure
- Segmented double-stranded RNA
- Replicate in cytoplasm
- Three genera of veterinary importance *Orthoreovirus, Orbivirus, Rotavirus*:
  —Orthoreoviruses cause arthritis and tenosynovitis in poultry
  —Rotaviruses cause enteritis in neonatal farm animals
  —Orbiviruses are arthropod-borne infections that cause African horse sickness in horses and bluetongue in sheep and in other domestic and wild ruminants

---

to heat, organic solvents and non-ionic detergents. Orthoreoviruses and rotaviruses are stable over a wide range of pH values unlike orbiviruses which lose infectivity at low pH values.

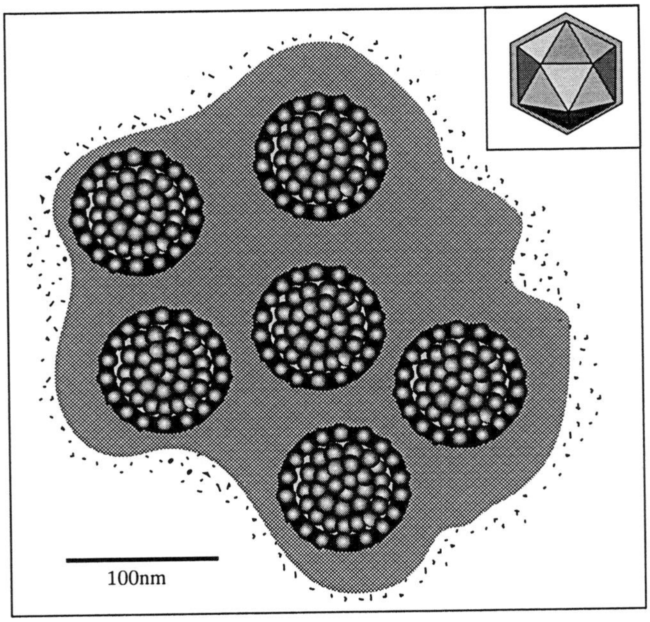

Clinical infections

Orthoreoviruses, which are widespread in nature, have been isolated from many animal species (Table 62.1). Mammalian and avian orthoreoviruses possess distinct group antigens. Avian orthoreoviruses have been implicated in arthritis, tenosynovitis, chronic respiratory disease and enteritis. Rotaviruses cause acute diarrhoea in young intensively-reared farm animals. Transmission of orthoreoviruses and rotaviruses is through contact with contaminated faeces.

Within the 19 currently recognized serogroups (species) of orbiviruses, there are defined serotypes and, in addition, antigenic complexes. The main serogroup-specific antigen is the immunodominant outer core protein VP7. Individual serotypes are distinguished by serum neutralization assays utilizing antibodies against outer capsid

Figure 62.1 Rotavirus particles as they appear in an electron micrograph and a diagrammatic representation (inset).

100nm

Family	Genus	Virus

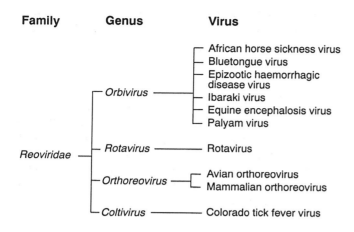

Figure 62.2 Viruses of veterinary importance in the family *Reoviridae*.

proteins. African horse sickness and bluetongue are particularly important diseases caused by orbiviruses. Epizootic haemorrhagic disease of deer and Ibaraki disease in cattle, both caused by closely-related orbiviruses, have clinical effects in these species similar to those of bluetongue in sheep. Infection with equine encephalosis virus has been recognized only in South Africa. Serological evidence suggests that this infection is widespread but acute disease occurs only sporadically. African

horse sickness, bluetongue and epizootic haemorrhagic disease of deer are transmitted by arthropods, especially by *Culicoides* species.

Diseases caused by avian orthoreoviruses

Infections caused by avian orthoreoviruses are usually inapparent. In certain circumstances, however, they may either cause primary disease or contribute to the severity of mixed infections. Using serum neutralization tests, at least nine serotypes are recognized. Although transmission is mainly by the faecal-oral route, transfer to developing chicks *in ovo* can occur. Arthritis/tenosynovitis, caused by orthoreoviruses in chickens between four and 16 weeks of age, has been reported worldwide. Lameness is a prominent feature of this disease and rupture of the tendon of the gastrocnemius muscle may occur. Affected birds have limited mobility and may die of starvation. Morbidity is usually less than 10%. The synovial lesions resemble those caused by infection with *Mycoplasma synoviae* or with *Staphylococcus aureus*. Orthoreovirus involvement can be confirmed by virus isolation. Specimens suitable for virus isolation are affected articular cartilage and tendon sheaths. Synovial fluid is not a reliable source for virus isolation. Suspensions of macerated tissues are inoculated into the yolk sac of embryonated eggs or onto monolayers of chick embryo

Table 62.1 Viruses of veterinary importance in the family *Reoviridae*.

Genus	Virus	Comments
Orbivirus	African horse sickness virus	Arthropod-borne infection of *Equidae*, principal vector *Culicoides* species. Endemic in Africa. High mortality rate
	Bluetongue virus	Arthropod-borne infection of sheep, cattle, goats and wild ruminants. Principal vector *Culicoides* species. Severe disease in some species of deer. Teratogenic effects. Clinical disease rare in cattle
	Epizootic haemorrhagic disease virus	Arthropod-borne infection of deer, cattle and buffalo. Principal vector *Culicoides* species. Clinically similar to bluetongue. Important disease of deer in North America. Subclinical infection occurs in cattle. Eight serotypes recognized
	Ibaraki virus	Member of the epizootic haemorrhagic disease virus serogroup. Acute febrile disease of cattle similar to bluetongue. Probably arthropod-borne. Present in south-east Asia
	Equine encephalosis virus	Reported in South Africa. Majority of infections subclinical. Sporadic cases of acute fatal disease. Cerebral oedema, fatty liver and enteritis are prominent features
	Palyam virus	Arthropod-borne disease of cattle. Causes abortion and teratogenic effects. Recorded in southern Africa, southeast Asia and Australia. Many viruses in the serogroup
Rotavirus	Rotaviruses	Occur in intensively-reared neonatal animals. Mild to severe diarrhoea, severity influenced by virulence of viral strain, age, colostral intake and management factors
Orthoreovirus	Avian orthoreoviruses	Important cause of viral arthritis/tenosynovitis in chickens. Multiple serotypes described. Turkeys and other avian species susceptible
	Mammalian orthoreoviruses	Associated with mild enteric and respiratory disease in many species, severity dependent on secondary infections. Three serotypes recognized
Coltivirus	Colorado tick fever virus	Rodent species act as reservoirs. Arthropod-borne, mainly ticks and also mosquitoes. Primarily of significance in humans, may cause encephalitis in children

liver cells. Viral antigen may be detectable by immuno-fluorescence in cryostat sections of tissues. Although serological testing is not particularly useful because of the high prevalence of subclinical infections, it may be employed to determine the immune status of a flock. Both inactivated and modified live vaccines have been used in parent flocks to stimulate high levels of maternally-derived antibody in chicks. However, vaccines may induce protection only against homologous serotypes (Meanger *et al.*, 1997). Control measures include total depopulation at the end of a production cycle followed by thorough cleansing and disinfection of premises.

Enteric disease caused by rotaviruses in young animals

Rotaviruses cause diarrhoea in intensively-reared young farm animals worldwide. Isolates are divided into seven antigenically-distinct serogroups (A to G), also termed species, based on reactions with the major capsid protein, VP6. Most isolates belong to serogroup A. Fourteen serotypes (G1-G14) are recognized within serogroup A on the basis of the antigenicity of VP7, an outer capsid glyco-protein which is highly immunogenic and induces type-specific neutralizing antibodies. Field infections with rotaviruses are considered to be species specific. However, virus isolates from one species can be transmitted experimentally to other species.

Epidemiology

High titres of virus (10^9 virus particles per gram of faeces) are excreted by clinically affected animals. Horizontal transmission occurs following ingestion of contaminated feed. Because the virus is stable in the environment, premises may be heavily contaminated and intensively-reared animals are those most often affected. Buildings can remain contaminated for long periods if thorough cleansing and disinfection procedures are not implemented.

Pathogenesis

The severity of infection is largely determined by the virulence of the infecting viral strain, the amount of virus ingested and the level of maternally-derived immunity. Other factors which influence the outcome of infection include age of the animal at the time of exposure, over-crowding and the presence of other enteric pathogens. The virus, which can survive gastric acidity, passes through the stomach and infects enterocytes at the tips of villi in the small intestine. Because the rate of enterocyte replacement is relatively slow in young animals, affected villi become stunted and covered by cuboidal cells. These immature replacement cells have reduced levels of disaccharidases and defective glucose-coupled sodium transport. Undigested lactose provides an ideal substrate for bacterial proliferation in the intestinal lumen. In addition, it exerts an osmotic effect which results in the retention of fluid in the lumen and, along with impaired fluid absorption, contributes to the development of diarrhoea.

Clinical signs

The incubation period is short, usually less than 24 hours. Affected animals are anorexic and depressed, and produce light-coloured, semi-liquid or pasty faeces. In uncompli-cated cases, animals frequently recover within four days without treatment. Concurrent infection with other enteric pathogens such as *Escherichia coli*, *Salmonella* species and *Cryptosporidium* species may add to the severity of the diarrhoea and deaths may occur.

Diagnosis

- Specimens suitable for laboratory examination include faeces and intestinal contents.
- Although negative-contrast electron microscopy is rapid, large numbers of virus particles (10^6 per gram of faeces) must be present for reliable confirmation. Immunoelectron microscopy increases the sensitivity of the procedure. Mixed viral infections can be detected by negative-contrast electron microscopy.
- Viral antigen can be demonstrated in faeces by ELISA and latex agglutination. The antisera employed in these tests is usually specific for serogroup A rotaviruses. Reagents for these assays are commercially available. Immunofluorescence can be used to detect viral antigen in smears or in cryostat sections of affected small intestines.
- Sodium dodecyl sulphate-polyacrylamide gel electrophoresis (SDS-PAGE) has been used success-fully to demonstrate RNA segments of rotaviruses in clinical samples. The sensitivity of this procedure is comparable with electron microscopy. The electrophoretic patterns permit differentiation of rotavirus serogroups.
- Rotaviruses are difficult to isolate in tissue culture from clinical samples. The addition of low concentrations of trypsin to the growth medium facilitates viral uncoating and improves viral replication.

Treatment

In mildly affected animals, water should be substituted for milk in the diet. Oral electrolyte solutions may be beneficial in some cases. Intravenous fluid replacement and antibiotic administration are required in severe cases complicated by bacterial infection.

Control

Measures aimed at reducing the levels of virus challenge in young animals are essential. These must be combined with management procedures which ensure that neonatal animals receive adequate amounts of colostrum. Local immunity is more important than circulating antibody; ingestion of colostrum provides protective antibodies in the intestinal lumen. Vaccination of pregnant dams enhances antibody levels in mammary secretions. Oral vaccination of newborn animals using modified live vaccine is of questionable value. Stressful environmental conditions should be minimized.

African horse sickness

This is a non-contagious disease of horses, mules and donkeys caused by African horse sickness virus (AHSV). Nine serotypes of this orbivirus, which can be distinguished by neutralization tests, constitute the African horse sickness serogroup. The disease is endemic in subtropical and tropical Africa. Although serious outbreaks have occurred in the Middle East, India and Pakistan, the disease has not persisted in these regions. Outbreaks have been recorded in Spain, Portugal and Morocco in recent years. African horse sickness is classified as a list A disease by the Office International des Epizooties.

Epidemiology
The virus is transmitted by haematophagous insects. The principal vector is *Culicoides imicola*, a species of Afro-Asian midge, which remains infected for life. This midge prefers a warm climate; it aestivates at temperatures below 10°C and replication of the virus in the midge ceases (Mellor *et al.*, 1998). *Culicoides imicola* is distributed as far north as latitude 41°N. Endemic disease occurs only in regions where *C. imicola* is constantly present. Epidemics of African horse sickness periodically occur outside these regions following climatic conditions which allow wind-borne transfer of infected midges for up to 700 km. Outbreaks of the disease are seasonal, usually occurring in late summer. The virus may be isolated from clinically normal maintenance hosts such as the zebra and African donkey.

Pathogenesis and pathology
The primary sites of viral replication are believed to be regional lymph nodes, spleen and lungs. Viraemia persists throughout the febrile period. Endothelial cells are important sites of secondary viral replication, resulting in increased vascular permeability, oedema, haemorrhage and intravascular coagulation. Postmortem findings include diffuse pulmonary oedema, hydrothorax, ascites and hydropericardium

Clinical signs
The incubation period is up to seven days. Four forms of this febrile disease, all of which can occur in a particular outbreak, are recognized. A peracute pulmonary form is characterized by depression and nasal discharge with rapid progression to severe respiratory distress. Mortality rate may approach 100%. A subacute cardiac form manifests as conjunctivitis, abdominal pain and progressive

dyspnoea. Subcutaneous oedematous swellings of the head and neck are most obvious in the supraorbital fossae, palpebral conjunctiva and intermandibular space. In this form of the disease, the mortality rate is up to 70%. A third form of African horse sickness presents with both cardiac and pulmonary features. A mild or subclinical form, termed horse sickness fever, may be observed in zebras and donkeys.

Diagnosis
- Characteristic clinical signs, such as oedema of the supraorbital fossae, may allow a clinical diagnosis. Postmortem findings, including pericardial and pleural effusions, are consistent with a diagnosis of African horse sickness.
- Suitable samples for laboratory examination include blood, lymph node and spleen. Inoculation of embryonated eggs or cell cultures may be used to demonstrate the presence of virus. Inoculation of newborn mice intracerebrally may also be used for this purpose. Virus can be identified by immuno-fluorescence and typed using virus neutralization with monovalent antiserum or competitive ELISA.
- Viral antigen can be detected by ELISA in samples.
- Viral RNA can be detected by RT-PCR (Zientara *et al.*, 1998). This test may provide results within 24 hours.
- Suitable serological methods include CFT, AGID, ELISA and serum neutralization tests. In acute disease, infected animals may die before antibodies are produced. Seroconversion in donkeys, used as sentinel animals outside endemic areas, confirms the presence of the disease.

Control
Vector control, quarantine of affected animals and vaccination are the main methods of control. Insect vector control includes the use of repellents and insecticides, the elimination of insect breeding areas and housing of animals in insect-proof buildings at dawn and at dusk when insect activity is maximum. Attenuated vaccines, both monovalent and polyvalent containing up to four serotypes, are available. However, these vaccines fail to prevent viraemia. Moreover, the vaccine virus may revert to virulence and be transmitted by vectors. In addition, vaccinated animals cannot be differentiated serologically from those with field infections. Inactivated vaccines based on serotype 4 are effective in preventing both clinical disease and viraemia. A polyvalent vaccine must be used if there is a risk of exposure to different serotypes. Protective immune responses may be generated using recombinant expressed structural proteins as subunit vaccines (Roy and Sutton, 1998). Such vaccines should be safe and permit differentiation of vaccinated from infected animals. Adequate biocontainment facilities are mandatory for vaccine production outside endemic regions.

Bluetongue

This non-contagious viral disease of sheep and other domestic and wild ruminants is transmitted by biting insects, principally *Culicoides* species. Isolates of the causal agent, bluetongue virus (BTV) belong to a distinct serogroup in the *Orbivirus* genus. Twenty four serotypes of BTV have been described. Bluetongue (BT) is of greatest significance in sheep and deer. The severity of the disease is influenced by the serotype of the virus, the breed of sheep and prevailing environmental conditions. Bluetongue is classified as a list A disease by the Office International des Epizooties.

Epidemiology

Bluetongue is widely distributed between latitudes 40°N and 35°S, reflecting the distribution of *Culicoides* species. *Culicoides imicola* is the principal vector in Africa and the Middle East. In Australia, *C. fulvus*, *C. wadai* and *C. brevitarsis* are involved in transmission. Other *Culicoides* species of importance in transmission are *C. varipennis* var. *sonorensis* in North America and *C. insignes* in South America. Female midges feeding on viraemic animals become infected and virus replicates in their tissues. *Culicoides* species can transmit virus in saliva within seven to ten days and they remain infected for life. Temperatures of 18°C to 29°C along with high humidity favour insect activity, accounting for the seasonal occurrence of the disease in many parts of the world. *Culicoides* species are most active at dawn and dusk. In localized areas within endemic regions there may be an increased frequency of BT outbreaks. These areas are particularly suitable for the breeding of *Culicoides* species because of the accumulation of animal faeces in marshland. Extension of disease to contiguous areas occurs through the movement of viraemic animals or insect vectors. Although the flight range of *Culicoides* species is limited, they may be transported over long distances by wind movement resulting in BT outbreaks in susceptible ruminant populations outside endemic regions. Such events may precipitate epidemics which are usually self-limiting unless the climate is suitable for vector activity throughout the year.

In endemic areas, infection of cattle is common and usually inapparent. The viraemia in cattle commonly lasts several weeks facilitating acquisition of virus by insect vectors. Consequently, cattle are considered to be important reservoirs of virus (Barratt-Boyes and MacLachlan, 1995). During the viraemic phase, virus can be detected in the semen of a proportion of rams and bulls. Venereal transfer of infection is uncommon. Embryos collected from infected ewes may transmit infection to recipient ewes but this can be prevented by washing embryos (Singh *et al.*, 1997).

Pathogenesis and pathology

After experimental infection, the virus replicates initially in regional lymph nodes. It is then carried in blood or lymph to other lymphoid tissues where further replication takes place. Virus localizes and multiplies in the endothelium of small blood vessels producing vascular damage with stasis, exudation and tissue hypoxia. The initiation and development of surface lesions in areas of tissue hypoxia relate to minor trauma and may be complicated by secondary bacterial infection. Lesions are particularly evident in the oral cavity, around the mouth and on the coronet of the hoof. In the bloodstream the virus is highly cell-associated, particularly with erythrocytes. It has been suggested that this may protect virus from antibody. Sporadic cases of clinical disease in cattle are thought to involve type I hypersensitivity reactions with participation of IgE as a result of previous exposure to BTV or related orbiviruses.

Clinical signs

The clinical presentation is highly variable, from subclinical to severe disease with high mortality. Severe disease is generally confined to Merinos and European mutton breeds. Nutritional status, exposure to sunlight and age also appear to influence the severity of lesions. The incubation period in sheep is up to ten days. Affected animals are febrile and depressed with vascular congestion of the lips and muzzle. Oedema of the lips, face, eyelids and ears develops. Erosions and ulcers are evident on the oral mucosa. There is excessive salivation and a watery discharge that subsequently becomes mucopurulent and dries to form crusts around the nares. The tongue may be swollen and cyanotic. Lameness may result from coronitis and laminitis. Some animals develop torticollis. Abortion may occur and lambs may be weak or deformed at birth. Mortality rate may be up to 30% and, in some outbreaks, may be higher. Animals recovering may lose part of the fleece some weeks after infection. Rare clinical cases in susceptible cattle are characterized by fever, stiffness, ulceration of the oral mucosa, 'burnt muzzle' and dermatitis. Cattle infected during pregnancy may abort or give birth to malformed calves.

Diagnosis

A presumptive diagnosis of BT may be based on clinical findings and postmortem lesions. Confirmation requires isolation and identification of the virus or demonstration of BTV-specific antibodies.

- Samples suitable for virus isolation include unclotted blood from febrile animals or fresh spleen and lymph node collected at postmortem. Virus may be isolated by intravenous inoculation of embryonated eggs.
- A highly sensitive nested PCR has been developed for detecting BTV nucleic acid in clinical samples (Aradaib *et al.*, 1998).

- Antigen detection ELISA systems have also been described (Stanislawek *et al.*, 1996; Hamblin *et al.*, 1998).
- Serological tests for the detection of antibodies to the BTV serogroup include CFT, AGID, indirect immuno-fluorescence and competitive ELISA. Neutralization or HAI assays are used for demonstrating type-specific antibodies. In animals from endemic regions, a rising antibody titre must be demonstrated using paired serum samples.

Control

As bluetongue is a list A disease, it is subject to international regulations controlling trade. The discovery of a number of serotypes of BTV in the Northern Territory of Australia resulted in disruption of trade in animals, semen and embryos although clinical disease was not present (Muller, 1995). Populations of insect vectors may be reduced by the use of larvicides at breeding sites. Insecticides applied to susceptible animals may temporarily halt feeding by vectors. Live attenuated vaccines have been used successfully for many years and provide protection against virulent virus of homologous serotype. Polyvalent vaccines are essential in regions where a number of serotypes are present. Attenuated vaccines may be teratogenic when used in ewes during the first half of gestation. These vaccines should not be used during periods of vector activity because of the risk of transferring vaccinal virus to pregnant ewes and the possibility of genetic reassortment with field virus and reversion to virulence (Osburn *et al.*, 1996). Killed adjuvanted vaccines can induce protection but are more expensive to produce and require two inoculations. Recombinant virus-like particles, capable of inducing protective immunity, have been produced in insect cells infected with recombinant baculoviruses expressing BTV proteins. However, vaccines produced by this method are not yet available commercially (Murray and Eaton, 1996).

References

Aradaib, I.E., Schore, C.E., Cullor, J.S. and Osburn, B.I. (1998). A nested PCR for detection of North American isolates of bluetongue virus based on NS1 genome sequence analysis of BTV-17. *Veterinary Microbiology*, **59**, 99–108.

Barratt-Boyes, S.M. and MacLachlan, N.J. (1995). Pathogenesis of bluetongue virus infection of cattle. *Journal of the American Veterinary Medicine Association*, **206**, 1322–1329.

Hamblin, C., Salt, J.S., Graham, S.D. *et al.* (1998). Bluetongue virus serotypes 1 and 3 infection in Poll Dorset sheep. *Australian Veterinary Journal*, **76**, 622–629.

Meanger, J., Wickramasinghe, R., Enriquez, C.E. and Wilcox, G.E. (1997). Immune response to avian reovirus in chickens and protection against experimental infection. *Australian Veterinary Journal*, **75**, 428–432.

Mellor, P.S., Rawlings, P., Baylis, M. and Wellby, M.P. (1998). Effect of temperature on African horse sickness virus infection in *Culicoides*. In *African Horse Sickness*. Eds. P.S. Mellor, M.Baylis, C. Hamblin, C.H. Calisher and P.P.C. Mertens. Springer-Verlag, Wien. pp. 156–163.

Muller, M.J. (1995). Veterinary arbovirus vectors in Australia – a retrospective. *Veterinary Microbiology*, **46**, 101–116.

Murray, P.K. and Eaton, B.T. (1996). Vaccines for bluetongue. *Australian Veterinary Journal*, **73**, 207–210.

Osburn, B.I., De Mattos, C.A., De Mattos, C.C. and MacLachlan, N.J. (1996). Bluetongue disease and the molecular epidemiology of viruses from the western United States. *Comparative Immunology and Microbiology of Infectious Disease*, **19**, 181–190.

Roy, P. and Sutton, G. (1998). New generation of African horse sickness virus vaccines based on structural and molecular studies of the virus particles. In *African Horse Sickness*. Eds. P.S. Mellor, M. Baylis, C. Hamblin, C.H. Calisher and P.P.C. Mertens. Springer-Verlag, Wien. pp. 177–202.

Singh, E.L., Dulac, G.C. and Henderson, J.M. (1997). Embryo transfer as a means of controlling the transmission of viral infections. XV. Failure to transmit bluetongue virus through the transfer of embryos from viraemic sheep donors. *Theriogenology*, **47**, 1205–1214.

Stanislawek, W.L., Lunt, R.A., Blacksell, S.D. (1996). Detection by ELISA of bluetongue antigen directly in the blood of experimentally infected sheep. *Veterinary Microbiology*, **52**, 1–12.

Zientara, S., Sailleau, C., Moulay, S. *et al.* (1998). Use of reverse transcriptase-polymerase chain reaction (RT-PCR) and dot-blot hybridization for the detection and identification of African horse sickness virus nucleic acids. In *African Horse Sickness*. Eds. P.S. Mellor, M. Baylis, C. Hamblin, C.H. Calisher and P.P.C. Mertens. Springer-Verlag, Wien. pp. 317–327.

Chapter 63

Birnaviridae

Birnaviruses are so named because their genomes contain two segments of linear, double-stranded RNA. The icosahedral virions are about 60 nm in diameter (Fig. 63.1). Five polypeptides, designated VP1, VP2, VP3, VP4 and VP5, have been identified. The major capsid protein (VP2) contains epitopes which induce neutralizing antibodies. Replication occurs in the cytoplasm of host cells and involves a virion-associated RNA-dependent RNA polymerase. The family *Birnaviridae* contains three genera: *Avibirnavirus*, *Aquabirnavirus* and *Entomobirnavirus*, which infect chickens, fish and insects respectively. Virions are stable over a wide pH range and at a temperature of 60°C for 1 hour. They are resistant to treatment with ether and chloroform.

Clinical infections

Two economically important diseases associated with birnaviruses are infectious bursal disease of chickens and infectious pancreatic necrosis of salmonids. These

---

Key points

- Double-stranded RNA viruses with icosahedral symmetry
- Replicate in cytoplasm
- Stable in the environment
- The family is composed of three genera:
  —*Avibirnavirus* contains viruses which cause infectious bursal disease
  —*Aquabirnavirus* contains viruses which cause infectious pancreatic necrosis in salmonids
  —*Entomobirnavirus* contains viruses which infect insects

---

diseases occur worldwide and cause considerable losses in poultry units and in farmed salmon.

Infectious bursal disease

This condition is a highly contagious disease of young chickens which is caused by infectious bursal disease virus (IBDV). The causal agent was first isolated in Gumboro, Delaware and the disease was originally known as Gumboro disease. Although turkeys and ducks are susceptible to infection, clinical disease occurs only in chickens. Based on neutralization tests, isolates of IBDV are assigned to two serotypes. There is considerable variation in the virulence of isolates in serotype 1. Very virulent (VV) strains were first reported in Europe and Asia in the late 1980s. These strains, although antigenically similar to classical serotype 1 strains, can cause disease even when maternally-derived antibody against the classical vaccine strains is present. Serotype 2 isolates are not associated with clinical disease. A variety of antigenic variants are recognized within each serotype. In the United States, in recent years, variant serotype 1 isolates have been detected in flocks that had been vaccinated with classical strain vaccines. These antigenic variants, which are highly immunosuppressive in young chicks, cause rapid bursal atrophy.

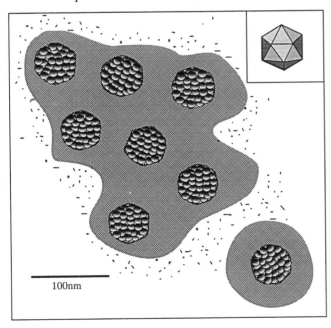

Figure 63.1 Birnavirus particles as they appear in an electron micrograph and a diagrammatic representation (inset).

100nm

Epidemiology

Infection, which is usually acquired by the oral route, occurs when maternally-derived antibody levels are waning at two to three weeks of age. Virus is shed in the faeces for up to two weeks after infection and can remain infectious in the environment of a poultry house for several months. Spread to other poultry units by fomites occurs. Neither a carrier state nor vertical transmission has been demonstrated.

Pathogenesis

Within hours of ingestion, virus can be detected in macrophages and lymphoid cells in the caeca, duodenum and jejunum. Virus reaches the liver via the portal circulation and infects Kupffer cells. Infection spreads to the bursa of Fabricius where rapid replication results in a pronounced secondary viraemia and dissemination to other tissues. The main target cells are B lymphocytes and their precursors in the bursa. The major antigenic protein VP2 has been shown to induce apoptosis in infected cells. Depletion of B lymphocytes in early life results in impaired immune responses, lowered resistance to infectious diseases and ineffective responses to vaccines. Bursal damage in chickens older than three weeks of age only marginally affects immune competence because many B lymphocytes are distributed peripherally before damage occurs.

Clinical signs

The severity of clinical signs is influenced by the virulence of the virus, the age of chicks at the time of infection, the breed of the chicks and the level of maternally-derived antibody. Chicks develop an acute form of the disease between three and six weeks of age following a short incubation period. Affected birds are depressed and inappetent and show evidence of diarrhoea and vent pecking. Morbidity ranges from 10% to 100% with a mortality rate up to 20% or, occasionally, higher. The course of the disease is short with surviving birds recovering in about four days. Many outbreaks are mild, detectable only by impaired weight gains. Although infections before three weeks of age are usually subclinical, severe depression of the humoral antibody response may result. Clinical signs in these birds are usually vague. Suboptimal growth, predisposition to secondary infections and poor response to vaccination may be encountered.

Diagnosis

- In acute disease, clinical signs and a swollen oedematous bursa at postmortem are often sufficient for diagnosis. Confirmation and identification of subclinical infection requires laboratory tests.
- Viral antigen can be detected in smears or frozen sections of the bursa using immunofluorescence. Macerated bursal tissue is suitable for detection of viral antigen by ELISA or by gel diffusion tests.
- Specimens of bursa, spleen or faeces are suitable for virus isolation. Most strains grow on the chorio-allantoic membrane of embryonated eggs.
- Recovered birds develop high antibody titres as mature peripheral B lymphocytes are unaffected. Suitable serological assays include ELISA and virus neutralization.

Control

Depopulation, thorough cleaning and effective disinfection programmes are required following an outbreak of disease in a unit. Most commercial units rely for control on vaccination. Both modified live and inactivated serotype 1 vaccines are available. Live vaccines can be administered by aerosol or in drinking water. To ensure high levels of maternally-derived antibody in chicks, breeding birds are usually vaccinated at four to ten weeks of age with a live vaccine and again, close to laying, with an inactivated oil-adjuvanted vaccine. Vaccines used in parent stock should contain both classical and variant strains of IBDV. Chicks can be actively immunized after maternally-derived antibody levels decline at about four weeks of age. In high risk flocks, vaccination may begin at one day of age to protect birds with little or no maternally-derived antibody, followed by booster inoculations at two and three weeks of age. Partially attenuated vaccines termed 'intermediate' and 'intermediate plus' ('hot') are generally used in this way in broilers and commercial layer replacements as they are capable of overcoming low levels of maternally-derived antibody. Recent vaccine developments include expression of VP2 gene by a baculovirus and by a recombinant fowlpox virus.

Further reading

Nagarajan, M.M. and Kibenge, F.S.B. (1997). Infectious bursal disease virus: a review of molecular basis for variations in antigenicity and virulence. *Canadian Journal of Veterinary Research*, **61**, 81–88.

Chapter 64

Orthomyxoviridae

The family *Orthomyxoviridae* (Greek *orthos*, proper and *myxa*, mucus) contains those viruses which cause influenza in humans and animals. Orthomyxoviruses are spherical or pleomorphic, enveloped viruses, 80 to 120 nm in diameter (Fig. 64.1). Long filamentous forms also occur. The envelope, which is derived from host cell membrane lipids, contains glycosylated and non-glycosylated viral proteins. Surface projections of glycoproteins form 'spikes' or peplomers which, in influenza A and B viruses, are of two types: a haemagglutinin (H) responsible for virus attachment and envelope fusion, and a neuraminidase (N) capable of cleaving viral receptors and promoting both entry of virus into cells and release of virions from infected cells.

Influenza viruses haemagglutinate erythrocytes from a wide range of species. Antibodies to the H glycoprotein are responsible for virus neutralization. The nucleocapsid has a helical symmetry. The genome, which is composed of six to eight segments, consists of linear, negative-sense, single-stranded RNA. Replication occurs in cell nuclei

> **Key points**
> - Enveloped viruses with helical nucleocapsids and spherical or pleomorphic morphology
> - Linear, negative-sense, single-stranded RNA
> - Replication occurs in the nucleus
> - Two important glycoproteins, one a haemagglutinin which binds to cell receptors and the other with neuraminidase activity, are present in the envelope
> - Genome is segmented facilitating genetic reassortment
> - Subtypes of Influenza A virus are important pathogens

with release of virions by budding from plasma membranes. Virions are labile in the environment and are sensitive to heat, lipid solvents, detergents, irradiation and oxidizing agents.

The family contains four genera namely *Influenzavirus A*, *Influenzavirus B*, *Influenzavirus C* and *Thogotovirus*. Influenza B and C viruses are pathogens of humans; Thogotovirus and Dhori virus are tick-borne arboviruses isolated from camels, cattle and humans in parts of Africa, Europe and Asia. Influenza A virus, the most important member of the family, is a significant pathogen of animals and humans.

Isolates of influenza A virus are grouped into subtypes on the basis of their H and N antigens. Currently, 15 H antigens and nine N antigens are recognized. New subtypes of influenza A virus emerge periodically. Two mechanisms, point mutation and genetic reassortment, are responsible for the emergence of new subtypes. Point mutations give rise to antigenic drift in which variation occurs within a subtype. Genetic reassortment, a more complex process producing antigenic shift, results in the development of new subtypes. To assess the risk posed by the emergence of new variant viruses, a precise classification of isolates has been adopted by the World Health Organization. This system is based on the influenza virus type, host, geographical origin, strain number, year of isolation and subtype. An example of this classification system, influenza virus A/equine/Prague/1/56 (H7N7),

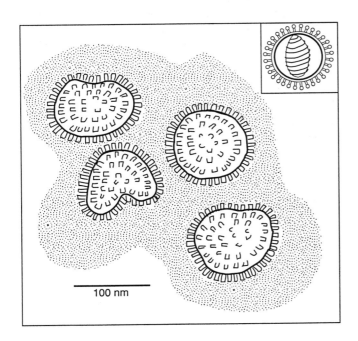

100 nm

Figure 64.1 Influenza A virus particles as they appear in an electron micrograph and a diagrammatic representation (inset).

indicates that this virus was isolated from a horse in Prague during 1956. Antigenic subtypes of influenza A virus which cause disease in humans and animals are presented in Table 64.1.

Clinical infections

Influenza A viruses cause significant infections in humans, pigs, horses and birds. Antibodies to influenza A virus have been detected in cattle in association with respiratory disease, but their significance is unclear (Brown *et al.*, 1998). Aquatic birds, particularly ducks which are reservoirs of influenza A virus, provide a genetic pool for the generation of the new subtypes capable of infecting mammals. Migratory waterfowl disseminate the virus across international borders. Although isolates of influenza A virus are usually species specific, there are well documented instances of transfer between species. The viruses replicate in the intestinal tract of birds and transmission is by the faecal-oral route. Human influenza pandemics have been attributed to the combined effects of poor hygiene and the close association of concentrated human populations with domestic fowl and pigs. The frequency of genetic reassortment in these animal populations can lead to the emergence of virulent influenza virus subtypes which are capable of infecting humans, thereby initiating pandemics (Fig. 64.2). Avian influenza viruses usually replicate poorly in humans. However, both human and avian influenza subtypes replicate in pigs, in which species genetic reassortment readily occurs. Because the genome of influenza A virus is segmented, mixed infections frequently give rise to genetic reassortment with the emergence of new subtypes. Such novel subtypes are often implicated in major pandemics which occur at about 20 year intervals. As there is limited

Table 64.1 Antigenic subtypes of influenza A virus isolated from humans and animals.

Hosts	Antigenic subtypes	Comments
Humans	H2N8 (1890)[a] H3N8 (1900) H1N1 (1918) H2N2 (1957) H3N2 (1967)	Subtypes which have been found in pigs such as H1N1 have been implicated in human pandemics
Birds	Many antigenic subtypes represented by different combinations of haemagglutinin (H) and neuraminidase (N) peplomers have been recognized	Disease is usually associated with subtypes expressing H5 or H7. Wild birds, especially migrating ducks, act as carriers
Pigs	Predominantly H1N1 and H3N2	Severity of disease is determined by the antigenic subtype
Horses	Usually H7N7 or H3N8	Subtypes associated with disease, which are widely distributed geographically, are absent from Australia, New Zealand and Iceland

a   year of recognition

immunity to the new subtypes in the human population, spread from country to country tends to occur rapidly. It is estimated that the pandemic of 'Spanish flu' in 1918 was responsible for more than 20 million human deaths worldwide.

Sporadic, less serious outbreaks of human influenza, which are of relatively frequent occurrence, can be attributed to subtle antigenic changes arising from errors

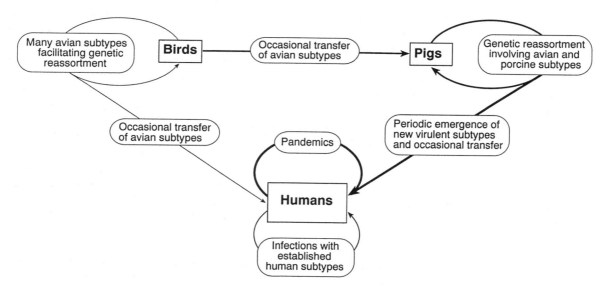

Figure 64.2 The circulation of subtypes of influenza A virus in bird and pig populations with the emergence of virulent subtypes which occasionally may be responsible for pandemics in the human population.

during replication of viral nucleic acid. If these subtypes exhibit antigenically distinct haemagglutinins, they are unaffected by existing neutralizing antibodies and a proportion of the susceptible population may become infected. Such outbreaks occur abruptly, typically in the winter months in temperate regions.

Subtypes of influenza A virus, which are well established as pathogens in animal populations, have also been implicated in human infections. In 1997, following a large epidemic of avian influenza in chickens, a H5N1 subtype was isolated from a fatal case in a young child in Hong Kong. This subtype had not previously been described outside of avian species. Human health fears prompted the destruction of 1.2 million birds. Fortunately human to human transmission did not occur to any significant extent, although other human cases did occur as a result of contact with infected poultry, By the end of 1997, 18 human cases had been confirmed resulting in 6 deaths.

Avian influenza (Fowl plague)

Many combinations of H and N antigens in influenza A virus are represented in isolates from avian species, particularly waterfowl. Influenza A virus subtypes are distributed worldwide and are frequently recovered from clinically normal birds. Outbreaks of severe clinical disease, usually caused by subtypes expressing H5 and H7 determinants, occur periodically in chickens and turkeys. In these species, acute infection is often referred to as fowl plague or highly pathogenic avian influenza and is categorised as a List A disease by the OIE.

Epidemiology

Infection is maintained in wild bird populations. Migrating waterfowl are considered to be responsible for spreading the virus to domestic birds. Although ducks become infected with influenza A virus, they rarely show signs of illness. A high level of subclinical infection occurs in susceptible young birds. Following replication in the intestinal tract, virus is shed in faeces. Live-bird markets may contribute to the spread of infection. Secondary spread can result from the movement of personnel and contaminated equipment between poultry farms.

Pathogenesis

Spread of influenza virus in tissues is dependent on the type of proteases present in a given tissue and the structure of the viral haemagglutinin molecule. The production of infectious virions requires cleavage of viral haemagglutinin. In the majority of influenza A virus subtypes, haemagglutinin cleavage takes place in the epithelial cells of the respiratory and digestive tracts. Because of the amino acid composition at their cleavage sites, haemagglutinins of virulent subtypes are susceptible to cleavage in many tissues, facilitating the development of generalized infection.

Clinical signs

The incubation period, which is variable, is up to seven days. Clinically, the disease may be inapparent, mild or, in some instances, severe with high mortality. Factors, such as overcrowding, poor ventilation and concurrent infections, may predispose to the development of severe disease. Highly virulent subtypes cause explosive outbreaks of disease with high mortality. Clinical signs are more apparent in birds which survive for a few days. Respiratory distress, diarrhoea, oedema in the cranial region, cyanosis, sinusitis and lacrimation are features of the clinical presentation. Infection of laying birds results in a dramatic drop in egg production.

Diagnosis

The severe form of the disease may be difficult to distinguish from velogenic viscerotropic Newcastle disease or from fowl cholera. Mild forms of the disease resemble other respiratory conditions in birds.

- Laboratory confirmation, which involves virus isolation and chacterization, is essential. Suitable specimens for laboratory examination include tracheal and cloacal swabs, faeces and pooled samples of organs.
- Tissue suspensions are inoculated into nine to 11 day old embryonated eggs. Allantoic fluid, harvested after incubation for four to seven days, is tested for haemagglutinating activity.
- The presence of influenza A virus can be confirmed by immunodiffusion using a suspension of chorioallantoic membrane from eggs inoculated with material from an outbreak and positive antiserum to the nucleocapsid or matrix antigens common to all influenza A viruses.
- Antisera with broad specificity may be used in haemagglutination inhibition (HI) or immunodiffusion tests to confirm that an isolate is influenza A virus. Definitive subtyping is carried out in reference laboratories using monospecific antisera prepared against the 15 haemagglutinins and nine neuraminidase determinants.
- All highly virulent avian influenza A subtypes possess either H5 or H7 antigens. However, numerous low virulence isolates expressing H5 and H7 determinants have been recorded. To assess pathogenicity, ten chickens should be inoculated intravenously at four to eight weeks of age. Isolates which cause more than 75% mortality within eight days are considered highly pathogenic.
- Genomic sequencing can be used to predict the amino acid composition at the cleavage site of the haemagglutinin molecule.
- Serological testing for antibodies to influenza virus can

be carried out using an agar gel immunodiffusion test or by competitive ELISA (Shafer *et al.*, 1998).

Control

Outbreaks of avian influenza in domestic species are notifiable to national regulatory authorities. In countries free of the disease, outbreaks are controlled by slaughter of affected flocks, imposition of movement restrictions and implementation of rigorous disinfection procedures. Imported birds are quarantined. In high risk areas along the migration routes of waterfowl, poultry should be housed in bird-proof buildings.

Vaccination is usually prohibited in those countries implementing a slaughter policy because of international trade restrictions and possible difficulties in establishing freedom from infection. Some countries accept the presence of mildly pathogenic subtypes because of the expense of implementing control measures. In such countries inactivated oil emulsion vaccines are available commercially and are used, particularly in turkeys, to protect against subtypes of low virulence. Recombinant haemagglutinin protein vaccines and recombinant fowlpox virus vector vaccines containing a haemagglutinin gene insert have been developed (Swayne *et al.*, 1997; Crawford *et al.*, 1999).

Vaccines, which are effective against a particular virulent influenza A subtype, may not be effective against new emerging subtypes. Due to the risk of reversion to virulence, live vaccines against influenza A virus are not used. However, clinical trials in humans with an attenuated cold-adapted, reassortant influenza virus vaccine have produced good results (Couch, 2000) and may lead to the development of similar vaccines for poultry.

Swine influenza

This highly contagious disease of pigs occurs worldwide. Swine influenza was first described in 1918, its occurrence coinciding with a major pandemic of human influenza. Two cocirculating subtypes, H1N1 and H3N2, are endemic in pig populations. In Europe during 1979, H1N1 isolates, clearly distinguishable from classical H1N1 subtypes and with haemagglutinins structurally similar to avian haemagglutinins, were identified. These H1N1 subtypes, which are more virulent than classical H1N1 isolates, now predominate in Europe. Acute respiratory disease of pigs in Japan (Ouchi *et al.*, 1996) and in the United Kingdom (Brown, 1998) has been attributed to the H1N2 subtype. There is convincing epidemiological evidence to support the view that transfer of virulent subtypes from pigs to humans is a major factor in the emergence of pandemics in the human population (Fig. 64.2).

Epidemiology

An outbreak of swine influenza is usually associated with the recent introduction of pigs into a herd. Virus, shed in high concentrations in the nasal secretions of infected pigs, spreads rapidly within a herd. The principal route of transmission is by direct contact. Airborne spread between farms may occur under suitable weather conditions in areas with high pig densities. Outbreaks of disease usually occur when environmental temperatures are low. Between outbreaks it is probable that virus circulates in herds without evidence of clinical disease and that some animals remain carriers for many months.

Pathogenesis and pathology

Infection is limited to the respiratory tract; the lungs are the major target organs. Following infection, virus multiplies in nasal, tracheal and bronchial epithelium. Spread of infection throughout the respiratory tract results in necrosis, extensive pneumonic change and consolidation. Lesions are often limited to the apical and cardiac lobes. The acute phase of the disease persists for more than 72 hours after which virus replication declines.

Clinical signs

Onset of the disease in a herd is often abrupt, many pigs becoming clinically ill simultaneously. The incubation period is up to three days. The severity of the illness ranges from subclinical to acute and is strongly influenced by the strain of the infecting virus. Secondary bacterial infections frequently complicate the course of the disease and delay recovery. Acute disease is characterized by huddling in groups, paroxysmal coughing, dyspnoea and fever. Some pigs may have a discharge from the eyes and nose. Most pigs recover within six days. Mortality is usually low except in very young pigs or when intercurrent infection is present. The economic impact of the disease is mainly attributable to loss of weight. In fully susceptible herds, abortion can occur in affected sows.

Diagnosis

- Samples suitable for virus isolation include nasal mucus and lung tissue from acute cases early in the disease. As the virus is labile, transport media should be used for rapid transfer of specimens to the laboratory. Isolation is usually carried out in embryonated eggs. After incubation for 72 hours, haemagglutinating activity is demonstrable in the allantoic fluid.
- Demonstration of a rise in antibody levels in paired serum samples using haemagglutination-inhibition test or ELISA procedures is indicative of infection.
- Viral antigen can be detected using immunofluorescence or ELISA.
- Viral nucleic acid can be detected with PCR.

Control

Good husbandry, including the elimination of stress

factors, may help to minimize losses from swine influenza. Measures should be implemented to prevent the introduction of infection. Inactivated vaccines are available commercially. Vaccination can be beneficial provided that the subtypes of virus incorporated in vaccines include those involved in the outbreaks.

Equine influenza

This economically important, acute respiratory disease of horses occurs worldwide except in Australia, New Zealand and Iceland. Two immunologically distinct subtypes of influenza A virus are described in horses. The virus, first isolated from horses in 1956, was designated A/equine/Prague/1/56 (H7N7) or influenza A/equine 1. In 1963, a second subtype was isolated in the USA and designated A/equine/Miami/2/63 (H3N8) or influenza A/equine 2. Infection or vaccination with one subtype does not induce protection against infection with the other subtype. Although the last outbreak of disease attributed to influenza A/equine 1 occurred in 1979, there is serological evidence that this subtype continues to circulate in the horse population.

Antigenic drift accounts for several variants of influenza A/equine 2 with two antigenically and genetically distinct lineages identified in Europe and the Americas (Oxburgh et al., 1998). In contrast, the H3N8 subtype isolated from horses in China was more closely related to avian strains than to the H3N8 subtype circulating in horses elsewhere.

Epidemiology

Outbreaks are associated with movement and assembly of horses for shows, sales, racing or training. The initial source of infection is often a partially immune horse shedding virus without showing clinical signs. Equine influenza is highly contagious and spreads rapidly among susceptible horses. Large quantities of virus are shed in aerosols by the frequent coughing of affected animals. Infection can be acquired at distances up to 30 metres. Indirect transmission through contamination of clothing, equipment and vehicles can also occur.

Pathogenesis

The virus replicates in the epithelium of the respiratory tract resulting in destruction of ciliated epithelium and hypersecretion from submucosal glands.

Clinical signs

The incubation period is up to two days. Affected animals develop a high temperature, nasal discharge and dry cough. Anorexia and depression, although common, can vary in intensity. Ocular discharge, limb oedema and stiffness may also be present. Age and previous exposure or vaccination status may influence the severity of the clinical signs and the likelihood of secondary bacterial infection with the development of respiratory complications. Exercise exacerbates the clinical signs (Gross et al., 1998). Animals with mild infections usually recover within three weeks. In severe cases, several months may be required for convalescence.

Diagnosis

Although clinical signs may be suggestive of equine influenza, laboratory confirmation is required.

- Nasopharyngeal swabs collected during the acute phase of the infection are suitable for isolation of the virus in embryonated eggs or in cell culture. New isolates should be closely monitored for antigenic drift.
- A commercial diagnostic kit, developed for the detection of the nucleoprotein of human influenza A virus, can be used for the diagnosis of equine influenza (Chambers et al., 1994).
- Serological diagnosis of equine influenza is possible. Haemagglutination inhibition or single radial haemolysis tests on paired serum samples can be used for diagnosis. Serum used in the HI test must be pretreated in order to remove non-specific inhibitors.

Treatment and control

Supportive therapy and rest is indicated for affected horses. The antiviral drugs, amantidine and rimantidine, which have been shown to be effective for inhibiting replication of influenza A virus in vitro, are being evaluated for therapeutic use (Rees et al., 1997). Several inactivated vaccines are commercially available. However, immunity is usually short-lived and booster injections are required in accordance with manufacturer's instructions. The incorporation of polymer adjuvants or Quil-A based immuno-stimulating complexes (ISCOMs) into vaccine preparations extends the duration of protective levels of immunity. Protective immunity generated by natural exposure is related both to a mucosal IgA immune response and to humoral IgGa and IgGb responses, a pattern of protective immunity not generated by conventional vaccines (Nelson et al., 1998). Vaccinated horses generally exhibit milder clinical signs and shed virus for shorter periods than unvaccinated animals. Vaccine manufacturers must update vaccinal strains regularly. Vaccines should include antigenic material representative of the influenza A virus subtypes prevalent in the horse population. In addition to vaccination, control of equine influenza requires isolation of affected horses and cleaning, disinfection and isolation of infected premises. Animal movement should cease until contaminated premises have been cleaned and disinfected.

References

Brown, I. (1998). Swine influenza - a disease of increasing importance? *State Veterinary Journal*, **8**, 2–4.

Brown, I.H., Crawshaw, T.R., Harris, P.A. and Alexander, D.J. (1998). Detection of antibodies to influenza A virus in cattle in association with respiratory disease and reduced milk yield. *Veterinary Record*, **143**, 637–638.

Chambers, T.M., Shortridge, K.F., Li, P.H. *et al.* (1994). Rapid diagnosis of equine influenza by the Directigen FLU-A enzyme immunoassay. *Veterinary Record*, **135**, 275–279.

Couch, R.B. (2000). Prevention and treatment of influenza. *New England Journal of Medicine*, **343**, 1778–1787.

Crawford, J., Wilkinson, B., Vosnesensky, A. *et al.* (1999). Baculovirus-derived haemagglutinin vaccines protect against lethal influenza infections by avian H5 and H7 subtypes. *Vaccine*, **17**, 2265–2274.

Gross, D.K., Hinchcliff, K.W., French, P.S. *et al.* (1998). Effect of moderate exercise on the severity of clinical signs associated with influenza virus infection in horses. *Equine Veterinary Journal*, **30**, 489–497.

Nelson, K.M., Schram, B.R., McGregor, M.W., *et al.* (1998). Local and systemic antibody responses to equine influenza virus infection versus conventional vaccination. *Vaccine*, **16**, 1306–1313.

Oxburgh, L., Akerblom, L., Fridberger, T. *et al.* (1998). Identification of two antigenically and genetically distinct lineages of H3N8 equine influenza virus in Sweden. *Epidemiology and Infection*, **120**, 61–70.

Ouchi, A., Nerome, K., Kanege, Y. *et al.* (1996). Large outbreak of swine influenza in southern Japan caused by reassortant (H1N2) influenza viruses: its epizootic background and characterization of the causative viruses. *Journal of General Virology*, **77**, 1751–1759.

Rees, W.A., Harkins, J.D., Woods, W.E. *et al.* (1997). Amantidine and equine influenza: pharmacology, pharmacokinetics and neurological effects in the horse. *Equine Veterinary Journal*, **29**, 104–110.

Shafer, A.L., Katz, J.B. and Eernisse, K.A. (1998). Development and validation of a competitive enzyme-linked immunosorbent assay for detection of type A influenza antibodies in avian sera. *Avian Diseases*, **42**, 28–34.

Swayne, D.E., Beck, J.R. and Mickle, T.R. (1997). Efficacy of recombinant fowlpox virus vaccine in protecting chickens against a highly pathogenic Mexican-origin H5N2 avian influenza virus. *Avian Diseases*, **41**, 910–922.

Further reading

Timoney, P.J. (1996). Equine influenza. *Comparative Immunology and Microbiology of Infectious Diseases*, **19**, 205–211.

Chapter 65

Paramyxoviridae

Paramyxoviruses and orthomyxoviruses were formerly grouped together as the 'myxoviruses' (Greek *myxa*, mucus), a name which describes their affinity for mucous membranes. Paramyxoviruses are pleomorphic, 150 nm or more in diameter and enveloped (Fig. 65.1). They contain a single molecule of negative-sense, single-stranded RNA. Two types of glycoprotein 'spikes' or peplomers are present in the envelope: an attachment protein and a fusion protein (F). The attachment protein may either be a haemagglutinin-neuraminidase protein (HN) or a protein without neuraminidase activity (G). The attachment proteins allow the virus to bind to cell surface receptors and the fusion protein causes the virus envelope to fuse with the host cell membrane. Both types of peplomers can induce production of virus neutralizing antibodies. There is also an envelope associated non-glycosylated membrane protein (M). Paramyxoviruses may exhibit haemagglutinating, haemolytic and neuraminidase activities. The nucleocapsid, which has helical symmetry, is 13 to 18 nm in diameter and has a characteristic herringbone appearance. Replication occurs in the cell cytoplasm. Virions

Key points
- Large pleomorphic enveloped viruses
- Negative sense single-stranded RNA
- Helically symmetrical nucleocapsid
- Replicate in the cytoplasm
- Subfamilies *Paramyxovirinae* and *Pneumovirinae* divided into five genera, each containing viruses of veterinary importance
- Cause rinderpest, peste des petits ruminants, canine distemper, Newcastle disease and a range of respiratory diseases in domestic animals

are released by budding from the plasma membrane at sites containing virus envelope proteins. The labile virions are sensitive to heat, desiccation, lipid solvents, non-ionic detergents and disinfectants.

Recently the classification of the *Paramyxoviridae* has been changed to include a new genus, *Metapneumovirus*, and renaming of the genus *Paramyxovirus* as *Respirovirus* (Fig. 65.2). Although paramyxoviruses are genetically stable and do not exhibit recombination, some antigenic variation may occur through mutation.

Clinical infections

Paramyxoviruses, which have a narrow host range, infect mainly mammals and birds (Table 65.1). Following transmission through close contact or by aerosols, replication occurs primarily in the respiratory tract. Infection is generally cytolytic but persistent infections are described *in vitro*. Formation of syncytia and intracytoplasmic, acidophilic inclusions are features of infection with these viruses. Serious diseases caused by paramyxoviruses include rinderpest, peste des petits ruminants, canine distemper, Newcastle disease, measles and mumps.

Rinderpest

This acute disease, which occurs primarily in ruminants and is also referred to as cattle plague, has been recognized for centuries as a major cause of mortality in cattle and

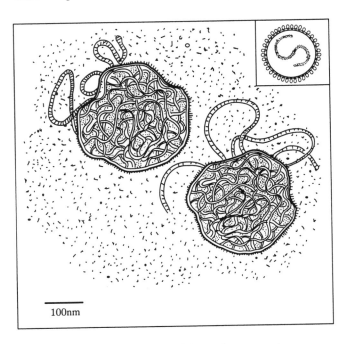

100nm

Figure 65.1 Paramyxovirus particles as they appear in an electron micrograph and a diagrammatic representation (inset).

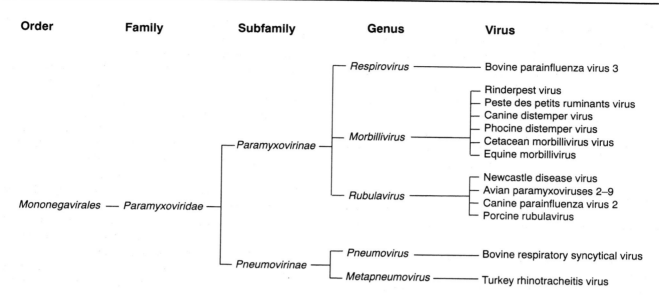

Figure 65.2 A classification of paramyxoviruses with emphasis on those of veterinary importance.

domestic buffalo. Rinderpest is endemic in parts of Africa, the Middle East and Asia. It is classed as a list A disease by the Office International des Epizooties (OIE).

Epidemiology
Although only one serotype of this morbillivirus is recognized, strains differ both in host range and in virulence. Individual host species exhibit differences in susceptibility to virus strains. Domestic cattle and buffalo

and several wildlife species including giraffe, warthog, Cape buffalo and eland are highly susceptible to infection. Gazelles and small domestic ruminants are less susceptible. Asiatic breeds of domestic pig develop disease whereas infection in European breeds is subclinical. Transmission, which occurs through aerosols, usually requires close contact as the virus is labile and remains viable in the environment for short periods only. Virus shedding in all secretions and excretions begins a few days

Table 65.1 Paramyxoviruses of veterinary importance.

Genus	Virus	Comments
Morbillivirus	Rinderpest virus	Causes highly contagious disease in domestic and wild ruminants characterized by high morbidity and high mortality
	Peste des petits ruminants virus	Causes severe disease in small ruminants, particularly sheep and goats, resembling rinderpest with high morbidity and high mortality rates
	Canine distemper virus	Causes acute disease in dogs and wild carnivores characterized by multisystemic involvement and variable mortality
Rubulavirus	Newcastle disease virus (Avian paramyxovirus 1)	Causes Newcastle disease in domestic and wild birds. Isolates vary in virulence: velogenic, mesogenic and lentogenic strains. Generalized infection characterized by respiratory, intestinal and nervous signs
	Porcine rubulavirus	Causes blue eye disease; described only in Mexico
	Canine parainfluenza virus 2	Causes inapparent or mild respiratory disease in dogs; sometimes associated with kennel cough; related to or possibly a subtype of simian virus 5 (SV5)
Respirovirus	Bovine parainfluenza virus 3	Causes subclinical or mild respiratory disease in cattle and sheep. Sometimes associated with shipping fever in cattle. Predisposes to secondary bacterial infection particularly with *Mannheimia haemolytica*
Pneumovirus	Bovine respiratory syncytial virus	Common subclinical infection in adult cattle. Associated with respiratory disease outbreaks of varying severity in young cattle. Sheep and goats are also susceptible
Metapneumo-virus	Turkey rhinotracheitis virus	Causes severe upper respiratory tract infection in turkeys with coryza and swollen sinuses. In chickens, the disease is referred to as swollen head syndrome

before clinical signs develop. In endemic areas, the disease is usually mild and is restricted to young cattle in which maternally-derived immunity has declined. As there is no carrier state, maintenance of infection requires continuous transmission to susceptible animals. Epidemics usually occur following movement of susceptible animals into an endemic area or the introduction of infected animals into susceptible populations. All ages of animals are affected in epidemics. Morbidity may reach 90% and mortality can approach 100%.

Pathogenesis
After inhalation of the virus, multiplication occurs in the pharyngeal and mandibular lymph nodes. Viraemia develops within three days resulting in spread to other lymphoid tissues and to the mucosae of the respiratory and digestive tracts. Leukopenia and immunosuppression follow necrosis in lymphoid tissues. Virus shedding, which continues throughout the acute phase of the disease, subsides a few days after body temperature returns to normal.

Clinical signs
After an incubation period of three to nine days, infected animals develop a fever and become anorexic and depressed. Mucosal erosions in the mouth and nasal passages become evident within five days . Profuse salivation is accompanied by an oculonasal discharge. About three days after the appearance of the mucosal ulcers, fever regresses and a profuse diarrhoea develops. The dark fluid faeces often contain mucus, necrotic debris and blood. Dehydration and wasting soon become evident. Severely affected animals may collapse and die within 12 days of the onset of clinical signs. In surviving animals, convalescence lasts several weeks. Secondary infections and activation of latent protozoal infections are frequent complications. Pregnant animals may abort during the convalescent period.

Diagnosis
Clinical and pathological findings may be sufficient for diagnosis in endemic areas. They may also be adequate in individual animals in outbreaks which have been confirmed by laboratory tests. In regions where rinderpest is uncommon or absent, laboratory confirmation is required to differentiate it from bovine viral diarrhoea, infectious bovine rhinotracheitis, malignant catarrhal fever and foot-and-mouth disease. When investigating an outbreak, specimens for laboratory examination should be collected from several febrile animals which have not developed diarrhoea.

- Specimens suitable for virus isolation include white cells from the buffy coat of heparinized blood samples, lymph node and spleen.
- The presence of rinderpest virus, which produces

cytopathic effects in cell cultures, can be confirmed by immunofluorescence.
- Agar gel immunodiffusion or a counter immuno-electrophoresis test are used as rapid antigen detection tests. Specimens suitable for these procedures include ocular discharge and mesenteric lymph nodes.
- A reverse transcription polymerase chain reaction method, which can detect rinderpest virus and differentiate it from the virus of peste des petits ruminants, has been developed (Forsyth and Barrett, 1995).
- A competitive ELISA for detecting serum antibodies to rinderpest virus is the test recommended by OIE for international trade.
- Postmortem enteric lesions are characteristic but not pathognomonic. Congestion of the folds of the colonic mucosa often produces a zebra-stripe pattern.
- Syncytia may form in stratified squamous epithelium of the upper alimentary tract and in crypts of the small intestine.

Control
The Food and Agricultural Organization aims to achieve worldwide eradication of rinderpest by 2010. Factors which render this achievable include the availability of a vaccine that induces lasting immunity, reliable diagnostic tests and the absence of carrier animals and wild life reservoirs.

In countries free of rinderpest, control is based on restriction of animal movement, quarantine of imported animals and slaughter of infected animals. In endemic areas, control is achieved by vaccination of domestic cattle and buffaloes with a modified live tissue culture-based vaccine that induces immunity lasting at least five years. This stable freeze-dried vaccine is thermolabile following reconstitution. Recombinant vaccinia and capripox virus vaccines expressing either haemagglutinin protein or fusion protein of rinderpest virus have high heat stability and have been used to protect cattle (Inui *et al.*, 1995; Ngichabe *et al.*, 1997). Control of animal movement is the single most important measure in preventing disease transmission.

Peste des petits ruminants

This condition, also referred to as goat plague, is an acute contagious disease of ruminants, particularly goats. It is caused by the morbillivirus, peste des petits ruminants virus (PPRV), which is closely related to other members of the genus. Peste des petits ruminants (PPR), which occurs in sub-Saharan Africa, the Middle East, India and Pakistan, is a list A disease.

Epidemiology
Close contact is required for transmission of this labile virus which occurs by aerosols. The introduction of infection into a flock is invariably associated with

movement of animals. Although a carrier state is not known to occur, subclinical infection and the onset of viral shedding before overt clinical signs facilitate spread of infection. In West Africa, epidemics tend to occur during the rainy season, when flocks are gathered together in preparation for sales. Infection rates are similar in sheep and goats but the disease is generally more severe in goats.

Pathogenesis

The pathogenesis of PPR is similar to that of rinderpest. Mucosal erosions and profuse diarrhoea are features of the condition. During the acute phase of the disease, virus is shed in all secretions and excretions.

Clinical signs

The incubation period is about four days. The disease is particularly severe in young animals. Affected goats exhibit fever, dry muzzle and a serous nasal discharge which becomes mucopurulent. Erosions on the mucous membrane of the buccal cavity are accompanied by marked salivation. Ulcers develop in the mucosae of the alimentary, respiratory and urinary tracts. Conjunctivitis with ocular discharge is a feature of the disease. A profuse diarrhoea, which results in dehydration, develops within days of infection. Signs of tracheitis and pneumonia are common. There is a severe leukopenia which facilitates secondary bacterial infection. Pulmonary infections caused by *Pasteurella* species are common in the later stages of the disease. Pregnant animals may abort. Mortality rates in severe outbreaks often exceed 70% and acutely affected goats may die within ten days of exposure to the virus.

In sheep, infection with PPRV is subacute and characterized by fever, nasal catarrh, mucosal erosions and intermittent diarrhoea. Affected animals usually recover after ten to 14 days.

Diagnosis

Specimens for laboratory examination should be taken from animals in the acute phase of the disease. Suitable specimens include nasal and ocular swabs, unclotted blood and scrapings of buccal and rectal mucosae. Samples of lung, spleen and lymph node from animals slaughtered early in the course of the disease are also suitable. Laboratory confirmation is based primarily on virus isolation in tissue culture and on antigen detection. Rapid antigen detection methods include ELISA, counter immunoelectrophoresis and agar gel immunodiffusion. Specific primers for use in PCR are available. Antibodies can be detected by virus neutralization or by competitive ELISA.

Control

Slaughter policies apply in countries free from PPR. Quarantine and vaccination are used in regions where the disease is endemic. Modified live rinderpest vaccine, which provides adequate protection against PPRV, has been used in sheep and goats for many years. A modified live PPRV vaccine has recently been developed.

Canine distemper

This highly contagious disease of dogs and other carnivores has a worldwide distribution. Canine distemper virus (CDV), a pantropic morbillivirus, produces a generalized infection involving many organ systems.

Epidemiology

The wide host range of CDV includes members of the families *Canidae, Ailuridae, Hyaenidae, Mustelidae, Procyonidae, Ursidae, Viverridae* and *Felidae*. Outbreaks of disease have been documented in several wildlife species including foxes, skunks, racoons, black-footed ferrets and lions (Appel and Summers, 1995; Roelke-Parker *et al.*, 1996). The virus is relatively labile, requiring transmission by direct contact or by aerosols. In urban dog populations, the virus is maintained by infection in susceptible animals. Infection spreads rapidly among young dogs, usually between three and six months of age when maternally-derived immunity declines. The number of dogs in populations in rural areas is often too low to maintain continuous infection with the result that, irrespective of age, unvaccinated dogs are susceptible and significant outbreaks of the disease can occur.

Pathogenesis

The virus, which replicates in the upper respiratory tract, spreads to the tonsils and bronchial lymph nodes. A cell-associated viraemia follows with spread to other lymphoreticular tissues. Viral replication produces lymphocytolysis and leukopenia resulting in immunosuppression and allowing a secondary viraemia to develop. The extent of spread to tissues and organs is determined by the rapidity and effectiveness of the immune response. In the absence of a sufficiently vigorous response, dissemination and replication of CDV occurs in the respiratory, gastrointestinal, urinary and central nervous systems. Spread to the skin may also occur.

Virus infects both neurons and glial cells within the CNS and may persist there for very long periods. Old dog encephalitis is apparently associated with prolonged persistence of the virus in the brain, possibly as a result of non-cytolytic spread from cell to cell without budding from the cell membrane thus evading immune detection (Stettler *et al.*, 1997). This mechanism appears to be analogous to that causing subacute sclerosing panencephalitis of children which is associated with persistent infection with defective measles virus. The presence of viral antigen in these conditions stimulates a low grade prolonged inflammatory response eventually leading to the development of neurological signs.

Clinical signs

The incubation period is usually about one week but may extend to four weeks or more when nervous signs appear without prior evidence of infection. The severity and duration of illness are variable and are influenced by the virulence of the infecting virus, the age and immune status of the infected animal and the rapidity of its immune response to infection. The pyrexic response to infection is biphasic although the initial elevation of temperature may not be noticed. During the second period of pyrexia, oculonasal discharge, pharyngitis and tonsillar enlargement become evident. Coughing, vomiting and diarrhoea are often consequences of secondary infections. A skin rash and pustules may be present on the abdomen. Some affected dogs have hyperkeratosis of the nose and footpads, referred to as 'hardpad'. Acute disease, which may last for a few weeks, is followed either by recovery and life-long immunity or by the development of neurological signs and, eventually, death. Common neurological signs include paresis, myoclonus and epileptiform seizures. A grave prognosis is indicated in animals displaying neurological disturbance. Residual neurological deficits are common in dogs that survive. Old dog encephalitis, characterized by motor and behavioural deterioration, is invariably fatal.

Diagnosis

A febrile, catarrhal illness with neurological sequelae in young dogs is highly suggestive of canine distemper.

- Viral antigen may be demonstrated by immunofluorescence in conjunctival or vaginal impression smears or in smears of cells from the buffy coat.
- Cryostat sections of lymph nodes, urinary bladder and cerebellum are also suitable for the demonstration of viral antigen.
- Eosinophilic inclusions can be demonstrated in nervous and epithelial tissues.
- Serological demonstration either of IgM antibodies or of a fourfold rise in antibody titre between acute and convalescent sera may be determined by virus neutralization, ELISA or indirect immunofluorescence. Antibody may be detected in cerebrospinal fluid.
- Virus isolation may prove difficult. Urinary bladder and brain are suitable postmortem specimens for virus isolation. Cells from the buffy coat of heparinized blood are also suitable.

Control

Modified live vaccines, which are available commercially, provide adequate protection when administered to pups after maternally-derived antibody has declined to negligible levels, usually after 12 weeks of age. Most CDV vaccines are produced from egg-adapted or avian cell culture-adapted virus (Onderstepoort strain) or from canine cell culture-adapted virus (Rockborn strain).

Because post-vaccinal encephalitis has been reported occasionally following the use of canine cell culture-adapted strains, the avian cell culture-adapted strain is considered to be safer. Heterotypic measles virus vaccines have been used in young pups to induce protection in the presence of moderate levels of maternally-derived antibody. Although many dogs remain immune for several years following vaccination, a proportion of vaccinated animals become susceptible after a year. Because of the labile nature of the virus, control can be achieved after an outbreak of disease in kennels by strict isolation and disinfection.

Infections caused by other morbilliviruses

During the late 1980s serious outbreaks of a disease, with clinical and pathological features similar to canine distemper, were recorded in the seal populations of the Baltic and the North Sea. The interest generated by these disease outbreaks of viral infections in marine mammals led to the recognition of several new morbilliviruses including phocine distemper virus, dolphin distemper virus and porpoise distemper virus. Serological evidence of morbillivirus infection has been recorded in several cetacean species.

Hendra virus, equine morbillivirus, was isolated during an outbreak of severe respiratory disease in Australia during 1994. Two humans in contact with infected horses were also affected. Fourteen horses and their trainer died. A related virus, Nipah virus, was isolated in Malaysia during 1999 following outbreaks of disease in pigs and humans working in affected pig units. The disease, which caused a febrile encephalitis, resulted in more than 100 deaths in humans. Although related to morbilliviruses, Hendra and Nipah viruses may be sufficiently different from them to warrant classification in a separate genus. It has been recently proposed that a new genus, *Henipavirus*, be created within the subfamily *Paramyxovirinae*.

Newcastle disease

A large number of avian paramyxovirus (APMV) isolates has been reported worldwide from a range of domestic and wild birds. Nine species of antigenically-distinct APMV are currently recognized in the genus *Rubulavirus*. New isolates are assigned to a species on the basis of antigenic relatedness in haemagglutination inhibition tests. Although infections with most avian paramyxovirses are associated with mild or inapparent disease, infections with APMV-2 and APMV-3 cause respiratory disease in turkeys.

The most important avian paramyxovirus is Newcastle disease virus (NDV), also designated avian paramyxovirus 1 (APMV-1), which causes Newcastle disease. This disease occurs in poultry worldwide. Newcastle disease was first described in 1926 when severe outbreaks were reported in Newcastle, England and in Java. Other major outbreaks of the disease occurred in the Middle East during the late 1960s and in the 1970s when pigeons were the species primarily affected.

Epidemiology

A wide range of avian species including chickens, turkeys, pigeons, pheasants, ducks and geese are susceptible. Infection with NDV is probably endemic in wild birds especially waterfowl (Takakuwa *et al.*, 1998). Strains of NDV differ in their virulence. Isolates are categorized into four groups or pathotypes on the basis of virulence and tissue tropism in poultry:

— viscerotropic velogenic isolates causing severe fatal disease characterized by haemorrhagic intestinal lesions (Doyle's form).
— neurotropic velogenic isolates causing acute disease characterized by nervous and respiratory signs with high mortality (Beach's form).
— mesogenic isolates causing mild disease with mortality confined to young birds (Beaudette's form).
— lentogenic isolates causing mild or inapparent infection (Hitchner's form).

Virus is shed in all excretions and secretions. Transmission usually occurs by aerosols or by ingestion of contaminated feed or water. The relative stability of the virus permits mechanical transfer of infective material through the movement of personnel and equipment. Virus, which can survive in carcases for some weeks, is present in all organs of acutely affected birds and in eggs.

Captive and wild birds can contribute to the spread of infection. Pigeons are susceptible to all strains of NDV and may play a role in the transmission of Newcastle disease. Mesogenic isolates, which can be distinguished from other NDV isolates using monoclonal antibodies, were obtained from racing pigeons in Europe during the early 1980s. These isolates, often referred to as 'pigeon' paramyxovirus 1, are associated with clinical disease in pigeons resembling the neurotropic form of Newcastle disease. Outbreaks of Newcastle disease in poultry in the United Kingdom during 1984 were linked to feed contaminated by infected feral pigeons.

Pathogenesis

Viral replication, which occurs initially in the epithelia of the respiratory and intestinal tracts, is followed by haematogenous spread to the spleen and bone marrow. Secondary viraemia results in infection of other organs including lungs, intestine and CNS. The extent of spread within the body relates to strain virulence which is determined by the amino acid sequence of the F glycoprotein. The fusion (F) glycoprotein of NDV is synthesized in an infected cell as a precursor molecule (F_0) which is cleaved by host cell proteases to F_1 and F_2 subunits. If cleavage fails to occur, non-infectious particles are produced. The F_0 molecules of virulent strains of NDV possess basic amino acids at critical positions which facilitate cleavage by proteases in a wide range of host tissues. In contrast, the replication of lentogenic strains is confined to the respiratory and intestinal epithelia where suitable proteases are produced.

Clinical signs

The incubation period is usually about five days. Respiratory, gastrointestinal and nervous signs occur in chickens. The particular clinical presentation relates to the virulence of the virus strain, its tissue tropism and the age and immune status of the host. Highly virulent strains may produce sudden high mortality in a flock in the absence of premonitory clinical signs. The mortality rate in fully susceptible flocks may be close to 100%. When present, signs in these flocks include listlessness, weakness and a decrease in egg production. Viscerotropic strains tend to produce respiratory signs such as gasping and rales, oedema of the head and neck and greenish diarrhoea. Birds that survive the acute phase may develop neurological signs. Infection with neurotropic velogenic strains results in respiratory disease followed by nervous signs such as wing paralysis, leg paralysis, torticollis and muscle spasms. Mesogenic strains usually cause respiratory disease. Lentogenic strains do not produce disease in adult birds but may produce respiratory signs in young birds. Pathogenicity of NDV isolates relates not only to their virulence but also to host susceptibility. Infection in turkeys, which usually involves the respiratory and central nervous systems, is less severe than that in chickens. Pigeons infected with 'pigeon' paramyxovirus 1 present with neurological signs and diarrhoea, and mortality in affected birds may approach 10%.

Humans may develop a transitory conjunctivitis if exposed to high concentrations of NDV.

Diagnosis

A presumptive clinical diagnosis may be made when the characteristic signs and lesions associated with virulent strains are present. Laboratory confirmation by isolation and identification of the virus is necessary.

- Tracheal and cloacal swabs from live birds are suitable for virus isolation. Suitable postmortem specimens for laboratory examination include faeces, intestinal contents and portions of trachea, intestine, spleen, brain and lung. Samples may be stored at 4°C for up to four days.
- Virus isolation is carried out in embryonated eggs from specific pathogen free (SPF) flocks, usually by inoculation into the allantoic cavity. After incubation, allantoic fluid is tested for haemagglutination activity.
- Haemagglutination-inhibition test using specific antiserum confirms the presence of NDV.

- Virulence of NDV isolates is assessed using *in vivo* tests including the intracerebral pathogenicity index and the intravenous pathogenicity index in SPF chicks. The mean death time (MDT) using embryonated eggs has been employed to classify isolates as velogenic (embryonic death (ED) in less than 60 hours), mesogenic (ED between 60 and 90 hours) and lentogenic (ED in more than 90 hours).

- Demonstration of antibody to NDV is of diagnostic value only in unvaccinated flocks. The haemagglutination-inhibition test is the most widely used assay. Commercial ELISA kits are available.

- Demonstration of viral antigen in tracheal sections or impression smears using immunofluorescence is a less sensitive technique than virus isolation.

Control

General control measures include locating poultry farms several kilometers apart, bird-proofing of houses and food stores, controlled access to farms, thorough cleaning and disinfection of vehicles and equipment and restriction of movement between poultry farms. National control policies for Newcastle disease differ from country to country and range from compulsory vaccination to slaughter of infected flocks. A combination of vaccination and slaughter policies is frequently employed. Vaccination is particularly important for birds in breeder flocks. Lentogenic or mesogenic strains of NDV propagated in eggs or tissue culture are used in live vaccines. They are administered as a spray, in drinking water or by intranasal or intraconjunctival instillation. The presence of maternally-derived antibodies interferes with the efficacy of live vaccines. In order to avoid this undesirable effect, vaccination should be delayed until two to four weeks of age or live vaccine should be administered to day old chicks by conjunctival instillation or by a coarse spray. This method, which may result in respiratory disease, establishes active infection in some birds that persists until maternally-derived immunity has waned in the rest of the birds. Revaccination is then carried out when chicks are three or four weeks of age. A schedule of vaccination employing both live and inactivated vaccines gives good results. Vaccinated birds, although protected from clinical disease, can be infected with wild type virus and become shedders.

Blue eye disease in pigs

This condition, caused by porcine rubulavirus, was first observed in pigs during 1980 in Mexico. Blue eye disease is characterized by neurological signs, corneal opacity and reproductive failure. Morbidity and mortality is highest in young pigs. Diagnosis is based on clinical signs, histopathological changes and serological testing of paired serum samples. Suitable tests for the detection of antibodies include haemagglutination-inhibition, ELISA

and virus neutralization. Methods aimed at preventing the introduction of the infection include strict isolation procedures combined with serological testing of replacement animals. Inactivated vaccines have been produced. The disease has not been reported outside Mexico.

Infection caused by bovine parainfluenza virus 3

Infection with bovine parainfluenza virus 3 (BPIV-3), occurs worldwide and is often subclinical. Transmission occurs by aerosols and direct contact. It is facilitated by overcrowding in poorly ventilated conditions. Although uncomplicated infections are frequently subclinical, mild respiratory disease may be seen. The virus is commonly isolated from animals during outbreaks of serious respiratory disease such as enzootic calf pneumonia and shipping fever, conditions in which other respiratory viruses and bacteria are often involved. Various stress factors such as transportation or adverse environmental conditions may contribute to the severity of the disease.

The virus infects ciliated epithelium of the respiratory tract, alveolar epithelium and macrophages. Infection causes destruction of ciliated epithelium resulting in interference with the mucociliary clearance mechanism. In addition, phagocytosis and intracellular destruction of bacteria by alveolar macrophages are depressed, predisposing to secondary bacterial infection in the lungs. Most uncomplicated infections with BPIV-3 are mild and are characterized by fever, nasal discharge and coughing. Most affected animals recover within a few days. The virus can be isolated in suitable bovine cell lines from nasal swabs or lung tissue. Samples should be taken from several animals in the early stages of the disease and transferred immediately to the laboratory in viral transport medium. Direct immunofluorescence for detecting viral antigen can be carried out on samples of nasal mucus or on cryostat sections of lung. Haemagglutination-inhibition tests, virus neutralization, ELISA and indirect immunofluorescence are commonly used to demonstrate a four-fold rise in antibody titre between acute and convalescent sera.

Both inactivated and modified live BPIV-3 vaccines are available, often combined with other respiratory viruses. Modified live vaccines are designed either for intranasal administration or for intramuscular injection. Immunity tends to be shortlived and reinfection may occur after some months.

Infection caused by bovine respiratory syncytial virus

Pulmonary disease, caused by bovine respiratory syncytial virus (BRSV), is recorded in beef and dairy calves worldwide. Infections occur in cattle, sheep and goats. The virus is named for the characteristic syncytia which it induces in infected cells *in vivo* and *in vitro*.

Epidemiology

Infection in cattle is common. Moderate to severe respiratory signs often develop in infected calves. Infection in adult animals is usually mild or subclinical but severe disease may occasionally occur (Ellis *et al.*, 1996; Elvander, 1996). Persistent infection in individual animals is considered to be responsible for the maintenance of infection in herds. Transmission occurs through aerosols or through direct contact with infected animals. Most clinical cases are recorded during autumn and winter months. Transportation, overcrowding or adverse weather conditions can precipitate outbreaks of the disease. Concurrent infection with bovine viral diarrhoea virus results in more severe clinical signs than those encountered in infection with each individual virus (Pollreiz *et al.*, 1997).

Pathogenesis

The virus replicates in the epithelia of the respiratory system. Destruction of bronchiolar epithelium results in necrotizing bronchiolitis. Multinucleate cells are occasionally formed by fusion of infected type 2 pneumocytes. Bovine respiratory syncytial virus is considered to be immunosuppressive. This effect along with the accumulation of cellular debris and exudate in pulmonary airways facilitates bacterial proliferation.

Clinical signs

Affected animals are typically between three and nine months old. Clinical signs, which range from mild to severe, include fever, nasal and lacrimal discharge, coughing and polypnoea. As the disease progresses, open-mouth and abdominal breathing may be present. The course of the disease is usually up to two weeks. A biphasic pattern is commonly observed in outbreaks among beef calves. Mild respiratory disease is followed by apparent recovery and, within a few days, dyspnoea and pulmonary emphysema develop. Mortality in these outbreaks may reach 20 %.

Diagnosis

Clinical signs and pathological findings may permit a presumptive diagnosis. Laboratory confirmation is necessary for definitive diagnosis.

- Suitable specimens for laboratory examination include nasal swabs, bronchoalveolar lavage fluid, lung tissue and paired serum samples. Specimens should be collected from several animals in the affected group.
- As the virus is thermolabile, specimens must be transferred to the laboratory rapidly in a suitable transport medium.
- Virus isolation is not attempted routinely as it is difficult and requires several blind passages in cell culture.
- Commercial ELISA kits are available for the detection of viral antigen. Immunofluorescence is a rapid and useful technique. Viral antigen can be detected more readily in specimens from the lower respiratory tract than in nasal swabs.
- Polymerase chain reaction procedures have been described for the detection of specific viral nucleic acid (Valarcher *et al.*, 1999).
- Suitable serological tests for demonstrating a rising antibody titre include virus neutralization and ELISA. Serum samples should be taken early in the course of the disease as antibody levels tend to rise rapidly.

Control

Suitable control measures include reducing stress factors, maintaining good hygiene in calf pens, raising calves away from older age groups and implementing a closed herd policy. Modified live and inactivated vaccines, which are safe, are administered parenterally and tend to induce systemic antibody responses, mainly to the fusion surface glycoprotein. Although vaccination tends to reduce the likelihood of clinical disease in exposed animals, the duration of protection is short and frequent boosters may be required. An intranasal recombinant herpes-1 vaccine expressing the attachment (G) glycoprotein and a subunit fusion glycoprotein vaccine expressed in recombinant baculovirus-infected insect cells have recently been developed (Taylor *et al.*, 1998; Sharma *et al.*, 1996).

References

Appel, M.J.G. and Summers, B.A. (1995). Pathogenicity of morbilliviruses for terrestrial carnivores. *Veterinary Microbiology*, **44**, 187–191.

Ellis, J.A., Philibert, H., West, K. *et al.* (1996). Fatal pneumonia in adult dairy cattle associated with active infection with bovine respiratory syncytial virus. *Canadian Veterinary Journal*, **37**, 103–105.

Elvander, M. (1996). Severe respiratory disease in dairy cows caused by infection with bovine respiratory syncytial virus. *Veterinary Record*, **138**, 101–105.

Forsyth, M.A. and Barrett, T. (1995). Evaluation of polymerase chain reaction for the detection and characterization of rinderpest and peste des petits ruminants viruses for epidemiological studies. *Virus Research*, **39**, 151–163.

Inui, K., Barrett, T., Kitching, R.P. and Yamanouchi, K. (1995). Long term immunity in cattle vaccinated with a recombinant rinderpest vaccine. *Veterinary Record*, **137**, 669–670.

Ngichabe, C.K., Wamwayi, H.M., Barrett, T. *et al.* (1997). Trial of a capripoxvirus-rinderpest recombinant vaccine in African cattle. *Epidemiology and Infection*, **118**, 63–70.

Pollreiz, J.H., Kelling, C.L., Brodersen, B.W. *et al.* (1997). Potentiation of bovine respiratory syncytial virus infection in calves by bovine viral diarrhoea virus. *Bovine Practitioner*,

31, 32–38.

Roelke-Parker, M.E., Munson, L., Packer, C. *et al.* (1996). A canine distemper virus epidemic in Serengeti lions (*Panthera leo*). *Nature*, **379**, 441–445.

Sharma, A.K., Woldehiwet, Z., Walrevens, K. and Letteson, J. (1996). Immune responses of lambs to the fusion (F) glycoprotein of bovine respiratory syncytial virus expressed on insect cells infected with a recombinant baculovirus. *Vaccine*, **14**, 773–779.

Stettler, M., Beck, K., Wagner, A., Vandevelde, M. and Zurbriggen, A. (1997). Determinants of persistence in canine distemper viruses. *Veterinary Microbiology,* **57**, 83–93.

Taylor, G., Rijsewijk F.A.M., Thomas L.H. *et al.* (1998). Resistance to bovine respiratory syncytial virus (BRSV) induced in calves by a recombinant bovine herpesvirus-1 expressing the attachment glycoprotein of BRSV. *Journal of General Virology*, **79**, 1759–1767.

Takakuwa, H., Toshihiro I., Takada, A. *et al.* (1998). Potentially virulent Newcastle disease viruses are maintained in migratory waterfowl populations. *Japanese Journal of Veterinary Research,* **45**, 207–215.

Valarcher J.F., Bourhy H., Gelfi J. and Schelcher F. (1999). Evaluation of a nested reverse transcription-PCR assay based on the nucleoprotein gene for diagnosis of spontaneous and experimental bovine respiratory syncytial virus infections. *Journal of Clinical Microbiology*, **37**, 1858–1862.

Further reading

Alansari, H., Duncan R.B., Baker J.C. and Potgeiter L.N.D. (1999). Analysis of ruminant respiratory syncytial virus isolates by RNAase protection of the G glycoprotein transcripts. *Journal of Veterinary Diagnostic Investigation*, **11**, 215–220.

Chapter 66

Rhabdoviridae

Members of the family *Rhabdoviridae* (Greek *rhabdos*, rod) have characteristic rod shapes (Fig. 66.1). This family, along with the families *Paramyxoviridae*, *Bornaviridae* and *Filoviridae,* belongs to the order *Mononegavirales* (Fig. 66.2). Viruses in this order possess a linear, non-segmented RNA genome of negative polarity encased in a ribonucleoprotein complex. Rhabdoviruses of vertebrates are bullet- or cone-shaped while those infecting plants are generally bacilliform. It is a large family, containing viruses of vertebrates, invertebrates and plants. The family *Rhabdoviridae* comprises six genera; *Vesiculovirus, Lyssavirus, Ephemerovirus, Cytorhabdovirus, Novirhabdovirus* and *Nucleorhabdovirus.* Moreover, a large number of rhabdoviruses have yet to be assigned to a genus. *Vesiculovirus, Lyssavirus* and *Ephemerovirus* genera contain viruses which infect vertebrates. Infectious haematopoietic necrosis virus and related rhabdoviruses of fish are included in the genus *Novirhabdovirus.*

Rhabdoviruses usually contain five major proteins: a large RNA-dependent RNA polymerase (L), a surface

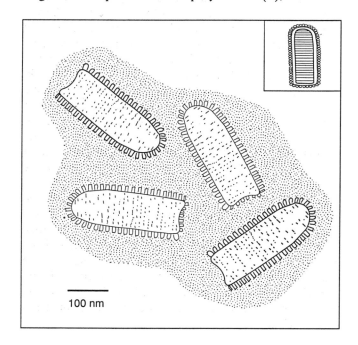

Key points
- Enveloped RNA viruses with helical symmetry and rod-shaped morphology
- Rabies virus and related lyssaviruses
  —present in saliva; transmitted by biting carnivores and bats
  —cause encephalitis in mammals which is invariably fatal
- Vesicular stomatitis viruses
  —transmitted by direct contact and environmental contamination or by arthropod vectors
  —cause febrile disease with vesicular lesions especially in cattle, horses and pigs
- Bovine ephemeral fever virus
  —transmitted by biting arthropods
  —causes febrile transient illness with ill-defined clinical signs

glycoprotein (G), a nucleoprotein (N), a protein component of the viral polymerase (P) and a matrix protein (M). The G protein forms the surface peplomers which interact with host cell receptors, facilitating endocytosis of the virion. In addition, the G protein induces virus-neutralising antibodies and cell-mediated immunity. Replication occurs in the cytoplasm (with the exception of nucleorhabdoviruses). Newly synthesized nucleocapsids acquire envelopes from the plasma membrane as virions bud from the cell. Virions (100 to 430 nm x 45 to 100 nm) are stable in the pH range of 5 to 10. They are rapidly inactivated by heating at 56°C, by treatment with lipid solvents and by exposure to UV light.

Clinical infections

Rhabdoviruses of veterinary importance are presented in Tables 66.1 and 66.2. They can be transmitted by bites of mammals, arthropod vectors or direct contact. Infection may also be acquired through environmental contamination.

The best known and most important member of the

Figure 66.1 Rhabdovirus particles as they appear in an electron micrograph and a diagrammatic representation (inset).

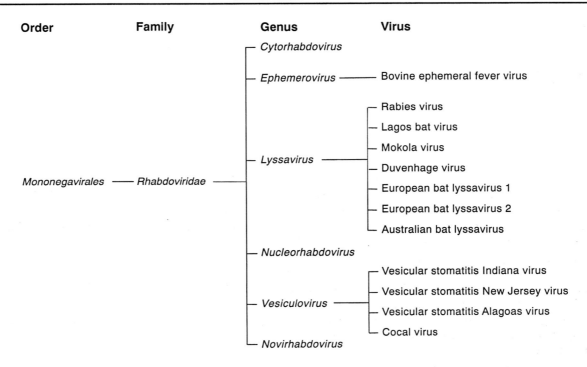

Figure 66.2 A classification of rhabdoviruses with emphasis on those of veterinary importance

Rhabdoviridae is rabies virus, a *Lyssavirus* (Greek *lyssa*, rage or fury). A number of distinct *Lyssavirus* genotypes produce clinical signs indistinguishable from rabies. More than 25 viruses isolated from animals have been classified in the genus *Vesiculovirus*. The most important vesiculoviruses which infect domestic animals are the vesicular stomatitis Indiana virus and the vesicular stomatitis New Jersey virus (Table 66.2). Bovine ephemeral fever virus, of significance in some countries, is the type species of the genus *Ephemerovirus*. Some fish diseases, such as infectious haematopoietic necrosis, viral haemorrhagic septicaemia and spring viraemia of carp are also caused by rhabdoviruses.

Rabies

This viral infection, which affects the central nervous system of most mammals including man, is invariably fatal. However, mammalian species vary widely in their susceptibility. Most clinical cases are due to infection with rabies virus (genotype 1). A number of other neurotropic lyssaviruses, closely related to the rabies virus, produce clinical signs indistinguishable from rabies (Table 66.1). Genetic sequencing and antigenic studies have been used to categorize lyssaviruses into seven genotypes and four serotypes (Smith, 1996; Gould *et al.*, 1998). Each genotype is assigned separate species status. Classical rabies caused by genotype 1 lyssavirus is endemic on continental land masses with the exception of Australia and Antarctica. Many island countries are also free of the disease.

Epidemiology

Several species-adapted strains of rabies virus have been described. Strains affecting a particular species are transmitted more readily to members of that species than to other animal species. In a given geographical region, rabies is usually maintained and transmitted by particular mammalian reservoir hosts. Two epidemiologically important infectious cycles are recognised, urban rabies in dogs and sylvatic rabies in wildlife. More than 95% of human cases are the result of bites from rabid dogs. Racoons, skunks, foxes and bats are important reservoirs of rabies virus in North America (Krebs *et al.*, 1998). In continental Europe, the principal reservoir is the red fox. The vampire bat is an important reservoir of the virus in Central and South America and in the Caribbean islands. In developed countries, the control of stray dogs and vaccination programmes have reduced the importance of urban rabies and have focused attention on wildlife reservoirs.

Species susceptibility to rabies virus is important epidemiologically. Domestic animals and man are considered to be moderately susceptible to the virus, whereas foxes, wolves, coyotes and jackals are considered to be highly susceptible. Although virus may be transmitted through scratching and licking, transmission usually occurs through bites. Infected animals may excrete virus in their saliva for some time before the onset of clinical signs.

Pathogenesis

Following introduction into the tissues, virus enters

Table 66.1 Lyssaviruses which cause rabies and rabies-like diseases.

Virus	Genotype	Serotype	Geographical distribution	Comments
Rabies virus	1	1	Apart from Australia and Antartica, rabies virus (genotype 1) occurs on all continents. Many island countries are free of the disease	Causes fatal encephalitis in many mammalian species. Transmitted by wildlife species including foxes, racoons and bats; domestic carnivores also involved in transmission. Rabies is a major zoonotic disease
Lagos bat virus	2	2	Africa	Isolated initially from fruit bats; also isolated from domestic animals with encephalitis
Mokola virus	3	3	Africa	Isolated initially from shrews; also isolated from domestic animals. Human infection reported
Duvenhage virus	4	4	Africa	Originally isolated from a human bitten by an insectivorous bat; additional cases reported in humans. Not reported in domestic animals
European bat lyssavirus 1	5	–	Europe	Identified with increasing frequency in insectivorous bats. Human infection reported
European bat lyssavirus 2	6	–	Europe	Isolated initially from a human with symptoms of rabies; present in insectivorous bats. Additional human cases reported; not reported in domestic animals
Australian bat lyssavirus	7	–	Australia	Identified in fruit bats and in insectivorous bats; human infection reported

peripheral nerve endings. There may be limited replication locally in myocytes or other tissue cells. The virus is transported to the central nervous system by retrograde axoplasmic flow and becomes widely disseminated in nervous tissue by intra-axonal spread. Clinical signs develop following neuronal damage caused by viral replication. Virus spreads centrifugally within nerve cell processes and is released at axon terminals where it infects many non-nervous tissues including the salivary glands. The presence of virus in saliva, especially in carnivores, is an important factor in rabies transmission.

Although rabies viral antigens are highly immunogenic, immune detection is delayed because intracellular transport prevents contact with the cells of the immune system in the early stages of infection.

Clinical signs
The incubation period, which is highly variable and can be as long as six months, is influenced by various factors including host species, virus strain, the amount of inoculum and the site of introduction of the virus. Large amounts of virus introduced into deep bite wounds in the head region are usually associated with short incubation periods. The clinical course in domestic carnivores, which usually lasts for days or for a few weeks, may encompass prodromal, furious (excitative) and dumb (paralytic) phases. In certain rabid animals, some of these phases may not be observed. In the prodromal phase, affected

animals are often confused and disorientated; wild animals may lose their natural fear of humans. The furious phase is charaterized by an increase in aggressiveness and hyperexcitability, and there is a tendency to bite at inanimate objects and at other animals. Affected animals may roam over long distances. The furious form is observed more often in cats than in dogs. Foxes rarely exhibit this form of the disease. In dumb rabies, muscle weakness, difficulty in swallowing, profuse salivation and dropping of the jaw are the usual features. These clinical signs may be mistaken for those caused by a foreign body in the mouth or throat. The term hydrophobia, a synonym for rabies in humans, relates to the inability to swallow water because of pharyngeal paralysis.

Diagnosis
Ante-mortem diagnostic tests for rabies are not generally used. In endemic areas, suspect domestic carnivores which have bitten humans should be isolated and observed for up to 14 days. The brains of animals which develop clinical signs should be examined for the presence of virus. Rapid laboratory confirmation is essential for the implementation of appropriate treatment of human patients.

- Non-suppurative encephalitis characterized by perivascular lymphoid cuffing and intracytoplasmic inclusions (Negri bodies) may be demonstrable histologically.
- The direct fluorescent antibody test (FAT), which provides a rapid and specific diagnosis, may yield false-

negative results with autolysed brain specimens. The conjugated antisera usually used for diagnosis are specific for rabies virus (serotype 1).

- Rabies virus can be cultured in neuroblastoma cells or in baby hamster kidney cells. Culture of the virus is of value when results of the FAT are uncertain. Rabies virus, which is non-cytopathic, can be detected in tissue culture using conjugated antisera.
- Suckling mice, inoculated intracerebrally with brain tissue from suspect rabies cases, should be observed over several days for the development of disease. The FAT is used to confirm the presence of rabies virus in infected mice.
- Reverse transcriptase polymerase chain reaction (RT-PCR) has been used to detect viral RNA in brain samples. This test can distinguish rabies virus (genotype 1) from rabies-related lyssaviruses. The sensitivity of RT-PCR can be enhanced by combining the technique with ELISA which aids detection of amplified product (Whitby et al., 1997).

Control

Most countries which are free of rabies rely on rigorous quarantine measures to prevent the introduction of disease. Movement of vaccinated domestic carnivores is permitted between some countries provided that strict identification and testing procedures are in place. In countries where rabies is endemic, control methods are aimed mainly at reservoir species. Urban rabies can be effectively controlled by vaccination and restriction of movement of dogs and cats and by the elimination of stray animals. Control of sylvatic rabies requires special measures. Regional depopulation of reservoir species, which has rarely been successful, is ecologically unacceptable. Vaccination of red foxes with live oral vaccines delivered in baits has eliminated sylvatic rabies from several regions of western Europe. Although attenuated virus vaccines were used initially, there was uncertainty about their ultimate safety. A vaccinia-rabies virus glycoprotein (VRG) vaccine was developed and has proved effective for vaccinating foxes (Pastoret and Brochier, 1999), coyotes (Fearneyhough et al., 1998) and racoons (Hanlon et al., 1998). The rapid increase in racoon rabies in the USA has proved difficult to control through vaccination (Smith, 1996). Laboratory based studies with recombinant rabies vaccines indicate that these vaccines are likely to be effective in the control of rabies in most wildlife species.

Commercial vaccines available for the immunization of domestic carnivores by parenteral inoculation contain inactivated virus (genotype 1) and are potent and safe. These inactivated rabies vaccines are considered to be effective against strains of genotype 1 virus. Their ability to induce protection against infection with other lyssavirus genotypes is variable and, in some instances, cross-protection may not occur.

Vesicular stomatitis

This febrile disease affects mainly horses, cattle and pigs. Other susceptible species include camels, several wildlife species and humans. Vesicular stomatitis is clinically similar to foot-and-mouth disease and is classified as a list A disease by the Office International des Epizooties. A number of closely related, antigenically distinct members of the genus Vesiculovirus, of which the type species is vesicular stomatitis Indiana virus, can cause the disease. Most outbreaks are associated with vesicular stomatitis Indiana virus or with vesicular stomatitis New Jersey virus, a more virulent virus. Cocal virus and vesicular stomatitis Alagoas virus, also referred to as subtypes 2 and 3 of vesicular stomatitis Indiana virus, have been isolated from outbreaks in horses and cattle in South America (Table 66.2).

Epidemiology

Infection is endemic in Central America and in regions of South America and the USA. Outbreaks of the disease occur every two to three years in tropical and subtropical regions, with clinical cases most common at the end of the rainy season and early in the dry season. Rapid spread from endemic areas to other regions may occur during some summer seasons. Disease outbreaks in temperate regions, which occur every five to ten years, usually cease abruptly with the onset of winter.

Table 66.2 Viruses of veterinary significance in the genera Vesiculovirus and Ephemerovirus.

Genus / Virus	Hosts	Comments
Vesiculovirus		
Vesicular stomatitis Indiana virus	Cattle, horses, pigs, humans	Causes febrile disease with vesicular lesions; resembles foot-and-mouth disease clinically. Occurs in North and South America
Vesicular stomatitis New Jersey virus	Cattle, horses, pigs, humans	Causes febrile disease with vesicular lesions; infection more severe than that caused by the Indiana virus. Occurs in North and South America
Vesicular stomatitis Alagoas virus (Brazil virus)	Horses, mules, cattle, humans	Originally isolated from mules in Brazil
Cocal virus (Argentina virus)	Horses	Isolated initially from mites in Trinidad; occurs in South America
Ephemerovirus		
Bovine ephemeral fever virus	Cattle	Causes febrile illness of short duration; occurs in Africa, Asia and Australia

Although the mode of transmission is incompletely understood, direct contact and insect vectors have been implicated. Virus is shed in saliva and can contaminate water and feed troughs. The involvement of insect vectors is inferred from the seasonal occurrence of cases and from the pattern of spread with clustering of cases along river valleys and in irrigated areas. Virus has been isolated from many insect species including blackflies, mosquitoes, sandflies and houseflies. Viral replication in blackflies has been demonstrated experimentally. It is unclear how biting insects acquire the virus from domestic animals as a viraemic phase has not been demonstrated in these species.

Pathogenesis

Virus probably enters the body through abrasions on the skin or mucous membranes or following an insect bite. Vesicles which develop at the site of infection may coalesce. Spread may occur locally by extension from primary lesions. Although secondary lesions at distant sites may develop, it is unclear how transfer of the virus occurs and if these lesions result from viraemia or following environmental contamination (Clarke *et al.*, 1996).

Clinical signs

The incubation period is up to five days. Subclinical infection is common. Affected animals, which are usually more than one year old, become febrile. Vesicles develop on the tongue and on oral mucous membranes, often accompanied by profuse salivation. Secondary lesions may occur on the coronary band and teats. Lameness is often a prominent feature of the disease in pigs. Mastitis may develop in cows with severe teat lesions. In the absence of secondary infection, lesions generally heal within two weeks.

The economic impact of the disease relates to production losses, culling and other disease control measures (Hayek *et al.*, 1998). Following infection, animals develop high levels of neutralising antibodies but the duration of protection is variable. Cross-protection between vesicular stomatitis Indiana virus and vesicular stomatitis New Jersey virus is limited.

Diagnosis

Prompt laboratory confirmation is required because of similarities between vesicular stomatitis, foot-and-mouth disease and swine vesicular disease. If horses present with vesicular lesions, infection with vesicular stomatitis virus should be considered.

- Suitable specimens for isolation of virus or the detection of viral antigen include epithelium from lesions and vesicular fluid.
- Viral antigen can be detected by CFT or ELISA.
- Virus may be isolated in suitable cell lines, in embryonated eggs or in suckling mice by intracerebral inoculation. The virus is cytopathic. The fluorescent

antibody test, ELISA, CFT or the virus neutralization test are suitable procedures for identification of isolates.
- Electron microscopy can be used to identify virus in specimens or tissue culture.
- Antibody levels in recovered animals may be assayed by CFT, the virus neutralization test, competitive ELISA or IgM-specific capture ELISA. Because levels of complement-fixing and IgM antibodies persist for only short periods, assays based on procedures involving these antibodies can be used to confirm recent infections in endemic areas.

Treatment and control

- Specific treatment is not available. Measures aimed at minimising secondary infections may be beneficial.
- Suspected cases should be notified to the relevant authorities. Movement restrictions and a 30-day quarantine period following the last clinical case are recommended for infected premises. International trade restrictions are generally instituted following an outbreak.
- Insect-proof buildings and avoidance of habitats associated with insect vectors reduce the likelihood of infection.
- Although both inactivated and attenuated vaccines have been used, they are not commercially available.
- Vesicular stomatitis is a zoonotic disease.

Bovine ephemeral fever

This arthropod-borne viral disease of cattle and water buffalo occurs in tropical and subtropical regions of Africa, Asia and Australia. The virus causes subclinical infection in many other ruminant species including Cape buffalo, wildebeest, waterbuck and deer.

Epidemiology

Epidemiological evidence suggests that *Culicoides* species are involved in transmission of the virus. In tropical areas where bovine ephemeral fever is endemic, subclinical infections are common. Outbreaks often follow periods of rainfall. In more temperate regions, epidemics occur during summer months and tend to decline with the onset of winter. Transmission does not occur by direct contact or by fomites. There is no evidence that the virus persists in animals following recovery from acute illness. It is probable that virus persistence occurs in arthropod vectors.

Pathogenesis

Blood-sucking insects acquire the virus when feeding on animals during the brief viraemic stage of the disease. The virus, which multiplies in the insect vector, is shed in its saliva and is transmitted to a new host through wounds during feeding. Many of the changes observed in infected animals are attributed to host response rather than to direct viral damage.

Clinical signs

The incubation period is up to eight days. The severity of the clinical signs is influenced by the immune status of infected animals and the virulence of the virus strain. The disease tends to be more severe in well-fed animals and high-yielding dairy cows. A biphasic high fever is commonly observed. Affected animals become depressed, anorexic, lame and constipated. Milk production drops dramatically. Muscle stiffness and ruminal stasis may develop. Pregnant animals may abort. Recumbency may be accompanied by salivation and ocular and nasal discharge. Muscular fibrillation and paresis frequently occur, reflecting the accompanying hypocalcaemia. The disease is of short duration and affected animals usually recover after a few days. Most recovered animals develop a solid immunity.

Diagnosis

Diagnosis of bovine ephemeral fever is usually based on clinical signs. Virus neutralization tests or ELISA should be carried out on paired serum samples to detect a rise in virus-specific antibody. Other serological tests such as immunofluorescence are less useful as interpretation is complicated by cross-reacting antibodies induced by infections with related non-pathogenic ephemeroviruses such as Kimberley virus. Neutrophilia, increased plasma fibrinogen and decreased plasma calcium levels are commonly present. Isolation of bovine ephemeral fever virus is difficult.

Treatment

Affected animals should be rested. Anti-inflammatory drugs such as phenylbutazone, flunixin meglumine and ketoprofen have proved useful for treatment (Fenwick and Daniel, 1996). Intravenous or subcutaneous administration of calcium borogluconate is recommended. Oral drenching should be avoided during the acute phase of the illness because swallowing may be impaired.

Control

Vector control is usually impractical in endemic areas. Control is based on the use of vaccines, both inactivated and attenuated. Trials have been carried out using a subunit vaccine based on the envelope glycoprotein (Uren et al., 1994). A recombinant virus-vectored glycoprotein vaccine has been developed.

References

Clarke, G.R., Stallknecht, D.E. and Howerth, E.W. (1996). Experimental infection of swine with a sandfly (*Lutzomyia shannoni*) isolate of vesicular stomatitis virus, New Jersey serotype. *Journal of Veterinary Diagnostic Investigation,* **8**, 105–108.

Fearneyhough, M.G., Wilson, P.J., Clark, K.A., *et al.* (1998). Results of an oral rabies vaccination program for coyotes. *Journal of the American Veterinary Medical Association*, **212**, 498–502.

Fenwick, D.C. and Daniel, R.C.W. (1996). Evaluation of the effect of ketoprofen on experimentally induced ephemeral fever in dairy heifers. *Australian Veterinary Journal*, **74**, 37–41.

Gould, A.R., Hyatt, A.D., Lunt, R. *et. al.* (1998). Characterization of a novel lyssavirus isolated from *Pteropid* bats in Australia. *Virus Research*, **54**, 165–187.

Hanlon, C.A., Niezgoda, M., Hamir, A.N., *et. al.* (1998). First North American field release of a vaccinia-rabies glycoprotein recombinant virus. *Journal of Wildlife Diseases*, **34**, 228–239.

Hayek, A.M., McCluskey, B.J., Chavez, G.T. and Salman, M.D. (1998). Financial impact of the 1995 outbreak of vesicular stomatitis on 16 beef ranches in Colorado. *Journal of the American Veterinary Medical Association*, **212**, 820–823.

Krebs, J.W., Smith, J.S., Rupprecht, C.E. and Childs, J.E. (1998). Rabies surveillance in the United States during 1997. *Journal of the American Veterinary Medical Association*, **213**, 1713–1728.

Pastoret, P.P. and Brochier, B. (1999). Epidemiology and control of fox rabies in Europe. *Vaccine*, **17**, 1750–1754.

Smith, J.S. (1996). New aspects of rabies with emphasis on epidemiology, diagnosis, and prevention of the disease in the United States. *Clinical Microbiology Reviews*, **9**, 166–176.

Uren, M.F., Walker, P.J., Zakrzewski, H., St. George, T.D. and Byrne, K.A. (1994). Effective vaccination of cattle using the virion G protein of bovine ephemeral fever as antigen. *Vaccine*, **12**, 845–850.

Whitby, J.E., Heaton, P.R., Whitby, H.E. *et al.* (1997). Rapid detection of rabies and rabies-related viruses by RT-PCR and enzyme-linked immunosorbent assay. *Journal of Virological Methods*, **69**, 63–72.

Further reading

Bridges, V.E., McCluskey, B.J., Salman, M.D. *et al.* Review of the 1995 vesicular stomatitis outbreak in the western United States. *Journal of the American Veterinary Medical Association,* **211**, 556–560.

Ministry of Agriculture, Fisheries and Food, UK (1998). *Quarantine and rabies, a reappraisal.* MAFF Publications, London.

Vanselow, B.A., Walthall, J.C. and Abetz, I. (1995). Field trials of ephemeral fever vaccines. *Veterinary Microbiology*, **46**, 117–130.

Chapter 68

Bunyaviridae

The name of this family is derived from Bunyamwera, the place in Uganda where the type species Bunyamwera virus was first isolated. The family *Bunyaviridae* contains more than 300 viruses. Virions, (80 to 120 nm in diameter), are spherical and enveloped. Glycoprotein peplomers project from the surface of the envelope which encloses three circular, helical nucleocapsid segments (Fig. 68.1). The viruses are sensitive to heat, acid pH levels, lipid solvents, detergents and disinfectants. The genera in the family are *Bunyavirus, Phlebovirus, Nairovirus, Hantavirus* and *Tospovirus*. Based on antigenic relatedness, viruses within each genus are placed in serogroups. The genome consists of three single-stranded RNA segments designated small (S), medium (M) and large (L). Genetic reassortment occurs between closely-related viruses. Replication takes place in the cytoplasm of host cells. In the final stages of assembly, virions acquire envelopes by budding into the Golgi network. They are then transported through the cytoplasm in secretory vesicles and released by exocytosis at the cell surface.

> **Key points**
> - Medium-sized, enveloped, single-stranded RNA viruses
> - Replicate in the cytoplasm
> - Labile in the environment
> - More than 300 viruses in the family, the majority are arthropod-borne
> - The family is composed of five genera:
>   —*Bunyavirus* contains viruses which cause congenital defects in cattle and sheep
>   —*Phlebovirus* contains the virus which causes Rift Valley fever
>   —*Nairovirus* contains the virus which causes Nairobi sheep disease
>   —*Hantavirus* contains many viruses which cause haemorrhagic fever in humans; rodents act as reservoirs
>   —*Tospovirus* contains viruses of plants

Viruses in the genera *Bunyavirus, Phlebovirus, Nairovirus* and *Hantavirus* infect vertebrates; those in the genus *Tospovirus* infect plants.

Clinical infections

With the exception of viruses in the genus *Hantavirus*, bunyaviruses are arthropod-borne. These arboviruses are maintained in nature in complex life cycles involving replication in both arthropod vectors and vertebrate hosts. Infection of mammalian cells often results in cytolysis while infection of invertebrate cells is non-cytolytic and persistent. Mosquitoes are the most important vectors. Ticks, sandflies and midges may act as vectors for some bunyaviruses. Arthropod vectors acquire virus from vertebrate hosts during viraemic periods. Each bunyavirus species replicates in a limited number of vertebrate and invertebrate hosts.

Hantaviruses, which are primarily human pathogens, are maintained in nature by persistent infections in rodents

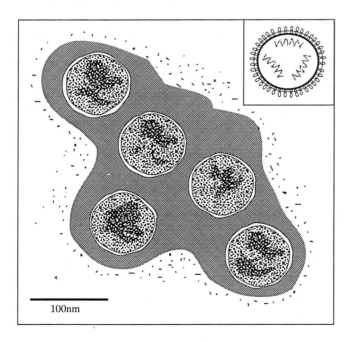

100nm

Figure 68.1 Bunyavirus particles as they appear in an electron micrograph and a diagrammatic representation (inset).

which shed virus in urine, faeces and saliva. Transmission between rodent hosts can occur by aerosols and biting. Individual hantaviruses are associated with particular rodent species. Many bunyaviruses infect humans and frequently cause serious diseases including California encephalitis, haemorrhagic fever with renal syndrome, hantavirus pulmonary syndrome and Crimean-Congo haemorrhagic fever. Such human infections are generally considered to be incidental and do not usually result in disease transmission.

Three important ruminant diseases, Rift Valley fever, Nairobi sheep disease and Akabane disease are caused by bunyaviruses (Table 68.1).

Rift Valley fever

This peracute or acute disease of domestic ruminants in Africa is characterized by abortion and also by high mortality rates in newborn animals. Although a wide range of ruminant species is susceptible to infection, Rift Valley fever occurs primarily in sheep, cattle and goats. Indigenous African ruminants are less susceptible to infection than imported species. Rift Valley fever is also an important zoonotic disease.

Epidemiology
Outbreaks of the disease tend to occur unpredictably in eastern and southern Africa at intervals of five or more years and are associated with abnormally heavy rains and a dramatic rise in vector populations. In exceptional years, large-scale epidemics have occurred in west Africa and in the Nile valley and delta. Transovarial transmission of Rift Valley fever virus (RVFV) occurs in *Aedes* species. During inter-epidemic periods, the virus is maintained in the eggs of floodwater species of mosquito laid in undrained shallow depressions at the edge of temporary pools. Eggs of these species must remain dry for a period before they hatch following re-immersion in water. During epidemics, RVFV replicates in both wild and domestic ruminants and can be transmitted by many species of mosquitoes. Humans are frequently infected during these epidemics. Infected ruminants develop marked viraemia for up to five days after infection. During this period, blood and tissues of affected animals are infectious. Direct and indirect transmission can occur through aerosols, contact with infected placentae or aborted foetuses, fomites or mechanical transfer on the mouthparts of flies. Abattoir workers and veterinarians are particularly at risk of acquiring infection.

Pathogenesis and pathology
Following infection and local replication, viraemia leads to invasion of the liver and other major organs. Cell necrosis is widespread, particularly in the liver. Extensive cytolysis results in foetal death.

Clinical signs
In mature sheep and goats, clinical signs include regurgitation of ingesta, foetid diarrhoea, blood-tinged mucopurulent nasal discharge and, occasionally, icterus. Pregnant ewes can abort. Abortion rates approaching 100% are not uncommon. Mortality rates in adult sheep may be up to 60%. In lambs the incubation period is up to 36 hours. Affected animals are pyrexic, listless and disinclined to move; they may show signs of abdominal pain. Affected lambs rarely survive more than 36 hours after the onset of clinical signs. The mortality rate in lambs less than one week old approaches 90%.

In cattle, mortality rates are usually below 10% and abortion rates range from 15 to 40%.

Human infections with RVFV are often inapparent or may present as a moderate to severe influenza-like illness. The haemorrhagic and encephalitic forms of the disease, which occur in a small number of patients, can be fatal.

Diagnosis
- The histopathological lesions, particularly in the livers of lambs, are considered pathognomonic.

Table 68.1 Bunyaviruses of veterinary importance.

Genus	Virus	Hosts	Comments
Phlebovirus	Rift Valley fever virus	Sheep, cattle, goats	Causes high mortality rates in neonatal animals and abortion in pregnant animals. Endemic in southern and eastern Africa, transmitted by mosquitoes. Important zoonotic disease
Nairovirus	Nairobi sheep disease virus	Sheep, goats	Causes severe, often fatal disease in susceptible animals. Present in central and eastern Africa. Transmitted by ticks
Bunyavirus	Akabane virus, Aino virus, Peaton virus	Cattle, sheep	Viruses belonging to the Simbu serogroup, transmitted by mosquitoes and midges. Widely distributed geographically in tropical and subtropical regions of the Old World. Associated with congenital defects and abortion
	Cache Valley virus	Sheep	Belongs to the Bunyamwera serogroup; transmitted by mosquitoes. Occasionally associated with congenital defects in sheep flocks in North America

Demonstration of viral antigen in fixed tissues by immunohistochemical methods is confirmatory.

- Virus can be isolated in suitable cell cultures, susceptible laboratory animals or embryonated eggs. Specimens for laboratory examinations include blood from viraemic animals, foetal organs and postmortem specimens of liver, spleen and brain. Because the virus can infect laboratory personnel, it should be handled only in properly equipped laboratories.
- Rapid confirmatory tests include detection of viral antigen in serum by ELISA or in impression smears by immunofluorescence.
- Demonstration of antibodies by ELISA in a serum sample or of seroconversion in paired serum samples by virus neutralization, ELISA or hamagglutination inhibition may be used for confirmation of the disease.

Control

Although vector control and environmental management can assist in limiting the spread of Rift Valley fever, such measures are often not feasible. Modified live vaccine containing Smithburn's attenuated strain of RVFV is widely used in endemic regions and during outbreaks. This vaccine is unsafe in pregnant animals because it may cause congenital defects or abortion. A mutagen-attenuated vaccine, developed for use in humans, is effective and appears to be safe for use in pregnant animals (Morrill *et al.*, 1997). Inactivated vaccines prepared from highly immunogenic virulent strains of RVFV are suitable for use in pregnant animals and may be used in Rift Valley fever-free countries bordering endemic regions.

Nairobi sheep disease

This severe, tick-borne viral infection of sheep and goats occurs in central and eastern Africa. The causal agent, Nairobi sheep disease virus (NSDV) is closely related to Ganjam virus of sheep and goats in India. Although humans are susceptible to NSDV, infection appears to be uncommon.

Epidemiology

The brown ear tick (*Rhipicephalus appendiculatus*) is the principal vector of the virus. Transovarial and trans-stadial infection occurs with transmission by all stages of the tick. In endemic areas, lambs and kids exposed to infection while protected by maternally-derived antibody develop active immunity. Outbreaks of disease arise from movement of susceptible animals into endemic areas or from the introduction of infected ticks into Nairobi sheep disease-free areas.

Pathogenesis

Following inoculation by an infected tick, virus replicates in the endothelium, in liver, spleen, lungs and other organs.

Clinical signs

The incubation period is up to six days. There is marked pyrexia and depression followed within 48 hours by foetid dysentery. A mucopurulent nasal discharge and conjunctivitis may be observed. Pregnant animals often abort. The mortality rate ranges from 30% to 90%; death may occur up to 11 days after the onset of clinical signs. The disease is more severe in native breeds of sheep than in Merinos. Clinical signs are milder in goats than in sheep.

Diagnosis

A history of a high mortality rate in a flock recently introduced into an endemic area may point to Nairobi sheep disease. Specimens suitable for virus isolation in cell culture include blood, mesenteric lymph nodes and spleen. Direct immunofluorescence is useful for identification of the virus in tissue culture cells. Viral antigen can be detected directly in tissue specimens by AGID. The indirect immunofluorescent test is recommended for the detection of antibodies to NSDV.

Control

Dipping is used to control the tick vector and animals at risk should be vaccinated. Modified live and inactivated vaccines have been used experimentally but the limited demand has not justified commercial production.

Akabane disease

Bunyaviruses, which belong to the Simbu serogroup and include Akabane, Aino and Peaton viruses, cause congenital defects, such as arthrogryposis and hydranencephaly, and abortion in cattle and sheep. One of the most important and virulent viruses in this group is Akabane virus. Serological studies indicate a widespread distribution in tropical and subtropical regions in the Middle East, Asia, Australia and Africa.

Sporadic epidemics, associated with developmental defects, have been described in Japan, Australia, Israel and parts of Africa. Viruses in the group are transmitted by midges and mosquitoes. Disease outbreaks appear to coincide with movements of the vectors or following the introduction of susceptible animals into endemic areas. Encephalomyelitis and polymyositis develop in foetuses infected with Akabane virus. The extent and degree of the pathological change relate to the stage of gestation at which infection occurred. The most severe damage, involving neurological defects, is evident in calves born to cows infected at about 28 weeks of gestation. Clinical signs are not observed in the dam. Diagnosis is based on gross pathological findings in the foetal CNS and the detection of specific neutralizing antibody in the sera of aborted calves or of newborn animals prior to suckling.

Vector control and vaccination are the methods used to prevent outbreaks of the disease. An inactivated vaccine is available in Japan and Australia. In order to minimize the occurrence of congenital defects in cattle and sheep, breeding stock should be introduced into endemic areas in advance of the breeding season.

Reference

Morrill, J.C., Mebus, A. and Peters, C.J. (1997). Safety and efficacy of a mutagen-attenuated Rift Valley fever virus vaccine in cattle. *American Journal of Veterinary Research*, **58**, 1104–1109.

Chapter 69

Picornaviridae

Picornaviruses (Spanish *pico*, very small), which are icosahedral and non-enveloped, contain a molecule of single-stranded RNA. Virions are 30 nm in diameter (Fig. 69.1). The capsid is composed of 60 identical subunits, each containing four major proteins VP1, VP2, VP3 and VP4. The VP4 protein is located on the inner surface of the capsid. Viral replication occurs in the cytoplasm in membrane-associated complexes and infection is usually cytolytic. Picornaviruses are resistant to ether, chloroform and non-ionic detergents. Individual genera differ in their thermal lability and pH stability. The family comprises six genera: *Enterovirus, Rhinovirus, Cardiovirus, Aphthovirus, Hepatovirus* and *Parechovirus*. It has recently been proposed by the ICTV to create three new genera: *Erbovirus, Kobuvirus* and *Teschovirus* (Pringle, 1999).

Viruses of veterinary importance in the family *Picornaviridae* are presented in Fig. 69.2. Apthoviruses are unstable at pH values below 6.5 and rhinoviruses are unstable below pH 5.0. Viruses in the other genera are stable at acid pH values. Some viruses in the genera

> **Key points**
> - Non-enveloped, positive-sense, single-stranded RNA viruses with icosahedral symmetry
> - Replicate in cytoplasm
> - Resistant to many organic solvents; individual members differ in their susceptibility to pH change
> - Four genera, *Aphthovirus, Enterovirus, Cardiovirus* and *Hepatovirus* contain viruses of veterinary significance
> - Aphthoviruses cause foot-and-mouth disease
> - Enteroviruses cause swine vesicular disease, Teschen/Talfan disease, reproductive problems and enteritis in pigs
> - Cardioviruses cause encephalomyocarditis in young pigs
> - Hepatoviruses cause encephalomyelitis in chickens

Hepatovirus and *Parechovirus*, including hepatitis A virus, are important human pathogens. Poliomyelitis virus which causes serious neurological disease in humans is an enterovirus.

Clinical infections

With the exception of foot-and-mouth disease virus and encephalomyocarditis virus, picornaviruses typically infect a single, or a limited number of, host species. Transmission usually occurs by the faecal-oral route but may also occur by fomites or by aerosols. Some picornaviruses, notably foot-and-mouth disease virus (Bergmann *et al.*, 1996; Mezencio *et al.*, 1999) and swine vesicular disease virus (Lin *et al.*, 1998), can produce persistent infections. Antigenic variation, which may contribute to the development of persistent infection (Woodbury, 1995), has been attributed to a number of molecular mechanisms including genetic recombination. Mixed infections with different serotypes of foot-and-mouth disease virus are known to occur in individual

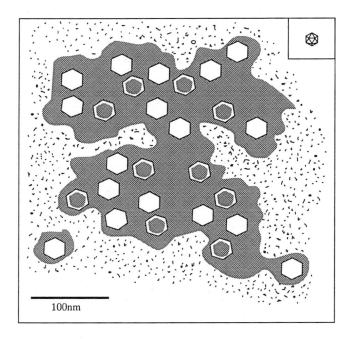

100nm

Figure 69.1 Picornavirus particles as they appear in an electron micrograph and a diagrammatic representation (inset).

Family   Genus   Virus

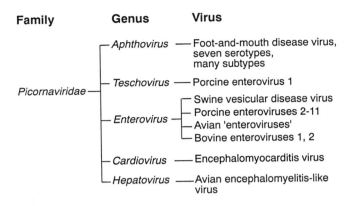

Figure 69.2 Viruses of veterinary importance in five genera of the family *Picornaviridae*.

animals, particularly in African Cape buffaloes. Although infections with enteroviruses are common in many vertebrate species, significant disease occurs only in pigs, poultry and humans (Table 69.1). Rhinoviruses, which are associated with the common cold in humans, are considered to be minor pathogens in cattle.

Swine vesicular disease

This mild vesicular disease of pigs occurs sporadically in parts of Europe and Asia. Because it is indistinguishable clinically from foot-and-mouth disease, accurate laboratory diagnosis of swine vesicular disease (SVD) is essential. Swine vesicular disease virus (SVDV), an enterovirus, is closely related to human coxsackievirus B5. The pig is the natural host for the virus. Laboratory workers handling contaminated material can become infected.

Epidemiology
In the presence of organic matter, SVDV is stable for long periods in the environment and transmission can occur directly or indirectly. Spread of disease from farm to farm is dependent on the movement of infected pigs or contaminated vehicles or fomites. Tissues of infected pigs, which contain large quantities of virus, remain infective despite the low pH values associated with rigor mortis. The virus exhibits prolonged survival in refrigerated pork.

Pathogenesis
Following entry through damaged skin or by ingestion, the virus replicates locally and subsequently spreads via the lymphatics to the blood stream. During a viraemia of short duration, many organs and tissues become infected. Virus shedding, which is greatest during the first week following infection, begins before clinical signs become evident. The faeces and tissue material from infected pigs may contain viable virus for months (Lin *et al.*, 1998).

Clinical signs
The incubation period is up to seven days. Infection is usually characterized by a mild febrile illness. Subclinical disease is common. Transient fever is followed by the development of vesicular lesions on the feet, particularly on the coronary bands. Less commonly, vesicles appear on the lips, tongue and snout. Lameness, dullness and inappetence may be present. Lameness is exacerbated by penning on concrete floors. Affected animals remain in good condition and the lesions heal within a few weeks.

Diagnosis
Laboratory tests are essential for differentiating SVD from other important vesicular diseases of pigs.

- An ELISA is available for the rapid detection of viral antigen in vesicular fluid or in epithelial tissues.
- Samples should be inoculated onto monolayers of susceptible cells. The virus produces cytopathic effects.
- Several serological procedures are suitable for herd screening for antibodies to SVDV. Virus neutralization and ELISA are the tests most frequently used. Virus neutralization, although the standard test, requires tissue culture procedures and takes longer to complete than ELISA. A limitation of ELISA is that it may occasionally yield false-positive results.

Control
Effective vaccines against SVD have been prepared. Commercial vaccines are not available because vaccination is not considered suitable as a control measure in countries free of the important vesicular diseases. In most countries, SVD is a notifiable disease and eradication

Table 69.1 Enteroviruses of veterinary importance.

Virus	Comments
Swine vesicular disease virus	Produces mild vesicular disease, indistinguishable from foot-and-mouth disease
Porcine enterovirus 1 (Porcine teschovirus)	Virulent strains which occur in eastern Europe and the Malagasy Republic cause Teschen disease; widely distributed mild strains cause Talfan disease
Porcine enteroviruses 2 to 11	Infection usually asymptomatic; occasionally cause mild posterior paresis of hind limbs, reproductive problems, diarrhoea or pneumonia
Avian 'enteroviruses'	Virulent strains cause avian encephalomyelitis, nephritis in chickens and hepatitis in ducks and turkeys
Bovine enteroviruses 1 and 2	Isolated from both normal cattle and animals with enteric, respiratory and reproductive disease

policies are enforced with restrictions on the importation of pigs and pork. Control measures, applied following an outbreak of SVD, include thorough cleaning and disinfection of premises, control of pig movement and boiling of waste food fed to pigs.

Porcine enteroviral encephalomyelitis

This condition, also referred to as Teschen/Talfan disease, was first described in Teschen, Czechoslovakia during 1929 and, subsequently, caused significant losses in several European countries. The clinical presentation varies in accordance with the virulence of the infecting strain of porcine enterovirus (PEV). Severe clinical disease is now rare and is largely confined to eastern Europe and the Malagasy Republic.

Epidemiology
Thirteen serotypes of porcine enteroviruses are recognized. Most important neurotropic strains belong to serotype PEV1, which includes both the highly virulent isolates associated with Teschen disease and the less virulent but more widely-distributed strains which cause endemic posterior paresis (Talfan disease). It has recently been proposed to rename PEV1 as porcine teschovirus, type species in the newly created genus *Teschovirus*. Other enterovirus serotypes associated with encephalomyelitis include PEV2, PEV3, PEV4, PEV5, PEV6, PEV8, PEV12 and PEV13. In common with swine vesicular disease, transmission occurs by the faecal-oral route either directly or indirectly. Clinical disease is most severe in young pigs in herds which have not been previously exposed to infection. In herds which are endemically infected, sporadic clinical disease tends to occur after mixing of weaned pigs when maternally-derived immunity has declined.

Pathogenesis
Following ingestion, virus replicates in the tonsils, intestines and associated lymph nodes. Viraemia and invasion of the central nervous system may follow, particularly when virulent strains are involved. Faecal excretion of virus may continue for several weeks.

Clinical signs
Fever, depression and listlessness may be followed about one week after infection by neurological signs. Weakness and incoordination progress to paraplegia and paralysis. Pigs with posterior paralysis may adopt a dog-sitting posture. Severely affected animals exhibit nystagmus, opisthotonos, convulsions and coma. Mortality rate in these animals is high. Mildly affected pigs usually recover.

Diagnosis
- A mild to severe non-suppurative encephalomyelitis is demonstrable histologically.

- Virus can be isolated in porcine kidney cell lines from specimens of brain and spinal cord. The virus produces a cytopathic effect.
- Virus neutralization and ELISA are the most frequently used serological methods for demonstrating antibodies to PEV1. Because antibodies to PEV1 strains are common in pig populations, it is necessary to demonstrate a four-fold rise in titre between acute and convalescent sera for disease confirmation.

Control
Both inactivated and modified live vaccines are effective. Inactivated vaccines are available commercially. Teschen disease is notifiable in many countries. Outbreaks can be controlled by slaughter, strict sanitary measures and ring vaccination.

Reproductive disorders caused by porcine enteroviruses

Several enterovirus serotypes including PEV1, PEV3, PEV6 and PEV8 are associated with the SMEDI syndrome (stillbirths, mummification, embryonic death and infertility) in pigs. Although enteroviruses capable of causing the SMEDI syndrome are widely distributed in commercial pig herds, they are pathogenic only for embryos and foetuses. Clinical disease follows infection of naive, pregnant animals. Cross-protection between serotypes does not occur. Transmission is by the faecal-oral route. Infection of the alimentary tract is followed by viraemia and transplacental spread to developing foetuses. The clinical effects of infection depend on the stage of gestation. Infection during early to mid-gestation results in embryonic death and mummification, whereas infection during the later stages of pregnancy may result in stillbirths or the birth of live piglets. A susceptible sow, therefore, may give birth to mummified, stillborn and live piglets, reflecting the stage of foetal development at the time of infection. The clinical presentation is indistinguishable from porcine parvovirus infection, a more common cause of the SMEDI syndrome. Laboratory confirmation requires either isolation of the virus from lung tissues of stillborn piglets or demonstration of antibody in the serum of stillborn or newborn piglets prior to ingestion of colostrum. Commercial vaccines are not available. Gilts should be exposed to PEV prior to breeding by contact with older sows, faeces or mummified foetuses.

Avian encephalomyelitis

This viral disease of young birds has been recorded in domestic fowl, pheasants, quail and turkeys. Avian encephalomyelitis (AE) is of considerable economic importance in chickens. Although avian encephalomyelitis-like virus (AEV) was formerly considered to be an enterovirus, it has been recently shown to be most closely related to hepatitis A virus and tentatively assigned to the genus *Hepatovirus* (Todd *et al.*, 1999). Horizontal and vertical transmission occurs. The virus produces enteric infection and is shed in the faeces. A proportion of the eggs of infected hens are infected. Chicks infected *in ovo* hatch normally but shed virus and infect other chicks in the incubator shortly after hatching. Infection of the intestinal tract is followed by viraemia, and a competent immune response is required to prevent infection of the central nervous system. Clinical signs, which usually become evident within two weeks, include ataxia and fine tremors of the head and neck. Progressive paralysis leads to death due to inanition or following trampling. Non-suppurative encephalomyelitis and lymphocytic accumulations in viscera, particularly the pancreas, are characteristic. Demonstration of viral antigen in tissues by immunofluorescence or by virus isolation from brain or pancreas is confirmatory. Serological testing of paired sera may be of diagnostic value. Control is achieved by vaccination of breeding flocks with a modified live vaccine to ensure the presence of maternally-derived antibodies in chicks.

Foot-and-mouth disease

This highly contagious disease of even-toed ungulates is characterized by fever and the formation of vesicles on epithelial surfaces. Foot-and-mouth disease (FMD) is a List A disease of major importance internationally on account of its rapid spread and the dramatic economic losses which it causes in susceptible animals. Isolates of foot-and-mouth disease virus (FMDV) are grouped in seven serotypes, recognised as separate species, with differing geographical distributions (Table 69.2). Infection with one serotype does not confer immunity against the other serotypes. A large number of subtypes is recognized within each serotype. Nucleotide sequencing of the VP1 gene, which encodes for a capsid protein, is used for

Table 69.2 The geographical distribution of foot-and-mouth disease virus serotypes. Australia, New Zealand, North and Central America, the Carribean countries and the countries of western Europe are free from the disease[a].

Foot-and-mouth disease virus serotypes	Geographical distribution
O, A and C	South America
O, A and C	Eastern European countries
O, A, C, SAT1, SAT2 and SAT3	Africa
O, A, C and Asia1	Asia

a large outbreak in UK during 2001

comparing an isolate from an outbreak with other isolates of the same serotype in order to determine possible sources of infection.

Epidemiology

Cattle, sheep, goats, pigs and domesticated buffalo are susceptible to FMD. Several wildlife species including African buffalo, elephants, hedgehogs, deer and antelopes are also susceptible. Large numbers of virus particles are shed in the secretions and excretions of infected animals. Virus shedding begins during the incubation period, about 24 hours before the appearance of clinical signs. Transmission can occur by direct contact, by aerosols, by mechanical carriage by humans or vehicles, on fomites and through animal products such as meat, offal, milk, semen or embryos. Infected groups of animals, particularly pigs, shed large quantities of virus in aerosols (Donaldson *et al.*, 2001). Under favourable conditions of low temperature, high humidity and moderate winds, virus in aerosols may spread up to 10 km over land. Turbulence is generally less marked over water than over land. In 1981, virus was carried a distance of more than 200 km from France to the south coast of England.

The virus, which is moderately resistant to environmental factors, is sensitive to acid and alkaline conditions outside the range pH of 6.0 to 9.0. Virus can remain infective on soil for three days in summer and for up to 28 days in the winter. Following death, lactic acid production in muscle inactivates the virus but it may survive in offal and in bone marrow. Foot-and-mouth virus can persist in the pharyngeal region of carrier animals which have recovered from FMD. It can also persist in vaccinated animals infected with a subtype different from the vaccinal subtype. Infection may persist for up to three years in cattle, for many months in sheep and for up to five years in the African Cape buffalo. Transmission of infection from persistently-infected African Cape buffalo to domestic cattle has been recorded. Because of their large respiratory volume and the low dose of virus required to establish infection, cattle are highly suseptible. It is unclear if virus can persist in pigs (Bergmann *et al.*, 1996; Mezencio *et al.*, 1999).

Pathogenesis

Although infection usually occurs through inhalation, virus can also gain entry to tissues through ingestion, insemination and inoculation, and through contact with abraded skin. Primary viral replication, after inhalation, takes place in the mucosal and lymphatic tissues of the pharynx. Viraemia follows primary multiplication with further viral replication in lymph nodes, mammary glands and other organs as well as the epithelial cells of the mouth, muzzle, teats, interdigital space and coronary band. In these areas of stratified squamous epithelium, vesicle formation results from swelling and rupture of keratinocytes in the stratum spinosum.

Clinical signs

The incubation period ranges from 2 to 14 days, but is generally shorter than a week. Infected cattle develop fever, inappetence and a drop in milk production. Profuse salivation, with characteristic drooling and smacking of lips, accompanies the formation of oral vesicles which rupture, leaving raw, painful ulcers. Ruptured vesicles in the interdigital cleft and on the coronary band lead to lameness. Vesicles may also appear on the skin of the teats and udders of lactating cows. Although the ulcers tend to heal rapidly, there may be secondary bacterial infection which exacerbates and prolongs the inflammatory process. Infected animals lose condition. Mature animals seldom die. Calves may die from acute myocarditis. Although the virus does not cross the placenta, abortion probably relates to the pyrexial response.

In pigs, foot lesions are severe and the hooves may slough. Marked lameness is the most prominent sign in this species. The disease in sheep, goats and wild ruminants is generally mild, presenting as fever accompanied by lameness which spreads rapidly through groups of animals.

Human infection, usually mild, has been described on rare occasions in laboratory personnel working with the virus and in individuals handling infected animals.

Diagnosis

Foot-and-mouth disease clinically resembles other vesicular diseases of domestic animals including vesicular stomatitis in cattle and pigs, swine vesicular disease and vesicular exanthema in pigs (Table 69.3). Consequently, FMD requires laboratory confirmation. Laboratory procedures involving FMDV must be carried out in purpose-built laboratories.

- Diagnosis is based on the demonstration of FMDV antigen in samples of tissue or in vesicular fluid.
- Epithelium collected from an unruptured or recently ruptured vesicle is suitable for antigen demonstration.

- In convalescent animals and in persistent or subclinical infections, samples of oesophageal/pharyngeal fluid can be obtained with a probang (sputum) cup.
- Appropriate serological tests include ELISA and CFT. The preferred test is ELISA which is sensitive and specific, and is available in kit form.
- The polymerase chain reaction has been adapted for the amplification of genome fragments of FMDV.
- Virus isolation is carried out in special cell lines such as primary bovine thyroid or kidney cells.
- Demonstration of specific antibody by virus neutralization or ELISA can be used to confirm a diagnosis in unvaccinated animals. In endemic areas, interpretation of antibody titres may prove difficult.

Control

In countries which are free from FMD, it is notifiable and affected and in-contact animals are slaughtered. Following an outbreak, movement restrictions are applied and infected premises must be thoroughly cleaned and disinfected. Mild acids, such as citric acid and acetic acid, and alkalis such as sodium carbonate are effective disinfectants. Reserves of inactivated virus are maintained in several countries to provide an adequate supply of vaccine at short notice in the event of a major outbreak of the disease. Although ring vaccination around an affected premises may help to limit the spread of the disease, it may also allow the development of the carrier state in animals subsequently exposed to the virus.

In countries where FMD is endemic, efforts are generally directed at protecting high-yielding dairy cattle by a combination of vaccination and control of animal movement. Vaccines for FMD, incorporating adjuvant, are derived from tissue culture-propagated virus which has been chemically inactivated. They are usually multivalent, containing three or more virus strains. Protection against antigenically similar strains of virus is satisfactory and lasts for up to six months. Research is continuing into the

Table 69.3 Susceptibility of farm animals to viruses which cause vesicular diseases.

Virus	Species			
	Cattle	Sheep / goats	Pigs	Horses
Foot-and-mouth disease virus	Susceptible	Susceptible	Susceptible	Resistant
Swine vesicular disease virus	Resistant	Resistant	Susceptible	Resistant
Vesicular exanthema of swine virus	Resistant	Resistant	Susceptible	Resistant
Vesicular stomatitis virus	Susceptible	Resistant	Susceptible	Susceptible

development of improved vaccines based principally on peptide synthesis or recombinant DNA technology (Doel, 1996).

Infections caused by equine rhinoviruses

Genomic and other studies have shown that equine rhinovirus 1 is closely related to foot-and-mouth disease virus. It has been renamed equine rhinitis A virus and has been placed in the genus *Aphthovirus*. Infection with rhinoviruses appears to be widespread and most horses are exposed early in life. Although equine rhinitis A virus and equine rhinitis B virus (equine rhinovirus 2) have been associated with acute respiratory disease (Carman *et al.*, 1997; Klaey *et al.*, 1998), they are generally considered to be minor respiratory pathogens. They may contribute to the development of disease following surgery or strenuous exercise or when present in mixed infections with bacteria or other viruses. Viraemia and prolonged shedding of virus in urine occurs in infection with equine rhinitis A virus.

Infection with encephalomyocarditis virus

Rodents are considered to be the natural hosts of encephalomyocarditis virus (EMCV). However, this cardiovirus has a wide host range including humans, monkeys and pigs. Infection in pigs is usually subclinical but sporadic deaths and minor outbreaks have been described. Rats and mice, the principal reservoirs, excrete virus in faeces and urine. The virus is stable in the environment. Pigs acquire infection by ingesting contaminated feed. Pig-to-pig transmission may also occur (Koenen *et al.*, 1999). Following ingestion, viraemia develops within a few days. Subsequently, high titres of virus can be demonstrated in the myocardium, spleen and mesenteric lymph nodes. Transplacental infection may occur. Virus isolates associated with myocardial disease are apparently distinct from those responsible for reproductive disease (Koenen *et al.*, 1999).

Outbreaks of disease are generally restricted to one particular age group. The severity of the disease relates to the strain of virus and the age of the infected pigs. Piglets may die suddenly as a result of heart failure. Hydrothorax, hydropericardium and ascites may be demonstrated at postmortem examination. Areas of myocardial necrosis with associated lymphoid infiltration may be demonstrable histologically. Changes in the CNS are minimal.

Reproductive failure in sows is characterized by mummified foetuses and stillbirths. Laboratory confirmation relies on virus isolation and identification. Virus neutralization and haemagglutination tests can be used to detect specific antibodies. Control of rodents is important in reducing the likelihood of infection. An inactivated vaccine is available commercially in the USA.

References

Bergmann, I.E., Malirat, V., de Mello, P.A. and Gomes I. (1996). Detection of foot-and-mouth viral sequences in various fluids and tissues during persistence of the virus in cattle. *American Journal of Veterinary Research*, **57**, 134–137.

Carman, S., Rosendal, S., Huber, L. *et al.* (1997). Infectious agents in acute respiratory disease in horses in Ontario. *Journal of Veterinary Diagnostic Investigation*, **9**, 17–23.

Doel, T.R. (1996). Natural and vaccine-induced immunity to foot-and-mouth disease: the prospects for improved vaccines. *Revue scientifique et technique Office International des Epizooties*, **1**, 883–911.

Donaldson, A.I., Alexandersen, S., Sorensen, J.H. and Mikkelsen, T. (2001). Relative risks of the uncontrollable (airborne) spread of FMD by different species. *Veterinary Record*, **148**, 602–604.

Klaey, M., Sanchez-Higgins, M., Leadon, D.P. *et al.* (1998). Field case study of equine rhinovirus 1 infection: clinical signs and clinicopathology. *Equine Veterinary Journal*, **30**, 267–269.

Koenen, F., Vanderhallen, H., Castryck, F. and Miry, C. (1999). Epidemiologic, pathogenic and molecular analysis of recent encephalomyocarditis outbreaks in Belgium. *Journal of Veterinary Medicine, Series B*, **46**, 217–231.

Lin, F., MacKay, D.K.J. and Knowles N.J. (1998). The persistence of swine vesicular disease virus infection in pigs. *Epidemiology and Infection*, **121**, 459-472.

Mezencio, J.M.S., Babcock, G.D., Kramer, E. and Brown, F. (1999). Evidence for the persistence of foot-and-mouth disease virus in pigs. *Veterinary Journal*, **157**, 213–217.

Pringle, C.R. (1999). Virus taxonomy — 1999. *Archives of Virology*, **144**, 421–429.

Todd, D., Weston, J.H., Mawhinny, K.A. and Laird, C. (1999). Characterization of the genome of avian encephalomyelitis virus with cloned cDNA fragments. *Avian Diseases*, **43**, 219–226.

Woodbury, E.L. (1995). A review of the possible mechanisms for the persistence of foot-and-mouth disease virus. *Epidemiology and Infection*, **114**, 1–13.

Chapter 70

Caliciviridae

Caliciviruses (Latin *calix*, cup) have cup-shaped depressions, demonstrable by electron microscopy, on the surface of virions. The virions, 27 to 40 nm in diameter, are icosahedral and non-enveloped (Fig. 70.1). The genome consists of a single molecule of linear, positive-sense, single-stranded RNA. Replication takes place in the cytoplasm of infected cells and virions are released by cell lysis. Many caliciviruses have not yet been cultured. The virions are resistant to ether, chloroform and mild detergents. They are relatively resistant to heat but are sensitive to acid pH values.

Caliciviruses, which are closely related to picornaviruses, were formerly grouped within the *Picornaviridae*. Currently, the family *Caliciviridae* is divided into four genera: *Vesivirus*, *Lagovirus* and two unnamed genera of human caliciviruses referred to as 'Norwalk-like viruses' and 'Sapporo-like viruses'. The genus *Vesivirus* contains vesicular exanthema of swine virus, the type virus of the family, San Miguel sea lion virus and feline calicivirus. The *Lagovirus* genus contains two viruses of lagomorphs, rabbit haemorrhagic disease virus and European brown

Key points

- Small, non-enveloped, single-stranded RNA viruses with icosahedral symmetry
- Replicate in the cytoplasm
- Stable in the environment
- Four genera:
  —*Vesivirus* contains viruses which cause vesicular exanthema of swine and feline calicivirus infection
  —*Lagovirus* contains viruses which cause rabbit haemorrhagic disease and European brown hare syndrome
  —Two genera contain human caliciviruses which cause gastroenteritis

hare syndrome virus. The human caliciviruses cause gastroenteritis. 'Norwalk-like viruses' are also referred to as small, round, structured viruses groups 1 and 2 because of the absence of surface detail and their fuzzy appearance when viewed by electron microscopy. Hepatitis E virus of humans, formerly classified in the *Caliciviridae*, has been placed in a newly-created genus 'Hepatitis E-like viruses' which has yet to be assigned to a new family.

Clinical infections

Caliciviruses have been recovered from many species including humans, cats, pigs, marine mammals, rabbits, hares, cattle, dogs, reptiles, amphibians and insects. They are associated with a wide range of conditions including respiratory disease, vesicular lesions, necrotizing hepatitis and gastroenteritis (Table 70.1). Infections with caliciviruses, which are frequently persistent, may be inapparent, mild or acute. Transmission occurs directly or indirectly without vector involvement.

Vesicular exanthema of swine

First reported in southern California in 1932, vesicular exanthema of swine (VES), an acute, highly contagious disease, became widespread throughout the USA during

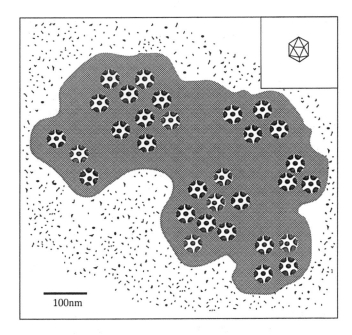

100nm

Figure 70.1 Calicivirus particles as they appear in an electron micrograph and a diagrammatic representation (inset).

Table 70.1 Caliciviruses of veterinary importance.

Virus	Hosts	Comments
Vesicular exanthema of swine virus (13 serotypes)	Pigs	Acute, contagious vesicular disease, clinically similar to foot-and-mouth disease. Occurred in the U.S.A. before 1956. May have arisen from feeding sea lion and seal meat contaminated with San Miguel sealion virus
San Miguel sea lion virus (17 serotypes)	Marine mammals, Opal eye fish	Associated with cutaneous vesicles and premature parturition in pinnipeds; when inoculated into pigs, causes vesicular exanthema
Feline calicivirus	Domestic and wild cats	Important cause of upper respiratory tract infection in cats worldwide
Rabbit haemorrhagic disease virus	European rabbits	Acute fatal disease in European rabbits over two months of age
European brown hare syndrome virus	European brown hare	Related to rabbit haemorrhagic disease virus. Causes hepatic necrosis and widespread haemorrhages with high mortality
Canine calicivirus	Dogs	Occasionally associated with diarrhoea

the 1950s. An eradication campaign included rigorous implementation of laws relating to the cooking of garbage. The last outbreak of VES was recorded in 1956 and the country was declared free of the disease in 1959. A reservoir of the virus exists in marine mammals. In 1972, the San Miguel sea lion virus (SMSV) was isolated from California sea lions, which had developed vesicles on their flippers. Premature parturition occurred in infected animals. Subsequently, SMSV has been isolated from a number of other marine mammals and from the opal eye fish. Strains of SMSV produce VES when inoculated into pigs and it is thought that the original outbreak of VES arose through the feeding of uncooked swill containing meat from infected marine mammals. These vesicular viruses show antigenic heterogeneity. There are 13 serotypes of vesicular exanthema of swine virus and 17 serotypes of SMSV.

The incubation period of VES is up to 72 hours and the course of the disease is approximately two weeks. Vesicles appear on the tongue, lips, snout, interdigital spaces and coronary bands. Affected pigs are febrile and acutely lame. Although morbidity is high, mortality is low. The disease is clinically indistinguishable from foot-and-mouth disease, vesicular stomatitis and swine vesicular disease. Because of its similarity to foot-and-mouth disease, vesicular exanthema of swine is an

important disease. Weight loss in fattening pigs and mortality in neonatal pigs are economically important consequences of the infection.

Vesicular fluid and the overlying flap of epithelium are rich in virus. Isolates can be identified by ELISA, CFT, immunoelectron microscopy and virus isolation in pig kidney cell lines.

Feline calicivirus infection

Infections caused by feline calicivirus (FCV) account for about 40% of upper respiratory tract inflammatory disease in cats worldwide. All species of *Felidae* are considered to be susceptible but natural disease tends to be confined to domestic cats and to cheetahs in captivity. There is a high degree of antigenic heterogeneity among FCV isolates. Sequence analysis studies have shown that individual isolates of FCV exist as quasispecies which evolve and exhibit antigenic drift. Significant alterations in the antigenic profiles of sequential virus isolates from carrier cats are thought to be influenced by immune selection and may play an important part in viral persistence (Radford *et al.*, 1998).

Epidemiology
Although cats of all ages are susceptible to infection with FCV, acute disease occurs most commonly in kittens as maternally-derived antibody wanes between two and six months of age. Infected cats excrete large amounts of virus in oronasal secretions. Many cats remain persistently infected after recovery from acute infection or following subclinical infection while protected by maternally-derived antibody or by vaccination. Infection is maintained in the cat population by these carriers which shed virus continuously from the oropharynx for months and, occasionally, for years.

Pathogenesis
Virus replication occurs primarily in the oropharynx with rapid spread throughout the upper respiratory tract and to the conjunctivae. A transient viraemia occurs. Infections range from subclinical to severe, reflecting differences in strain virulence. Virulent strains of FCV can cause interstitial pneumonia in young kittens. The virus has been recovered from the joints of lame cats.

Clinical signs
The incubation period is up to five days. Clinical signs, which are usually confined to the upper respiratory tract and the conjunctivae, are often less severe than those caused by feline herpesvirus 1 infection. Fever, oculonasal discharge and conjunctivitis are accompanied by the development of characteristic vesicles on the tongue and oral mucosa. These vesicles rupture leaving shallow ulcers. Morbidity may be high but mortality is usually low. Stiffness and shifting lameness, which usually

resolve within a few days, are sometimes seen during the acute phase of FCV infection or following inoculation with FCV vaccine. An association between infection with FCV and chronic gingivitis and stomatitis, when infection with feline immunodeficiency virus is also present, has been suggested.

Diagnosis
* Upper respiratory tract signs along with ulcers on the oral mucosa are suggestive of infection with FCV. Differentiation from feline herpesvirus 1 infection requires laboratory testing.
* Feline calicivirus can be isolated in feline cell lines from oropharyngeal swabs or from lung tissue. Isolation of FCV may not be aetiologically significant because of the large numbers of carrier animals in cat populations.
* Demonstration of a rising antibody titre in paired serum samples is required for laboratory confirmation.

Control
Vaccination and management practices aimed at reducing exposure to the virus are the main methods of control. Inactivated vaccines for parenteral administration and modified live vaccines for either parenteral or intranasal administration are available. Although vaccination protects effectively against clinical disease, it does not prevent subclinical infection or the development of a carrier state. Vaccines are based on a limited number of FCV isolates which cross-react with a broad spectrum of field isolates. An increasing number of recent field isolates are not neutralized by vaccine-induced antisera *in vitro* (Lauritzen *et al.*, 1997). Live vaccines for administration by injection may cause clinical signs if given by other routes.

Rabbit haemorrhagic disease

This is a highly contagious, acute and often fatal disease of European rabbits (*Oryctolagus cuniculus*). Rabbits under two months of age are not susceptible. Rabbit haemorrhagic disease (RHD) was first reported in China during 1984 and has since been encountered in many parts of the world. This virus (RHDV) is considered to be a mutant form of a non-pathogenic virus, termed rabbit calicivirus, which has been endemic in commercial and wild rabbits in Europe for many years. Rabbit haemorrhagic disease virus has been used for biological control of rabbits in Australia and New Zealand.

Epidemiology
Virus is shed in all excretions and secretions. Among rabbits in close contact, transmission is mainly by the faecal-oral route. Infection may also occur by inhalation or through the conjunctiva. Mechanical transmission by a variety of insects including mosquitoes and fleas has been demonstrated. The virus survives in the environment and indirect transmission through contaminated foodstuff or fomites may occur. Spread of virus between units and between countries may result from uncontrolled movement of infected rabbits or from contact with infected rabbit meat, insects or fomites. The virus was inadvertently released from a research facility in Australia during 1995 and, subsequently, was illegally introduced into New Zealand in 1997. In Europe, outbreaks of RHD have been variable in severity and this has been attributed to the presence of rabbit calicivirus infection.

Pathogenesis and pathology
Cells of the mononuclear phagocyte lineage are considered to be the major targets of the virus (Ramiro-Ibanez *et al.*, 1999). Rabbits under two months of age do not develop clinical signs. The reason for this resistance is unclear but it may have a physiological basis.

Severe hepatic necrosis is the most obvious lesion in affected rabbits. In addition, there may be evidence of disseminated intravascular coagulation.

Clinical signs
The incubation period is up to three days. The disease is characterized by high morbidity and high mortality. The course is short with death occurring within 36 hours of the onset of clinical signs. Acutely affected animals are pyrexic and depressed and have an increased respiratory rate. A serosanguineous nasal discharge, haematuria and neurological signs including convulsions may be present. Rabbits may be found dead or die in convulsions. A few rabbits may present with milder, subacute signs during the later stages of an epizootic. Some animals may survive for a few weeks with jaundice, weight loss and lethargy.

Diagnosis
High mortality in rabbits along with characteristic gross lesions including necrotic hepatitis and congestion of spleen and lungs are suggestive of RHD. Culture of RHDV has been unsuccessful. High concentrations of virus are present in affected livers. Confirmation is based on detection of virus by electron microscopy or of viral antigen by ELISA, immunofluorescence or haemagglutination using human erythrocytes. Reverse transcriptase PCR has been developed for the detection of RHDV nucleic acid. Suitable serological tests for the detection of specific antibodies to the virus include haemagglutination-inhibition and ELISA.

Control
In countries where RHD is endemic, control is achieved by vaccination. Inactivated and adjuvanted vaccines prepared from clarified liver suspensions of experimentally-infected rabbits are usually administered at about 10 weeks of age. Novel vaccines, based on recombinant myxoma virus expressing RHDV capsid protein or on virus-like particles

from capsid protein produced in baculovirus expression systems, are being developed.

References

Lauritzen, A., Jarrett, O. and Sabara, M. (1997). Serological analysis of feline calicivirus isolates from the United States and United Kingdom. *Veterinary Microbiology*, **56**, 55–63.

Radford, A.D., Turner, P.C., Bennett, M. *et al.* (1998). Quasispecies evolution of a hypervariable region of the feline calicivirus capsid gene in cell culture and in persistently infected cats. *Journal of General Virology*, **79**, 1–10.

Ramiro-Ibanez, F., Martin-Alonso, J.M., Garcia-Palencia, P. *et al.* (1999). Macrophage tropism of rabbit haemorrhagic disease virus is associated with vascular pathology. *Virus Research*, **60**, 21–28.

Chapter 71

Astroviridae

The family *Astroviridae* (Greek *aster*, star) contains viruses with a surface structure which imparts a star-like appearance. Astroviruses, 28 to 30 nm in diameter, are non-enveloped with icosahedral symmetry (Fig. 71.1). The genome consists of a single molecule of positive-sense, linear, single-stranded RNA. These viruses are resistant to low pH values, various detergents and heating at 60°C for 5 minutes. Replication occurs in the cytoplasm of host cells and virions are released by cell lysis. Trypsin is required for cultivation of these viruses. *Astrovirus* is the only genus in the family.

Key points

- Small, single-stranded RNA viruses with icosahedral symmetry
- Replicate in the cytoplasm
- Single genus *Astrovirus* contains viruses which produce mild gastroenteritis in most domestic species; in ducks serious disease may occur

---

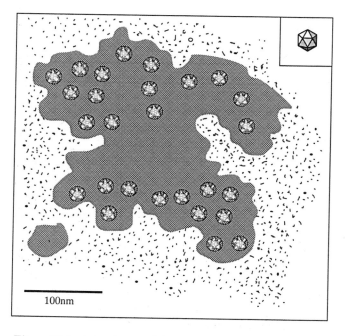

Figure 71.1 Astrovirus particles as they appear in an electron micrograph and a diagrammatic representation (inset).

Clinical infections

Astroviruses, which are distributed worldwide, are associated with self-limiting gastroenteritis in animals and humans. These viruses have been detected in the faeces of humans, cattle, pigs, sheep, dogs, cats, deer, mice, ducks and turkeys. Isolates from different host species are antigenically distinct and species-specific. Two serotypes of bovine astrovirus are recognised. Transmission occurs by the faecal-oral route. Following an incubation period of up to four days, diarrhoea may develop. Infections are mild in most species; in ducklings a severe hepatitis may develop.

Diagnosis is based on the detection of astroviruses in faeces using electron microscopy or ELISA. Detection of viral RNA using reverse transcriptase PCR and virus isolation in primary cell lines or embryonated eggs are also possible. Because astrovirus infections are generally mild, vaccines have not been developed except for duck astrovirus. Control is based on husbandry practices appropriate for the prevention of neonatal enteritis.

Chapter 72

Coronaviridae

Members of the family *Coronaviridae* (Latin *corona*, crown) are large, pleomorphic, enveloped viruses. They contain a single molecule of linear, positive-sense, single-stranded RNA. Club-shaped glycoprotein peplomers projecting from the envelope impart a crown-like appearance to the virus (Fig. 72.1). Each peplomer is composed of a large viral glycoprotein (spike or S protein) which is responsible for attachment to cells. The S protein is the main antigenic component which induces the production of neutralizing antibodies during natural infection. Hypervariable domains in the S protein facilitate the production of virus escape mutants, capable of evading the host immune response. Along with the family *Arteriviridae*, the family *Coronaviridae* belongs to the order *Nidovirales*. There are two genera in the family, *Coronavirus* and *Torovirus*. Coronaviruses, which are almost spherical with a diameter of 120 to 160 nm, have helical nucleocapsids. Toroviruses, which have a tubular nucleocapsid, may be disc-shaped, kidney-shaped or rod-shaped and are 120 to 140 nm in diameter.

Key points
■ Enveloped, pleomorphic, single-stranded RNA viruses
■ Replicate in the cytoplasm
■ Labile in the environment
■ Two genera:
—*Coronavirus*, helical nucleocapsid
—*Torovirus*, tubular nucleocapsid
■ Coronaviruses:
—Systemic disease in cats
—Enteric and systemic disease in pigs
—Respiratory disease in poultry
—Enteric disease in cattle

Coronaviruses replicate in the cytoplasm of cells. Newly synthesized virions acquire their envelopes from the membranes of the endoplasmic reticulum and the Golgi complex. They are incorporated into vesicles and transported to the cell surface where the virions are released following fusion of the vesicles with the plasma membrane. Genetic recombination can occur at high frequency between related coronaviruses.

With the exception of infectious bronchitis virus, coronaviruses are usually difficult to grow in cell culture. The virions are sensitive to heat, lipid solvents, formaldehyde, oxidizing agents and non-ionic detergents. The stability of coronaviruses at low pH values is variable; some are stable at values as low as pH 3.0.

Clinical infections

Coronaviruses can infect a number of mammalian and avian species and many display tropisms for respiratory and intestinal epithelium. The coronaviruses of veterinary importance and the clinical consequences of infection are indicated in Table 72.1. Infections, which are usually mild or inapparent in mature animals, may be severe in young animals. Coronaviruses are aetiologically important in humans as a cause of the common cold.

Although evidence of torovirus infection has been

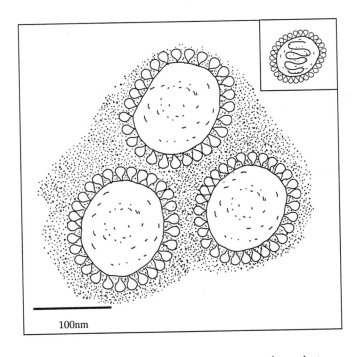

100nm

Figure 72.1 Coronavirus particles as they appear in an electron micrograph and a diagrammatic representation (inset).

Table 72.1 Coronaviruses of veterinary significance.

Virus	Consequences of infection
Feline coronavirus (FCoV)	Replicates in enterocytes; subclinical infection common. May produce mild gastroenteritis in young kittens; also referred to as feline enteric coronavirus (FECV). Feline infectious peritonitis virus (FIPV) is considered to have derived from strains of FCoV which initially replicated in enterocytes and subsequently in macrophages; causes sporadic fatal disease of young cats often presenting clinically as an effusive peritonitis
Transmissible gastroenteritis virus (TGEV)	Highly contagious infection with vomiting and diarrhoea in piglets; high mortality in newborn piglets. A deletion-mutant of TGEV, porcine respiratory coronavirus, induces partial immunity to TGEV
Porcine epidemic diarrhoea virus	Causes enteric infection similar to that caused by TGEV but with lower neonatal mortality
Porcine haemagglutinating encephalomyelitis virus	Nervous disease or vomiting and emaciation (vomiting and wasting disease) in young pigs. Infection is widespread but clinical disease is uncommon
Infectious bronchitis virus	Acute, highly contagious respiratory infection in young birds; causes a drop in egg production in layers
Turkey coronavirus	Infectious enteritis (bluecomb disease)
Bovine coronavirus	Diarrhoea in calves; associated with winter dysentery in adult cattle
Canine coronavirus	Asymptomatic infection or diarrhoea in dogs

found in pigs, sheep, goats and cats (Muir *et al.*, 1990), the clinical significance of these infections is questionable. Two toroviruses have been implicated in enteric diseases of domestic animals (Table 72.2).

Feline infectious peritonitis

This disease, feline infectious peritonitis (FIP), caused by certain strains of feline coronavirus, is a worldwide and invariably fatal, sporadic disease of domestic cats and other *Felidae*. Strains of feline coronavirus vary in pathogenicity. The term feline enteric coronavirus (FECV) has been used to describe strains that cause mild or inapparent enteritis, while the term feline infectious peritonitis virus (FIPV) was applied to those strains aetiologically implicated in FIP. It is believed that FIPV arises as a mutant of the widely distributed FECV resulting in an alteration in tropism from enteric epithelial cells to macrophages (Pedersen and Floyd, 1985; Poland *et al.*, 1996). Current

thinking envisages a single virus termed feline coronavirus (FCoV) which encompasses strains of varying virulence. Although genomic studies have so far failed to demonstrate consistent genetic changes distinguishing enteric from peritonitis strains, they have shown a high degree of genetic relatedness between isolates of the two strains from the same locations (Vennema *et al.*, 1998). Two serotypes of FCoV are described. Serotype 1 accounts for most field infections whereas serotype 2 is thought to have arisen due to a recombinational event between FCoV and canine coronavirus (Herrewegh *et al.*, 1998).

Epidemiology

Feline infectious peritonitis occurs sporadically in catteries or multicat households. The incidence is reported to be higher in pedigree cats (Sparkes *et al.*, 1992). Although cats of any age may be affected, those less than one year of age appear to be most susceptible. A second peak of disease in cats over ten years of age has been noted (Barr, 1998). Infected cats shed virus in faeces and oronasal secretions. Transmission is mainly by ingestion or inhalation. Infection is acquired by young kittens from their mothers or from other adult cats (Addie and Jarrett, 1992). In infected households about 15% of cats are persistently infected carriers, responsible for maintaining the infection. The majority of cats are transiently infected but reinfection can occur.

Pathogenesis

The pathogenesis of FIP is outlined in Fig. 72.2. Infection with FIPV does not always result in clinical disease. Factors which may influence the development of the disease include the age, immune status and genetic characteristics of the host and the emergence of virulent virus strains (Addie *et al.*, 1995). In some instances, probably due to mutational changes in the virus, the emergence of a virulent FIPV strain results in systemic invasion with replication in macrophages. In most infected kittens, the development of effective cell-mediated immunity (CMI) restricts viral replication and ultimately eliminates infection. Some individual animals with less effective CMI may shed virus intermittently while remaining clinically normal. When CMI is severely impaired or defective, virus replication continues leading to B cell

Table 72.2 Toroviruses of veterinary significance.

Virus	Hosts	Comments
Equine torovirus (Berne virus)	Horses	Isolated from rectal swab of a horse with diarrhoea in Berne, Switzerland. Clinical disease appears to be uncommon
Bovine torovirus (Breda virus)	Calves	Diarrhoea in newborn calves, particularly if deprived of colostrum

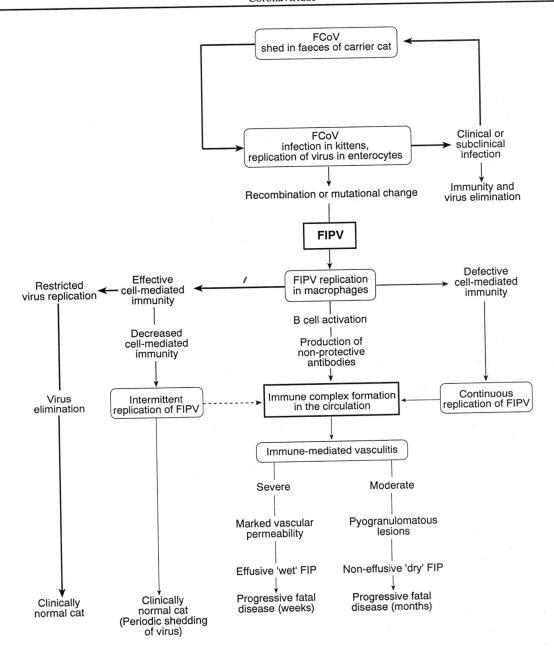

Figure 72.2 Proposed relationship between infection with feline enteric coronavirus and the emergence of feline infectious peritonitis virus leading to the development of feline infectious peritonitis.

FCoV, feline coronavirus; FIPV, feline infectious peritonitis virus; FIP, feline infectious peritonitis

activation and the production of non-protective antibodies. The immune complexes, formed from these antibodies and FIPV, activate complement leading to immune-mediated vasculitis. The severity of this vasculitis influences the clinical presentation and the rate of progression of the disease. In addition to type III hypersensitivity, there is evidence of type IV hypersensitivity in FIPV-induced lesions (Paltrinieri *et al.*, 1998a; Paltrinieri *et al.*, 1998b).

Clinical signs

The incubation period ranges from weeks to months. The

onset of clinical signs may be either sudden or slow and insidious. Early signs, which are generally non-specific, include anorexia, weight loss, listlessness and dehydration. Affected cats often present with icterus.

Cats with the effusive form of the disease have fibrin-rich exudates in the abdominal or thoracic cavities. If the pleural effusion is marked, dyspnoea develops. The effusive form of the disease usually leads to death within eight weeks.

In the non-effusive form of FIP, clinical findings are less characteristic. Signs referable to lesions in organs or tissues in the abdominal cavity are present in about 50% of affected cats. Anterior uveitis, chorioretinitis and neurological signs may be evident in up to 30% of cases. The course of the disease is usually protracted with animals surviving for weeks or months. Infection with feline leukaemia virus or with feline immunodeficiency virus may increase susceptibility to FIPV and contribute to the severity of the clinical signs.

Diagnosis

- Currently, histological examination of affected tissues is the only procedure available for the definitive diagnosis of FIP.
- Pleural or peritoneal fluid, which may contain fibrin strands, clots on standing. It has a high protein content. A gamma globulin content exceeding 32% of total protein is suggestive of FIP (Weiss, 1991).
- Typical haematological changes include neutrophilia, lymphopenia and, in chronic cases, a normocytic, normochromic, non-regenerative anaemia.
- A serum hyperproteinaemia is frequently present due to a hypergammaglobulinaemia. Serum liver enzymes and total bilirubin may also be raised.
- Diagnostic serological tests, including IFA and ELISA do not distinguish between cats infected with FCoV and FIPV. In indirect immunofluorescence, antibody titres may be very high in some FIP cases. In other cases antibody titres are negligible (Sparkes *et al.*, 1991).
- RT-PCR can be used to detect virus shed in the faeces and for the identification of carriers (Addie and Jarrett, 2001).

Treatment and control

There is no specific treatment for FIP. Supportive therapy and broad spectrum antibiotics may be useful for treating affected cats in good physical condition (Weiss, 1994).

An intranasal vaccine employing a temperature-sensitive mutant strain of FIPV has recently been developed. Although some efficacy and safety test results have been favourable (Postorino Reeves *et al.*, 1992; Hoskins *et al.*, 1994; Fehr *et al.*, 1997), other studies have failed to demonstrate significant protective immunity.

The creation and maintenance of coronavirus-negative catteries is an effective method of control but is extremely difficult to achieve. Measures aimed at reducing the incidence of the disease include breeding from bloodlines free of FIP, rearing litters of kittens in isolation (Addie and Jarrett, 1990) and reducing stress in the catteries.

Canine coronavirus infection

The importance of canine coronavirus (CCV) as a cause of disease is uncertain as the agent can be isolated from normal dogs and those with diarrhoea (Tennant *et al.*,

1993). This virus is related antigenically to the feline coronaviruses.

Epidemiology

Serological studies indicate that infection is common (Tennant *et al.*, 1991). Infections with CCV may spread rapidly among susceptible dogs at shows and in kennels. Seroprevalence may approach 100% in kennels and range from 6% to 75% in pet dog populations.

Infection is acquired from the faeces of infected animals. Infected dogs usually shed the virus for up to 9 days and intermittent shedding may continue for months. The virus is not particularly resistant in the environment and carrier dogs are required for its maintenance. Mucosal immunity appears to be more important than circulating antibody for protection of dogs from reinfection. In the absence of frequent re-exposure to the virus, the duration of immunity may be relatively short.

Pathogenesis

Canine coronaviruses withstand the acid environment of the stomach and infect enterocytes in the duodenum. Infection spreads rapidly to involve other parts of the small intestine. Diarrhoea may follow loss of digestive and absorptive capacity in the small intestine as a result of damage to mature enterocytes at the tips of villi. Recovery is rapid in uncomplicated cases.

Clinical signs

Although clinical disease has been recorded in dogs, foxes and coyotes, infection with CCV is often asymptomatic. Dogs of all ages can become infected; serious illness is most likely to occur in pups. The incubation period is up to three days. Clinical signs, which are variable and non-specific, include anorexia, depression, vomiting and diarrhoea. Most animals recover in seven to ten days. Occasionally, illness may be protracted due to secondary bacterial, parasitic or other viral infections. The mortality rate is low.

Diagnosis

- Virus may be detected in faeces by electron microscopy.
- Virus can be isolated in a number of cell lines but the procedure is slow and unreliable.
- Serum neutralization or indirect immunofluorescence tests can be used to demonstrate an increasing antibody titre.

Treatment and control

- Supportive treatment, including fluid replacement therapy and antibiotic administration, should be instituted when required.
- Although inactivated vaccines are available and can be used in pregnant bitches to boost colostral immunity, the degree of protection induced by these vaccines is

uncertain.

- Contact with infected animals and faeces should be minimized.
- Effective disinfection of premises and utensils can be achieved with 3% sodium hypochlorite or 2% formalin.

Transmissible gastroenteritis

Transmissible gastroenteritis (TGE) is a highly contagious, coronaviral disease of young pigs which occurs worldwide. There is one serotype of transmissible gastroenteritis virus (TGEV) which is closely related antigenically to feline coronavirus and canine coronavirus. A relatively non-pathogenic respiratory variant of TGEV, referred to as porcine respiratory coronavirus (PRCV), was first recognized in 1984. This virus spread to pig populations in many European countries and has now been identified in the USA and in some Asian countries. Infection with PRCV is usually subclinical.

Epidemiology

Transmission of TGEV is usually by the faecal-oral route. The virus is moderately stable in the presence of proteolytic enzymes and at pH 3.0, ensuring survival in the stomach and small intestine. Viral shedding in faeces can persist for up to two weeks. Outbreaks of TGE tend to occur in winter. In fully susceptible herds, the virus spreads rapidly infecting animals of all ages. The disease, however, is most severe in newborn piglets. Outbreaks usually terminate in a few weeks if no new susceptible animals are introduced into the herd.

Pathogenesis

Following ingestion, the virus replicates mainly in mature enterocytes at the tips of the villi in the small intestine. Viral replication results in villous atrophy throughout the length of the small intestine. Digestion and cellular transport of nutrients and electrolytes are severely disrupted resulting in the accumulation of fluid in the intestinal lumen and diarrhoea. Young piglets are particularly susceptible to the ensuing dehydration and metabolic acidosis.

Clinical signs

The incubation period is up to three days. Vomiting and watery diarrhoea may be evident in affected piglets less than seven days old. Rapid dehydration and weight loss follow. Mortality may approach 100% in newborn piglets and is usually confined to animals under three weeks of age. Inappetence and transient diarrhoea may be observed in older pigs. Subclinical infections also occur. Sows quickly become immune and maternally-derived immunity reduces the severity of clinical signs in piglets. Outbreaks usually last a few weeks. However, TGE infection may become endemic in a herd if consecutive litters become infected as maternally-derived immunity wanes. Clinically, such infections are usually mild.

Diagnosis

The sudden onset and rapid spread of diarrhoea among newborn pigs along with almost 100% mortality is highly suggestive of TGE. Postmortem examination of washed small intestine discloses paper-thin walls, due to villous atrophy. The walls of the jejunum and ileum are affected while those of the duodenum are usually normal.

- Viral antigen can be detected in mucosal smears or cryostat sections of the small intestine by immunofluorescence. It may be necessary to euthanize some piglets in the early stages of the disease in order to obtain suitable specimens for laboratory examination. Viral antigens can be demonstrated in faeces by ELISA.
- Virus can be isolated from faeces in a swine testis cell line.
- Serological testing for antibodies can be carried out using virus neutralization. However, virus neutralization does not distinguish antibodies to TGEV from those induced by PRCV infection. A blocking ELISA, which is based on the use of monoclonal antibody directed against a glycoprotein epitope present in TGEV but absent from PRCV, can be used to distinguish infections caused by these two viruses.

Treatment and control

- There is no specific treatment but fluid replacement therapy may be beneficial. Maintaining the farrowing house at an optimal temperature may enhance survival.
- In acute outbreaks of TGE, deliberate exposure of pregnant sows to the virus may reduce neonatal mortality. After exposure, sows due to farrow should be moved to clean premises. Newborn piglets born to exposed sows will usually receive passive antibody protection following suckling.
- Modified live and inactivated vaccines are available. Modified live vaccines are administered orally to sows five to seven weeks before farrowing and a booster inoculation is administered parenterally one week before parturition. Vaccination reduces mortality but does not eliminate infection.
- Serious outbreaks of TGE have become rare in European pig populations endemically infected with PRCV. Porcine respiratory coronavirus is spread in pig herds by aerosols. Sows infected with PRCV usually transfer substantial colostral protection to their litters (Wesley and Woods, 1993).

Porcine epidemic diarrhoea

This porcine disease, which is clinically similar to TGE, is described in Europe and Asia but not in America. There is only one serotype of porcine epidemic diarrhoea virus (PEDV), a coronavirus serologically unrelated to TGEV.

Epidemiology

The virus is transmitted by the faecal-oral route. Spread of the virus to susceptible herds occurs directly through infected pigs and indirectly through contaminated fomites or vehicles. The rate of spread of infection within a farm is slower than that of TGEV.

Pathogenesis

Virus replication, which occurs in enterocytes in the small intestine and colon, results in shortening of villi. The rate and severity of cell destruction is less marked than with TGEV.

Clinical signs

The incubation period is up to four days. The age of animals affected and the associated morbidity and mortality are variable. On some farms, animals of all ages become sick and the mortality rate in piglets under one week may approach 50%. Watery diarrhoea, which may be preceded by vomiting, is the main clinical presentation. Occasionally a few animals die suddenly, with back muscle necrosis evident at postmortem. The virus may persist on large breeding farms by infecting consecutive litters of pigs. Most affected pigs recover after about one week and mortality rates are usually low.

Diagnosis

- Direct immunofluorescence, using cryostat sections of small intestine from pigs euthanized during the phase of acute diarrhoea, is sensitive and reliable, particularly in specimens from newborn piglets.
- Viral antigen may be detected by ELISA in faecal material or intestinal contents collected during the acute phase of the disease.
- Antibodies can be detected in paired serum samples using a blocking ELISA or by indirect immuno-fluorescence on PEDV-positive cryostat sections of intestine.

Treatment and control

- There is no specific treatment and vaccines are not available.
- Appropriate hygienic measures and the control of animal and human movement onto a farm are necessary for disease prevention.
- During an outbreak of the disease on a breeding farm, good hygiene slows the spread of infection. Deliberate spread of the virus to pregnant sows using infected faecal material stimulates colostral immunity and shortens the course of the disease outbreak.

Porcine haemagglutinating encephalomyelitis virus infection

This coronavirus disease of young pigs, also known as vomiting and wasting disease, is caused by haem-agglutinating encephalomyelitis virus of which there is only one serotype. The virus agglutinates red cells of several animal species.

Epidemiology

Infection is common and probably worldwide. The virus is shed in nasal secretions and readily transmitted by aerosols. Infection persists on breeding farms as a sub-clinical respiratory condition. In herds where infection is endemic, immune sows transfer protective antibodies to their offspring and piglets are protected until they have developed an age-related resistance. Pigs which become subclinically infected develop an active immunity at eight to 16 weeks of age.

Pathogenesis

The virus replicates locally in the upper respiratory tract and tonsils before spreading via the peripheral nervous system to the medulla oblongata. It then spreads to various other parts of the central nervous system. Viral damage to the vagal sensory ganglion and to the intramural plexus of the stomach are considered to be responsible for vomiting and delayed gastric emptying.

Clinical signs

Clinical signs develop in pigs less than three weeks of age after an incubation period of up to seven days. Signs of acute encephalomyelitis, vomiting and wasting are the predominant clinical features. Newborn piglets become severely dehydrated and may die. The mortality rate is often 100% in young pigs. Older pigs continue to vomit and become emaciated. Survivors may be permanently stunted.

Diagnosis

- For the isolation of virus or demonstration of viral antigen in cryostat sections by immunofluorescence, samples of brain stem must be collected within two days of the onset of clinical signs. Porcine thyroid cells are suitable for isolation.
- Lesions of non-suppurative encephalomyelitis may be evident.
- A significant rise in antibody titre may be demonstrable in paired serum samples by virus neutralization or haemagglutination inhibition tests.

Treatment and control

- No specific treatment is available.
- Due to the sporadic nature of the disease, vaccination is unwarranted.
- Appropriate measures should be taken to prevent the

introduction of infection into breeding units. If infection is introduced, it is important to ensure that infection of sows results in an adequate antibody response for the protection of litters.

Infectious bronchitis

Infectious bronchitis, caused by infectious bronchitis virus (IBV), is a highly contagious, economically important, worldwide disease of poultry which affects the respiratory, reproductive and renal systems. Many serotypes, often with different virulence and tissue tropisms probably as a result of mutation or recombination, are recognised.

Epidemiology

The chicken is the main host although IBV has been isolated from pigeons and pheasants. The most important route of transmission is by aerosols and spread of infection occurs rapidly among susceptible birds. Morbidity may approach 100%. Virus, shed from the respiratory tract for a few weeks after infection, may be recovered over a period of weeks from the faeces and from eggs of infected birds. Infection may persist in the digestive tract of individual birds.

Pathogenesis

The respiratory system is the primary site of virus replication. Viraemia follows within one to two days of exposure. The virus becomes widely distributed throughout the body, particularly in the oviducts, kidneys and bursa of Fabricius. The distribution and severity of lesions in these tissues are influenced by the virulence of the infecting strain.

Clinical signs

The incubation period is up to 48 hours. Age, immune status and strain of virus strongly influence the nature and severity of disease observed in a flock. In general, disease is most severe in young birds, particularly when secondary infections are present. In chickens less than three weeks of age there is gasping and nasal exudate. Infection may result in stunting and some birds may die suddenly from occluded bronchi. In older birds, rales and gasping are usually observed. Mortality rates are generally low in the absence of secondary infections. The course of the disease is up to seven days in individual birds and outbreaks last about ten to 14 days in flocks. Layers show signs of rales followed by a marked reduction in egg production which slowly returns to normal. Egg quality, with soft-shelled and mis-shaped eggs, may be poor for several weeks. Infection with nephrotropic strains of IBV are associated with interstitial nephritis and mild respiratory signs with moderate to high levels of mortality.

Diagnosis

- Virus isolation is often feasible in the acute stage of the disease. Although specimens from the respiratory tract are those most suitable for virus isolation, samples from kidney, oviduct and faeces can also be used. Material is usually inoculated into the allantoic sac of nine to ten day old embryonated eggs. A number of passages may be required to produce the characteristic stunting and curling of the embryo. Tracheal explants from day-old specific-pathogen-free chicks may also be used for virus isolation.
- Serological tests, including virus neutralization, agar gel immunodiffusion, haemagglutination inhibition and ELISA, can be used to demonstrate a rise in antibody titre between acute and convalescent serum samples.

Treatment and control

- There is no specific treatment. The administration of antibiotics may reduce mortality due to secondary bacterial infections.
- Both live and killed vaccines with adjuvant are available. Live vaccines are usually administered in the drinking water or by aerosol to chicks up to 14 days of age and again at about 4 weeks of age. A high-passage vaccinal virus, which is less pathogenic, is used for primary immunization. A more virulent strain of virus is used for booster vaccination. Following primary immunization with live vaccines, killed vaccines are useful in layer and breeder flocks to prevent losses in egg production and to ensure a high level of yolk sac-derived immunity in chicks.

Bovine coronavirus infection

Bovine coronavirus (BCV) is one of the causes of calf diarrhoea and is also associated with winter dysentery in adult housed cattle. There is evidence of its involvement in the bovine respiratory disease complex (Kapil and Goyal, 1995). The virus, which exists as a single serotype, haemagglutinates red cells of mice, rats and hamsters.

Epidemiology and pathogenesis

Virus is mainly transmitted by the faecal-oral route. However, coronaviruses have also been recovered from the respiratory tract of calves (McNulty *et al.*, 1984) and infected calves often harbour BCV in both the enteric and respiratory tracts. Infection is usually endemic on farms, maintained by clinically-affected calves and persistently-infected, clinically normal, calves and cows. The virus replicates and destroys mature enterocytes in the small intestine and colon, resulting in a malabsorptive diarrhoea. The severity of disease is influenced by the age of the animal at the time of infection and type of management. Risk factors, which include changes in diet, cold temperatures, close confinement and the presence of other microorganisms such as *Campylobacter jejuni*, appear to be particularly important in the development and pathogenesis of winter dysentery.

Clinical signs

In calves, the incubation period is up to two days and clinical signs are usually observed between three to 21 days of age. There is profuse diarrhoea which may result in dehydration, acidosis and death. If milk is withdrawn and the calves are fed oral electrolytes, the diarrhoea usually ceases in a few days. Respiratory tract infections are generally mild but may predispose to more severe secondary infections.

In adult animals the incubation period of winter dysentery is three to seven days. There is a sudden onset of diarrhoea accompanied by a dramatic drop in milk yield. The faeces of some animals may contain blood or blood clots. A nasolacrimal discharge and cough may accompany the diarrhoea. Herd outbreaks can last for two weeks.

Diagnosis

- Faeces or intestinal contents for laboratory examination should be collected early in the course of the disease.
- Typical coronavirus particles can be demonstrated in faecal samples by direct electron microscopy (EM). Immune EM is preferable as it is more sensitive and specific. Alternative diagnostic methods of detection include ELISA and reverse passive haemagglutination.
- Immunofluorescence can be used to detect viral antigen in cryostat sections of distal small intestine or colon.
- Isolation of virus in tissue culture is difficult.

Treatment and control

Treatment is supportive but non-specific. Control of the disease in calves is based on vaccination and good management practices. Both live and inactivated vaccines have been developed and can be used orally in calves to stimulate active immunity. They may also be administered parenterally in cows to increase the level of antibody in colostrum and milk. However, no vaccine is available for the prevention of winter dysentery.

References

Addie, D.D. and Jarrett, O. (1990). Control of feline coronavirus infection in kittens. *Veterinary Record*, **126,** 164.

Addie, D.D. and Jarrett, O. (1992). A study of naturally occurring feline coronavirus infections in kittens. *Veterinary Record*, **130**, 133–137.

Addie, D. and Jarrett, O. (2001). Use of reverse-transsciptase polymerase chain reaction for monitoring the shedding of feline coronavirus by healthy cats. *Veterinary Record*, **148**, 649–653.

Addie, D.D., Toth, S., Murray, G.D. and Jarrett, O. (1995). Risk of feline infectious peritonitis in cats naturally infected with feline coronavirus. *American Journal of Veterinary Research*, 56, 429–434.

Barr, F. (1998). Feline infectious peritonitis. *Journal of Small Animal Practice*, **39**, 501–504.

Fehr, D., Holznagel, E., Bolla, S. *et al.* (1997). Placebo-controlled evaluation of a modified live virus vaccine against feline infectious peritonitis: Safety and efficacy under field conditions. *Vaccine*, **15**, 1101–1109.

Herrewegh, A.A.P.M., Smeenk, I., Horzinek, M.C. *et al.* (1998). Feline coronavirus type II strains 79–1683 and 79–1146 originate from a double recombination between feline coronavirus type 1 and canine coronavirus. *Journal of Virology*, **72**, 4508–4514.

Hoskins, J.D., Taylor, H.W. and Lomax, T.L. (1994). Challenge trial of an intranasal feline infectious peritonitis vaccine. *Feline Practice*, **22**, 9–13.

Kapil, S. and Goyal, S.M. (1995). Bovine coronavirus-associated respiratory disease. *Compendium on Continuing Education for the Practicing Veterinarian*, **17**, 1179–1181.

McNulty, M.S., Bryson, D.G., Allan, G.M. and Logan, E.F. (1984). Coronavirus infection of the bovine respiratory tract. *Veterinary Microbiology*, **9**, 425–434.

Muir, P., Harbour, D.A., Gruffydd-Jones, T.J. *et al.* (1990). A clinical and microbiological study of cats with protruding nictitating membranes and diarrhoea: isolation of a novel agent. *Veterinary Record*, **127**, 324–330.

Paltrinieri, S., Cammarata, M.P., Cammarata, G. and Mambretti, M. (1998a). Type IV hypersensitivity in the pathogenesis of FIPV-induced lesions. *Journal of Veterinary Medicine, Series B*, **45**, 151–159.

Paltrinieri, S., Cammarata, M.P., Cammarata, G. and Comazzi, S. (1998b). Some aspects of humoral and cellular immunity in naturally occurring feline infectious peritonitis. *Veterinary Immunology and Immunopathology*, **65**, 205–220.

Pedersen, N.C. and Floyd, K. (1985). Experimental studies with three new strains of feline infectious peritonitis virus: FIPV-UCD2, FIPV-UCD3 and FIPV-UCD4. *Compendium on Continuing Education for the Practicing Veterinarian*, **7**, 1001–1011.

Poland, A., Vennema, H., Foley, J.E. and Pedersen, N.C. (1996). Two related strains of feline infectious peritonitis virus isolated from immunocompromised cats infected with a feline enteric coronavirus. *Journal of Clinical Microbiology*, **34**, 3180–3184.

Postorino Reeves, N.C., Pollock, R.V.H. and Thurber, E.T. (1992). Long-term follow-up study of cats vaccinated with a temperature-sensitive feline infectious peritonitis vaccine. *Cornell Veterinarian*, **82**, 117–123.

Sparkes, A.H., Gruffydd-Jones, T.J. and Harbour, D.A. (1991). Feline infectious peritonitis: a review of clinico-pathological changes in 65 cases, and a critical assessment of their diagnostic value. *Veterinary Record*, **129**, 209–212.

Sparkes, A.H., Gruffydd-Jones, T.J., Howard, P.E. and Harbour, D.A. (1992). Coronavirus serology in healthy pedigree cats. *Veterinary Record*, **131**, 35–36.

Tennant, B.J., Gaskell, R.M., Jones, R.C. and Gaskell, C.J. (1991). Prevalence of antibodies to four major canine viral diseases in dogs in a Liverpool hospital population. *Journal of Small Animal Practice*, **32**, 175–179.

Tennant, B.J., Gaskell, R.M., Jones, R.C. and Gaskell, C.J. (1993). Studies on the epizootiology of canine coronavirus. *Veterinary Record*, **132**, 7–11.

Vennema, H., Poland, A., Foley, J. and Pedersen, N.C. (1998). Feline infectious peritonitis viruses arise by mutation from endemic feline enteric coronaviruses. *Virology*, **243**, 150–157.

Weiss, R.C. (1991). The diagnosis and clinical management of feline infectious peritonitis. *Veterinary Medicine*, **86**, 308–319.

Weiss, R.C. (1994). Feline infectious peritonitis virus: advances in therapy and control. In *Consultations in Feline Internal Medicine 2*. Ed. J.R. August. W.B. Saunders, Philadelphia. pp. 3–12.

Wesley, D. and Woods, R.D. (1993). Immunization of pregnant gilts with PRCV induces lactogenic immunity for protection of nursing piglets from challenge with TGEV. *Veterinary Microbiology*, **38**, 31–40.

Further reading

Clark, M.A. (1993). Bovine coronavirus. *British Veterinary Journal*, **149**, 51–70.

Gamble, D.A., Lobbiani, A., Gramegna, M. *et al.* (1997). Development of a nested PCR assay for detection of feline infectious peritonitis virus in clinical specimens. *Journal of Clinical Microbiology*, **35**, 673–675.

Olsen, C.W. (1993). A review of feline infectious peritonitis virus: molecular biology, immunopathogenesis, clinical aspects, and vaccination. *Veterinary Microbiology*, **36**, 1–37.

Siddell, S.G. (1995). *The Coronaviridae*. Plenum Press, New York.

Chapter 73

Arteriviridae

Arteriviruses, formerly classified as members of the family *Togaviridae*, have recently been assigned to the family *Arteriviridae*. Their genome organization and mode of replication are similar to those of members of the *Coronaviridae* and these two families make up the order *Nidovirales*. In the family *Arteriviridae* there is a single genus, *Arterivirus*. The name of the genus derives from the disease, equine arteritis, which is caused by the type species. Arteriviruses are spherical, 40 to 60 nm in diameter and possess a lipid-containing envelope which has ring-like surface structures (Fig. 73.1). The icosahedral nucleocapsid contains a molecule of linear single-stranded RNA. Replication takes place in the cytoplasm of infected cells. Arteriviruses, which are relatively labile, are sensitive to heat, low pH, lipid solvents, detergent treatment, UV irradiation and many disinfectants.

Key points

- Medium-sized, enveloped, single-stranded RNA viruses
- Icosahedral symmetry
- Replicate in cytoplasm of macrophages and endothelial cells
- Cause equine viral arteritis and porcine respiratory and reproductive syndrome

Clinical infections

Members of the genus are host-specific and antigenically unrelated. Infections have been described in horses, pigs, mice and monkeys. The primary target cells are macrophages. Infection is spread horizontally by aerosol, by biting or by venereal transmission. Infections are frequently persistent.

Equine viral arteritis

Although infection with equine arteritis virus (EAV) occurs worldwide, outbreaks of clinical disease are comparatively rare. Upper respiratory tract infection, ventral oedema and abortion are prominent clinical features. Biological and genomic differences have been demonstrated in isolates of EAV but antigenic variation is limited. Only one serotype has been recognized.

Epidemiology

Horses, donkeys and mules are susceptible to infection. The percentage of seropositive animals is higher in Standardbreds than in Thoroughbreds. Whether this reflects differences in susceptibility or in degree of exposure as a result of management practices is unclear. Although infection is prevalent in some horse populations, outbreaks of disease are sporadic. The frequency of confirmed outbreaks of equine viral arteritis has increased in recent years. Factors which may have contributed to this increase include increased international movement of horses, more extensive use of artificial insemination and greater awareness of the disease.

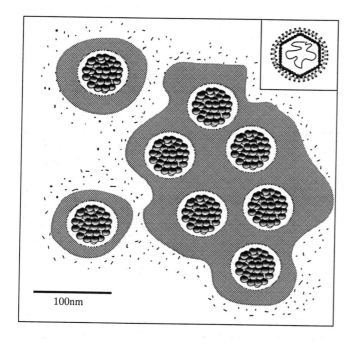

100nm

Figure 73.1 Arterivirus particles as they appear in an electron micrograph and a diagrammatic representation (inset).

During the acute phase of infection, virus is spread primarily by aerosols from the respiratory tract. Virus is also shed in faeces, urine and vaginal secretions. Close contact facilitates spread of infection. Virus is usually eliminated from mares and geldings within one to two months but may persist in about 35% of infected stallions. Carrier stallions are asymptomatic and shed virus continuously in semen. More than 80% of mares covered by carrier stallions may become infected. Persistent infection, which does not impair the fertility of stallions, appears to be testosterone-dependent (McCollum et al., 1994). Mares infected venereally may spread virus horizontally to in-contact susceptible animals. Abortion or infection of the foal may result when pregnant mares are infected.

Pathogenesis and pathology

Following aerosol transmission, replication occurs in pulmonary macrophages. There is subsequent spread to the bronchial lymph nodes and viraemia. Pathological changes, arising from infection of endothelial cells and widespread necrotic arteritis, include oedema, congestion and haemorrhage in many tissues. Aborted foetuses, which often exhibit autolysis, rarely display characteristic lesions.

Clinical signs

The incubation period ranges from three to 14 days. Many infections are subclinical. The disease tends to be more severe in very young and aged animals and in those subjected to stress. Affected animals present with fever, anorexia, depression, conjunctivitis, rhinitis and stiff gait. Oedema, which is usually prominent, may involve the eyelids, ventral abdomen and limbs, particularly the hind limbs. Urticarial-type lesions commonly affect the skin of the neck. Acute, often fatal, respiratory disease has been recorded in foals (Del Piero et al., 1997). Clinical signs in donkeys are similar to those in horses but generally milder. Animals which recover are usually immune for several years.

Diagnosis

Because equine viral arteritis resembles a number of other equine diseases in its clinical presentation, definitive diagnosis requires laboratory confirmation. Internationally accepted testing procedures have been published (Timoney, 1996).

- Virus isolation is carried out in appropriate cell lines such as rabbit or equine kidney cells. Samples suitable for isolation procedures include nasopharyngeal and conjunctival swabs, placental tissue and foetal tissue and fluids.
- Viral RNA can be detected in semen and other specimens using the reverse transcriptase polymerase chain reaction.
- Acute and convalescent blood samples can be submitted

for serology. Several serological tests including virus neutralization, complement fixation, indirect fluorescent antibody, agar gel immunodiffusion and ELISA have been used. The virus neutralization test, considered to be sensitive and highly specific, is the most widely used test.

- Carrier stallions can be identified by serological testing. If stallions are seropositive, virus isolation from semen should be attempted. The sperm-rich fraction of semen is suitable for virus isolation. Alternatively, carrier animals can be mated to seronegative mares which are monitored for seroconversion.

Treatment

Supportive therapy is indicated in severe cases. The carrier state in stallions cannot be eliminated by chemotherapy.

Control

Persistently-infected stallions should be identified and their breeding activities confined to seropositive or vaccinated mares. In order to reduce the risk of colt foals becoming carriers, vaccination at six to 12 months of age is recommended (Timoney and McCollum, 1996). Two types of vaccine are available:

— A modified live tissue culture-adapted vaccine induces good protection against clinical disease but not against infection. Use of this vaccine is contraindicated in pregnant mares and in foals under six weeks of age.
— An inactivated whole-virus vaccine with adjuvant is reported to be safe for pregnant mares but requires booster injections at six to 12 month intervals (Fukunaga, 1994).

Porcine respiratory and reproductive syndrome

This economically important condition is characterized by reproductive failure in sows and pneumonia in young pigs. The syndrome was first described in the USA in 1987. Despite attempts at controlling spread, the disease is now endemic in many countries. The aetiological agent, originally called Lelystad virus, was first isolated in the Netherlands (Wensvoort et al., 1991). It was characterized as an arterivirus and renamed porcine respiratory and reproductive syndrome virus (PRRSV). Significant antigenic and genomic differences between American and European isolates of the virus are evident.

Epidemiology

Natural infection occurs in pigs and wild boars. Virus, which is shed in saliva, urine, semen and faeces, is highly infectious. Nose-to-nose contact is considered to be the most likely route of transmission. Airborne transmission between farms was important during the early acute outbreaks of the disease when large quantities of virus were excreted. Now it appears to be important only when pig population densities are high and when weather conditions are suitable. Virus survival, which is prolonged in winter months when low temperature and high humidity prevail, facilitates transmission. Infection is generally introduced onto farms by infected pigs or by infected semen. On endemically infected farms, virus is transmitted either continuously or in waves. Maintenance of infection on farms is multifactorial (Albina, 1997). Maternally-derived immunity is of such short duration that piglets become susceptible to infection at four to 10 weeks of age. Susceptible replacement pigs maintain infection in endemic herds. Infection may spread in a slow and unpredictable manner with the result that some animals in infected herds remain susceptible. Immunocompetent pigs, which display a progressive decline in antibody levels over a period of several months, may become susceptible to reinfection. In experimentally infected pigs, infection persisted for up to 157 days (Wills *et al.*, 1997).

Pathogenesis and pathology

Infection occurs most frequently by the respiratory route. The virus has an affinity for pulmonary alveolar macrophages and the lungs are probably the target organs (Van Reeth, 1997). Early antibody responses are not effective in clearing virus infection. Antibody-dependent enhancement of infection of pulmonary alveolar macrophages has been described in the disease. After transportation to regional lymph nodes, virus spreads to tissue macrophages throughout the body. Transplacental infection of foetuses occurs. For reasons which are unclear, reproductive failure is more difficult to induce experimentally in early gestation than in late gestation (Kranker *et al.*, 1998). Foetal and placental abnormalities are not consistently present and the mechanism of foetal death and reproductive failure is uncertain. Although the virus does not appear to have a systemic immunosuppressive effect, it predisposes to infection with other microorganisms such as *Streptococcus suis*, porcine respiratory coronavirus and *Haemophilus parasuis* (Albina *et al.*, 1998).

Clinical signs

Introduction of PRRSV to a breeding herd is usually followed by reproductive failure which may take the form of abortions, early farrowing, increased numbers of stillborn and mummified foetuses, weak neonatal pigs and delayed return to service in affected sows. A 'rolling inappetence', progressively affecting animals in an infected herd, has been described. In some cases, cyanosis of the ears and vulva along with erythematous plaques on the skin ('blue-eared disease') have been described. Respiratory distress and increased preweaning mortality are important features of the disease in neonatal pigs.

Subclinical infection is common. Factors which may exacerbate clinical disease include concentrated numbers of pigs, the virulence of the strain of PRRSV and the presence of slatted floors. Although sporadic respiratory and reproductive problems are the main clinical manifestations in most affected herds, in a few endemic herds, chronic disease problems predominate (Zimmermann *et al.*, 1997).

Diagnosis

- Laboratory confirmation is usually required because the clinical presentation, particularly in endemic herds, is variable.
- Serology is the most widely used diagnostic method. Several serological tests are available including ELISA, virus neutralization, indirect fluorescent antibody and immunoperoxidase monolayer assay. However, these tests do not distinguish carrier from vaccinated animals.
- The presence of PRRSV may be demonstrated by virus isolation, direct FA staining, *in situ* hybridization or reverse transcriptase polymerase chain reaction. Suitable samples for submission include serum, foetal fluids and lung tissue.

Treatment

There is no specific treatment. Supportive therapy and antibiotic administration to suppress secondary infections may be beneficial.

Control

Vaccination and effective hygiene and health management are important for controlling infection.

- A commercial modified live vaccine is available for use in pigs 3 to 18 weeks of age and is suitable for use in non-pregnant sows before breeding. It is not suitable for use in boars and pregnant sows or in herds free from PRRSV infection. An inactivated vaccine with adjuvant is also available (Plana-Duran *et al.*, 1997). Vaccination provides reasonable protection from the clinical effects of infection.
- Stabilization of the sow herd is required to avoid subpopulations of non-immune sows and to break the cycle of reinfection. Replacement sows should be introduced to the herd only when effective isolation and acclimatization procedures are instituted. Other control measures, relating to the weaning and rearing of piglets on infected premises and to strategies for the elimination of infection from herds, have been proposed (Dee and Joo, 1997; Dee and Molitor, 1998).

References

Albina, E. (1997). Epidemiology of porcine reproductive and respiratory syndrome (PRRS): an overview. *Veterinary Microbiology*, **55**, 309–316.

Albina, E., Piriou, L., Hutet, E. *et al.* (1998). Immune response in pigs infected with porcine reproductive and respiratory syndrome virus (PRRSV). *Veterinary Immunology and Immunopathology*, **61**, 49–66.

Dee, S.A. and Joo, H. (1997). Strategies to control PRRS: a summary of field and research experience. *Veterinary Microbiology*, **55**, 347–353.

Dee, S.A. and Molitor, T.W. (1998). Elimination of porcine reproductive and respiratory syndrome virus using a test and removal process. *Veterinary Record*, **143**, 474–476.

Del Piero, F., Wilkins, P.A., Lopez, J.W. *et al.* (1997). Equine viral arteritis in newborn foals: clinical, pathological, serological, microbiological and immunohistochemical observations. *Equine Veterinary Journal*, **29**, 178–185.

Fukunaga, Y. (1994). Equine viral arteritis: diagnostic and control measures. *Journal of Equine Science*, **5**, 101–114.

Kranker, S., Nielsen, J., Bille-Hansen, V. and Botner, A. (1998). Experimental inoculation of swine at various stages of gestation with a Danish isolate of porcine reproductive and respiratory syndrome virus (PRRSV). *Veterinary Microbiology*, **61**, 21–31.

McCollum, W.H., Little, T.V., Timoney, P.J. and Swerczek, T.W. (1994). Resistance of castrated male horses to attempted establishment of the carrier state with equine arteritis virus. *Journal of Comparative Pathology*, **111**, 383–388.

Plana-Duran J., Bastons, M., Urniza, A. *et al.* (1997). Efficacy of an inactivated vaccine for prevention of reproductive failure induced by porcine reproductive and respiratory syndrome virus. *Veterinary Microbiology*, **55**, 361–370.

Timoney, P.J. (1996). Equine viral arteritis. In *Manual of Standards for Diagnostic Tests and Vaccines*. Third Edition. Office International des Epizooties (OIE), Paris. p.p. 440–448.

Timoney, P.J. and McCollum, W.H. (1996). Equine viral arteritis. *Equine Veterinary Education*, **8**, 97–100.

Van Reeth, K. (1997). Pathogenesis and clinical aspects of a respiratory porcine reproductive and respiratory syndrome virus. *Veterinary Microbiology*, **55**, 223–230.

Wensvoort, G., Terpstra, C., Pol, T.J.M. *et al.* (1991). Mystery swine disease in the Netherlands: the isolation of Lelystad virus. *Veterinary Quarterly*, **13**, 121–130.

Wills, R.W., Zimmermann, J.J., Yoon, K.-J. *et al.* (1997). Porcine reproductive and respiratory syndrome virus: a persistent infection. *Veterinary Microbiology*, **55**, 231–240.

Zimmermann, J.J., Yoon, K.-J., Wills, R.W. and Swenson, S.L. (1997). General overview of PRRSV: a perspective from the United States. *Veterinary Microbiology*, **55**, 187–196.

Further reading

Glaser, A.L., Chirnside, E.D., Horzinek, M.C. and de Vries, A.A.F. (1997). Equine arteritis virus. *Theriogenology*, **47**, 1275–1295.

Chapter 74

Flaviviridae

The family name of the *Flaviviridae* (Latin *flavus*, yellow) is derived from yellow fever, a disease of humans caused by a flavivirus, with jaundice as a major clinical feature. Members of the family are 40 to 60 nm in diameter with icosahedral capsids and tightly adherent envelopes which contain either two or three virus-encoded proteins, depending on the genus (Fig. 74.1). The genome is composed of positive-sense single-stranded RNA. Replication of virus occurs in the cytoplasm with maturation in cytoplasmic vesicles and release by exocytosis. The mature virions are generally labile, being sensitive to heat, detergents and organic solvents.

The family comprises three genera namely *Flavivirus*, *Pestivirus* and *Hepacivirus* (Fig. 74.2). Two genera, *Flavivirus* and *Pestivirus* contain viruses of veterinary importance. The genus *Flavivirus* contains approximately 70 members assigned to several serologically defined groups. Most members of the genus are arboviruses, which require either mosquitoes or ticks as vectors.

Key points
- Enveloped labile viruses
- Positive-sense, single-stranded RNA
- Replicate in the cytoplasm
- Two genera of veterinary importance, *Flavivirus* and *Pestivirus*
- Most viruses in the genus *Flavivirus* are transmitted by arthropods and cause encephalitis
- Pestiviruses, which are transmitted directly or indirectly, cause bovine viral diarrhoea, border disease and classical swine fever

Viruses in the genus agglutinate goose red cells. The genus *Pestivirus* contains three viruses of veterinary importance namely bovine viral diarrhoea virus, border disease virus and classical swine fever virus. Pestiviruses possess four structural proteins: a capsid protein and three envelope glycoproteins designated E^{rns} (soluble ribonuclease), E1 and E2. The immunodominant major glycoprotein, E2 (gp53) induces neutralizing antibodies.

Clinical infections

In the genera *Flavivirus* and *Pestivirus* there are several viruses of particular veterinary importance (Table 74.1). Three members of the genus *Flavivirus*, louping ill virus, Japanese encephalitis virus and Wesselsbron virus, cause disease in domestic animals. In addition, infection with West Nile virus, an important human pathogen, causes fatal disease in horses. Other members of the genus which are important human pathogens include yellow fever virus, dengue virus, Japanese encephalitis virus, tick-borne encephalitis virus and St. Louis encephalitis virus. The sole member of the *Hepacivirus* genus, hepatitis C virus, is an important cause of hepatitis in humans.

The four recognised members of the *Pestivirus* genus which infect domestic species are closely related antigenically. Bovine viral diarrhoea virus can infect both cattle and sheep, as well as other ruminants and pigs. Six distinct genotypes have recently been defined within the

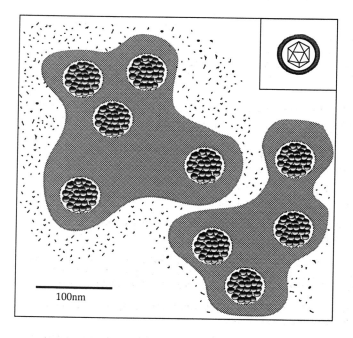

Figure 74.1 Flavivirus particles as they appear in an electron micrograph and a diagrammatic representation (inset).

Family	Genus	Virus

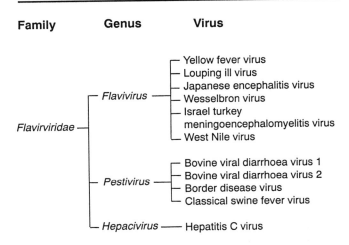

Figure 74.2 Viruses in the family *Flaviviridae*, with emphasis on those of veterinary importance.

genus on the basis of sequence differences in the gene coding for the envelope glycoprotein E2 (gp53) of various isolates (van Rijn *et al.*, 1997): classical swine fever virus, border disease virus, classical bovine viral diarrhoea virus (isolates predominantly from cattle), atypical bovine viral diarrhoea virus (isolates from cattle, sheep and pigs), deer pestivirus and giraffe pestivirus. Pestivirus infections may be inapparent, acute or persistent and are economically important worldwide.

Louping ill

The name 'louping ill' derives from the Scottish vernacular for 'leaping' or 'bounding', an allusion to the abnormal gait of some affected animals. Louping ill is a viral disease primarily of sheep. Although the virus is pathogenic for humans, infection is rare. The disease, which is largely confined to Britain and Ireland, has also been described in Norway, Spain, Bulgaria and Turkey. Isolates from Spain and Turkey are distinct from each other and also from isolates in Britain, Ireland and Norway (Marin *et al.*, 1995). Louping ill virus belongs to a group of serologically related viruses, the tick-borne encephalitis group or complex. The members of this group are distributed in northern temperate latitudes and are mainly human pathogens.

Epidemiology

Louping ill virus is transmitted by the tick *Ixodes ricinus* and the seasonal incidence and regional distribution of the disease reflect periods of tick activity in a suitable habitat such as upland grazing. Two main periods of tick activity occur, the first in spring and a second in late summer or early autumn. The host range of *I. ricinus* is wide and infection with louping ill virus can occur in many vertebrate species including sheep, cattle, horses, deer, red grouse and humans. Red grouse are particularly susceptible to infection with mortality reaching 80% in experimental infections. In areas where louping ill is

Table 74.1 Viruses of veterinary importance in the genera *Flavivirus* and *Pestivirus*.

Genus	Virus	Hosts	Comments
Flavivirus	Louping ill virus	Sheep, cattle, horses, red grouse and humans	Present in defined regions of Europe. Transmitted by the tick *Ixodes ricinus* and produces encephalitis in sheep and other species
	Japanese encephalitis virus	Waterfowl, pigs, horses and humans	Widely distributed in Asia. Transmitted by mosquitoes. Waterfowl are reservoir hosts. Infection in pigs results in abortion and neonatal mortality
	Wesselsbron virus	Sheep	Occurs in parts of sub-Saharan Africa. Transmitted by mosquitoes. Produces generalized infection, hepatitis and abortion
	Israel turkey meningo-encephalomyelitis virus	Turkeys	Reported in Israel and South Africa. Transmitted by mosquitoes. Progressive paresis and paralysis
	West Nile virus	Birds, humans, horses	Birds are the natural hosts. Transmitted by mosquitoes. Serious nervous disease reported sporadically in humans and horses
Pestivirus	Bovine viral diarrhoea virus types 1 and 2	Cattle (sheep, pigs)	Occurs worldwide. Causes inapparent infection, bovine viral diarrhoea and mucosal disease. Congenital infection may result in abortion, congenital defects and persistent infection due to immunotolerance
	Border disease virus	Sheep	Occurs worldwide. Infection of pregnant ewes may result in abortion and congenital abnormalities
	Classical swine fever (hog cholera) virus	Pigs	Highly contagious, economically important disease with high mortality. Generalized infection with nervous signs and abortion; congenital tremors in piglets

endemic, infection can result in a dramatic reduction in the population of red grouse. They are, therefore, not considered to be important maintenance hosts. Louping ill virus is maintained in endemic areas through a sheep-tick cycle. Trans-stadial but not transovarial transmission of the virus occurs in the tick. Rarely, contaminated instruments may be responsible for virus transmission. On farms where infection is endemic, losses occur mainly in sheep under two years of age. Most sheep acquire life-long immunity. Young lambs are protected by colostral antibody.

Pathogenesis

Viral replication occurs initially in lymph nodes draining sites of inoculation. Viraemia follows with dissemination to other lymphatic organs and sometimes to the brain and spinal cord. The speed and onset of the immune response are important in preventing spread of virus to the central nervous system. Immunosuppression caused by infection with *Ehrlichia phagocytophila*, the agent of tickborne fever, is considered to be responsible for increased mortality in sheep with louping ill.

Clinical signs

Following infection, sheep develop a febrile response which may go unnoticed. The temperature then returns to normal and, in a proportion of animals, rises again as neurological signs develop. These signs include hyperexcitability, fine muscular tremor, incoordination and exaggerated limb movements. Most affected animals develop convulsions prior to coma and death. Some sheep recover but exhibit mild, residual neurological signs. In cattle, the course of louping ill is more protracted. Affected animals may become recumbent but usually remain bright and many eventually recover. In humans, influenza-like clinical signs are followed, in most cases, by mild neurological disturbance.

Diagnosis

- A history of neurological signs or unexplained deaths in sheep in endemic areas during periods of tick activity may indicate louping ill. Laboratory confirmation is usually required.
- A non-suppurative encephalomyelitis is usually detectable histologically. Lesions are most pronounced in the brain stem and spinal cord. A specific diagnosis may be possible using an immunoperoxidase technique to detect viral antigen.
- Specimens of brain, collected aseptically into 50% glycerol saline, may be inoculated into tissue culture or intracerebrally into baby mice in order to isolate the virus.
- Antibody to the virus can be detected using complement fixation, gel diffusion, haemagglutination inhibition or IFA tests. The virus agglutinates goose red cells. The detection of IgM antibodies is indicative of acute infection.

Treatment

No specific treatment is available. Careful nursing and sedation may aid recovery.

Control

- Inactivated vaccines are protective. In the past, formalized vaccines produced from infected sheep brains were responsible, in some instances, for causing scrapie in vaccinated animals. Tissue culture-derived virus is now used for inactivated vaccines.
- Animals to be retained for breeding are vaccinated at six to 12 months of age. Colostrum from vaccinated ewes protects lambs during the first year of life. A booster injection may be advisable for ewes in their second pregnancy to enhance colostral antibody levels.
- Land improvement may help to reduce tick populations. Dipping of sheep may also reduce risk of infection.

Japanese encephalitis

This disease, which mainly affects humans, has a wide geographical distribution in Asia. Infection can occur in a number of animal species including horses and pigs. The virus is transmitted by mosquitoes and is maintained by a mosquito-aquatic bird cycle. The disease is of reduced importance in horses because of their declining numbers in endemic areas and the use of effective vaccines. The pig is an important amplifying host because of its close association with human populations in parts of Asia. Infection can cause reproductive failure in sows. Litters of infected sows may contain mummified and stillborn foetuses, weak piglets with neurological signs and clinically normal piglets. Confirmation is based either on virus isolation or on the demonstration of specific antibody. Both inactivated and live attenuated vaccines have been used to control the disease.

Wesselsbron disease

This disease, caused by a flavivirus, has a wide host range including domestic species, wild mammals and humans. However, clinical disease is usually encountered in sheep; infections in other species tend to be mild or subclinical. Infection in humans may result in febrile influenza-like symptoms. The virus is transmitted by mosquitoes. Infection is widespread in sub-Saharan Africa. The disease in sheep is similar to Rift Valley fever but is clinically less severe. It is characterized by abortion, neonatal mortality and congenital abnormalities such as hydranencephaly and arthrogryposis. The disease is most severe in newborn lambs which present with fever, depression, general weakness and polypnoea. Confirmation is based on virus isolation, intracerebral inoculation of baby mice and the demonstration of specific antibody. An attenuated vaccine which provides life-long immunity is available. Pregnant animals should not be vaccinated because of the risk of abortion.

Bovine viral diarrhoea and mucosal disease

Infection with bovine viral diarrhoea virus (BVDV), also known as bovine virus diarrhoea virus, is common in cattle populations throughout the world. The virus can cause both acute disease, bovine viral diarrhoea (BVD), and a protracted form of illness, mucosal disease, arising from persistent infection. Using cell culture, cytopathic and non-cytopathic biotypes are recognized. The biotype most often isolated from cattle populations is non-cytopathic. Cytopathic isolates can arise from non-cytopathic BVDV as a result of recombination events including incorporation of host RNA and duplication of viral RNA sequences (Meyers et al., 1996). Two genotypes now considered separate species, BVDV 1 (classical BVDV isolates) and BVDV 2 (atypical BVDV isolates), are recognized on the basis of differences in the 5' untranslated region of the viral genome. Both genotypes contain cytopathic and non-cytopathic isolates, and produce similar clinical syndromes in cattle. However, only type 2 isolates have been associated with thrombocytopenia and a haemorrhagic syndrome, first described in North America (Rebuhn et al., 1989). Isolates of BVDV used in vaccines and for diagnostic tests generally belong to the type 1 genotype.

Epidemiology

When cattle are infected initially with BVDV, they shed virus for a short period and may transmit virus to other animals. Persistently-infected animals, which shed virus in secretions and excretions, are particularly important sources of infection. Persistent infection develops when infection of the foetus with a non-cytopathic strain occurs before day 120 of gestation. About 1% of animals in an infected population are persistently-infected and viraemic. Although persistently-infected cows may breed successfully, they can transmit virus transplacentally to calves during successive gestations. This form of disease transmission is relatively common. The presence of cattle with persistent infection in a herd results in constant exposure of the other cattle to virus, producing a high level of herd immunity. In such herds, more than 80% of animals are serologically positive.

Virus is excreted in the semen of both persistently-infected and transiently-infected bulls. Infection may be transmitted through natural service or by artificial insemination. Embryo transfer from animals with persistent or transient infection can lead to infection in recipient cows. If pregnant animals are inoculated with live vaccines, their calves may develop persistent infection. Due to the instability of the virus, indirect transmission rarely occurs through farm workers, equipment and biting flies. Although cattle are the primary hosts, the virus can infect most even-toed ungulates. Interspecies spread of bovine and ovine pestiviruses has been demonstrated under natural conditions but its epidemiological significance is uncertain.

Pathogenesis

The virus is usually acquired by the oronasal route and initial replication occurs in the oronasal mucosa. In the subsequent viraemia, virus spreads throughout the body either free in the serum or in association with leukocytes. Both B and T lymphocyte numbers decrease. As the virus has an immunosuppressive effect, infection may predispose calves to respiratory and enteric disease. The outcome of transplacental spread depends on the age of the foetus at the time of infection. During the first 30 days of gestation, infection may result in embryonic death with return of the dam to oestrus. The effects of foetal infection between 30 and 90 days of gestation include abortion, mummification and congenital abnormalities of the CNS, often cerebellar hypoplasia. Foetuses, which become infected after day 120 of gestation, can mount an active immune response and are usually normal at birth. If virus invades the foetus before the development of immune competence, immunotolerance to the agent develops with persistent infection for the lifetime of the animal. The virus involved in this persistent infection is non-cytopathic. Later, usually between six months and two years of age, a cytopathic biotype emerges as a consequence of mutation of the non-cytopathic virus or of recombination with nucleic acid of the host cell or other non-cytopathic biotypes. These may lead to the development of mucosal disease in some animals.

Cytopathic isolates differ from their non-cytopathic counterparts by producing an 80 kDa non-structural protein (NS3). The role of NS3 in the pathogenesis of mucosal disease is unclear. Cytopathic isolates have a particular tropism for gut-associated lymphoid tissues.

Clinical signs

Most BVDV infections are subclinical. Outbreaks of BVD are usually associated with high morbidity and low mortality. When present, clinical signs include inappetence, depression, fever and diarrhoea. Significant mortality has been described in some outbreaks of BVD (David et al., 1994). Peracute BVD is characterized by high fever, severe diarrhoea and dehydration. Ulceration of the oral mucous membrane and the epithelia of the interdigital cleft and coronary band may also be present. In some cases thrombocytopenia results in bloody diarrhoea, epistaxis and petechiae in the mouth, conjunctiva and sclera.

Although a significant proportion of persistently-infected animals are clinically normal, some are born undersized and demonstrate retarded growth rate and poor viability. Increased susceptibility to enteritis and pneumonia has been reported. Mucosal disease is usually sporadic in occurrence. The condition affects persistently-infected animals, usually between six months and two years of age. Clinical signs include depression, fever, profuse watery diarrhoea, nasal discharge, salivation and lameness. Ulcerative lesions are present in the mouth and interdigital clefts. Case fatality rate is 100%; death usually occurs within weeks of the onset of clinical signs. A few animals may survive for several months before dying from severe debilitation.

Diagnosis

A tentative diagnosis may be possible on the basis of clinical signs and pathological findings. Laboratory confirmation requires demonstration of antibody, viral antigen or viral RNA. Seroconversion and the presence of viraemic animals are necessary for confirmation of established infection in a herd.

- Specimens suitable for laboratory examinations include the buffy coat from whole blood, spleen, lymph node and lesions from the gastrointestinal tract.
- Virus can be isolated in cell cultures. Sequential samples taken three weeks apart should be used to confirm persistent infection. Before foetal calf serum is used in cell culture medium, it should be screened for the presence of virus and antibody.
- Viral antigen can be detected in frozen sections or buffy coat smears by immunofluorescence. An ELISA or immunoperoxidase technique may also be used.
- Dot blot, *in situ* hybridization and PCR techniques for the detection of viral RNA have been described.
- Virus neutralization and ELISA are the most commonly used methods for the detection of antibodies to BVDV. Demonstration of a four-fold increase in antibody titre of paired serum samples is necessary to confirm recent infection.

Treatment and control

Supportive therapy may be of benefit in outbreaks of bovine viral diarrhoea. Treatment of animals with mucosal disease is of no benefit. Most losses arising from BVDV infections in herds result from the effects of prenatal infections and mucosal disease. Control strategies are directed at preventing infections which can lead to the birth of persistently-infected animals.

- Killed, attenuated live and temperature-sensitive mutant virus vaccines have been developed. Live vaccines may cause foetal infections and immunosuppression. In addition, they may precipitate mucosal disease in some persistently-infected animals. Killed vaccines may be used in pregnant animals but require regular boosters to maintain protection. Vaccines produced from a single strain or genotype of virus may not be fully protective due to antigenic variation, a feature of BVDV isolates. Vaccines have generally been evaluated for their ability to prevent acute disease and manufacturers do not claim that vaccination prevents foetal infection (van Campen

and Woodard, 1997). Exposure of replacement stock before breeding commences to a persistently-infected animal may help to maintain herd immunity.

- The elimination of BVDV from a herd requires the identification and removal of persistently-infected animals. The dam, sire and progeny of persistently-infected animals should be tested since the virus can be passed from parent to offspring.
- Herd immunity wanes following the removal of persistently-infected animals. Therefore, all newly-acquired cattle should be tested before being introduced to the herd.
- Systematic testing of bulk milk or pooled blood samples for antibodies is important in national eradication programmes.

Border disease

This congenital disorder of lambs, also known as hairy shaker disease, occurs worldwide. Border disease, which was first reported from the Welsh-English border, is caused by infection of the foetus with a non-cytopathic pestivirus. Border disease virus (BDV) is closely related to bovine viral diarrhoea virus and it has been suggested that they may be a single species. Pestivirus isolates from sheep can infect other domestic ruminants and pigs. Moreover, pestivirus isolates from a number of domestic species can infect pregnant sheep causing border disease in their offspring.

Epidemiology

Persistently-infected animals shed virus continuously in excretions and secretions. These animals tend to have a low survival rate under field conditions, although some may survive for several years without developing clinical signs. Persistently-infected ewes may give birth to persistently-infected lambs. Acute infections in susceptible sheep are transient and result in immunity to challenge with homologous strains of BDV. Infected rams shed virus in semen and may infect susceptible ewes. In addition to sheep-to-sheep contact, transmission can occur through contaminated needles during flock vaccination. Other ruminant species shedding pestivirus are potential sources of infection for sheep.

Pathogenesis

Virus is probably acquired by the oronasal route. In susceptible pregnant ewes, infection results in placentitis and invasion of the foetus. The immune response of the ewe does not protect the developing foetus. The age of the foetus at the time of infection ultimately determines the outcome. The foetus develops immune competence between 60 and 80 days of gestation. Foetal death may follow infection prior to the development of immune competence, the outcome being resorption, abortion or mummification. Foetuses which survive become immunotolerant and remain persistently infected. These animals may be clinically normal at birth or may display tremors and hairy birthcoat, consequences of viral interference with organogenesis. Congenital defects in affected lambs include skeletal growth retardation, hypomyelinogenesis and enlarged primary hair follicles with reduced numbers of secondary follicles. Infection after day 80 of gestation induces an immune response with elimination of the virus and the birth of a healthy lamb. Foetal infection during mid-gestation when the immune system is developing may result in lesions in the central nervous system including cerebral cavitation and cerebellar dysplasia. Immune-mediated reactions have been suggested as the possible explanation for these severe lesions. Some persistently-infected sheep may develop a condition similar to mucosal disease of cattle. Cytopathic isolates of BDV have been recovered from the intestines of such affected animals.

Clinical signs

In flocks infected with BDV, there may be an increase in the number of abortions and weak neonatal lambs. Characteristic signs of infection in newborn lambs include altered body conformation, changes in fleece quality and tremors. Hairs projecting above the wool, particularly along the neck and back, impart a halo effect that is most noticeable in fine coated breeds. Affected lambs are often small and their survival rate is poor. The survival rate is influenced not only by the severity of the neurological dysfunction but also by the standard of animal care. In well-nursed lambs, the neurological signs gradually abate and such animals may eventually become clinically normal.

Diagnosis

- The characteristic clinical signs are diagnostic.
- Dysmyelination may be demonstrable histologically in the central nervous system. Immunocytochemical staining can be used to demonstrate virus in brain tissue.
- Virus isolation is possible in susceptible bovine or ovine cell lines. Immunocytochemical staining is used to demonstrate the presence of non-cytopathic virus.
- Samples suitable for virus isolation include whole blood and tissues from affected lambs. Pre-colostral blood from lambs is preferable because antibody acquired from colostrum may interfere with virus isolation.
- Viral antigen can be detected by immunofluorescence staining of frozen sections or by immunoperoxidase staining of fixed sections. An ELISA is used for detecting viral antigen in blood.
- Serological testing, employing methods such as serum neutralization and ELISA, can be used to determine the extent of infection in a flock.

Control

Control should be based on identification and removal of persistently-infected animals and precautions to avoid introduction of infected animals into a flock. Where such a policy is not feasible, breeding stock should be deliberately mixed with persistently-infected animals at least two months before mating. A commercial inactivated, adjuvanted vaccine is available, containing BDV and BVDV-1 (Nettleton *et al.*, 1998).

Classical swine fever (Hog cholera)

This highly contagious, potentially fatal disease of pigs, although still present in many countries, has been eradicated from North America, Australia and most European countries. It is classed as a List A disease by the Office International des Epizooties. In recent years, sporadic outbreaks have occurred in the United Kingdom, Italy, Belgium, the Netherlands and Germany. Isolates of classical swine fever virus (CSFV), the causal agent of the disease, can be placed in two major groups on the basis of nucleotide sequence data. Recent European isolates, placed in Group 2, are distinct from those which caused swine fever outbreaks during the 1940s and 1950s (Lowings *et al.*, 1996). Isolates, although conforming to a single major antigenic type and being mostly non-cytopathic, differ substantially in virulence.

Epidemiology

Pigs, both domestic and feral, are the natural hosts of CSFV and direct contact between infected and susceptible animals is the main means of transmission. In endemic areas, the disease is spread principally by movement of infected pigs. Shedding of virus may begin before clinical signs become evident. Virulent virus is shed in all excretions and secretions until the time of death at about 20 days post infection. Virus strains of moderate virulence may result in chronic infection with continuous or intermittent shedding by infected pigs. In addition, congenital infections with strains of low virulence may result in the birth of persistently-infected piglets. Although infected animals have been found in the wild boar populations in Europe, their significance as reservoirs of infection is unclear. Spread between premises can occur indirectly, particularly in regions with a high density of pig farms. The virus can be transmitted mechanically by personnel, vehicles and biting arthropods. The virus, which is relatively fragile and does not persist in the environment, is not spread over long distances by air movement. Despite its lability, CSFV can survive for long periods in protein-rich biological materials such as meat or body fluids, particularly if chilled or frozen. Although legislation is in place in most European countries prohibiting the feeding of uncooked swill, recent outbreaks of classical swine fever can still be traced to waste food fed to pigs.

Pathogenesis and pathology

Pigs are usually infected by the oronasal route. The tonsil is the primary site of viral multiplication. Virus spreads to regional lymph nodes and viraemia develops after further viral multiplication. Virus, which has an affinity for vascular endothelium and reticuloendothelial cells, can be isolated from all major organs and tissues. In acute swine fever, vascular damage in conjunction with severe thrombocytopenia results in widespread petechial haemorrhages. A non-suppurative encephalitis with prominent perivascular cuffing is present in most CSFV-infected pigs. Virus strains of reduced virulence can cause a mild form of the disease. In pregnant sows, virus may be transmitted to foetuses. The outcome of transplacental infection is determined by the age of the foetus and the virulence of the invading strain of virus. Infection early in gestation results in foetal death with resorption or abortion. *In utero* infection may also result in stillbirths, weak newborn piglets with congenital tremors and, occasionally, clinically normal piglets. Piglets with immune tolerance to the virus remain persistently-infected and excrete virus continuously. Animals, which are clinically normal when born, may subsequently develop late-onset disease. The factors which precipitate late-onset disease are unclear.

Clinical signs

Following an incubation period of up to ten days, affected animals develop high fever and become inappetent and depressed. Sick pigs are inclined to huddle together. Vomiting and constipation are followed by diarrhoea. Some animals may die soon after developing convulsions. A swaying gait usually precedes posterior paresis. Most cases of acute classical swine fever succumb within 20 days after infection.

Signs of disease are milder in infections caused by strains of low virulence. Partial recovery from an initial phase of acute illness may be followed by relapse and death. Some pigs may survive for several months but exhibit marked growth retardation. Abortion, mummification, malformations and stillbirths may be encountered in breeding herds. Live-born infected piglets, often exhibiting tremors, may die soon after birth. Some affected piglets may present with haemorrhages in the skin. Congenital malformations include deformities of the head and limbs and cerebellar hypoplasia.

Diagnosis

Although clinical signs and history may provide evidence for a tentative diagnosis, laboratory confirmation is essential, particularly with infections caused by strains of reduced virulence.

- In acute disease, haemorrhages are present in many internal organs and on serosal surfaces. Petechiae are often present on kidney surfaces and in lymph nodes. Other gross pathological features of diagnostic significance are splenic infarction and 'button' ulcers in the mucosa of the terminal ileum near the ileocaecal valve.

- Rapid confirmation is possible using direct immunofluorescence on frozen sections of tonsillar tissue, kidney, spleen, distal ileum and lymph nodes. As pigs can be infected with BVDV, monoclonal antibodies specific for CSFV may be required to reach a definitive diagnosis.

- Virus isolation can be carried out in porcine cell lines using homogenates of spleen and tonsil. As most isolates are non-cytopathic, immunostaining is necessary for the demonstration of viral antigen.

- Serological testing is useful on farms infected with strains of low virulence or for serological surveys. Virus neutralization and ELISA are the tests most widely used. A blocking ELISA has been developed for distinguishing CSFV from BVDV (Wensvoort *et al.*, 1988).

Control

- The disease is notifiable in many countries which have adopted slaughter policies and banned vaccination. Pigs and pig products should not be imported from countries where infection with CSFV is present. Swill must be boiled before being fed to pigs.

- In countries where the disease is endemic or during the early stages of an eradication programme, vaccination may be used. Live vaccines attenuated either by serial passage in rabbits (Chinese strain) or in tissue culture (Japanese guinea pig strain or French Thiverval strain) are currently used. These vaccines are safe and effective. Vaccinated animals cannot be distinguished serologically from naturally-infected animals. The recently-developed recombinant E2 marker vaccine used in conjunction with a specific ELISA capable of detecting antibodies to the other main envelope glycoprotein, E^{rns}, may offer a way of distinguishing vaccinated from naturally infected pigs (Baars *et al.*, 1998).

References

Baars, J., Bonde Larsen, A. and Martens, M. (1998). Porcilis pestis: the missing link in the failing non-vaccination policy for classical swine fever. *The Pig Journal*, **41**, 26–38.

David, G.P., Crawshaw, T.R., Gunning, R.F. *et al.* (1994). Severe disease in adult dairy cattle in three UK dairy herds associated with BVD virus infection. *Veterinary Record*, **134**, 468–472.

Lowings, P., Ibata, G., Needham, J. and Paton, D. (1996). Classical swine fever virus diversity and evolution. *Journal of General Virology*, **77**, 1311–1321.

Marin, M.S., McKenzie, J., Gao, G.F. *et al.* (1995). The virus causing encephalomyelitis in sheep in Spain: a new member of the tick-borne encephalitis group. *Research in Veterinary*

Science, **58**, 11–13.

Meyers, G., Tautz, N., Dubovi, E.J. and Thiel, H.J. (1996). Origin and diversity of cytopathogenic pestiviruses. In *International Symposium Bovine Viral Diarrhoea Virus. A 50 Year Review.* Cornell University, New York. pp. 24–34.

Nettleton, P.F., Gilray, J.A., Russo, P. and Dlissi, E. (1998). Border disease of sheep and goats. *Veterinary Research*, **29**, 327–340.

Rebuhn, W.C., French, T.W., Perdrizet, J.A. *et al.* (1989). Thrombocytopenia associated with acute bovine virus diarrhoea infection in cattle. *Journal of Veterinary Internal Medicine*, **3**, 42–46.

van Campen, H. and Woodard, L. (1997). Fetal infection may not be preventable with BVDV vaccines. *Journal of the American Veterinary Medical Association*, **210**, 480.

van Rijn, P.A., Gennip, H.G.P., Leendertse, C.H. *et al.* (1997). Subdivision of the *Pestivirus* genus based on envelope glycoprotein E2. *Virology*, **237**, 337–348.

Wensvoort, G., Bloemraad, M. and Terpestra, C. (1988). An enzyme immunoassay employing monoclonal antibodies and detecting specifically antibodies to classical swine fever virus. *Veterinary Microbiology*, **17**, 129–140.

Further reading

Brownlie, J., Thompson, I. and Curwen, A. (2000). Bovine virus diarrhoea virus — strategic decisions for diagnosis and control. *In Practice*, **22**, 176–187.

Chapter 75

Togaviridae

Viruses in the family *Togaviridae* (Latin *toga*, cloak) are enveloped RNA viruses, approximately 70 nm in diameter, with icosahedral symmetry. The envelope, which contains glycoprotein spikes, is closely bound to an icosahedral capsid (Fig. 75.1). Togaviruses agglutinate goose and chick erythrocytes. There are two genera, *Alphavirus* and *Rubivirus*, in the family. The sole member of the genus *Rubivirus* is rubella virus, which causes German measles in children and young adults.

The genus *Alphavirus* includes more than 25 species, a number of which are important animal pathogens. Alphaviruses are divided, on the basis of genomic composition, into a number of groups including Venezuelan equine encephalitis virus (VEEV) complex, eastern equine encephalitis virus (EEEV) complex, Semliki forest virus complex and western equine encephalitis virus (WEEV) complex. Western equine encephalitis virus has been shown to have arisen by recombination between EEEV and Sindbis-like viruses, probably between 1,300 and 1,900 years ago (Weaver *et al.*, 1997).

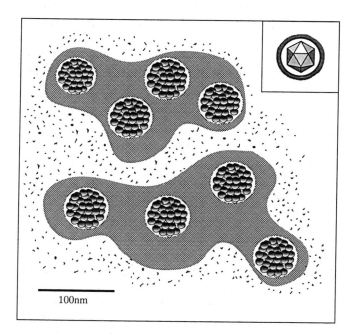

Figure 75.1 Togavirus particles as they appear in an electron micrograph and a diagrammatic representation (inset).

Key points
■ Enveloped, RNA viruses with icosahedral symmetry
■ Replicate in cell cytoplasm
■ Labile in the environment
■ Genus *Alphavirus*
—arthropod-borne
—cause eastern equine encephalitis, western equine encephalitis and Venezuelan equine encephalitis
—major cause of zoonotic infections

Replication of alphaviruses, which contain positive-sense single-stranded RNA, occurs in the cytoplasm and nucleocapsids are assembled in the cytosol. In vertebrates, alphavirus infection results in cytolysis. The viral envelope is acquired as the nucleocapsid buds into the plasma membrane which contains virus-derived glycoprotein spikes. Viral infection of invertebrate cells is usually non-cytolytic and is persistent. In this instance virus assembly occurs in association with intracellular membranes rather than through the plasma membrane.

Mature virions of alphaviruses are sensitive to pH changes, heat, detergents and disinfectants, and are not stable in the environment. Alphaviruses, in common with certain members of the *Flaviviridae*, *Reoviridae*, *Rhabdoviridae* and *Bunyaviridae*, are termed arboviruses indicating that they are **arthropod-borne**. This term, however, has no taxonomic significance.

Clinical infections

Domestic animals and humans are usually considered to be 'dead-end' hosts of alphaviruses because they do not develop a sufficiently high titre of circulating virus to act as reservoir hosts. A number of important equine diseases are caused by infection with members of the genus *Alphavirus* (Table 75.1). The three equine encephalitis viruses (Venezuelan, eastern and western), which are confined to the western hemisphere, are transmitted by mosquitoes. Getah virus occurs mainly in south-east Asia and in Australia. A number of outbreaks of disease caused by this virus have been recorded in Japan.

Table 75.1 Alphaviruses of veterinary significance.

Virus	Vector	Comments
Eastern equine encephalitis virus	Mosquito (*Culiseta melanura*, *Aedes* species)	Infection endemic in passerine birds which frequent freshwater swamps of eastern North America, Caribbean Islands and parts of South America. Causes disease in horses, humans and pheasants
Venezuelan equine encephalitis virus	Mosquito (*Culex* species)	Infection endemic in small mammals in Central and South America. Causes outbreaks of disease in horses, donkeys and humans in endemic regions, occasionally spreading to southern USA
Western equine encephalitis virus	Mosquito (*Culex tarsalis* and other *Culex* species, *Aedes* species)	Infection of passerine birds widespread in the Americas. Causes mild disease in horses and humans
Getah virus	Mosquito	Causes sporadic disease in horses in south-east Asia and Australia characterized by fever, urticaria and oedema of the limbs. Subclinical infection occurs in pigs

Equine encephalitides

The viruses which cause Venezuelan, eastern and western encephalitis are important in the Americas. These three viruses produce similar clinical signs although infections caused by the virus of western equine encephalitis tend to be milder.

Epidemiology

The equine encephalitides share some common epidemiological features. The peak periods of these diseases coincide with times of maximum vector numbers usually in late summer following heavy rainfall. The regional distribution of the viruses is related to that of mosquito vectors. Numbers of clinical cases drop dramatically when vector numbers decrease due to cold or drought.

Eastern equine encephalitis virus (EEEV) occurs principally in Atlantic coast areas of North America. However, EEEV has also been isolated in Michigan, the Caribbean islands and South America. The virus is maintained in cycles of infection involving passerine birds and the irrigation ditch mosquito (*Culiseta melanura*), which inhabits freshwater swamps (Fig. 75.2). Following infection, a high titre of virus develops in many wild birds without evidence of disease. High mortality rates have, however, been recorded in pheasants, emus and whooping cranes. Virus can be transmitted between pheasants by pecking and cannibalism. Periodic epidemic outbreaks of infection in wild birds, which may lead to infection of humans and horses, involve additional mosquito species such as *Aedes sollicitans* and *Coquillettidia perturbans* which feed both on birds and on mammals. Infection usually results in sporadic disease in man, horses and pheasants. Epizootics, which tend to occur in the autumn, disappear with the arrival of the first frosts. Overwintering mechanisms for virus maintenance are unclear, although wild birds are considered to be possible reservoirs. Transovarial transmission in mosquitoes has not been demonstrated.

Isolates of Venezuelan equine encephalitis virus (VEEV) comprise a complex of six subtypes. Epidemic forms of Venezuelan equine encephalitis (VEE) are caused by two highly virulent subtype I serotypes of the virus (I-AB and I-C). Other subtypes are considered to be either non-pathogenic or of low pathogenicity for horses. The viruses are maintained in sylvatic cycles involving rodents and mosquitoes (*Culex* species) in swampy habitats. Phylogenetic studies suggest that the viruses implicated in epizootics are derived from mutation of viruses involved in enzootic cycles (Weaver *et al.*, 1992). Epizootics of VEE occurred regularly between 1962 and 1972 in the northern part of South America and in Central America, extending at one stage as far as Texas. Following a quiescent period of 20 years, a limited outbreak of disease occurred in Venezuela in 1992 followed by an extensive epizootic in Venezuela and Columbia in 1995 (Weaver *et al.*, 1996). Horses inoculated with a virulent subtype of VEEV develop a viraemia of sufficiently high titre to allow transmission by feeding mosquitoes.

Although western equine encephalitis (WEE) has traditionally occurred in the USA west of the Mississippi, it is also present in many other parts of the American continent. Infections tend to recur in certain areas. The cycle of infection involves mosquitoes, usually *Culex tarsalis*, and indigenous wild birds in which infection is inapparent. Horses are infected incidentally and are 'dead-end' hosts because levels of virus in the blood remain low. Epizootics are rare. Overwintering mechanisms of the virus are unclear but may involve birds, reptiles or mosquitoes.

Pathogenesis

Following inoculation by a feeding mosquito, viral replication occurs near the site of entry and in the regional lymph nodes. Viraemia, ranging from barely detectable to high levels, is accompanied by fever. When disease is severe, the virus invades the central nervous system resulting in neuronal necrosis and perivascular lymphoid cuffing.

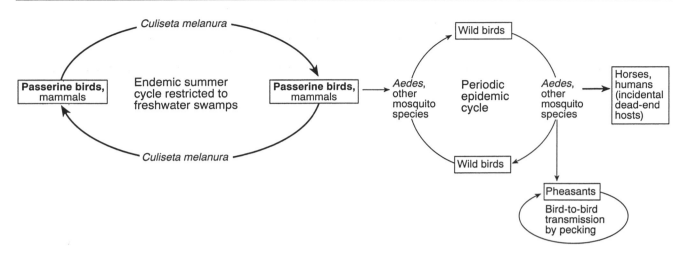

Figure 75.2 Endemic and epidemic transmission cycles of eastern equine encephalitis virus in North America. The endemic cycle which occurs in summer, is restricted to swampy regions. The epidemic cycle, which occurs periodically, involves mosquito species and wild birds not usually associated with swamps. Infection in horses and humans, which are 'dead-end' hosts, is a 'spill over' from the epidemic cycle. In farmed pheasants, bird-to-bird transmission may occur through pecking.

Clinical signs

Diseases caused by the three equine encephalitis viruses are clinically similar. The incubation period may be up to nine days. Clinical signs, which usually last from four to nine days, range from mild fever and depression to fatal febrile encephalomyelitis. Neurological signs include photophobia, blindness, head pressing, circling, ataxia and inability to swallow. Affected horses exhibit severe depression with low carriage of the head and a wide-based stance. Terminally, animals become recumbent and semi-comatose with convulsions prior to death. The case fatality rate is 90% for EEE, 50%-80% for VEE and 20%-40% for WEE.

Diagnosis

Clinical signs along with a history of previous cases of equine encephalitis in the same region may be suggestive of the disease. However, laboratory confirmation is usually required. Due to the possibility of human infection, care must be taken during specimen collection.

- Virus isolation provides a definitive diagnosis. Isolation is carried out in cell culture or in suckling mice. Whole blood or serum, collected during the pyrexic phase of the disease, is suitable for virus isolation. Brain or cerebrospinal fluid can be collected at postmortem. When VEE is suspected, isolates should be typed in order to distinguish virulent from non-virulent subtypes.
- An immunohistochemical staining technique for the detection of EEEV antigen in fixed brain sections has been described (Patterson *et al.*, 1996).
- Diagnosis of WEE or EEE is usually based on serology. Paired serum samples should be collected to demonstrate a rising titre. Suitable testing methods include

ELISA, plaque reduction neutralization assay, haemagglutination inhibition and complement fixation. An IgM capture ELISA has been used to provide evidence of infection in single serum samples. The vaccination status of an animal must be considered in interpreting the results of serological tests. The interpretation of serological results for VEEV is complicated by the presence of antibodies produced in response to inapparent infections with non-virulent subtypes.

Treatment and control

Although supportive palliative treatments may be beneficial, the prognosis is generally poor. Control is based on vaccination of horses and implementation of measures aimed at reducing mosquito populations.

- Monovalent, bivalent and trivalent vaccines are available. Vaccines for EEE and WEE are inactivated. A live attenuated TC-83 VEEV vaccine provides effective protection and has been used successfully to prevent epizootics of VEE.
- Vector control measures include spraying of vector habitats, destruction of mosquito breeding areas, use of insect repellants and stabling of horses at night in insect-proof buildings.

References

Patterson, J.S., Maes, R.K., Mullaney, T.P. and Benson, C.L. (1996). Immunohistochemical diagnosis of eastern equine encephalomyelitis. *Journal of Veterinary Diagnostic Investigation*, **8**, 156–160.

Weaver, S.C., Bellew, L.A. and Rico-Hesse, R. (1992).

Phylogenetic analysis of alphaviruses in the Venezuelan equine encephalitis complex and identification of the source of epizootic viruses. *Virology*, **191**, 282–290.

Weaver, S.C., Salas, R., Rico-Hesse, R. *et al.* (1996). Re-emergence of epidemic Venezuelan equine encephalomyelitis in South America. *Lancet,* **348**, 436–440.

Weaver, S.C., Kang WenLi, Shirako, Y. *et al.* (1997). Recombinational history and molecular evolution of western equine encephalomyelitis complex alphaviruses. *Journal of Virology*, **71**, 613–623.

Chapter 76

Prions: unconventional infectious agents

At present, conventional infectious agents have not been implicated aetiologically in the transmissible spongiform encephalopathies (TSEs), a unique group of neurodegnerative diseases. Intensive research efforts to elucidate the cause of TSEs have been inconclusive. It has been proposed that these diseases are caused by unconventional infectious agents termed prions (Prusiner, 1982). These infectious agents are 'unconventional' because they appear to be devoid of nucleic acid, unlike viruses and other microbial agents. In addition, they are non-immunogenic and are extremely resistant to inactivation by heating, exposure to chemicals and irradiation. The 'prion theory' proposes that they are derived from a native glycoprotein (Prusiner *et al.*, 1999). This native glycoprotein, PrP^C, (cellular prion protein) is associated with the plasma membrane of many cell types particularly neurons and lymphocytes. Structurally, PrP^C is composed of more α-helices than β-sheets. Following exposure to abnormal prion protein (PrP^{Sc}, scrapie prion protein), PrP^C is altered post-translationally to a structure similar to that of the PrP^{Sc} in which the β-sheet content predominates. As more PrP^C is converted to PrP^{Sc}, this protease-resistant molecule gradually accumulates especially in the long-lived cells of the CNS (Fig. 76.1). Recent studies suggest that PrP^{Sc} is formed from PrP^C on cell membranes in caveolae-like structures before these fuse with endosomes. During normal metabolic turnover in cells, most membrane glycoproteins are transported in endosomes to lysosomes for degradation. However, because it is protease-resistant, PrP^{Sc} accumulates in cytoplasmic vesicles particularly lysosomes (Prusiner *et al.*, 1999).

The mechanism by which PrP^{Sc} induces the structural alteration in native PrP^C has not yet been defined. However, the newly formed PrP^{Sc} closely resembles in its three dimensional structure the 'infecting' PrP^{Sc}, implying that the latter has a central role in the initiation of the chain reaction which results in the intracellular accumulation of large amounts of PrP^{Sc}.

Experimentally, mild acidification and reduction procedures induce structural rearrangement in PrP^C producing a highly soluble monomeric form of PrP (β-PrP) which is rich in β-sheets (Jackson *et al.*, 1999). This β-PrP can revert to an α-configuration or, alternatively, it can act as a stable 'seed' inducing polymerization with the *in vitro* formation of insoluble fibrillar structures similar to the

> **Key points**
> - Prions are proteinaceous particles apparently devoid of nucleic acid
> - Aetiologically implicated in the transmissible spongiform encephalopathies, fatal neurodegenerative diseases with long incubation periods
> - Neuropathological changes, which include vacuolation of both neurons and neuropil without evidence of an inflammatory response, are associated with the accumulation of abnormally-folded host-derived prion protein
> - Transmissible spongiform encephalopathies include:
>   —Scrapie in sheep
>   —Bovine spongiform encephalopathy
>   —Feline spongiform encephalopathy
>   —Transmissible mink encephalopathy
>   —Kuru and Creutzfeldt-Jakob disease in humans

prion fibrils which can be recovered from detergent-treated extracts of the brains of animals with TSEs. These experiments demonstrate that binding of several β-PrP molecules together can lead to the formation of an irreversible β-sheet configuration, the probable basis of PrP^{Sc} accumulation in TSEs.

The formation of PrP^{Sc} from PrP^C in TSEs may be initiated following exposure to an external source of PrP^{Sc}, usually by ingestion (Fig. 76.2). Rarely, random spontaneous conversion of native PrP^C to PrP^{Sc} may initiate the process in an individual. A third mechanism which predisposes to configurational change in PrP^C relates to mutation in the *PrP* gene as occurs in the Gerstmann-Sträussler-Scheinker syndrome in humans.

The *PrP* gene of an infected animal determines the primary amino acid sequence of the prion protein in that animal. The resistance of some species to infection by prions derived from another species is termed the 'species barrier'. This barrier is attributed to differences between the amino acid sequences of the prion proteins in the two species. On initial transfer of PrP^{Sc} between species, the

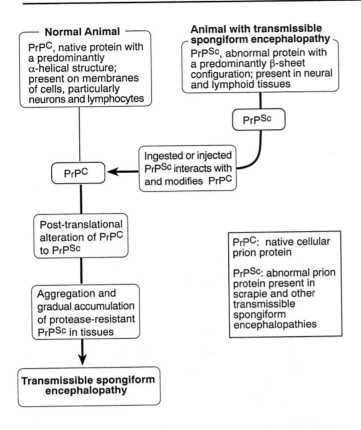

Normal Animal

PrP^C, native protein with a predominantly α-helical structure; present on membranes of cells, particularly neurons and lymphocytes

Animal with transmissible spongiform encephalopathy

PrP^{Sc}, abnormal protein with a predominantly β-sheet configuration; present in neural and lymphoid tissues

PrP^{Sc}

Ingested or injected PrP^{Sc} interacts with and modifies PrP^C

PrP^C

Post-translational alteration of PrP^C to PrP^{Sc}

Aggregation and gradual accumulation of protease-resistant PrP^{Sc} in tissues

Transmissible spongiform encephalopathy

PrP^C: native cellular prion protein

PrP^{Sc}: abnormal prion protein present in scrapie and other transmissible spongiform encephalopathies

Figure 76.1 Outline of the proposed mechanisms involved in the pathogenesis of transmissible spongiform encephalopathies

incubation period tends to be relatively long. Subsequent transfer between members of the recipient species leads to shorter incubation periods. The presence of a 'species barrier' may explain the resistance of humans to infection with PrP^{Sc} derived from sheep with scrapie. Prion strains from infected sheep have been described on the basis of bioassays in mice. Strain differentiation is based on incubation periods, mortality patterns, lesion profiles and titratable infectivity in the brains of mice of known genotypes. Prion diversity is thought to be determined by the conformation and glycosylation patterns of PrP^{Sc} and may account for the observed differences in prion strains. The 'protein only' theory of prion composition is contested (Chesebro, 1998). The existence of strains has been cited as evidence which supports a requirement for nucleic acid in prions.

Prions are stable at a wide pH range and are remarkably resistant to most methods of biological inactivation. Early evidence of the resistance of these agents to chemical inactivation was provided by retrospective studies on 18,000 sheep, which had been inadvertently exposed to infection when inoculated with a formalized louping ill vaccine. The vaccine, prepared from brains, spinal cords and spleens of sheep, contained the scrapie agent which was not inactivated by treatment with formaldehyde (Greig, 1950). Approximately 10% of the vaccinated

animals developed scrapie. Treatment of prions with alcohols and aldehydes that fix proteins may help to stabilize rather than inactivate these agents. Physical methods for inactivating the agents of bovine spongiform encephalopathy (BSE) and scrapie have been intensively investigated because safe disposal of infected carcases is mandatory. Although autoclaving at temperatures of 132°C has been recommended, it does not ensure prion inactivation. Paradoxically, autoclaving at temperatures above 138°C may increase the resistance of prions to inactivation. It has recently been shown that high concentrations of sodium hypochlorite or hot solutions of sodium hydroxide inactivate a thermostable strain of scrapie agent (Taylor, 2000). The inclusion of a formic acid step in formaldehyde fixation of brain tissue reduces the infectivity of the agents of scrapie, BSE and Creutzfeldt-Jacob disease without adversely affecting the quality of histological sections.

Clinical infections

Diseases attributed to prions occur sporadically and are significantly influenced by the genome of the affected animal. These slowly progressive neurodegenerative diseases, which are characterized by long incubation periods and spongiform changes in the brain, have been described in many animal species and in humans. Transmissible spongiform encephalopathies have been recognized in both ruminants and carnivores (Table 76.1).

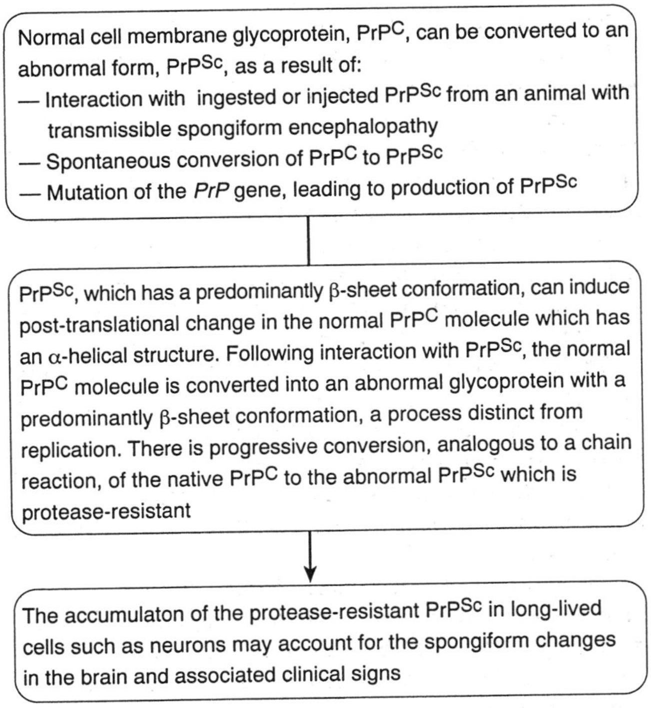

Normal cell membrane glycoprotein, PrP^C, can be converted to an abnormal form, PrP^{Sc}, as a result of:
— Interaction with ingested or injected PrP^{Sc} from an animal with transmissible spongiform encephalopathy
— Spontaneous conversion of PrP^C to PrP^{Sc}
— Mutation of the *PrP* gene, leading to production of PrP^{Sc}

PrP^{Sc}, which has a predominantly β-sheet conformation, can induce post-translational change in the normal PrP^C molecule which has an α-helical structure. Following interaction with PrP^{Sc}, the normal PrP^C molecule is converted into an abnormal glycoprotein with a predominantly β-sheet conformation, a process distinct from replication. There is progressive conversion, analogous to a chain reaction, of the native PrP^C to the abnormal PrP^{Sc} which is protease-resistant

The accumulaton of the protease-resistant PrP^{Sc} in long-lived cells such as neurons may account for the spongiform changes in the brain and associated clinical signs

Figure 76.2 An outline of the probable mechanisms which lead to the accumulation of PrP^{Sc} in neurons.

Table 76.1 Transmissible spongiform encephalopathies of animals.

Disease	Comments
Scrapie	Recognized in sheep in parts of Europe for 300 years; apart from Australia and New Zealand, now occurs worldwide. Occurs also in goats
Bovine spongiform encephalopathy	First reported in England in 1986; developed into a major epidemic over a ten year period. Prevalence declined with the implementation of effective control measures. Occurs at lower frequency in many other European countries
Feline spongiform encephalopathy	First recorded during the bovine spongiform encephalopathy epidemic in the early 1990s. Most cases reported in the UK
Transmissible mink encephalopathy	First recognized in caged mink in Wisconsin in 1947; attributed to the feeding of scrapie-infected sheep meat
Spongiform encephalopathy in captive ruminants	First recorded during the bovine spongiform encephalopathy epidemic in 1986. Reported in greater kudu, nyala, oryx and some other captive ruminants in zoological collections
Chronic wasting disease	First recognized in captive mule deer in Colorado in 1980. Occurs in deer and elk populations in the wild in North America

Similarities in the neuropathological features of scrapie in sheep and kuru in humans suggested that the two diseases had a similar aetiology (Hadlow, 1959). Subsequently, it was established that kuru, like scrapie, was caused by an unconventional transmissible agent. A number of other similar neurodegenerative diseases of humans, some of which are genetically determined, are classified as TSEs. The TSEs which have been described in humans are presented in Table 76.2. In humans, these TSEs may occur as infectious, genetic or sporadic diseases. In scrapie, there is convincing evidence for the importance of the genetic constitution of certain breeds of sheep in determining susceptibility to the disease.

Scrapie

This insidious, fatal, neurological disease of adult sheep and goats occurs worldwide except in Australia and New Zealand.

Epidemiology

The mode of transmission of scrapie is not clearly understood. Potential modes for natural infection include ingestion, entry through superficial abrasions and transmission from ewe to lamb. There is evidence that transmission tends to occur during the perinatal period and that exposure to placental material from affected ewes may

be important. Pastures grazed by affected animals appear to remain contaminated for years.

Particular polymorphisms of the *PrP* gene are associated with an increased incidence of scrapie in certain breeds of sheep. Some research workers have inferred from breeding experiments that scrapie is an exclusively genetic disease. However, Australia and New Zealand are free of scrapie despite the presence of animals with scrapie-associated *PrP* alleles (Hunter *et al.*, 1997). The *PrP* gene-coding sequence in sheep is highly polymorphic. Polymorphisms at codons 136, 154 and 171 of the *PrP* gene, producing amino acid substitutions in PrP, are important in influencing susceptibility to scrapie. In many breeds, the valine 136 glutamine 171 arginine 154 (denoted VRQ) allele is strongly associated with susceptibility to scrapie (Laplanche *et al.*, 1999).

Pathogenesis and pathology

Following natural infection, PrP^{Sc} is usually first detected in tissues of the lymphoreticular system including the spleen, the palatine tonsil and the retropharyngeal and mesenteric lymph nodes. In lymph nodes, replication apparently occurs in follicular dendritic cells. After oral exposure it is thought that the portal of entry to neural tissues is in the duodenum and ileum. The agent then spreads through fibres of the autonomic nervous system to the spinal cord and the medulla oblongata (van Keulen *et al.*, 1999). Neuronal and neuropil vacuolation and astrogliosis are associated with accumulation of PrP^{Sc} in the CNS.

Clinical signs

The disease has a long incubation period. Neurological signs develop predominantly in sheep of breeding age with a peak incidence between three and four years of age. Initially, affected animals may present with restlessness or nervousness, particularly after sudden noise or movement. Fine tremors of the head and neck and incoordination with a tendency to exhibit jerky movements are characteristic signs. Pruritis may result in loss of wool. In some affected sheep, a nibbling reflex can be elicited by scratching the back. Progression of the disease leads to emaciation. Death usually occurs within six months from the onset of clinical signs.

Diagnosis

Clinical signs and histopathological examination of the CNS form the basis for diagnosis. Characteristic microscopic changes include neuronal vacuolation and degeneration, vacuolar change in the neuropil and astrocytosis, particularly in the medulla. No obvious inflammatory response is evident. Confirmatory methods include immunohistochemical staining for PrP^{Sc}, immunoblotting to detect proteinase-K-resistant PrP^{Sc} and electron microscopy to detect scrapie-associated fibrils in detergent-treated extracts of brain. Antemortem detection

Table 76.2 Transmissible spongiform encephalopathies of humans.

Disease	Comments
Kuru	Described in members of the Fore population in Papua New Guinea. Acquired through ritualistic cannibalism; brain tissue was the primary source of infection.
Creutzfeldt-Jakob disease (CJD)	
Sporadic CJD	Attributed to somatic mutation in *PrP* gene or to random conversion of PrP^C into PrP^{Sc}
Iatrogenic CJD	Transmitted by medical or surgical procedures which utilized contaminated human tissues
Variant CJD	Considered to be a consequence of exposure to PrP^{Sc} from cattle with bovine spongiform encephalopathy
Familial CJD	Germline mutations in *PrP* gene
Gerstmann-Sträussler-Scheinker syndrome	Germline mutations in *PrP* gene
Fatal familial insomnia	Germline mutation in *PrP* gene

methods, based on demonstration of PrP^{Sc} in lymphoid tissues of the palatine tonsil and nictitating membrane by histochemical methods, are being developed.

Control

In the European Union, scrapie has been designated a notifiable disease. Countries free of the disease impose strict quarantine procedures. Slaughter policies have been enforced with different degrees of success in several countries. In Australia and New Zealand an eradication policy, implemented soon after the introduction of the disease, was successful. Eradication was abandoned in the United States because of the cost and difficulties in implementation. A control policy involving flock certification and movement restrictions is now in place. Breeding scrapie-resistant sheep may be a realistic method for reducing the frequency of the disease (Parry, 1983).

Bovine spongiform encephalopathy

This condition is a progressive, neurodegenerative disease of adult cattle, first recognized in England in 1986 (Wells *et al.*, 1987). More than 170,000 cases of the disease were subsequently confirmed and an estimated one million animals were infected. This common source epidemic peaked in 1993 when more than 300 new cases were identified each week. Since then, there has been a steady decline in numbers of confirmed cases. The disease has been reported in several countries in animals imported from Great Britain. In addition, indigenous cattle in a number of European countries, including Switzerland, Ireland, France and Portugal, have developed the disease.

The prion strain causing bovine spongiform encephalopathy (BSE) is not considered to be species-specific; infection has been reported in exotic ungulates in zoological collections following ingestion of feed derived from contaminated bovine tissues. In addition, feline spongiform encephalopathy was first recorded in the early 1990s in association with the BSE epidemic. In 1996, a novel form of human prion disease termed variant Creutzfeldt-Jakob disease (vCJD) was recognized in Great Britain. Molecular strain-typing studies and experimental transmission in transgenic and conventional mice indicated that vCJD and BSE are caused by indistinguishable prion strains. The extent of exposure of the human population to the agent cannot be accurately estimated because of uncertainties about risk factors and about the length of the incubation period in vCJD (Collinge, 1999).

Epidemiology

The BSE epidemic, which started simultaneously at several geographical locations in Great Britain, was attributed to contaminated meat-and-bone meal (MBM) prepared from slaughterhouse offal and fed as a protein dietary supplement to cattle. It is postulated that the scrapie agent crossed the species barrier into cattle in the early 1980s following changes in the rendering process which allowed survival of increased amounts of scrapie PrP (PrP^{Sc}) in the MBM. Recycling of infected tissues from animals with BSE, prior to the recognition of the disease and the imposition of control measures, resulted in extension of the epidemic. Because of the high ratio of sheep to cattle, the frequency of endemic scrapie and the heavy reliance on MBM as a supplement for dairy cattle in Great Britain, the epidemic has been largely confined to that country (Nathanson *et al.*, 1999). As a result of the banning of ruminant-derived MBM in 1988, there was a marked decline in the prevalence of BSE in Great Britain after 1993. Despite this decline, animals born after imposition of the ban have developed BSE. This was ascribed to the continued use of ruminant-derived MBM and also to cross-contamination in feed mills by rations specified for pigs and poultry. Additional stringent regulations, introduced in 1996, banned the inclusion of mammalian-derived MBM from farm animal feed.

Horizontal transmission of BSE does not appear to occur and, although maternal transmission may occur at a low rate, it is considered to be of minimal importance in the spread of disease. Susceptibility of cattle to BSE appears to be independent of sex, breed and genotype.

Pathogenesis and pathology

The pathogenesis of BSE is poorly defined. The agent of

BSE has been found in the distal ileum following experimental oral exposure. In naturally occuring cases of the disease, the agent has not been demonstrated in lymphoreticular tissues or peripheral nodes. Accumulation of PrP^{Sc} in the CNS is associated with vacuolation and glial proliferation.

Clinical signs

The mean incubation period is about five years. Neurological signs, which are highly variable, include changes in behaviour and deficits in posture and movement. Loss of weight and decreased milk production also occur. Other clinical signs include tremors, hyperaesthesia, apprehension, bruxism, exaggerated menace reflex and head shyness. Ataxia, hypermetria and a tendency to fall become increasingly evident in the later stages of the disease. The clinical course may extend over many days or months.

Diagnosis

Bovine spongiform encephalopathy can be confirmed by histopathological examination of brain tissue and appropriate additional methods. Examination of brain tissue may be confined to a coronal section of the medulla at the obex. Characteristic neuropathological changes including neuropil vacuolation and astrocytosis are consistently present at this site. Additional confirmatory methods include immunohistochemical staining for PrP^{Sc}, immunoblotting to demonstrate proteinase K-resistant PrP^{Sc} and electron microscopy to detect prion fibrils in detergent-treated extracts of brain.

Control

Bovine spongiform encephalopathy is a notifiable disease in countries of the European Union. In some countries, the entire herd, in which an affected animal is detected, is slaughtered. In other countries, clinically affected animals only are slaughtered. Ruminant-derived protein should be excluded from ruminant rations. Carcases of infected animals should be incinerated at high temperatures to ensure destruction of the thermostable agent. Buildings and equipment can be decontaminated by the application of high concentrations of sodium hypochlorite or of heated strong solutions of sodium hydroxide (Taylor, 2000).

References

Chesebro, B. (1998). BSE and prions: uncertainties about the agent. *Science*, **279**, 42–43.

Collinge, J. (1999). Variant Creutzfeldt-Jakob disease. *Lancet,* **354**, 317–323.

Greig, J.R. (1950). Scrapie in sheep. *Journal of Comparative Pathology*, **60**, 263–266.

Hadlow, W.J. (1959). Scrapie and kuru. *Lancet,* **ii**, 289–290.

Hunter, N., Cairns, D., Foster, J.D. *et al.* (1997). Is scrapie solely a genetic disease? *Nature*, **386**, 137.

Jackson, G.S., Hosszu, L.L.P., Power, A. *et al.* (1999). Reversible conversion of monomeric human prion protein between native and fibrillogenic conformations. *Science*, **283**, 1935–1937.

Laplanche, J.L., Hunter, N., Shinagawa, M. and Williams, E. (1999). Scrapie, chronic wasting disease and transmissible mink encephalopathy. In *Prion Biology and Diseases*. Ed. S.P. Prusiner. Cold Spring Harbor Laboratory Press, New York. pp. 393–429.

Nathanson, N., Wilesmith, J., Wells, G.A. and Griot, C. (1999). Bovine spongiform encephalopathy and related diseases. In *Prion Biology and Diseases*. Ed. S.B. Prusiner. Cold Spring Harbor Laboratory Press, New York. pp. 431–463.

Parry, H.B. (1983). *Scrapie disease in sheep*. Academic Press, New York.

Prusiner, S.B. (1982). Novel proteinaceous infectious particles cause scrapie. *Science*, **216**, 136–144.

Prusiner, S.B., Peters, P., Kaneko, K. *et al.* (1999). Cell biology of prions. In *Prion Biology and Diseases*. Ed. S.B. Prusiner. Cold Spring Harbor Laboratory Press, New York. pp. 349–391.

Taylor, D.M. (2000). Inactivation of transmissible degenerative encephalopathy agents: a review. *Veterinary Journal*, **159**, 1–7.

van Keulen, L.J.M., Schreuder, B.E.C., Vromans, M.E.W. *et al.* (1999). Pathogenesis of natural scrapie in sheep. In *Proceedings of Characterization and Diagnosis of Prion Diseases in Animals and Man*, Tubingen.

Wells, G.A.H., Scott, A.C., Johnson, C.T. *et al.* (1987). A novel progressive spongiform encephalopathy in cattle. *Veterinary Record*, **121**, 419–420.

Further reading

Chin, J. (2000). *Control of Communicable Diseases Manual*. Seventeenth Edition. American Public Health Association, Washington, D.C. pp. 183–186.

Prusiner, S.B. (1999). *Prion Biology and Diseases*. Ed. S.B. Prusiner. Cold Spring Harbor Laboratory Press, New York.

Prusiner, S.B. (1997). Prion diseases and the BSE crisis. *Science,* **278**, 245–251.

Prusiner, S.B. (2001). Shatuck lecture – neurodegenerative diseases and prions. *New England Journal of Medicine*, **344**, 1516–1526.

Raeber, A.J. and Aguzzi, A. (2000). Engulfment of prions in the germinal centre. *Immunology Today*, 21, 66–67.

Wilesmith, J.W. (1993). Epidemiology of bovine spongiform encephalopathy and related diseases. *Archives of Virology*, 7, 245–254.

Section VI

Microbial Agents and Disease Production

Viral infections which cause developmental anomalies

Viruses which cause developmental anomalies in the CNS of domestic animals are listed in Box 77.1. The susceptibility of the developing nervous tissues to the destructive effects of these viruses is closely related to the stage of gestation at the time of infection. Destruction of germinal cells by these viruses results in teratological defects such as cerebral cavitation and cerebellar hypoplasia. Teratological changes may follow intrauterine infection with pestiviruses such as classical swine fever virus, bovine virus diarrhoea virus and border disease virus. Hypomyelinogenesis, another developmental defect in lambs with Border disease, is attributed to delayed maturation of oligodendrocytes. Lambs with tremors typical of the condition can recover with careful management.

Box 77.1 Viruses with teratogenic effects on nervous tissues.

- Akabane virus
- Border disease virus
- Bovine herpesvirus 5
- Bovine virus diarrhoea virus
- Cache Valley virus
- Feline panleukopenia virus
- Swine fever virus

Transmissible spongiform encephalopathies (TSE)

Spongiform encephalopathies are so called because of the characteristic vacuolation of the neural parenchyma seen in affected animals. These neurodegenerative diseases have been described in a number of domestic and captive animal species (*see* Chapter 76). They have many features in common including the nature of the aetiological agent, transmissibility, and prolonged incubation periods and clinical courses.

It is widely accepted that the aetiological agents, prions, are structurally-modified forms of protein normally present on cell membranes. The structural change, initiated post-translationally in the normal protein through association with abnormal prion protein, results in accumulation of these abnormal molecules. In the abnormal protein, α-helices are largely replaced by β-sheets which resist enzymatic digestion. This conformational change allows polymerization, often demonstrable as amyloid plaques in the brain tissue of some affected species. Scrapie-associated fibrils containing the abnormal protein can be demonstrated in extracts of brain tissues from animals with spongiform encephalopathy and serve as markers of the disease.

There is strong experimental evidence in mice and sheep to support the view that, after ingestion and processing in regional lymph nodes, spread of the aetiological agent to the spinal cord is via the splanchnic nerves. Although there are differences in lesion distribution between the various spongiform encephalopathies, major vacuolar changes are found in the brain stem, particularly in the medulla, in all affected animals. In the later stages of the disease diffuse astrogliosis may be present. Clinical signs, though somewhat variable, usually relate to loss of motor control and to behavioural changes.

Algal, bacterial and fungal neurotoxicity

Diseases caused by bacterial agents which elaborate toxins affecting neurological function are listed in Table 77.6. In the clostridial diseases, botulism and tetanus, the toxins affect neuromuscular function. In botulism, following ingestion of preformed toxin, there is flaccid paralysis as a result of blocking of acetylcholine release at neuromuscular junctions. The tetanus toxin, elaborated by organisms in an infected wound, blocks inhibitory signals from the CNS with resultant muscular spasms. Morphological tissue changes are absent in botulism and tetanus.

Focal symmetrical encephalomalacia and oedema

Table 77.6 Neurological diseases produced by bacterial toxins.

Disease	Bacterium / method of exposure	Toxic effects	Species affected
Botulism	*Clostridium botulinum* / ingestion of preformed toxin — toxigenic form. Toxin produced in infected wound or intestine — toxicoinfectious form (rare)	Blocking of acetylcholine release at neuromuscular junctions	Many species
Focal symmetrical encephalomalacia	*Clostridium perfringens* type D / enterotoxaemia	Vasculopathy, encephalomalacia in midbrain and basal ganglia	Sheep (lambs), goats
Oedema disease (cerebrospinal angiopathy)	*Escherichia coli* (oedema strains) / enterotoxaemia	Vasculopathy, fibrinoid necrosis of arteriolar walls, encephalomalacia	Pigs
Tetanus	*Clostridium tetani* / toxin produced locally in infected tissue	Blocking of presynaptic transmission of inhibitory signals from neurons in CNS	Most species, especially horses and sheep

Table 77.7 Neurological diseases caused by algal and fungal toxins.

Disease	Microbial agent / method of exposure	Toxic effects	Species affected
Blue green algal toxicoses	Cyanobacteria / preformed toxins ingested with water	Mimics action of acetylcholine	Many species
Aspergillus clavatus toxicosis	*A. clavatus* / feed containing preformed toxins	Chromatolysis in neurons of brainstem, spinal ganglia and cord, Wallerian degeneration in cord	Cattle, sheep
Equine leukoencephalo-malacia	*Fusarium moniliforme* / corn-based feed containing preformed toxins	Vasculitis, perivascular oedema, malacia	Horses
Tremorgen intoxication			
Paspalum staggers	*Claviceps paspali* / ingestion of sclerotia on paspalum grasses	Interference with neuromuscular function causing tremors	Ruminants, horses
Penitrem staggers	*Penicillium cyclopium* and other *Penicillium* species / ingestion of contaminated pasture	Clinical effects similar to paspalum staggers	Cattle, sheep
Perennial ryegrass staggers	*Acremonium loliae* / ingestion of contaminated ryegrass stubble	Clinical effects similar to paspalum staggers	Ruminants, horses

disease, are caused by toxins elaborated in the intestinal tract by replicating *Clostridium perfringens* type D and certain strains of *Escherichia coli* respectively. These toxins usually produce acute disease with sudden or rapid death. Degenerative lesions relating to vascular damage develop in animals which survive the acute phase and there is progressive neurological disturbance.

Ingestion of preformed neurotoxin is the main method of exposure in toxicoses of algal and fungal origin (Table 77.7). Neurological signs may follow ingestion of fungal toxins in grasses of the *Paspalum* genus on which *Claviceps paspali* is growing. Similar neurological signs follow the ingestion of lolitrems in perennial rye grass contaminated with *Acremonium loliae* and feed or pasture contaminated by tremorgens produced by other fungi. Affected animals have fine head tremors at rest and may show incoordination, stiffness or muscular spasms if forced to move. Mortality is low and recovery occurs shortly after removal from affected pasture or withdrawal of contaminated feed. The clinical signs in equine leukoencephalomalacia are more severe and include depression, blindness, pharyngeal paralysis and staggering. Death follows within a few days.

> ### Box 77.2 Algal and fungal infections which may affect the nervous system.
>
> - Aspergillosis
> - Blastomycosis
> - Coccidioidomycosis
> - Cryptococcosis
> - Histoplasmosis
> - Protothecosis

Algal and fungal infections

Algal and fungal infections which may affect the nervous system are listed in Box 77.2. Although lesions produced by the fungi are generally located in the respiratory tract, infection of the CNS may occasionally occur. A defective immune response, immunosuppressive therapy or prolonged administration of antibiotics predispose to tissue invasion by fungi. Infection with the algal agent, *Prototheca zopfii*, may occasionally spread to the CNS from a primary site in the intestines.

Further reading

Barlow, R. (1983). Neurological disorders of cattle and sheep. *In Practice*, **5**, 77–84.

Barlow, R. (1989). Differential diagnosis of bovine neurological disorders. *In Practice*, **11**, 64–73.

Done, S. (1995). Diagnosis of central nervous system disorders in the pig. *In Practice*, **17**, 318–327.

Kitching, P. (1997). Notifiable viral diseases and spongiform encephalopathies of cattle, sheep and goats. *In Practice*, **19**, 51–63.

Luttgen, P.J. (1988). Inflammatory disease of the central nervous system. *Veterinary Clinics of North America: Small Animal Practice*, **18**, 623–640.

Pattison, I.H. (1988). Fifty years with scrapie: a personal reminiscence. *Veterinary Record*, **123**, 661–666.

Sargison, N. (1995). Scrapie in sheep and goats. *In Practice*, **17**, 467–469.

Scott, P.R. (1995). The collection and analysis of cerebrospinal fluid as an aid to diagnosis in ruminant neurological disease. *British Veterinary Journal*, **151**, 603–614.

Chapter 78

Interactions of microbial pathogens with the male and female reproductive systems

Microbial agents represent a relatively small proportion of the aetiological factors which can affect reproductive performance in domestic animals (Box 78.1). Protozoal diseases, such as ovine toxoplasmosis and bovine neosporosis can be a greater threat to foetal survival than bacterial, fungal or viral infections. When taken together, microbial and protozoal agents account for less than 30% of the diagnoses recorded in many surveys of abortion in farm animals. Chromosomal, hormonal, nutritional, toxic and physical factors may account for large numbers of unspecified embryonic and foetal deaths. Certain microbial infections are, nevertheless, important causes of reduced reproductive performance in many countries.

Male and female reproductive systems in domestic animal species are dependent on delicately balanced hormonal interactions for their development and for their functional integrity. In male animals, the clinical effects of microbial infections on reproductive performance relate largely to tissue destruction and associated anatomical alterations. In contrast, microbial infections of the female tract can disrupt the hormonal interactions which influence tissue and behavioural changes during oestrous cycles, and those which are essential for the maintenance of pregnancy.

Infection of the male reproductive system

Microbial infections of the male reproductive system in domestic animals may lead to the development of lesions which adversely affect fertility. In addition, venereal spread of infection by an infected male may have a serious impact on the reproductive performance of susceptible females. In some venereal infections, such as those involving bovine herpesvirus 1 (infectious pustular vulvo-vaginitis) and equine herpesvirus 3 (equine coital exanthema), lesions are usually confined to the mucosal surfaces of the penis, vulva and vagina. Other, more serious venereal infections may cause metritis or abortion.

Infections which produce inflammation of the penis and prepuce (balanoposthitis) are rarely of major clinical significance. Balanoposthitis caused by herpesvirus infections in bulls and stallions, can result in ulcerative lesions which may be extensive but resolve spontaneously within a few weeks. A diverse population of bacterial, fungal and protozoal species is present in the prepuce in many domestic animals. Some of these microorganisms are potentially pathogenic and, in a suitable micro-environment, selective overgrowth of a species can result in clinical disease. The development of ulcerative balanoposthitis due to the activity of *Corynebacterium renale* in wethers and rams on high protein diets is an example of the effect of this type of microenvironmental influence.

Primary testicular infections are usually haematogenous in origin, whereas those involving the epididymis generally originate in the urogenital tract. Infection, once established in the scrotal sac, may spread to involve both testis and epididymis. Inflammation of the testis (orchitis) and of the epididymis (epididymitis) are often concurrent. Among the bacterial pathogens which affect the male reproductive system, *Brucella* species have a particular predilection for testicular and epididymal tissues in the bull, boar, ram and dog. In bulls, infection with *B. abortus* produces an acute orchitis leading to tissue necrosis. In rams, infection with *B. melitensis* also results in orchitis, whereas epididymitis is the main effect of infection with *B. ovis*. The epididymis is also the primary target of *Actinobacillus seminis* and 'Haemophilus somnus' infections in rams. Multifocal suppurative orchitis in boars, caused by *B. suis*, is often accompanied by lesions in the epididymis. Concurrent orchitis and epididymitis are present also in *B. canis* infection in dogs. In addition to *Brucella* species other bacterial agents which produce

---

Box 78.1 Factors which may adversely affect reproductive performance in domestic animals.

- Microbial agents
  — Bacteria
  — Fungi
  — Viruses
- Parasitic agents
  — Protozoa
- Anatomical defects
- Genetic factors and developmental defects
- Hormonal imbalance, constitutive or induced
- Nutritional deficiencies
- Physical injury
- Toxic agents including mycotoxins

orchitis and epididymitis in bulls include *Escherichia coli, Haemophilus* species and *Salmonella* serotypes. *Burkholderia mallei* can produce testicular lesions in boars and dogs, and *Arcanobacterium pyogenes* is an important cause of orchitis in bulls, boars and rams. Lesions involving testicular tissues of stallions have been described in glanders and in infections with *Salmonella* Abortus-equi. Viral infections in stallions in which orchitis may be a feature include equine viral arteritis and equine infectious anaemia. Orchitis and epididymitis have been reported in canine distemper virus infection in dogs.

In bulls, microbial infections caused by *Arcanobacterium pyogenes*, staphylococci, streptococci and *Brucella abortus* often result in seminal vesiculitis. The seminal vesicles of the bull are also considered to be a major site for the localization of *Leptospira interrogans* serovar *hardjo*. In the dog, urinary pathogens such as *E. coli* and *Proteus* species can invade the prostate as part of an ascending infection through the urethra.

Infection of the non-pregnant uterus

Although the non-pregnant uterus is relatively resistant to infection, susceptibility to pathogens varies during the oestrous cycle. In early oestrus, uterine motility increases under the influence of oestrogens, contributing to mechanical expulsion of potential pathogens. In addition, neutrophils in the uterine lumen appear to be particularly active during this phase of the cycle. The uterus becomes more vulnerable to infection in dioestrus when progesterone secretion from the corpus luteum (CL) increases. During this phase, the phagocytic activity of neutrophils in the uterine lumen is reduced and immunosuppressive products are secreted into the lumen. Moreover, experimental studies have demonstrated an increased susceptibility of the progesterone-stimulated endometrium to opportunistic pathogens.

Many of the microbial agents which invade the non-pregnant uterus can be transmitted by venereal contact (Box 78.2). The outcome of postcoital infection, even if caused by agents specifically capable of inducing uterine disease, is usually a mild short-lived endometritis. Opportunistic pathogens, such as *A. pyogenes*, *E. coli* and streptococci, are transient inhabitants of the vagina in many species and are often associated with postcoital endometritis. The mare appears to be particularly susceptible to postcoital endometritis because the marked relaxation of the cervix during oestrus facilitates the introduction of opportunistic pathogens from the vulva, the vagina or the external genitalia of the stallion.

The uterus and uterine tubes are especially vulnerable to infection immediately following parturition. Retention of the placenta and trauma resulting from difficult parturitions are important factors contributing to the development of post-partum metritis and salpingitis. Abortion, both infectious and non-infectious, is often followed by

Box 78.2 Microbial pathogens which can be transmitted by venereal contact.

- **Cattle**
  — Bovine herpesvirus 1
  — *Brucella abortus* (rare)
  — *Campylobacter fetus* subsp. *venerealis*
  — *Chlamydophila abortus*
  — *Leptospira interrogans* serovars
  — *Mycoplasma bovigenitalium*
  — *Ureaplasma diversum*
- **Horses**
  — Equine herpesvirus 3
  — Equine viral arteritis virus
  — *Klebsiella pneumoniae*
  — *Pseudomonas aeruginosa*
  — *Taylorella equigenitalis*
- **Sheep**
  — *Brucella ovis*
  — *Brucella melitensis* (rare)
  — *Chlamydophila abortus*
- **Pigs**
  — *Brucella suis*
  — Porcine reproductive and respiratory virus
  — Porcine herpesvirus 1
  — Porcine parvovirus
- **Dogs**
  — *Brucella canis*
  — Canine herpesvirus 1

retention of the placenta and delayed uterine involution which allow access for opportunistic pathogens through the cervix. Post-partum metritis can follow infection with a wide range of bacteria, some of which may also be responsible for placentitis and abortion (Box 78.3). These infections, which may be mixed, often resolve spontaneously. However, when severe, infection can result in death from toxaemia. Moreover, a chronic metritis may develop, characterized by persistent inflammatory exudation into the uterine lumen.

Pyometra

In cattle, post-partum bacterial metritis can progress to pyometra, the accumulation of pus in the uterus. In this condition the diseased endometrium produces insufficient prostaglandin $F_{2\alpha}$ (PGF$_{2\alpha}$), a luteolytic factor normally responsible for regression of the CL. The persistent CL continues to secrete progesterone which stimulates hyperplasia of the endometrium and increases its susceptibility to infection. In addition, myometrial activity is inhibited, the cervix remains closed and pus and uterine secretions accumulate.

The sequence of events leading to pyometra in domestic carnivores is somewhat different. Canine pyometra usually occurs in unbred, mature bitches. The disease

Table 78.2 Microbial agents implicated in ovine abortion.

Agent	Comments
Bacillus licheniformis	Placentitis. Oral infection from poor-quality silage or mouldy hay, bedding or feed
Border disease virus	Effects, ranging from embryonic and foetal death to congenital defects and weak newborn lambs, relate to gestational age when infected. Intrauterine growth retardation. Placentitis
Brucella melitensis	Abortion may be the only evidence of infection. Uterine discharges heavily contaminated. Successive abortions may occur in infected ewes
Brucella ovis	Venereal transmission important. Sporadic abortion. Intercotyledonary tissue thickened and oedematous. Mummification or autolysis of foetus. Epididymitis in affected rams
Campylobacter fetus subsp. *fetus* *Campylobacter jejuni*	Faecal-oral transmission. Localisation in pregnant uterus from bacteraemia. Abortion late in gestation. Placentitis and mild enteritis. Umbilicated, pale, necrotic lesions in some foetal livers
Chlamydophila abortus	Enzootic abortion of ewes. Abortion commonly in last month of gestation. Placentitis. Thickening and oedema in intercotyledonary tissue. Foetal livers may be swollen with pinpoint necrotic lesions
Coxiella burnetii	Rare abortion late in gestation. Diffuse placentitis. Persistent infection. Shedding of organisms in milk
Listeria monocytogenes	Infection *per os*. Silage often the source. Abortion usually sporadic. Placentitis. Multifocal hepatitis in foetus. Abortion late in gestation may be followed by metritis and septicaemia
Salmonella serotypes	Some *Salmonella* serotypes cause abortion with minor clinical disturbance in the dam. Those due to *Salmonella* Dublin and *Salmonella* Typhimurium can produce systemic signs and abortion. Abortion occurs late in gestation

hepatic necrosis is present in infected foetuses.

Abortion caused by *Listeria monocytogenes* appears to be dependent on the ingestion of large numbers of organisms and, in cattle and sheep, is commonly associated with the feeding of poor quality silage which can contain large numbers of these bacteria. Placentitis and foetal infection are recorded in both species, and abortion occurs in the last third of gestation. Infection and retention of a dead foetus close to term can result in dystocia, with subsequent septicaemia or metritis in the dam. Aborted lambs occasionally have numerous small, pale areas of microabscessation throughout the liver.

Abortion associated with *Bacillus licheniformis* is an emerging problem in cows and ewes in Scotland, the north of England and Ireland. The infection is associated with feeding of poor quality silage and mouldy hay. The thickened, leathery appearance of the placenta resembles that observed in mycotic abortion.

Bovine brucellosis, caused by *Brucella abortus*, is the most extensively studied reproductive disease in cattle. The disease is recorded in most parts of the world and, in regions where control measures are ineffective, is usually endemic. Reproductive performance in affected herds is severely impaired, and there is the possibility of zoonotic transfer to the human population. Sexually-immature cattle are relatively refractory to infection. In susceptible mature animals, especially females, infection may persist in lymph nodes and other tissues for prolonged periods, producing no clinical disturbance. Because *B. abortus* has a predilection for endometrial and placental tissues, spread of the organism and replication in these tissues occurs during pregnancy. Abortion, the main clinical manifestation of the infection, usually occurs during the seventh or eighth month of gestation. There may be extensive necrotic lesions in cotyledons with oedema of intercotyledonary areas. Organisms can be demonstrated in smears from affected cotyledons and can be cultured from uterine fluids, cotyledons and the abomasal contents of aborted calves.

Of the microbial pathogens capable of causing abortion in sows, viruses are particularly significant (Table 78.3). Viral infections spread readily under intensive husbandry conditions operating in breeding herds and often result in serious economic loss from reproductive failure. The spectrum of clinical presentations has already been mentioned. The SMEDI syndrome of stillbirths, mummification, embryonic death and infertility is a major indicator of viral infection in affected herds. Latency or subclinical infection may allow viral persistence in a herd.

Microbial causes of equine abortion are listed in Table 78.4. Equine herpesvirus 1 (EHV-1) is important worldwide as a cause of abortion, sometimes resulting in abortion storms. A related virus, equine herpesvirus 4 which is mainly responsible for rhinopneumonitis, has also been isolated from aborted foals. Abortions due to EHV-1 usually occur after 7 months of gestation. Multifocal pinpoint necrotic lesions may be evident in the livers of aborted foals. Latent carriers may act as reservoirs of infection.

Brucella canis causes abortion in bitches and is the only

Table 78.3 Microbial pathogens implicated in porcine abortion.

Agent	Comments
Brucella suis	Mainly venereal transmission. Foci of infection in male and female genitalia, in joints and in bones. Chronic metritis with multiple granulomatous nodules in mucosa. Abortion in second half of pregnancy. Stillborn and weak piglets
Classical swine fever virus (Porcine pestivirus)	Stillbirths, mummification, embryonic death and infertility (SMEDI) syndrome in affected breeding herds. Foetal growth retardation. Congenital defects in central nervous system. Vaccine strains can produce congenital defects
Encephalomyocarditis virus	One of the main causes of SMEDI syndrome in the USA. Myocarditis in young pigs
Leptospira species (particularly serovars *pomona*, *tarassovi* and *bratislava*)	Abortions late in gestation may be the only indication of infection in a herd. Subclinical infections. Bacteria infect uterus and foetus during leptospiraemia. Stillbirths, mummification, autolysis and weak newborn piglets
Porcine enteroviruses 2–11	First viruses to be associated with SMEDI syndrome, but role in abortion probably minor
Porcine herpesvirus 1 (Aujeszky's disease virus)	Abortion secondary to fever and systemic disease. Some strains invade placenta and foetus. Multifocal necrosis of placenta and foetal organs. SMEDI syndrome in affected breeding herds
Porcine herpesvirus 2 (cytomegalovirus)	Subclinical infections in sows. Foetal death and mummification. Necrotizing rhinitis in neonates
Porcine parvovirus	Oral and veneral transmission. SMEDI syndrome in susceptible sows introduced into infected herds. Virus invades rapidly-dividing cells in foetus
Porcine respiratory and reproductive virus (porcine arterivirus)	First described in 1987. Pneumonia and reproductive wastage. SMEDI syndrome in affected breeding herds

microbial pathogen which primarily affects the male and female canine reproductive systems.

Abortions may occur incidentally during many generalized bacterial and viral infections as a consequence of the direct effects of viraemia, septicaemia or toxaemia on maternal and foetal tissues and, indirectly, on the hormonal regulation of pregnancy. Those microorganisms which may induce abortion during generalized infections are listed in Table 78.5.

Table 78.4 Microbial pathogens implicated in equine abortion.

Agent	Comments
Equine herpesvirus 1 (EHV1)	EHV 1 most common cause of equine abortion, EHV 4 causing sporadic cases. Abortion after 8 months of gestation. Foetus usually fresh, indicating recent death. Multifocal hepatitis, icterus and pulmonary oedema in foetus
Equine viral arteritis virus (equine arterivirus)	Over half infected mares abort or have stillborn offspring. Autolysis and excess pleural and peritoneal fluid in foetus
Leptospira interrogans serovars	Abortion is often a sequel to acute leptospirosis. Large multinucleate hepatocytes in foetal livers
Taylorella equigenitalis	Implicated in abortion at about 7 months gestation

Table 78.5 Infectious agents which induce abortion in association with systemic disease.

Infectious agents	Hosts
Bacteria	
Coxiella burnetii	Sheep, goats
Ehrlichia phagocytophila	Sheep, cattle
Erysipelothrix rhusiopathiae	Pigs
Streptococcus suis type 2	Pigs
Viruses	
African swine fever virus	Pigs
Akabane virus	Cattle, sheep
Bluetongue virus	Sheep, cattle
Canine herpesvirus 1	Dogs
Ephemeral fever virus	Cattle
Nairobi sheep disease virus	Sheep, goats
Rift Valley fever virus	Sheep, cattle
Wesselsbron disease virus	Sheep, cattle

Further reading

Barr, B.C. and Anderson, M.L. (1993). Infectious diseases causing bovine abortion and foetal loss. *Veterinary Clinics of*

North America: Food Animal Practice **9**, 343–368.

Buergelt, C.D. (1997). *Colour Atlas of Reproductive Pathology of Domestic Animals.* Mosby-Year Book Inc., St. Louis.

Caffrey, J.F., Dudgeon, A.M., Donnelly, W.J.C., Sheahan, B.J. and Atkins, G.J. (1997). Morphometric analysis of growth retardation in foetal lambs following experimental infection of pregnant ewes with border disease virus. *Research in Veterinary Science,* **62**, 245-248.

Carson, R.L., Wolfe, D.F., Klesius, P.H., Kemppainen, R.J. and Scanlan, C.M., (1988). The effects of ovarian hormones and ACTH on uterine defense to *Corynebacterium pyogenes* in cows. *Theriogenology* **30**, 91–97.

Ellis, W.A. (1994). Leptospirosis as a cause of reproductive failure. *Veterinary Clinics of North America: Food Animal Practice* **10**, 463–478.

Goyal, S.M. (1993). Porcine reproductive and respiratory syndrome. Review article. *Journal of Veterinary Diagnostic Investigation* **5**, 656–664.

Kirkbride, C.A (1992). Viral agents and associated lesions detected in a 10-year study of bovine abortions and stillbirths. *Journal of Veterinary Diagnostic Investigation* **4**, 374–379.

Kirkbride, C.A. (1993). Bacterial agents detected in a 10-year study of bovine abortions and stillbirths. *Journal of Veterinary Diagnostic Investigation* **5**, 64–68.

Lander Chacin, M.F., Hansen, P.J. and Drost. M. (1990). Effects of the stage of the estrous cycle and steroid treatment on uterine immunoglobulin content and polymorphonuclear leukocytes in cattle. *Theriogenology* **34**, 1169–1184.

Potter, K, Hancock, D.H. and Gallina, A.M. (1991). Clinical and pathological features of endometrial hyperplasia, pyometra and endometritis in cats. *Journal of the American Veterinary Medical Association* **198**, 1427–1431.

Chapter 79

The role of microbial pathogens in intestinal disease

The digestive system is constantly bombarded by organisms derived from environmental sources. In the anterior part of the tract, members of all of the major groups of microorganisms are capable of colonizing the oral and pharyngeal mucosae and, in some instances, can produce defined clinical conditions. Some of these conditions, such as canine oral papillomatosis, are caused by particular infectious agents; others like acute necrotizing ulcerative gingivitis are associated with overgrowth of some members of the resident microbial flora, often as a result of immunosuppression. Other parts of the upper digestive system are less susceptible to microbial colonization. The stratified squamous epithelium of the oesophageal mucosa and the acidity of the secretion from gastric mucosal glands, along with the layer of mucus covering both oesophageal and gastric or abomasal mucosae, are inimical to microbial colonization. In contrast, the environment of the intestinal tract is particularly suitable for microbial colonization. Moreover, many enteric organisms have evolved superficial structures which allow attachment to the surface of enterocytes.

Intestinal structure and function

The intestinal tract is the portion of the digestive system which is largely responsible for digestion of food and for absorption of nutrients, water and electrolytes. Although there are considerable species differences in the length and anatomical positioning of the tract, its general structure and function are similar in all domestic animals. The two main parts of the tract, the small and large intestines, differ functionally with regard to digestion and absorption; These functional differences are reflected in structural differences in their mucosal surfaces. In the small intestine, where most digestion and absorption of organic compounds takes place, the mucosal surface area is greatly increased by folds, villi and microvilli of the lining enterocytes. In the large intestine, mucosal folding is less prominent, villi are absent and microvilli are less numerous. In carnivores, the functions of the large intestine are mainly confined to the absorption of water and electrolytes. In herbivores, the metabolic activities of members of the normal microbial flora of the caecum and colon produce nutrients which are absorbed along with the water and electrolytes. Goblet cells, which are present in the

mucosal epithelium throughout the intestine, are particularly numerous in the large intestine where mucus secretion is important for faecal lubrication. In all species, after a storage period of 24 to 36 hours, the solid or semi-solid contents of the rectum are expelled as faeces.

The integrity of the mucosal epithelium is maintained by replication of undifferentiated cells in the glandular crypts. The immature enterocytes differentiate as they migrate onto mucosal surfaces, replacing effete epithelial cells which are constantly shed from the tips of villi in the small intestine and from the surface of the large intestine.

In addition to participation in the digestion and absorption of nutrients, enterocytes have an important role in controlling water and electrolyte transfer between the intestinal lumen and the lamina propria. The end result of this activity is the absorption of water from the lumen and the production of formed faecal material. Disturbance of the mechanisms involved in this process is a major factor in diseases produced by some enteropathogenic microorganisms.

In the small intestine, absorption of sodium and chloride ions and non-electrolytes, such as glucose and amino acids, occurs mainly by transcellular transport. Ionic balance in the cells is maintained by loss of intracellular hydrogen and bicarbonate ions. Transfer of water from the intestinal lumen into intercellular spaces occurs through the tight junctions between enterocytes. This paracellular transport is induced by an osmotic gradient between intestinal contents and the fluid in the intercellular space. The gradient is produced by energy-dependent transfer of sodium ions into the space through the basolateral parts of enterocyte plasma membranes. Because tight junctions in the small intestine are relatively permeable, especially in the duodenum and jejunum, backflow occurs. The overall balance is in favour of absorption with diffusion into the capillaries of the lamina propria. Because the tight junctions in the large intestine are more impermeable than those in the small intestine, a high osmotic pressure is maintained in intercellular spaces and in the lamina propria, contributing to water absorption. Moreover, absorption of volatile fatty acids in the colon results in further water absorption.

Solute movement across enterocyte plasma membranes is controlled by peptide hormones acting through the intracellular secondary messengers adenyl cyclase and guanyl cyclase. Activation of these enzymes produces increased cellular levels of cyclic AMP and cyclic GMP, which depress sodium absorption and promote chloride secretion by crypt cells.

Normal flora

The intestinal tract is bacteriologically sterile at birth. Within hours, the tract is colonized by a range of bacteria including *Lactobacillus* species, *Escherichia coli* and strict anaerobes such as *Clostridium* species, *Peptostreptococcus* species and *Fusobacterium necrophorum*. Because the ingesta in the anterior small intestine tends to retain the acidity derived from the secretion of gastric acid, these bacterial populations usually establish in the terminal part of the small intestine and in the large intestine where they persist throughout the life of the host. In ruminants, the resident microflora of the rumen, caecum and colon, which includes yeasts and protozoa along with bacteria, is responsible for the degradation of cellulose and for metabolic processes involving other carbohydrates and nitrogenous compounds. Similar digestive functions are performed by the normal microflora of the caecum and colon in monogastric herbivores, thereby contributing to their nutritional requirements.

Following establishment of a resident microflora, antigenic stimulation promotes expansion of the gut-associated lymphoid tissue (GALT), allowing local production of immunoglobulins, an important factor in preventing colonization by pathogenic microorganisms. Components of GALT include intraepithelial lymphocytes and Peyer's patches, localized aggregates of lymphocytes and plasma cells in the mucosa and submucosa of the small intestine. The epithelial cells (M cells) covering Peyer's patches are actively pinocytotic and appear to be able to sample, process and present antigen to the underlying lymphocytes. The immunoglobulins produced by GALT are predominantly IgA. They are secreted onto the surface of the intestinal epithelium where they protect against pathogen adhesion to enterocytes.

Short chain fatty acids produced by certain members of the resident flora inhibit growth of exogenous bacteria. Moreover, competition between bacterial species for energy-producing nutrients and for receptors on enterocytes influences the composition of the intestinal microbial population.

Pathogenetic mechanisms in enteritis

The specific intestinal niches occupied by the various resident bacteria are determined by the affinity of surface structures on the microorganisms for specific receptors on the enterocytes. Changes in the normal microflora may allow access of pathogenic microorganisms to epithelial cell receptors leading to the establishment of infection. Factors which contribute to changes in the normal

---

Box 79.1 Some microbial pathogens associated with intestinal disease in cattle.

- *Escherichia coli*
- *Salmonella* serotypes
- *Mycobacterium avium* subsp. *paratuberculosis*
- *Clostridium perfringens* types B and C
- Rotavirus
- Bovine coronavirus
- Bovine viral diarrhoea virus
- Rinderpest virus

---

microflora include antimicrobial drug therapy and stress related to changes in feeding or management practices. Moreover, animals are particularly susceptible to infection with pathogenic microorganisms during the neonatal period before the resident microflora becomes fully established. The significant pathogenic microorganisms associated with intestinal disease in large animals are listed in Boxes 79.1 to 79.4.

Pathogenic microorganisms utilize a number of mechanisms to produce the metabolic and structural changes in the intestinal epithelium which lead to diarrhoea and to dysentery. Because of the complex microenvironment in the intestine and the possibility of synergism between pathogens, categorization of the functional and structural changes produced by individual pathogens is not always possible. Nevertheless, certain pathological alterations, including hypersecretion, villous atrophy, mucosal distortion and necrosis, may result from infection with particular enteric pathogens.

Hypersecretion

Functional disturbance of intestinal epithelial cells is exemplified by infection with enterotoxigenic strains of *E. coli*, a common aetiological agent of diarrhoea in neonatal calves, pigs and lambs. The toxic mechanisms involved in this type of enteric infection are detailed in Chapter 18. These enterotoxigenic strains of *E. coli* possess fimbrial adhesins which allow attachment to enterocytes in the small intestine. The hypersecretion induced by the enterotoxins relates to the activation of adenylate cyclase or guanylate cyclase in enterocytes. Hypersecretory diarrhoea results from a combination of increased chloride and water secretion and inhibition of

---

Box 79.2 Some microbial pathogens associated with intestinal disease in sheep and goats.

- *Escherichia coli*
- *Clostridium perfringens* types B and C
- *Salmonella* serotypes
- Rotavirus
- Peste des petits ruminants virus

Box 79.3 Some microbial pathogens associated with intestinal disease in pigs.

- *Escherichia coli*
- *Clostridium perfringens* types A and C
- *Brachyspira hyodysenteriae*
- *Lawsonia intracellularis*
- *Salmonella* serotypes
- Rotavirus
- Transmissible gastroenteritis virus
- Porcine epidemic diarrhoea virus
- Classical swine fever virus
- African swine fever virus

---

sodium and water absorption. The excess fluid entering the large intestine overloads its absorptive capacity. Morphological and inflammatory changes in the mucosa of the small intestine are absent or negligible.

Villous atrophy

Destruction of the epithelial cells on the surface of villi or in the crypts of the small intestine results in changes in the size and shape of the villi and enterocytes. The villi, which become stunted and often fuse, are covered by cuboidal epithelium. This villous atrophy is encountered in the terminal small intestine during some infections with bacteria such as attaching-effacing *E. coli*. However, it is most commonly encountered in enteric viral infections. The degree of epithelial damage and subsequent villous change ranges from the relatively mild alterations encountered in rotavirus infections of neonatal farm animals to the marked structural disruption produced by infection with canine parvovirus type 2. These differences relate not only to viral virulence but also to the cells targeted by the particular virus. In rotavirus infections, the mature epithelial cells near the tips of villi are affected. Replacement cells, produced from the pool of undifferentiated replicating cells in the crypts of Lieberkühn, may be immature and cuboidal. In uncomplicated infections, epithelial replacement with clinical recovery may occur within a few days. Nevertheless, interference with digestive and absorptive processes, due to stunting of villi

---

Box 79.4 Some microbial pathogens associated with intestinal disease in horses.

- *Salmonella* serotypes
- *Clostridium perfringens* types A and C
- *Clostridium difficile*
- *Ehrlichia risticii*
- *Rhodococcus equi*
- *Actinobacillus equuli*
- *Escherichia coli* (role unclear)
- Rotavirus

---

and incomplete differention of replacement epithelial cells, can result in fluid overload of the colon with consequent diarrhoea. The coronavirus of pigs, transmissible gastroenteritis virus, also targets enterocytes on villi. However, villous damage is much more extensive than that encountered in rotavirus infections and may be permanent. In affected newborn piglets, severe diarrhoea may result in rapid dehydration and high mortality.

Canine parvovirus type 2 targets actively dividing cells. In enteric infection, the virus invades and destroys the progenitor cells in the crypts of Lieberkühn interfering with the mechanism for replacement of villous epithelium and leading to widespread villous atrophy in the jejunum and ileum. Dilation and collapse of glandular structures may produce irreparable mucosal damage. If stem cells survive, restoration of the mucosa occurs. Because rapidly dividing cells in the germinal centres of lymphoid tissues including GALT are also targeted by the virus, secondary bacterial infection often exacerbates the condition.

Infiltrative and proliferative distortion of the mucosa

Paratuberculosis (Johne's disease), a chronic, progressive, cell-mediated immunoinflammatory disease of adult ruminants, is caused by *Mycobacterium avium* subspecies *paratuberculosis*. The condition is characterized by the recruitment of large numbers of macrophages and T lymphocytes into the lamina propria and the submucosa mainly in the terminal part of the ileum and large intestine. The large numbers of infiltrating cells produce crypt compression and villous distortion and atrophy. As a result, the absorptive surface area in the ileum is markedly reduced and there is interference with fluid resorption in the large intestine. Lymphatic drainage from the intestinal wall may be partially impeded by granulomatous lymphadenitis and lymphangitis which are constant features of the disease. Lymphatic blockage may be a contributory factor to the protein loss, which occurs in bovine paratuberculosis. Increased permeability of vascular endothelium and of the tight junctions between enterocytes may heighten protein loss. Moreover, loss of plasma albumin into the intestine and the consequent hypoalbuminaemia can result in further loss of fluid from the circulation. The protein-losing enteropathy of paratuberculosis accounts in part for the fact that affected animals become emaciated while usually retaining their appetite.

The effects of proliferative mucosal changes are evident in the intestinal adenomatosis complex in growing pigs. The various clinicopathological syndromes within this complex are considered to be caused by a campylobacter-like organism, *Lawsonia intracellularis*. As its name implies, this organism is present and replicates in the cytoplasm of enterocytes in the crypts, especially in the ileum. Mitosis of infected enterocytes results in glandular hyperplasia and the production of a population of enterocytes which remain undifferentiated. These

to the effects of deleterious environmental and other stress factors (Box 80.2). Cold air temperatures, uraemia or dehydration can affect mucociliary function by reducing ciliary activity, slowing the rate of clearance of foreign material. The rate is slower also in hot dry atmospheric conditions as a result of fluid evaporation from the mucus component of the clearance mechanism. Immunodeficient animals are particularly prone to pulmonary infection, an indication of the importance of local immunity as a pulmonary defence mechanism. Moreover, immunosuppression may increase susceptibility to pulmonary infection which often involves both viral and bacterial pathogens. Bacterial species commonly implicated in mixed pulmonary infections in young animals are indicated in Box 80.3.

Box 80.2   Factors predisposing to the development of pneumonia in calves.

- Close confinement at markets or shows
- Transportation and other stress factors
- Poorly ventilated and overcrowded housing conditions
- Decline of maternally-derived antibody levels
- Intercurrent infections

Patterns of pulmonary inflammation

The significant pneumonic conditions affecting large animals are presented in Tables 80.1 to 80.4. Two main patterns of pneumonia, namely bronchopneumonia and interstitial (proliferative) pneumonia, are recognized.

Bronchopneumonia

Usually aerogenous in origin, bronchopneumonia is commonly caused by bacterial infection. Predisposing factors, including viral or mycoplasmal infection of the respiratory tract and environmental stress, can interfere with respiratory clearance mechanisms and with immune competence. These are almost always involved in the pathogenesis of the condition. Lesions, characteristically located in the anteroventral regions of the lungs, consist of irregular areas of consolidation. Affected regions of lung, which are reddened and swollen during the acute inflammatory phase of the pneumonia, collapse as it resolves. Inflammatory lesions develop initially at the

---

Box 80.3   Bacteria commonly implicated in mixed respiratory infections in young animals.

- *Escherichia coli*
- *Streptococcus* species
- *Actinobacillus* species
- *Pasteurella multocida*
- *Bordetella bronchiseptica*

Table 80.1   Important pathogens associated with pneumonia in cattle.

Pathogen	Comments
Mannheimia haemolytica type A1	Associated with acute fibrinonecrotic bronchopneumonia. Often affects beef and store cattle after transportation in overcrowded conditions. It is also encountered in housed calves. May exacerbate viral pneumonia
'Haemophilus somnus'	Produces pulmonary lesions similar to those caused by infection with *Mannheimia haemolytica*
Pasteurella multocida	Occasionally isolated from lesions of acute fibrinonecrotic bronchopneumonia in adult cattle
Mycobacterium bovis	Causes chronic granulomatous lesions in lungs. In advanced lesions, caseation relates to cell-mediated hypersensitivity
Mycoplasma mycoides subsp. *mycoides* (small colony type)	Causes contagious bovine pleuropneumonia, an acute fibrinonecrotic pneumonia with serofibrinous exudation in alveoli and in thickened interlobular septa. The disease is notifiable in most countries
Mycoplasma bovis	Associated with the enzootic pneumonia complex in calves. Peribronchiolar and perivascular lymphoid hyperplasia is prominent in affected lungs
Mycoplasma dispar	Associated with enzootic pneumonia complex in calves. May cause low grade bronchiolitis
Parainfluenza virus 3	Associated with enzootic pneumonia complex in calves. Consolidation of ventral portions of cranial and middle lobes of lungs. Perivascular and peribronchiolar lymphoid cuffs. Eosinophilic intracytoplasmic inclusion bodies in bronchiolar epithelial cells
Bovine respiratory syncytial virus	Associated with enzootic pneumonia complex in calves. Syncytial giant cells, present in bronchioles and alveoli, may contain intracytoplasmic inclusions
Bovine herpesvirus 1	Causes infectious bovine rhinotracheitis, mainly affecting upper respiratory tract. Direct effect of virus on pulmonary tissues not clearly shown. Severe infections result in secondary bacterial pneumonia in calves
Bovine viral diarrhoea virus	May predispose to bacterial pneumonia by causing immunosuppression

bronchiolar-alveolar junction, a location where inhaled bacteria and aerosol droplet nuclei are often deposited. Neutrophil infiltration and serofibrinous exudation extend from the original nidus to surrounding alveoli and bronchioles within affected lobules. The outcome of bronchopneumonia depends on the virulence of the causal

Table 80.2 Microbial pathogens associated with pneumonia in sheep and goats.

Pathogen	Comments
Mannheimia haemolytica	Causes acute fibrinonecrotic pneumonia and pleurisy in lambs. Stress factors predispose to the development of the disease. Parainfluenza 3 virus and *Mycoplasma ovipneumoniae* may be implicated in lesion development
Mycoplasma capricolum subsp. *capripneumoniae* *Mycoplasma mycoides* subsp. *mycoides* (large colony type) *Mycoplasma mycoides* subsp. *capri*	*M. capricolum* subsp. *capripneumoniae* causes classical contagious caprine pleuropneumonia. Subspecies of *M. mycoides* cause pleuropneumonia. Lung lesions include serofibrinous bronchopneumonia with thickening of interlobular septa due to inflammatory exudate
Maedi/visna virus	A lentivirus (retrovirus) which causes maedi (ovine progressive pneumonia, zwoegerziekte), a chronic interstitial pneumonia of adult sheep. Affected lungs are grossly enlarged and weigh considerably more than normal lungs. Thickening of alveolar walls and marked lymphoproliferative changes around vessels and bronchioles occur
Caprine arthritis-encephalitis virus	A lentivirus closely related to maedi/visna virus. Chronic interstitial pneumonia with alveolar epithelialization and intra-alveolar exudation of proteinaceous fluid
Pulmonary adenomatosis virus	A retrovirus which causes jaagsiekte, a chronic proliferative pneumonia of sheep. The proliferative epithelial tissue, which occurs as multiple foci of columnar or cuboidal cells lining alveoli, has the characteristics of a low grade carcinoma; foci of these cells are occasionally present in the regional lymph nodes. There is marked fluid accumulation in the lungs

agent and on the severity and extent of the inflammatory reaction. When alveolar basement membranes remain intact and inflammatory exudates are cleared rapidly, complete restoration of structure and function can occur. More often, because of the extent of the original lesion, chronic suppuration and fibrosis develop. If pyogenic organisms such as *Arcanobacterium pyogenes* and *Rhodococcus equi* persist and proliferate in lesions, abscesses form. Clinical signs of respiratory involvement may be minimal in chronic bronchopneumonia, although there may be considerable economic loss due to poor productivity in affected herds and flocks. An acute

fibrinonecrotic form of pneumonia occurs in which the bronchopneumonic pattern of lesion development is not readily detected. The inflammatory reaction spreads rapidly through pulmonary tissues often involving entire lobes. Pneumonias of this type are caused by infection with virulent strains of *Mannheimia haemolytica* in ruminants, *Actinobacillus pleuropneumoniae* in pigs and *Pasteurella multocida* in a number of domestic animal species. Affected pulmonary tissue is swollen and dark red and exudes blood-stained fluid from cut surfaces, on which irregular pale areas of necrosis may be detected. The interlobular septa may be distended with serofibrinous exudate and fibrinous deposits are usually present on the overlying pleura. Septicaemia or toxaemia frequently develops and some animals may die suddenly.

Interstitial pneumonia

In contrast to the tissue reactions in bronchopneumonia, the exudative, infiltrative and proliferative reactions associated with interstitial pneumonia primarily involve

Table 80.3 Microbial pathogens associated with pneumonia in pigs.

Pathogen	Comments
Pasteurella multocida	Often involved as secondary invader in enzootic pneumonia of pigs caused by *Mycoplasma hyopneumoniae*. Produces acute fibrinous pneumonia
Actinobacillus pleuropneumoniae	Causes porcine contagious pleuropneumonia usually in young pigs. Haemorrhagic consolidation of dorsocaudal areas of lungs close to hilus. Necrotic foci in areas of consolidation
Mycoplasma hyopneumoniae	Causes porcine enzootic pneumonia, a non-fatal disease of young pigs. Secondary bacterial infections may cause death. Cranioventral pulmonary consolidation. Peribronchial and perivascular lymphoid accumulations and macrophage infiltration in alveolar lumen are prominent microscopic features
Influenzavirus A	Classical swine influenza is caused by subtype H_1N_1. All swine influenza virus subtypes are potentially zoonotic. Cranioventral consolidation. Secondary bacterial infections often associated with fatalities
Porcine herpesvirus 1	Causes Aujeszky's disease. Some strains associated with pneumonic lesions
Porcine respiratory and reproductive syndrome virus	This arterivirus has an affinity for pulmonary macrophages. Causes pneumonia in neonatal piglets. Predisposes to infection with *Streptococcus suis*, *Haemophilus suis* and porcine respiratory coronavirus

Table 80.4 Microbial pathogens associated with pneumonia in horses.

Pathogen	Comments
Rhodococcus equi	Causes suppurative bronchopneumonia in foals less than 6 months old
Burkholderia mallei	Causes glanders, an important zoonosis. Pyogranulomatous nodules develop in the lungs of chronically affected animals
Streptococcus equi subsp. *equi*	Causes strangles, an upper respiratory tract infection. Systemic dissemination occurs in bastard strangles; abscessation develops in the lungs and other internal organs
Equine herpesvirus 1 and 4	Cause pneumonia in neonatal and young foals. EHV-4 usually affects foals between two and 12 months of age. Pulmonary disease caused by EHV-1 is less important
Influenzavirus A	Equine subtypes A/equi 1, H7N7 and A/equi 2, H3N8 cause upper respiratory disease mainly in young horses. In severe disease, broncho-interstitial pneumonia may be exacerbated by secondary bacterial infection
Equine adenovirus A	Subclinical infection widespread in horses. Disease occurs in Arabian foals with severe combined immunodeficiency. Necrotizing bronchiolitis and intranuclear inclusions in hyperplastic bronchiolar epithelial cells are often present. Secondary infection with *Streptococcus zooepidemicus* may occur

alveolar walls. Although sometimes associated with the ingestion of toxic chemicals or with hypersensitivity responses, interstitial pneumonia is also a feature of a number of bacterial and viral infections. Spread of infection to the lungs is often haematogenous, particularly in acute systemic disease, resulting in a diffuse or multi-focal lesion distribution with no clearcut relationship to airways. This type of acute interstitial pneumonia occurs, for example, in canine distemper and in septicaemic salmonellosis in calves and pigs. Although transmission of canine distemper virus is generally through aerosol, lung involvement results from viraemia following viral replication in the tonsils and other lymphoid tissues. The alveolar walls are infiltrated with lymphoid cells, and multinucleate giant cells, derived from type 2 pneumo-

cytes, may be present in alveoli along with alveolar macrophages. In the later stages of the disease, focal areas of alveolar epithelialization may be present. In septicaemic salmonellosis, alveolar walls are thickened as a result of leukocytic infiltration. Damage to capillary and alveolar walls, presumably due to endotoxin, is followed by fibrinohaemorrhagic exudation into the alveoli. Acute septicaemic infections of this type usually occur in young animals which succumb before further pathological changes can develop.

Chronic interstitial tissue changes occur in ovine progressive pneumonia caused by maedi-visna virus. This lentivirus is transmitted to adult sheep by aerosols and to lambs in the milk of infected dams. The virus, which targets monocytes and macrophages, persists and can replicate in the presence of the immune response of the host. Affected sheep may be clinically normal for several years after infection. Gradual loss of condition and hypernoea may then develop. At postmortem, the lungs do not collapse and may be up to four times the weight of normal lungs. Grey areas of consolidation can be detected on cut surfaces. The condition is characterized microscopically by infiltration of macrophages and lymphocytes into the alveolar walls and proliferative lymphoid nodules around bronchioles and blood vessels.

Further reading

Done, S.H. (1991). Environmental factors affecting the severity of pneumonia in pigs. *Veterinary Record,* **128**, 582–586.

Healy, A.M., Monaghan, M.L., Bassett, H.F., Gunn, H.M. *et al.* (1993). Morbidity and mortality in a large Irish feedlot: microbiological and serological findings in cattle with acute respiratory distress. *British Veterinary Journal,* **149**, 549–560.

Høie, S., Falk, K. and Lium, B.M. (1991). An abattoir survey of pneumonia and pleuritis in slaughter weight swine from 9 selected herds. IV. Bacteriological findings in chronic pneumonic lesions. *Acta Veterinaria Scandinavica,* **32**, 395–402.

Whitely, L.O., Maheswaran, S.K., Weiss, D.J. *et al.* (1992). *Pasteurella haemolytica* A1 and bovine respiratory disease: pathogenesis. *Journal of Veterinary Internal Medicine,* **6**, 11–22.

Zielinski, G.C. and Ross, R.F. (1993). Adherence of *Mycoplasma hyopneumoniae* to porcine ciliated respiratory tract cells. *American Journal of Veterinary Research,* **54**, 1262–1269.

Chapter 81

Bacterial causes of bovine mastitis

Mastitis is the most common infectious disease encountered in intensively-farmed dairy cattle. Although more than 100 microbial species have been isolated from the mammary gland of the cow, a relatively small number are responsible for most cases of clinical mastitis. It is usual to designate mastitis according to the origin of the organisms. Contagious mastitis is caused by bacteria which reside primarily in the mammary gland of cows whereas environmental mastitis is associated with micro-organisms which are present in the environment. Formerly, contagious mastitis accounted for most outbreaks of the disease but, following the implementation of mastitis control programmes during the past three decades, the incidence of contagious mastitis due to *Staphylococcus aureus* and *Streptococcus agalactiae* declined. Data from the UK show that the incidence of clinical mastitis decreased from approximately 150 cases per 100 cows per year in the 1960s to 35 to 40 cases per 100 cows per year in the early 1980s (Leigh, 1999). Mastitis control programmes are particularly effective against pathogens which reside in the mammary gland. Control measures for mastitis pathogens which are widespread in the environment are difficult to implement. Mastitis remains the most common and economically important infectious disease of dairy cows (Kossaibati and Esslemont, 1997).

With the exception of *Mycoplasma* species which can invade the mammary gland from the bloodstream, most organisms which cause mastitis enter the gland through the teat canal. Fungal and viral pathogens are occasionally implicated in mastitis. Five bacterial pathogens are responsible for most cases of bovine mastitis (Box 81.1).

Mammary gland defence mechanisms

The teat orifice and the teat canal are the first barriers to infection of the mammary gland. Some pathogens such as *S. aureus* colonize the teat skin and teat canal increasing the probability of intramammary infection. Desquamation of keratinized cells from the epithelial surface of the teat canal may contribute to the mechanical removal of bacteria from this location. In addition, fatty acids present in the keratinized layer exert a bacteriostatic effect. The flushing action of milk through the gland also acts as a natural defence mechanism and frequent stripping of the gland is

---

Box 81.1 Bacterial pathogens frequently isolated from cows with clinical mastitis.

- *Escherichia coli*
- *Streptococcus uberis*
- *Staphylococcus aureus*
- *Streptococcus dysgalactiae*
- *Streptococcus agalactiae*

---

recommended for treatment of mastitis caused by Gram-negative bacteria. Teat length may be important in determining susceptibility to infection; the short teats of heifers in association with oedema of mammary tissue at calving may predispose to mastitis due to the mechanical action of machine milking (Waage *et al.*, 2001). Superficial teat lesions also increase the likelihood of infection due to impairment of mechanical barriers. Even relatively mild hyperkeratosis of the teat orifice caused by incorrect milking machine function is associated with increased subclinical mastitis (Lewis *et al.*, 2000).

Non-specific antibacterial factors found in the mammary gland are listed in Box 81.2. Lactoferrin exerts a bacteriostatic effect by binding free ferric ions which are then unavailable for bacterial utilization. Because of the low concentration of lactoferrin in the lactating mammary gland, its principal function appears to relate to protection against coliform infection during the drying off period. Lysozyme is a bactericidal protein active against both Gram-positive and Gram-negative bacteria but, because it is present in low concentrations in bovine milk, its significance compared to other defence mechanisms is uncertain. The lactoperoxidase-thiocyanate-hydrogen peroxide system is bacteriostatic for Gram-positive bacteria and bactericidal for Gram-negative bacteria. This system

---

Box 81.2 Non-specific soluble factors in the mammary gland with antibacterial activity.

- Lactoferrin
- Lactoperoxidase-thiocyanate-hydrogen peroxide system
- Complement
- Lysozyme

depends on adequate concentrations of all components within the mammary gland. Lactoperoxidase is synthesized in mammary epithelium whereas thiocyanate levels are influenced by the dietary intake of certain green feeds. Hydrogen peroxide may be produced by a variety of enzymatic activities in milk and by the metabolic activity of streptococci if present. Complement, activated by the alternate pathway, may contribute to a limited extent to defence against Gram-negative bacteria.

Cell counts in the non-infected lactating mammary gland are usually less than 10^5 somatic cells per ml. The cell types include macrophages, with lesser numbers of lymphocytes and neutrophils and small numbers of epithelial cells. Cell counts tend to be higher during early and late lactation and the percentage of neutrophils increases late in lactation. The speed of recruitment of cells to the udder is an important factor in susceptibility to mastitis and cows with low somatic cell counts before infection are at greater risk of developing severe disease. Neutrophils are the principal cells involved in eliminating bacteria from the mammary gland. Recruitment of neutrophils from the blood to the site of infection in response to a number of inflammatory mediators such as cytokines and prostaglandins, is one of the first steps in the inflammatory response. Cell numbers in milk increase within hours of infection with counts of several hundred cells per ml common in subclinical infections. In clinical cases of mastitis, millions of cells per ml may be present. Neutrophils act by engulfing invading bacteria and subsequently killing them by oxygen-dependent or oxygen-independent systems. Oxidative damage is generally effective against Gram-negative bacteria but organisms such as *Staphylococcus aureus* which produce catalase can resist oxidative damage. Oxygen-independent killing is mediated through hydrolytic enzymes within lysosomes. However, the functioning of this mechanism may be less efficient in milk due to ingestion of casein and fat particles by neutrophils. Tissue damage and impaired mammary function may result from the respiratory burst and enzyme release by the activity of the accumulating neutrophils.

The role of lymphocytes in the protection of the mammary gland is the subject of much research. The proportion of T lymphocytes present, which varies with the stage of lactation, is greatest in late lactation and the ratio of T lymphocyte subpopulations also changes throughout lactation. The functional significance of these changes, which is unclear, appears to correlate with reduced resistance to infection in the postpartum period (Sordillo *et al.*, 1997).

The predominant immunoglobulin isotype in normal bovine milk, IgG_1, is selectively transferred into milk from serum. This isotype opsonizes bacteria for phagocytosis by macrophages. As neutrophils are recruited into the affected tissue, the importance of IgG_2 increases as this isotype can opsonize bacteria for phagocytosis by

neutrophils. IgM can also act as an opsonin. IgA agglutinates bacteria, prevents bacterial adherence to epithelium and neutralizes bacterial toxins. Cytokines, produced primarily by cells of the immune system, are glycoproteins which regulate the activity of cells participating both in specific and non-specific immune responses. Their role in the pathophysiology of bovine mastitis has been extensively studied in recent years. The research is aimed at modifying the inflammatory reaction by enhancing the immune response or by eliminating the undesirable effects of certain cytokines. The incorporation of interleukin-2 as an adjuvant in a bovine *Staphylococcus aureus* vaccine and attempts to limit production of tumour necrosis factor-alpha by monocytes are examples of this type of research (Sordillo *et al.*, 1995; DeRosa and Sordillo, 1997).

Contagious mastitis

The bovine mammary gland is the principal reservoir of infectious agents which cause contagious mastitis, namely *Staphylococcus aureus*, *Streptococcus agalactiae*, *Mycoplasma bovis* and *Corynebacterium bovis*. The source of infection is usually an infected mammary gland. Transmission of infection and appropriate control measures relate to factors such as the ability of a particular pathogen to survive the host. Because streptococci and mycoplasmas are susceptible to environmental influences they survive for much shorter periods outside the host than staphylococci. The severity of local systemic responses in mastitis depends directly on the virulence attributes of the pathogen.

Staphylococcus aureus

Infection with *S. aureus* is a common cause of clinical and subclinical mastitis in many modern dairy herds despite the implementation of mastitis control measures. *Staphylococcus aureus* can colonize the teat skin and teat canal and this may predispose to intramammary infection. However, the udder is considered to be the main source of infection with teat skin of lesser importance. Strain typing has shown that strains of *S. aureus* derived from the udder tend to be different from those isolated from other sites on the body. Although staphylococci are resistant organisms which can survive in the environment for weeks, transmission of infection occurs mainly at milking through contaminated milkers' hands, teat cup liners and udder cloths. The organism can adhere to the internal mucosal surfaces and produces a number of virulence factors which allow it to establish in spite of local immune responses. Enzymes such as hyaluronidase, staphylokinase and proteinases assist tissue invasion. Antiphagocytic factors such as a capsule allow staphylococci to resist phagocytosis and, even if phagocytosed, engulfed organisms are frequently not destroyed and can persist and multiply within phagocytes. When this occurs, *S. aureus* outlives the phagocytic cells and is periodically released into the tissues where it can cause further damage. Virulence factors such as haemolysins augment tissue damage.

Mastitis caused by *S. aureus* ranges in severity from peracute to subclinical. Chronic subclinical disease interspersed with periodic clinical episodes is the most common form observed. There are no apparent differences in virulence factor production between isolates from acute and chronic staphylococcal mastitis, and variation in disease manifestations is likely to be influenced by the stage of lactation at which infection occurs. Severe disease usually develops early in lactation. In the most severe form, peracute gangrenous mastitis, the infection causes venous thrombosis with local oedema and congestion of the udder leading to tissue necrosis. In this uncommon form of staphylococcal mastitis, onset is sudden and clinical signs include high fever, profound depression and anorexia. The affected quarter is swollen and sore on palpation. Udder discolouration becomes evident and gangrenous black areas are obvious within 24 hours. Toxaemia may result in death unless appropriate treatment is instituted early. The acute form is characterized by severe swelling of the affected gland and a purulent secretion which often contains thick clots. Extensive fibrosis is a common sequel.

In chronic or subclinical staphylococcal mastitis, episodes of bacterial shedding from affected quarters occur along with elevated somatic cell counts. Clinical detection of this form of mastitis relates to the extent of tissue damage. Bacterial multiplication occurs principally in the collecting ducts and, to a limited extent, in the alveoli. The inflammatory response results in duct blockage and atrophy of the associated alveoli. Influx of phagocytic cells may lead to abscess formation and fibrosis which further limits effective clearance of the organisms and also interferes with antibiotic penetration during treatment. Accordingly, although some *S. aureus* intramammary infections are cleared by immune mechanisms, the majority become chronic, low-grade or subclinical resulting in substantial production losses.

Streptococcus agalactiae

In recent years, *S. agalactiae* is encountered less frequently as a cause of mastitis. However, it continues to be a problem in individual herds with high cell counts. It is an obligate parasite of the bovine mammary gland which can also survive to a limited extent in the environment. In herds with poor hygiene, environmental sources of infection may be important. The course of infection is similar to that of chronic *S. aureus* infection with cycles of bacterial shedding and high somatic cell counts. Following introduction into the mammary gland, *S. agalactiae* multiplies and invades the lactiferous ducts. Passage through the duct walls into the lymphatic system and the supramammary lymph node occurs. An influx of neutrophils into the gland follows and the inflammatory

reaction results in blockage of the teat ducts and atrophy of secretory tissues. These inflammatory cycles occur periodically with progressive loss of secretory tissue. A relatively mild systemic reaction occurs coinciding with the first phase of replication and inflammation. Subsequently, clinical signs are usually mild and confined to the mammary gland. When the inflammation of the acini and ducts begins to resolve, the epithelial lining is shed contributing to clot formation in the milk. Most udder damage has already occurred before clinically detectable changes in milk are evident.

Mycoplasma species

Although a number of *Mycoplasma* species have been isolated from outbreaks of bovine mastitis, the most important pathogen is *Mycoplasma bovis*. Mycoplasmal mastitis is particularly common in large dairy herds. The reservoir of infection appears to be clinically healthy calves and young cattle which harbour *M. bovis* in the respiratory tract. Infection may initially be introduced into a herd by accidental inoculation of the organisms with teat syringes or cannulae. Once infection becomes established, transmission to other animals occurs during milking. Affected cows can shed 10^5 to 10^8 CFU per ml of milk contaminating milking machines, milkers' hands and cloths which are then important sources of infection for other animals in the herd. Haematogenous spread of infection between quarters occurs. *Mycoplasma bovis* can also cause congenital infection, thus maintaining the infection within a herd. The pathogenesis of mastitis caused by *Mycoplasma* species is unclear. A purulent interstitial exudate is present throughout the gland resulting in degeneration of alveolar epithelium. This is followed by epithelial hyperplasia with fibrosis and atrophy in the late stages of the disease.

Clinical signs do not develop in all affected cows and subclinical carriers are important sources of infection. When present, clinical signs include a dramatic alteration in milk consistency and a rapid decrease in milk yield within days of infection. The secretion appears normal but on standing, a deposit of sand-like or flocculent material settles out leaving a whey-like supernatant. Later in the disease, the secretion may be scanty and thick or serum-like containing curds. As response to treatment is variable, infection often results in agalactia.

Coagulase-negative staphylococci and *Corynebacterium bovis*

These bacteria are minor mastitis pathogens but they may cause subclinical infections or mild clinical disease. They can be classified as contagious pathogens because coagulase-negative staphylococci are considered to be part of the normal flora of animals and *C. bovis* is an inhabitant of the bovine mammary gland and teat ducts. Infections with these bacterial pathogens are more prevalent in herds which do not practise teat dipping or use dry cow therapy.

abort. The affected quarter is swollen, hard and painful and the secretion is watery with clots. Later it becomes purulent with a foetid odour. If the cow survives the toxaemia, an abscess may form and eventually discharge to the exterior. There is usually complete loss of function of the quarter and affected cows are culled.

Diagnosis

The quality of the milk sample submitted determines the reliability of the laboratory diagnosis. If more than one organism is isolated from a milk sample, such a sample is regarded as contaminated and the results are unreliable. An exception occurs when mastitis follows severe traumatic injury to the teats in which mixed infections are relatively common. The correct sampling procedure should be followed for milk collection:

- Teats which are obviously dirty should be washed and dried immediately.
- Each teat end should be treated with 70% ethyl alcohol and left for one minute before sampling.
- As the first milk expressed may be contaminated, it should be discarded.
- The sterile container used to collect the milk sample should be held almost parallel to the ground at an angle close to 90° to the teat being sampled. This minimizes the risk of contamination from the udder or abdomen.
- The container should be capped tightly, labelled with the cow number and date and submitted for immediate culture. If this is not possible, it should be stored at 4°C until it can be sent to the laboratory. Many mastitis pathogens survive freezing at -20°C and accordingly, samples can be frozen and submitted in batches for culture. Some bacteria may not survive freezing and if difficulty in isolating pathogens arises, samples should be submitted immediately for culture.

Most mastitis pathogens can be isolated easily using routine culture methods. Media used for primary culture are blood agar, Edward's medium which is selective for streptococci, and MacConkey agar. Colony morphology, patterns of haemolysis and growth characteristics on these media often allow a presumptive identification to be made. A definitive identification of a suspect pathogen can be made using tests specific for that organism as described in the chapters on individual pathogens. Diagnostic kits for the identification of the more common mastitis pathogens are available. These include miniaturized biochemical systems which test the ability of an organism to utilize different sugars. Other metabolic reactions can also be detected. These are frequently used for the identification of streptococci and members of the *Enterobacteriaceae*. Commercial agglutination test kits are also available for Lancefield grouping of streptococci and for agglutination assays to differentiate *S. aureus* from coagulase-negative staphylococci.

Occasionally, no bacteria can be isolated from mastitic milk samples. Reasons for this include:

- Treatment with antibiotics before sampling.
- Destruction of the bacteria in the course of the inflammatory reaction. In some forms of mastitis caused by *E. coli* or other environmental organisms, systemic effects of endotoxin continue in the absence of viable bacteria in the milk.
- Chronic mastitis in which the organisms have been eliminated but the pathological changes persist.
- Failure to isolate pathogens may relate to the media and cultural methods used. Some microorganisms such as *Mycoplasma* species, *Leptospira* serovar *hardjo* and fungi require specialized isolation procedures and suitable media.
- Traumatic mastitis.

The history accompanying the samples may provide background information relating to samples which are bacteriologically negative. Further investigation may be required if the history does not match the results obtained.

Treatment of mastitis

Antimicrobial agents are used extensively for the treatment and control of bovine mastitis. Intramammary antibiotic preparations are available to farmers in many countries and this easy access is likely to result in excessive antimicrobial chemotherapy. In countries such as Norway where antibiotic preparations are available only on prescription, indiscriminate use of these therapeutic agents is less likely to occur. It is important that the rationale for use of antibiotics in the treatment of mastitis is thoroughly understood by veterinarians prescribing treatment and that this information is communicated clearly to farmers. Antibiotics used in the treatment of mastitis can be administered by parenteral or intramammary routes. Intramuscular or intravenous injection is frequently used for the treatment of acute clinical mastitis. In acute mastitis, antimicrobial compounds given by the intramammary route may fail to reach the affected site due to occlusion of milk ducts by inflammatory exudates. Chemotherapeutic agents given by the parenteral route for the treatment of mastitis should, ideally, have certain characterisitcs which are listed in Box 81.5 (Sandholm, 1995; Ziv, 1980).

Interactions between host, pathogen and antimicrobial agent

In bovine mastitis, the choice of antimicrobial agent is influenced by the nature of the pathogen and its location within the mammary tissues, the host reaction to the pathogen and the pharmacokinetics and mechanism of action of the drug. Because individual cases of mastitis are usually caused by a single bacterial species, the therapeutic agent selected should be as specific as

---

Box 81.5 Desirable characteristics of drugs for parenteral administration in the treatment of mastitis.

- Low minimal inhibitory concentration for pathogens causing mastitis
- High bioavailability and distribution in mammary tissue after intramuscular or intravenous administration
- Chemical structure favouring accumulation in milk
- Low serum protein-binding activity
- Long half life

---

possible. Accordingly, antimicrobial combinations and broad-spectrum antibiotics should be avoided. Although the treatment of clinical mastitis usually begins before identification of the causal agent, the clinical signs and the herd history may indicate which agent is most likely to be involved. Treatment can be changed, if necessary, in the light of *in vitro* antibiotic sensitivity testing.

The effectiveness of antimicrobial drugs for treating mastitis caused by *Escherichia coli* is considered to be questionable because the main clinical manifestations of the condition relate to endotoxin activity and the subsequent release of inflammatory mediators. In experimental studies of acute *E. coli* mastitis, no significant improvement in recovery rates was demonstrable following antimicrobial therapy. Moreover, the rate of spontaneous recovery in subacute and mild infections with *E. coli* may approach 90%. Treatment with oxytocin along with frequent stripping of the mammary gland may be as beneficial as the administration of

antibiotics.

Antibiotics which accumulate in extracellular spaces are effective chemotherapeutic agents for treating streptococcal mastitis because streptococci are not intracellular pathogens. In contrast, staphylococcal infections are difficult to eliminate because *Staphylococcus aureus* can survive in phagocytes. Moreover, the abscess formation and fibrosis, features of these infections, limit penetration of antimicrobial agents. Furthermore, β-lactam antibiotics may be inactivated by the oxygen burst in phagocytes stimulated by the presence of staphylococci.

Antibiotic susceptibility testing can determine the therapeutic agent which is most effective *in vitro* against a particular pathogen. However, *in vitro* effectiveness may not match the results obtained *in vivo*. Moreover, many antimicrobial agents lose much of their activity when milk is incorporated into the medium used for antibiotic susceptibility testing. Macrolides are up to 90% less effective and tetracyclines up to 75% less effective against staphylococci when tested in a medium containing milk (Sandholm, 1995).

Although no ideal chemotherapeutic agents are available for the treatment of mastitis, some antimicrobial compounds currently used are presented in Table 81.1.

Antibiotic resistance

The resistance of staphylococci to antibiotics is a major obstacle to the successful treatment of mastitis in dairy cattle. Although there are many reasons for the failure of treatment in staphylococcal mastitis, production of beta-lactamase by certain staphylococcal strains is the principal

Table 81.1 Chemotherapy used for the treatment of bacterial pathogens which cause bovine mastitis.

Pathogen	Antimicrobial agents used for treatment	Comments
Staphylococcus aureus	Cephalosporins, cloxacillin, erythromycin, penicillin (if organism is susceptible), penicillin combined with novobiocin, tetracyclines, tylosin	Because of inadequate drug penetration at site of infection, clinical recovery is not assured and elimination of bacteria is unpredictable.
Streptococcus agalactiae	Cephalosporins, cloxacillin, macrolides, penicillin	Successful treatment can be carried out during lactation. Eradication of the organism from a herd, using intensive antibiotic therapy, is possible.
Mycoplasma bovis	Tetracyclines, tylosin	Because antibiotic treatment is usually unsuccessful, control is based on culling of infected animals.
Escherichia coli	Ampicillin-cloxacillin, cephalosporins, gentamicin, tetracyclines	Antibiotic usage is of questionable benefit but may improve recovery rates in animals with impaired immune defences. Supportive therapy is essential in acute disease.
Environmental streptococci	Ampicillin, cephalosporins, cloxacillin, novobiocin, penicillin, tetracyclines	Clinical cases respond well to treatment with antibiotics given by the intramammary route.
Arcanobacterium pyogenes	Penicillin, tetracyclines	The suppurative reaction induced by *A. pyogenes* infection results in poor antibiotic penetration and treatment is usually ineffective.

reason for failure. The prevalence of penicillin-resistant strains of *S. aureus* differs from country to country. Approximately 20% of strains isolated in Norway were resistant to penicillin (Brun, 1998); 36% of strains tested were resistant in a study conducted in a number of European countries, the U.S. and Zimbabwe (de Oliveira *et al.*, 2000). In a study conducted in Sudan, 73% of *S. aureus* isolates exhibited multiple resistance (Kuwajock *et al.*, 1999).

Antibiotic therapy in lactating cows

During lactation, antimicrobial therapy is generally used for treatment of clinical mastitis, whereas dry cow therapy is employed for controlling subclinical disease. Mastitis caused by *S. agalactiae* is exceptional as both clinical and subclinical disease can be successfully treated during lactation. *Streptococcus agalactiae* is usually treated by the intramammary route with success rates approaching 100%. Saturation therapy can be used to eradicate the disease from some herds. This entails identification and treatment of all infected cows combined with strict hygienic measures to prevent the spread of infection. Any cows still infected after this regime will require further treatment. A second option entails treating all lactating cows in the herd.

Treatment of *S. aureus* infections during lactation results in clinical recovery rates of 30 to 60%. However, complete elimination of the organism is rarely achieved during lactation and invariably requires dry cow therapy. Antibiotic treatment of mycoplasmal mastitis is not generally effective although a recent report documented the successful treatment of an outbreak of *M. californicum* and *M. canadense* mastitis with a combination of intramammary chlortetracycline and intramuscular tylosin. There is uncertainty about the value of antibiotic therapy for the treatment of *E. coli* mastitis. However, when treatment is given early enough to limit endotoxin production, antibiotics may improve recovery rates during the early postpartum period when a degree of immunosuppression may be present.

Dry cow therapy

Administration of intramammary antibiotics at the beginning of the dry period is used for the treatment of mastitis caused by contagious pathogens, principally *S. aureus*. Treatment of subclinical cases of mastitis due to environmental organisms such as *S. uberis*, which are detected late in lactation, may be deferred until the dry period. Rates of clearance of *S. aureus* achieved with dry cow therapy range from 25 to 75%. Treatment is unlikely to be successful in older cows, in cows with high somatic cell counts and when more than one quarter is infected.

Other therapeutic measures

To combat the effects of endotoxin, supportive therapy in the form of intravenous fluids and anti-inflammatory drugs is important in the treatment of peracute and acute *E. coli* mastitis. Oxytocin, in combination with hand stripping, assists in the removal of organisms, their toxins and inflammatory debris. In addition, oxytocin has been found to be as effective as antibiotics for treating experimentally-induced *S. aureus* mastitis (Knight *et al.*, 2000). Homeopathic, herbal and other remedies are used for the treatment of mastitis but their efficacy is difficult to assess due to lack of objective published data.

Prevention and control

The measures appropriate for the prevention and control of bovine mastitis differ depending on whether the causative organisms are contagious or environmental in origin. Although some measures such as a correctly functioning milking machine are useful in prevention of predisposing conditions, it is essential that the major pathogens causing mastitis on a farm are identified in order to formulate effective control strategies. A general plan for the control of bovine mastitis is presented in Box 81.6.

Box 81.6 Control plan for bovine mastitis.

- Properly maintained milking equipment
- Hygienic milking practices
- Post-milking teat disinfection
- Antibiotic therapy for clinical cases and for dry cows
- Culling of persistently-infected animals

Contagious mastitis

The reservoir of infection for contagious mastitis is infected cows and measures aimed at elimination of infection from the mammary glands are of major importance in control.

- The efficacy of dry cow antibiotic therapy depends on the susceptibility of the infecting pathogens. Dry cow therapy is effective against up to 80% of streptococcal infections but is is only effective against 50% of *S. aureus* infections.
- Elimination of teat lesions helps to reduce colonization of the teat skin, especially by *S. aureus*.
- Culling persistently-infected cows is important for the control of staphylococcal mastitis and for the control of mycoplasmal mastitis.

Prevention of new infections requires measures to exclude introduction of pathogens into the teat and to reduce exposure of the teats to pathogens.

- Correctly maintained milking equipment minimizes liner slip and incorrect vacuum levels. A properly functioning milking machine reduces the risk of introducing pathogens into the teat canal because of vacuum fluctuations and abnormal pressure gradients within the teats. In addition, milking machine performance can directly affect teat tissues. Prevention of minor lesions such as hyperkeratosis of the teat orifice helps to reduce the incidence of mastitis. The milking machine cluster can transmit contagious pathogens and efficient designs can reduce transmission. Research suggests that low volume claws, absence of air transmission and low milk flow-rates increase transfer of pathogens between teats (Woolford, 1995).

• Hygienic milking practices which include washing visibly dirty teats with a disinfectant solution, followed by drying with paper towels, and effective washing and disinfection of the milking machine reduces the likelihood of infection.

• Effective post-milking teat dipping or spraying is a major control measure for contagious mastitis. A limited number of chemical disinfectants can be used as teat dips. These include chlorine-releasing compounds, iodophors, quaternary ammonium compounds and chlorhexidine gluconate. The range of suitable disinfectants available is limited because teat dips should fulfil a number of criteria in order to be useful and safe. They should be non-irritating and non-toxic. In addition, they should remain active in the presence of organic matter such as milk and should not be absorbed

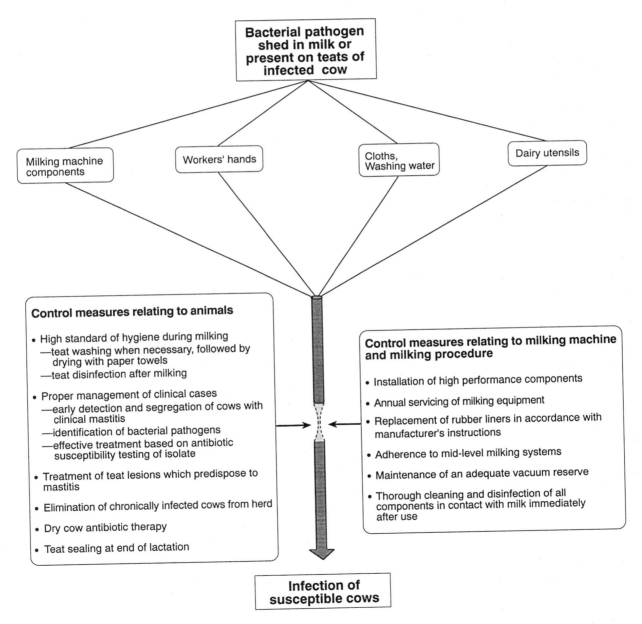

Figure 81.1 Transmission of contagious bacterial pathogens which cause mastitis in dairy cows and relevant control measures.

into the tissues or leave undesirable residues in milk.

- Milking clinically affected cows last reduces the likelihood of transmission of infection. If it is not possible to segregate clinically affected cows, disinfection of milk clusters immediately after removal from an affected cow or use of separate clusters for infected cows can help to reduce the spread of infection.

Control measures appropriate for the prevention of contagious bacterial pathogen transmission are summarized in Figure 81.1. Increasing the resistance of the cow through vaccination would be an obvious way of preventing and controlling pathogens causing contagious mastitis. Although research is continuing into vaccines against *S. aureus* and a commercial inactivated vaccine is available in the USA, efficacy of such vaccines is limited and their use is unlikely to be economically worthwhile where the prevalence of *S. aureus* mastitis has been reduced using other established control measures.

Environmental mastitis

Reduction of the number of pathogens in the environment depends on maintenance of satisfactory conditions while cows are housed or at pasture. Housing facilities should be correctly designed and well maintained for both lactating and dry cows. Facilities for dry cows and those which are calving are especially important for the control of *E. coli* mastitis as in many instances acquisition of infection occurs just before calving. Some measures important for reducing the reservoir of pathogens in the environment of the cow include:

- Provision of housing facilities designed to ensure correct lying behaviour with good cubicle usage to avoid teat injuries is essential.
- Clean, dry bedding minimizes the multiplication of pathogens. Bacterial numbers are lower in dry inorganic bedding such as sand or mats than in organic bedding such as straw or sawdust.
- Well ventilated buildings prevent wet conditions which encourage the build-up of potential pathogens.

Reduction of new infections can be achieved by using:

- Correctly functioning milking equipment to prevent the introduction of environmental pathogens into the teat canal and udder.
- Internal teat seals at drying off reduce the rate of new infections both during the dry period and at calving (Woolford *et al.*, 1998). Dry cow antibiotic therapy can also be helpful in the prevention of new infections but it has no effect on the reservoir of mastitis-producing bacteria of environmental origin.
- Keeping animals standing after milking until the teat sphincter has fully closed may decrease the risk of infection. This can be achieved by feeding animals after milking.
- Teat dipping before milking is reported to reduce new

infection rates with environmental pathogens by as much as 50% in some studies; in other studies no improvement was observed.

- A commercial vaccine is available for preventing mastitis caused by *E. coli*. Vaccination of cows during the dry period and early lactation reduces the incidence and severity of clinical coliform mastitis. However, it does not protect against infection. No commercial vaccines against streptococci causing bovine mastitis are available but research is ongoing into the development of a subunit vaccine for *S. uberis* based on the plasminogen activator, PauA.

References

Bradley, A.J. and Green, M. (2000). The importance of chronic infection and adaptation of *Escherichia coli* to the mammary environment – preliminary UK data. *Cattle Practice*, **8**, 233–237.

Brun, E. (1998). Use of antibiotics and antibiotic resistance in Norwegian animal husbandry. *Meierposten*, **87**, 216–218.

de Oliveira, A.P., Watts, J.L., Salmon, S.A. and Aarestrup, F.M. (2000). Antimicrobial susceptibility of *Staphylococcus aureus* isolated from bovine mastitis in Europe and the United States. *Journal of Dairy Science*, **83**, 855–862.

DeRosa, D.C. and Sordillo, L.M. (1997). Efficacy of a bovine *Staphylococcus aureus* vaccine using Interleukin-2 as an adjuvant. *Journal of Veterinary Medicine*, Series B, **44**, 599–607.

Green, L. (2000). Latest situation on low SCC and subsequent intramammary infection. *Cattle Practice*, **8**, 239–241.

Green, M.J., Green, L.E. and Cripps, P.J. (1996). Low BMSCC and endotoxin associated (toxic) mastitis: an association. *Veterinary Record*, **138**, 305–306.

Harmon, R.J., Clark, T., Ramesh, T. *et al.* (1992). Environmental pathogen numbers in pastures and bedding of dairy cattle. *Journal of Dairy Science*, **75**, 256.

Hill, A.W. (1981). Factors affecting the outcome of *Escherichia coli* mastitis in the dairy cow. *Research in Veterinary Science*, **31**, 107–112.

Knight, C.H., Fitzpatrick, J.L., Logue, D.N. and Platt, D.J. (2000). Efficacy of two non-antibiotic therapies, oxytocin and topical liniment, against bovine staphylococcal mastitis. *Veterinary Record*, **146**, 311–316.

Kossaibati, M.A. and Esslemont, R.J. (1997). The costs of production diseases in dairy herds in England. *Veterinary Journal*, **154**, 41–51.

Kuwajock, V.L., Bagadi, H.O., Shears, P. and Mukhtar, M.M. (1999). Prevalence of multiple antibiotic resistances among bovine mastitis pathogens in Khartoum State, Sudan. *Sudan Journal of Veterinary Science and Animal Husbandry*, **38**, 64–70.

Leigh, J.A. (1999). *Streptococcus uberis*: a permanent barrier to the control of bovine mastitis? *Veterinary Journal*, **157**, 225–238.

Lewis, S., Cockcroft, P.D., Bramley, R.A. and Jackson, P.G.G. (2000). The likelihood of subclinical mastitis in quarters with different types of teat lesions in the dairy cow. *Cattle Practice*, **8**, 293–299.

Menzies, F.D., McBride, S.H., McDowell, S.W.J. *et al.* (2000). Clinical and laboratory findings in cases of toxic mastitis in cows in Northern Ireland. *Veterinary Record*, **147**, 123–128.

Sandholm, M. (1995) A critical view on antibacterial mastitis therapy. In *The bovine udder and mastitis*. Eds. M. Sandholm,T. Honkanen-Buzalski, L. Kaartinen, and S. Pyorala, University of Helsinki, Finland. pp.169–186.

Shuster, D.E., Lee, E.K. and Kehril, M.E. (1996). Bacterial growth, inflammatory cytokine production and neutrophil recruitment during coliform mastitis in cows within ten days of calving compared with cows at midlactation. *American Journal of Veterinary Research*, **11**, 1569–1575.

Smith, K.L. and Hogan, J.S. (1993). Environmental mastitis. *Veterinary Clinics of North America, Food Animal Practice*, **9**, 489–498.

Sordillo, S.M., Pighetti, G.M. and Davis, M.R. (1995). Enhanced production of bovine tumor necrosis factor-alpha during the periparturient period. *Veterinary Immunology and Immunopathology*, **49**, 263–270.

Sordillo, S.M., Shafer-Weaver, K and De Rosa, D. (1997). Immunobiology of the mammary gland. *Journal of Dairy Science*, **80**, 1851–1865.

Waage, S., Odegaard, S.A., Lund, A., Brattgjerd, S. and Rothe, T. (2001). Case-control study of risk factors for clinical mastitis in postpartum dairy heifers. *Journal of Dairy Science*, **85**, 392–399.

Woolford, M.W. (1995). Milking machine effects on mastitis progress 1985–1995. In *Proceedings of the 3rd IDF International Mastitis Seminar, Session 7: Milking Machine and Udder Health.* May 28–June 1, 1995. Tel Aviv, Israel. pp.3–12.

Woolford, M.W., Williamson, J.H., Day, A.M. and Copeman, P.J.A. (1998). The prophylactic effect of a teat sealer on bovine mastitis during the dry period and the following lactation. *New Zealand Veterinary Journal*, **46**, 12–19.

Ziv, G. (1980). Drug selection and use in mastitis: systemic vs local drug therapy. *Journal of the American Veterinary Medical Association*, **176**, 1109–1115.

Further reading

Keefe, G.P. (1997). *Streptococcus agalactiae* mastitis: a review. *Canadian Veterinary Journal*, **38**, 429–437.

Chapter 82

Foot infections of cattle, sheep and pigs associated with microbial agents

Lameness, particularly foot lameness, can cause significant economic loss in farm animal production. The relative importance of foot lameness in various species differs; it is especially important in cattle and sheep. Footrot caused by infection with *Dichelobacter nodosus* and other bacterial pathogens is a major cause of lameness in sheep. Relative to sheep, infections of the foot in dairy cows are less common.

Although foot lameness in farm animals is mainly attributable to bacterial infections, it is also a significant clinical feature in a number of important viral diseases in which pedal lesions develop (Table 82.1). Lesions can develop in locations other than the foot in these systemic viral diseases. In contrast, bacterial infections are usually limited to pedal tissues. Bacteria, which affect the skin and horn of the digit in farm animals, include *Fusobacterium necrophorum*, *Arcanobacterium pyogenes* and *Prevotella* species, and these are often normal inhabitants of the gastrointestinal tract. Virulent strains of *Dichelobacter nodosus*, the primary cause of footrot in sheep, are not regarded as commensals. These pathogenic strains are maintained by clinically affected and recovered carrier sheep. Observations on the epidemiology of digital dermatitis in cattle also suggest that the putative causative organisms are maintained by carrier animals which can introduce infection into clean herds.

The aetiology and epidemiology of infectious digital disease are complex and definitive diagnosis is difficult. Isolation of anaerobic and other bacteria from pedal lesions is demanding and specific procedures must be followed (*see* Chapter 32). Moreover, contamination by opportunistic bacteria may render interpretation of the significance of isolates difficult. Infectious foot conditions of sheep and cattle and their associated aetiological agents are listed in Tables 82.2 and 82.3 respectively. The aetiological role of the bacteria commonly isolated from digital lesions is well established for some conditions but is unclear in others; the primary role of *Dichelobacter nodosus* in the aetiology of footrot in sheep is not disputed whereas its role in interdigital dermatitis is uncertain. In addition, synergism between two or more organisms is important in the aetiology of many foot conditions as illustrated by the relationship between *F. necrophorum* and *D. nodosus* in ovine footrot and between *F. necrophorum* and *Porphyromonas levii* in foul-of-the-foot in cattle.

Furthermore, the occurrence of disease may be dependent on the presence of certain environmental conditions or predisposing factors before bacterial invasion can occur. Because of the complex relationship between the causative organisms and predisposing factors, the most appropriate and effective control measures are not always evident or feasible.

Ovine footrot

Two clinical forms of footrot, virulent and benign, apparently relate to the invasiveness of the strain of *Dichelobacter nodosus* involved. Although *D. nodosus* is the principal pathogen in ovine footrot, a number of other organisms are commonly associated with the condition (Table 82.2). The bacterium largely responsible for the

Table 82.1 Systemic viral diseases of cattle, sheep and pigs in which foot lameness occurs.

Disease/ species affected	Virus/genus/family	Nature and extent of foot lesions
Blue tongue/ sheep, cattle	Blue tongue virus/ *Orbivirus*/ *Reoviridae*	Laminitis; inflammation of the coronary band (coronitis)
Foot-and-mouth disease/ cattle, sheep, pigs	Foot-and-mouth disease virus/ *Aphthovirus*/ *Picornaviridae*	Vesicles in the interdigital skin and on the coronary band; ulceration following vesicle rupture may lead to secondary bacterial invasion.
Mucosal disease/ cattle	Bovine viral diarrhoea virus/ *Pestivirus*/ *Flaviviridae*	Ulcerative lesions in the interdigital clefts; coronitis Lesions may occur in all four feet
Swine vesicular disease/ pigs	Swine vesicular disease virus/ *Enterovirus*/ *Picornaviride*	Vesicular or ulcerative lesions on the coronary bands may involve the entire coronet producing severe lameness
Vesicular stomatitis/ cattle, pigs, horses, rarely sheep	Vesicular stomatitis virus/*Vesiculovirus*/ *Rhabdoviridae*	Vesicular lesions on coronary bands progressing to ulceration complicated by secondary bacterial infection

Table 82.2 Infectious foot conditions of sheep.

Clinical condition	Bacteria implicated	Comments
Ovine footrot	*Dichelobacter nodosus*, *Fusobacterium necrophorum*, *Arcanobacterium pyogenes*, Spirochaetes (unclassified)	Severity of lesions determined by the virulence of *D. nodosus*; may occur as benign and virulent forms
Ovine interdigital dermatitis	*Fusobacterium necrophorum*, *Dichelobacter nodosus* (benign strains)	Superficial interdigital inflammation, caused primarily by *F. necrophorum*. Mild condition; also referred to as scald.
Heel abscess	*Fusobacterium necrophorum*, *Arcanobacterium pyogenes* together with opportunistic anaerobic bacteria	Associated with prolonged wet seasons; usually affects adult sheep. Painful pyogenic condition which often extends to the interphalangeal joints.
Erysipelas laminitis	*Erysipelothrix rhusiopathiae*	Occurs in sheep following immersion in contaminated dipping fluid. The bacteria enter through skin abrasions in the hoof regions causing cellulitis and laminitis.
Strawberry footrot	*Dermatophilus congolensis*	Proliferative, inflammatory lesions affecting the coronary band and the lower limb of sheep
Lamellar suppuration	Mixed bacterial infection with *Fusobacterium necrophorum*, *Arcanobacterium pyogenes*, *Dichelobacter nodosus*, *Prevotella* species and other opportunistic bacteria	Pyogenic infection located between the horn and sensitive lamina. Infection usually enters at the white line between the horn of the wall and the sole. Often associated with trauma. Referred to as toe abscess in sheep.

initiation of footrot is *Fusobacterium necrophorum*, which causes tissue necrosis with a subsequent inflammatory reaction. Damage to the inter-digital skin as a result of constant wetting and infection with *Arcanobacterium pyogenes* are also involved in lesion development. The local anaerobic microenvironment facilitates infection with *D. nodosus* which possesses pili allowing adherence to the epithelium of the foot. If the strain of *D. nodosus* has poor keratolytic activity, limited separation of horn from underlying matrix may occur at the heel. This benign form of footrot manifests as slight lameness which rapidly regresses after topical treatment or with the onset of dry weather. Virulent strains of *D. nodosus* cause extensive separation of horn from underlying matrix, extending from the heel to the sole and toe, with the formation of a foul-smelling necrotic exudate. Lameness, which is severe and persistent, usually involves more than one foot. Adult sheep are more commonly affected than lambs and the Merino breed appears to be more susceptible than other breeds. A recent report, which describes particularly virulent outbreaks of footrot in the UK, has recorded the apparent involvement of spirochaetes (Naylor *et al.*, 1998). These spirochaetes are genetically identical to those associated with digital dermatitis in cattle.

Dichelobacter nodosus, a Gram-negative anaerobic bacterium, is an obligate pathogen of the feet of clinically affected or chronic carrier ruminants. The organism can survive in warm, wet, muddy environmental conditions for about 4 days. During the summer, survival of the pathogen is favoured by grazing on lush pastures and wet underfoot conditions enhance survival when sheep are housed in the winter. Both of these environmental situations can contribute to maceration of interdigital skin. For transmission to occur daily mean temperatures must exceed 10°C.

Diagnosis of footrot is based primarily on clinical examination. A number of scoring systems have been devised to aid in the characterization and control of the disease (Whittington and Nichols, 1995). If microbiological confirmation of the strain virulence of *D. nodosus* is required, biochemical tests for virulence attributes can be used. However, tests for elastase production and gelatin liquefaction can take from one to five weeks to complete and are, therefore, of retrospective value only. Newer diagnostic methods based on PCR and detection of specific DNA products can be used for rapid detection of virulent and benign strains (Liu and Webber, 1995). Rapid detection of strain virulence is important because clinical differentiation between benign footrot and the early manifestations of the virulent form of the disease may be difficult.

Extensive studies on the control of footrot were carried out in Australia. They included comparisons of the economic return from different control options (Egerton *et al.*, 1989; Egerton and Raadsma, 1991). A number of control strategies are available including topical treatment of affected feet, identification and elimination of virulent strains of *D. nodosus*, vaccination and genetic selection for improved resistance to footrot. The conventional method of treatment and control of footrot is paring of affected feet to remove separated horn and establish drainage. This is followed by topical application of antibacterial solutions such as 10% zinc or copper sulphate or 5% oxytetracycline solution. This method of treatment is labour intensive and is often replaced by the use of a foot bath, usually after separation of affected sheep from the rest of the flock.

Table 82.3   Infectious foot conditions of cattle.

Clinical condition	Bacteria implicated	Comments
Bovine interdigital dermatitis	*Dichelobacter nodosus, Fusobacterium necrophorum Prevotella* species Spirochaetes (unclassified)	Benign condition with superficial lesions confined to the interdigital skin; usually subclinical
Bovine interdigital necrobacillosis	*Fusobacterium necrophorum, Porphyromonas levii*	Severe, necrotizing condition of interdigital skin; characteristic foetid odour. May extend to deeper tissues including joints. Also called foul-in-the-foot.
Digital dermatitis	Unclassified spirochaetes; other opportunistic invaders	Proliferative dermatitis affecting the bulbs of heels in cattle. Also termed verrucose dermatitis. Opportunistic, secondary bacterial infection may contribute to severity of lesions.
Lamellar suppuration	Mixed bacterial infection with *Fusobacterium necrophorum, Arcanobacterium pyogenes, Dichelobacter nodosus, Prevotella* species and other opportunistic bacteria	Pyogenic infection located between the horn and sensitive lamina. Infection usually enters at the white line between the horn of the wall and the sole. Often associated with trauma. Referred to as white line abscess in cattle.

After treatment, the affected animals are isolated from the rest of the flock to minimize the risk of spread of the infection while grazing. Affected animals can be removed from a problem flock in order to eradicate footrot. Carriers of benign strains of *D. nodosus* cannot be identified as the interdigital skin remains normal and they do not develop lameness.

Although natural infection with *D. nodosus* confers no appreciable immunity, vaccination can increase short-term resistance and is a useful adjunct to control and treatment. The antigens which evoke a protective immune response are pili. There are nine major serogroups of *D. nodosus* and immunity develops to the homologous strain only. Vaccines usually contain a number of different strains from the serogroups most commonly associated with footrot but protection cannot always be assured. Vaccination can be used therapeutically to reduce the severity and duration of infection. Two injections of vaccine are necessary; the effectiveness of the procedure varies.

Genetic selection may be aimed at increased resistance to virulent strains of *D. nodosus*. Alternatively, strategies might be directed towards increasing responsiveness to vaccination. Although considerable information is available on the genetic basis of susceptibility to footrot in Merino sheep, the practical application of selection for either increased resistance or responsiveness to vaccination has not yet been achieved.

Ovine interdigital dermatitis

In this mild disease, inflammation is confined to the interdigital skin. *Fusobacterium necrophorum*, which is the principal pathogen, invades the epidermis following maceration of the skin due to wet conditions underfoot or following local injury. The interdigital skin is erythematous and swollen, and there may be superficial greyish discolouration. Lameness is not usually apparent and affected animals recover when underfoot conditions improve. Ovine interdigital dermatitis is clinically indistinguishable from benign footrot.

Opportunistic suppurative conditions of the foot

In sheep, lamellar abscessation can occur at the heel or the toe. Horn defects may allow opportunistic infection which usually includes *F. necrophorum* and *A. pyogenes*. Increased weight in late gestation predisposes to heel abscessation in ewes. Extension of infection from ovine interdigital dermatitis may predispose to infection of the second interphalangeal joint. When abscess formation occurs at the toe, infection is usually confined to the corium of the hoof without joint involvement.

In cattle, lamellar abscessation is frequently termed white line disease. Infection of defective horn by opportunistic bacteria may occur at any point on the white line. In dairy cattle, the condition often affects the lateral claw of a hind foot. This site is particularly susceptible to a combination of mechanical stress and subclinical laminitis which may predispose to disruption of horn structure, facilitating entry of pyogenic bacteria. The subsequent suppurative process may extend along the sensitive laminae to discharge at the coronary band or at the skin-horn junction of the heel. If left untreated the inflammatory process may involve the deeper tissues of the foot leading to septic arthritis of the second interphalangeal joint.

In pigs, lamellar abscessation (bush foot) occurs when traumatic lesions of the white line or the sole become infected. Trauma, due to rough floor surfaces, produces erosions of the horn and haemorrhage in almost 100% of intensively-reared piglets. These minor lesions do not cause lameness unless they become infected and there is subsequent extension to the sensitive laminae. Progression of infection may be similar to that observed in other species with discharge at the coronary band. Serious sequelae such as arthritis and tenosynovitis can also occur.

Bovine interdigital necrobacillosis

This condition is an acute or subacute necrotizing interdigital dermatitis (Table 82.3). The infection results in necrosis with fissure formation in the interdigital skin and a purulent exudate. Extension of the process to underlying soft tissues is characterized by swelling. There is considerable pain and lameness. The tissue damage is a consequence of the synergistic action of *F. necrophorum* and *Porphyromonas levii*, formerly known as *Bacteroides melaninogenicus* subspecies *levii* (Berg and Loan, 1975; Berg and Franklin, 2000). In common with other bacterial infections of the digital skin and horn, predisposing factors are considered important in the pathogenesis of interdigital necrobacillosis. Trauma, maceration of the skin after prolonged wetting and nutritional deficiencies have been suggested as important contributory factors in the development of the condition. Bovine interdigital necrobacillosis usually affects one foot and extension to the second interphalangeal joint may occur. A particularly severe form of the disease, termed 'superfoul', in which there is rapid development of necrosis and spread to deeper tissues, has been reported (Cook and Cutler, 1995). Response to antibiotic therapy is poor. Isolates of *F. necrophorum* from these severe lesions are extremely virulent (Berg and Franklin, 2000). A possible relationship with digital dermatitis has been noted in herds affected with 'superfoul'. Spirochaetes were observed in lesions but their aetiological role was not clearly defined (Doherty *et al.*, 1998). Systemic antimicrobial therapy is the usual treatment for interdigital necrobacillosis. Early and sustained treatment is required for 'superfoul', including local debridement of necrotic tissue and high doses of parenteral antibiotics for five days.

Digital dermatitis

This condition was first described in Italy in 1974. Inflammatory lesions occur in the interdigital skin and may extend to the coronet. Two forms of the disease, erosive and verrucose, may reflect different stages in its development. The degree of lameness is variable and, on palpation, lesions may be tender. The aetiology of digital dermatitis is multifactorial. A number of infectious agents and environmental factors appear to be associated with the development of the disease. The condition is seen most frequently in first-calved heifers. There may be an increase in the occurrence of the disease in loose-housed herds when conditions are unhygienic. The prevalence of the disease decreases when animals are at pasture.

Current evidence supports the hypothesis that spirochaetes have an aetiological role despite the absence

of experimental proof. The spirochaetes which have been implicated appear to be closely related to human oral treponemes and are considered capable of invading the skin. Other bacteria isolated from the lesions include *F. necrophorum*, *Prevotella* species, *Porphyromonas* species and *Peptostreptococcus indolicus* (Döpfer, 2000). Topical applications of antibiotics are used for treatment. Herd outbreaks can be treated with antibiotic solutions, usually of lincomycin or oxytetracycline, in foot baths.

Bovine interdigital dermatitis

Dichelobacter nodosus is considered to be the principal aetiological agent in this condition. The strains involved differ from those which cause virulent footrot in sheep. In several investigations, *D. nodosus* was not isolated from the lesions; a number of anaerobes including *F. necrophorum* and *Prevotella* species were isolated and spirochaetes were demonstrated in the pedal lesion. Digital and interdigital dermatitis may be closely related. Lameness is uncommon in bovine interdigital dermatitis. Footbaths containing formalin or copper sulphate are used as part of a control programme.

References

Berg, J.N. and Franklin, C. L. (2000). Interdigital phlegmon a.k.a. interdigital necrobacillosis a.k.a. acute footrot of cattle: considerations in etiology, diagnosis and treatment. In *Proceedings of the XI International Symposium on Disorders of the Ruminant Digit and III International Conference on Bovine Lameness*, Parma, Italy 3–7 September 2000. Eds. C.M. Mortellaro, L. De Vecchis, and A. Brizzi. pp. 24–26.

Berg, J.N. and Loan, R.W. (1975). *Fusobacterium necrophorum* and *Bacteroides melaninogenicus* as etiologic agents of footrot in cattle. *American Journal of Veterinary Research*, **36**, 1115–1122.

Cook, N.B. and Cutler, K.L. (1995). Treatment and outcome of a severe form of foul-in-the-foot. *Veterinary Record*, **136**, 19–20.

Doherty, M.L., Bassett, H.F., Markey, B., Healy, A.M and Sammin, D. (1998). Severe foot lameness in cattle associated with invasive spirochaetes. *Irish Veterinary Journal*, **51**, 195–198.

Döpfer, D. (2000). Summary of research activities concerning (papillomatous) digital dermatitis in cattle published or developed since 1998. In *Proceedings of the XI International Symposium on Disorders of the Ruminant Digit and III International Conference on Bovine Lameness*, Parma, Italy 3–7. September 2000. Eds. Mortellaro, C. M., De Vecchis, L. and Brizzi, A. pp. 19–23.

Egerton, J.R. and Raadsma, H.W. (1991). Breeding sheep for resistance to footrot. In *Breeding for Disease Resistance in Farm Animals*. Eds. Owen, J.B. and Axford, R.F.E. CAB International, Wallingford. pp. 347–370.

Egerton J.R., Yong, W.K. and Riffkin, G.G. (1989). Footrot and

Foot Abscess of Ruminants. CRC Press, Boca Raton, Florida.

Liu, D. and Webber, J (1995). A polymerase chain reaction assay for improved determination of virulence of *Dichelobacter nodosus*, the specific causative pathogen for ovine footrot. *Veterinary Microbiology*, **42**, 197–207.

Naylor, R.D., Martin, P.K., Jones, J.R. and Burnell, M.C. (1998). Isolation of spirochaetes from an incident of severe virulent ovine footrot. *Veterinary Record*, **143**, 690–691.

Whittington, R. J. and Nicholls, P.J (1995). Grading the lesions of ovine footrot. *Research in Veterinary Science*, **58**, 26–34.

Further reading

Raadsma, H. W. (2000) Genetic aspects of resistance to ovine footrot. In *Breeding for Disease Resistance in Farm Animals*. Eds. Axford, R.F.E., Bishop, S.C., Nicholas, F. W. and Owen, J.B. Second Edition. CAB International, Wallingford. pp. 219–241.

Chapter 83

Disinfection and other aspects of disease control

Many infectious diseases of animals are spread not only directly by the infected animal but also indirectly through environmental contamination. Intensive management systems may contribute to the occurrence of enteric and respiratory diseases particularly in young animals. Effective control measures are required to minimize the spread of infectious agents in susceptible animal populations, especially when intensive production systems are used. Vaccination is one of the preferred methods for preventing infectious diseases caused by specific pathogens. However, many major diseases cannot as yet be controlled by vaccination. In addition, some 'complex' diseases of mixed or uncertain aetiology cannot be controlled by this method.

Measures for the control of infectious diseases in domestic animals include accurate identification of individual animals and restrictions on their movement either into a country or within a country. Following an outbreak of an infectious disease, isolation of infected and in-contact animals is used to limit spread. If the disease is exotic or subject to a national eradication programme, laboratory testing of clinically affected animals is followed by slaughter of infected and in-contact animals. For endemic infectious diseases, vaccination, disinfection, chemotherapy and chemoprophylaxis are employed selectively depending on the aetiological agents and the methods applicable for their control. In most countries, the control measures applied to a particular disease relate to its status within the country, its economic importance both nationally and internationally, and its public health significance. Preventive, treatment and control measures appropriate for particular infectious agents are presented in Table 83.1.

Despite the availability of a wide range of chemotherapeutic drugs and a large number of effective veterinary vaccines, infectious diseases still cause substantial losses in animal populations worldwide. In addition to losses as a result of mortality, there are costs arising from decreased productivity of meat, milk and eggs, reproductive failure and treatment programmes. Infected animals frequently shed pathogenic microorganisms, often in large numbers and the resulting environmental contamination is an important method of transmitting infection to healthy animals (Fig. 83.1). Salmonellosis, paratuberculosis, leptospirosis and parvovirus and rotavirus infections are examples of diseases in which extensive environmental contamination occurs.

Movement of animals for sale, breeding, restocking or competitive events often contributes to the spread of infectious agents. In addition to sick animals exhibiting clinical signs, subclinically affected animals may shed infectious agents. Carrier animals, which appear clinically normal can also shed pathogens intermittently. The role of animal feeds in disease transmission has become a topic of international importance following the unexpected appearance and persistence of bovine spongiform encephalopathy (BSE) in British cattle. The recognition of the extreme resistance of the agent of BSE to thermal and chemical inactivation renders recycling food of animal origin, especially if derived from ruminants, an undesirable practice.

Survival of infectious agents in the environment

Infectious agents shed in excretions or secretions of animals, or present in products of animal origin, may remain viable for long periods in the environment. Buildings, transport vehicles, soil, pasture, water and fomites may become contaminated by the faeces or urine of infected animals containing bacterial or viral pathogens.

Considerable variation in the survival times of animal pathogens under defined environmental conditions is recorded (Fig. 83.2). Survival times, however, are influenced by many factors including the number of infectious agents excreted by an infected animal, the availability of nutrients, competition from other microorganisms and other microenvironmental factors such as the type and amount of organic matter present, temperature, pH, humidity and exposure to ultraviolet light.

Lability in the environment is a feature of mycoplasmas, many enveloped viruses and spirochaetes. Because of their stability in the environment, pathogenic mycobacteria, salmonellae, fungal spores and parvoviruses remain viable in faeces, soil or contaminated buildings for many months and, in favourable circumstances, some of these pathogens may survive for more than one year (Quinn and Markey, 2001). Prions and bacterial endospores exhibit exceptional resistance to environmental factors. Scrapie-infected hamster brain homogenates

Table 83.1 Methods for the prevention, treatment and control of particular infectious agents.

Infectious agent	Disease/Hosts	Methods					Comments
		Movement[a] restriction	Vector control	Chemotherapy	Disinfection	Vaccination	
Bacillus anthracis	Anthrax/many species	+	−	+	++	++	Endospores survive for many years in soil; vaccination is permitted where disease is endemic
Streptococcus equi	Strangles/ horses	+	−	+	++	±	Efficacy of vaccines uncertain
Clostridium tetani	Tetanus/many species	−	−	+	±	++	Endospores of *C. tetani* are widely distributed in soil and in faeces of animals
Microsporum canis	Ringworm/ many species	+	−	++	+	−	*M. canis* is transmitted by direct and indirect contact
Histoplasma capsulatum	Histoplasmosis /many species	−	−	++	+	−	Soil-borne fungus which causes opportunistic infections
Foot-and-mouth disease virus	Foot-and-mouth disease/ many species	++	−	−	++	+	Vaccination is permitted where disease is endemic. Vaccinal strain must match field strain and duration of protection is limited
African swine fever virus	African swine fever/pigs	++	++	−	++	−	Soft ticks of the genus *Ornithodoros* are vectors of the virus.

++ effective method
+ effective under defined conditions
a exclusion from a country, quarantine or
   restriction of movement on affected farm

− not applicable
± of questionable value

mixed with soil and packed in perforated petri dishes retained infectivity for more than 3 years when buried in soil (Brown and Gajdusek, 1991). The endospores of *Bacillus anthracis* are considered to be among the most resistant microbial forms encountered in soil. Annual soil sampling on an island off the coast of Scotland, where endospores of *B. anthracis* were released in 1942 during biological weapons trials in World War II, showed that endospore numbers were declining slowly (Manchee *et al.*, 1994). More than 40 years after their release viable endospores were demonstrable in the top layer of soil. A solution of formaldehyde in seawater was used to decontaminate the island.

Thermal inactivation of microbial pathogens

Infectious agents vary widely in their susceptibility to thermal inactivation (Fig. 83.3). Although both moist and dry heat can be used for inactivating microorganisms, moist heat is more effective and requires less time to achieve inactivation than dry heat. Many vegetative bacteria are killed in less than 20 seconds by heating at 72°C. At temperatures above 80°C, most vegetative bacteria are killed within seconds. Bacterial endospores are remarkably thermostable and moist heat at 121°C for at least 15 minutes is required for their destruction. Many viruses are labile at temperatures close to 70°C. Canine parvovirus is a notable exception; a temperature of 100°C for 1 minute is required to inactivate this resistant virus. Foot-and-mouth disease virus in milk can survive pasteurization at 72°C for 15 seconds and further heating at 72°C for 5 minutes (Blackwell and Hyde, 1976). The virus also survives heating at 93°C for 15 seconds in cream. At temperatures close to 100°C, more than 20 minutes may be required to inactivate this resistant virus in milk (Walker *et al.*, 1984). Heat treatment of milk at 148°C for 3 seconds reliably inactivates the virus.

The prions that cause transmissible spongiform encephalopathies are extremely resistant to thermal inactivation. Dry heat at 160°C does not inactivate these agents. Autoclaving at 132°C for 4.5 hours is required for their inactivation.

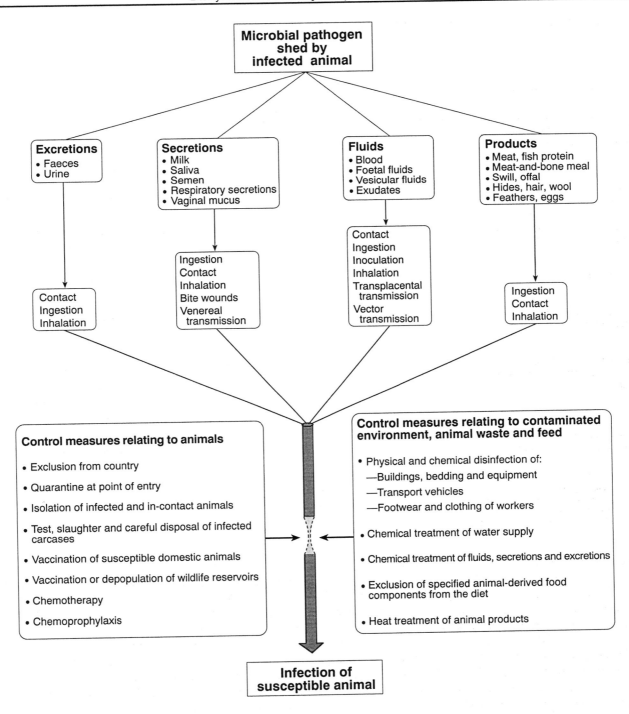

Figure 83.1 Modes of transmission of infectious agents from infected to susceptible animals and relevant control measures.

Disinfection, antisepsis and sterilization

There are a number of well-defined measures which can be applied for the prevention and control of infectious diseases within a country or in regions of a country. These include exclusion of susceptible animals, quarantine at point of entry and isolation and slaughter of infected animals if exotic disease is confirmed by clinical or laboratory tests. When infectious diseases are endemic in a country, control measures include vaccination, chemotherapy and chemoprophylaxis (Fig. 83.1, Box 83.1). During the implementation of disease eradication programmes, vaccination may be permitted alongside a slaughter policy in some circumstances. Effective control measures relating to the environment, animal waste and animal products are central to the success of disease

Infectious agent   **Estimated survival time**

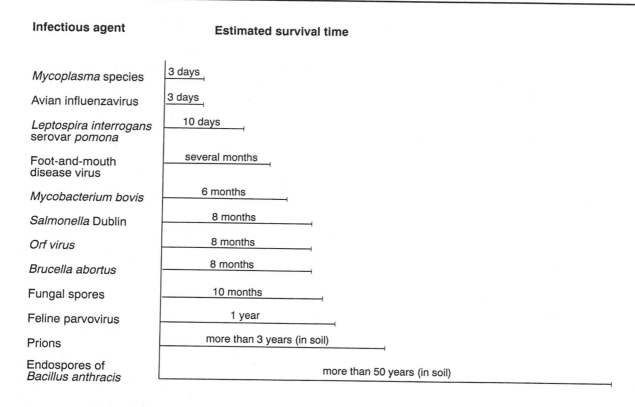

Figure 83.2 Estimated survival times of microbial pathogens under favourable environmental conditions

eradication programmes (Fig. 83.1, Box 83.2). Chemical decontamination can be used for buildings, equipment, transport vehicles, footwear and clothing. Heat treatment of milk, milk products and waste food of animal origin such as swill, and chemical treatment of fluids, secretions and excretions are also essential for effective disease control.

Disinfection implies the use of physical or chemical methods for the destruction of microorganisms, especially potential pathogens on the surfaces of inanimate objects or in the environment. Antisepsis can be defined as the destruction or inhibition of microorganisms on living tissues by chemicals which are non-toxic and non-irritating for the tissues. Disinfectants and antiseptics differ fundamentally from systemically-active chemotherapeutic agents in that they exhibit minimal selective toxicity. Most chemicals used as disinfectants are toxic not only for microbial pathogens but also for host cells. Disinfectants, therefore, are used only to reduce the microbial population on inanimate surfaces or in organic materials, whereas antiseptics can be applied topically to living tissues.

Because of the great diversity of microbial pathogens, complete destruction of bacteria, fungi and viruses by sterilization, requires carefully controlled conditions. Steam under pressure generating a temperature of 121°C for 20 minutes, dry heat at 160°C for 2 hours or ionizing radiation (gamma radiation) effectively inactivate conventional microbial pathogens. Glutaraldehyde and peracetic

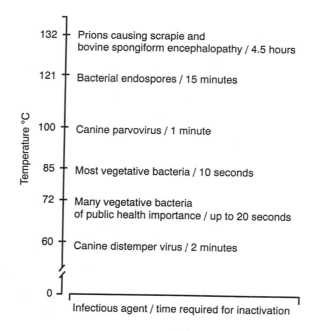

Figure 83.3 Thermal inactivation of infectious agents by moist heat. The number of infectious agents initially present influences the time required for inactivation. The system used to determine survival or inactivation may alter the reliability of the results. The temperature and time for inactivation of prions is not yet clearly established.

Box 83.1 Strategies for the prevention, treatment or control of infectious diseases in animal populations.

- Exclusion of animals from a country or continent
- Quarantine of imported animals at point of entry
- Accurate identification of farm animals, especially ruminants, using ear tags or microchip implantation; colour markings can be used for horse identification while dogs and cats may require detailed written descriptions with accompanying photographs
- Isolation of infected or in-contact animals on the farm of origin or on the premises being inspected
- Exclusion of animal-derived food components from the diet of ruminants
- Clinical or laboratory confirmation of exotic infectious disease followed by slaughter and careful disposal of infected carcases
- Vaccination of susceptible domestic animals before exposure to possible sources of endemic or exotic diseases
- Either vaccination or depopulation of wildlife reservoirs depending on the importance of the disease and the feasibility of implementing control measures
- Chemotherapy for animals with endemic disease
- Chemoprophylaxis for prevention of predictable infectious disease in animal populations when vaccination is either impractical or ineffective

acid at specified concentrations are used as sterilizing agents. Sterilization methods, which require strict adherence to well defined procedures, are used for surgical instruments, fluids for systemic administration, media for culture of microorganisms and for inactivation of microbial pathogens in specimens submitted for laboratory identification. In contrast, disinfection is a less exact method used for decontaminating buildings, equipment, transport vehicles, footwear and clothing.

Characteristics, modes of action and selection of chemical disinfectants

Although a number of potentially useful physical methods including dry and moist heat, ionizing radiation and mechanical methods may be used for disinfection in the laboratory, at farm level, in clinical facilities and in locations where animals are assembled for sporting events or for sale, chemical disinfection procedures find wider application than physical methods.

Many chemicals with antimicrobial activity can be used for the inactivation of microbial pathogens in buildings, stockyards, transport vehicles and on equipment. Chemicals used include acids, alkalis, alcohols, aldehydes, halogens, phenols and quaternary ammonium compounds.

Characteristics of an ideal disinfectant are presented in Box 83.3. None of the currently available compounds possess all of these characteristics. Selection of a disinfectant agent should be based on its spectrum of activity, its efficacy, and its susceptibility to inactivation by organic matter. Additional considerations include compatibility with soaps and detergents, toxicity for personnel and animals, contact time required, optimal temperature, residual activity, corrosiveness, effects on the environment and cost.

Selection and use of a disinfectant requires consideration of the infectious agents likely to be present and the conditions prevailing in the location where microbial contamination has occurred. If the pathogen that caused the disease outbreak has been identified, a disinfectant with known activity against that agent should be selected (Table 83.2). The activity of complex disinfectants may vary in accordance with their formulation, and the efficacy of individual compounds listed in Table 83.2 relates to their use under ideal conditions. Before the application of a disinfectant, surfaces should be thoroughly cleaned. This physical procedure, if properly carried out, removes a high percentage of accessible infectious agents. Staff training and proper supervision is essential for the successful implementation of a cleaning and disinfection programme. Effective cleaning should always precede disinfection of buildings, with the exception of those that have housed animals with major zoonotic diseases such as anthrax,

Infectious agents vary in their susceptibility to the chemical disinfectants (Fig. 83.4). Most vegetative bacteria and enveloped viruses are readily inactivated by disinfectants; fungal spores and non-enveloped viruses are less susceptible. Mycobacteria and bacterial endospores are resistant to many commonly used disinfectants. Prions are extremely resistant to chemical inactivation. High concentrations of sodium hypochlorite or heated strong solutions of sodium hydroxide are reported to inactivate these unconventional infectious agents.

Box 83.2 Control measures relating to the environment, animal waste and animal products.

- Chemical disinfection of:
  — buildings, bedding and equipment
  — transport vehicles
  — footwear and clothing of workers
- Chemical treatment of water supply following disinfection of building.
- Chemical treatment of fluids, excretions, secretions.
- Heat treatment of milk and milk products; mandatory boiling of waste food if swill feeding to pigs is permitted.

Box 83.3 Characteristics of an ideal chemical disinfectant.

- Broad antimicrobial spectrum with activity at low concentrations against vegetative bacteria, (including mycobacteria), bacterial endospores, fungal spores, enveloped and non-enveloped viruses and prions
- Absence of irritancy, toxicity, teratogenicity, mutagenicity and carcinogenicity
- Stability with a long shelf life at ambient temperatures
- Solubility in water to the concentration required for effective antimicrobial activity
- Compatibility with a wide range of chemicals including acids, alkalis, anionic and cationic compounds
- Retention of activity in the presence of organic matter
- Absence of corrosiveness or chemical interactions with metals or other structural materials
- Retention of antimicrobial activity over a wide range of temperatures
- Absence of tainting or toxicity after topical use in food-producing animals and following application to surfaces or equipment in dairies, meat plants or food preparation areas
- Moderately priced and readily available
- Non-polluting for ground water and biodegradable

Chemicals used as disinfectants in veterinary medicine

The modes of action of antibacterial disinfectants are illustrated in Fig. 83.5. Interactions with the bacterial cell wall, cytoplasmic membrane, nucleic acid and other cytoplasmic constituents have been demonstrated for some disinfectants (Hugo, 1999). Virucidal disinfectants may react with nucleic acid, structural or functional proteins, glycoproteins or, in the case of enveloped viruses, with the lipid envelope.

Acids

The antimicrobial activity of acids is related to the pH achieved and their modes of action is often uncertain. Acidic conditions tend to inhibit the growth of micro-organisms and many organic acids have been used as preservatives in the food industry.

Viruses show wide variation in their susceptibility to acids. Citric acid and phosphoric acid inactivate the virus of foot-and-mouth disease. Swine vesicular disease virus, however, is not inactivated by phosphoric acid. Peracetic acid, a strong oxidizing agent, is bactericidal, fungicidal, sporicidal and virucidal. Hydrochloric acid at 2.5% concentration has been used for inactivating the endospores of *Bacillus anthracis* on hides. Because they

are corrosive and also hazardous for workers, mineral acids such as sulphuric acid and hydrochloric acid have limited roles in disinfection programmes. In food processing industries, mineral acids are used extensively as cleaning agents for removing lime scale, milk stone and other alkaline deposits in pipes, milking machines and on surfaces. The choice of chemical is determined by the ability of the materials being treated to withstand acidity.

Alcohols

Of the many alcohols with antimicrobial activity, only two, ethyl alcohol and isopropyl alcohol, are widely used as disinfectants. The presence of water is essential for their antimicrobial activity. The most effective concentration of ethyl alcohol is approximately 70%. Alcohols exhibit rapid antimicrobial activity against vegetative bacteria, including mycobacteria, fungi and some viruses. They are not sporicidal and small, non-enveloped viruses are resistant.

Alcohols are often used alone; sometimes they are combined with other antimicrobial compounds such as chlorhexidine. In comparison with other disinfectants, alcohols are inexpensive, relatively non-toxic, non-tainting and colourless. Dried organic matter on surfaces interferes with the action of alcohols. Because they evaporate readily, they exert no residual effects following topical application. Due to their flammability, alcohols should be stored away from heat and should not be applied to surfaces close to naked flames.

Aldehydes

As a group, aldehydes are highly reactive chemicals that interact with protein, nucleic acid and other constituents of bacteria, fungi and viruses. Two aldehydes, formaldehyde and glutaraldehyde are widely used as disinfectants. Formaldehyde is a monoaldehyde that exists as a gas which is freely soluble in water. Formaldehyde solution (formalin), is an aqueous solution containing approximately 38% formaldehyde (w/w) with methyl alcohol added to delay polymerization. Glutaraldehyde is a dialdehyde with high microbiocidal activity against vegetative bacteria, fungal spores, bacterial endospores, and both enveloped and non-enveloped viruses.

Although glutaraldehyde is stable at acid pH, it is more active at alkaline pH values (approximately 7.5 to 8.5). Its activity is also enhanced by elevated temperatures. Glutaraldehyde is non-corrosive and usually does not damage rubber or plastic components. The antimicrobial activity of glutaraldehyde is affected minimally by the presence of organic matter. Even at low levels, glutaraldehyde vapour is irritating for the eyes and mucous membranes. Some workers exposed to glutaraldehyde develop allergic contact dermatitis, asthma and rhinitis.

Formaldehyde, which has a wide antimicrobial spectrum, acts more slowly than glutaraldehyde. It is used as an aqueous solution and also as a gas for fumigation of

Table 83.2 The antimicrobial spectrum of chemical disinfectants[a].

Disinfectant	Microbial Pathogens							
	Bacteria				Fungi Spores	Viruses		Prions
	Gram- positive	Gram- negative	Myco- bacteria	Endo- spores		Enveloped	Non-Enveloped	
Acids (mineral)	++	+	−	±	±	+	±[b]	−
Alcohols	++	++	++	−	+	+	−	−
Aldehydes	++	++	+	++	++	++	++	−
Alkalis	++	++	+	+	+	+	±[b]	±[c]
Biguanides	++	+	−	−	+	+	−	−
Halogens								
Chlorine compounds	++	++	+	+	+	++	++	±[d]
Iodine compounds	++	++	+	+	+	++	+	−
Peroxygen compounds								
Hydrogen peroxide	++	++	±	+	+	++	±	−
Peracetic acid	++	++	++	++	++	++	+	−
Phenolic compounds	++	++	+	−	+	+	−	−
Quaternary ammonium compounds	++	+	−	−	+	+	−	−

++ highly effective
+ effective
± limited activity
− no activity

a the antimicrobial activity of complex disinfectants may vary in accordance with their formulation. The data presented relate to the use of chemical compounds at appropriate concentrations under ideal conditions.
b acids and alkalis inactivate the virus of foot-and-mouth disease
c hot 1M NaOH is reported to be effective
d high chlorine concentrations are required for inactivation

buildings and equipment. When used for fumigation, a temperature close to 14°C and relative humidity near 70% is required for optimal efficiency. For fumigation of buildings, gas can be generated by heating paraformaldehyde or by adding formalin to potassium permanganate crystals.

Apart from its use as a disinfectant, formaldehyde is used in the preparation of veterinary vaccines and also in footbaths to prevent or treat foot lameness in cattle and sheep. Even at low levels, the irritating vapour and pungent odour of formaldehyde is evident. The use of formaldehyde as a broad-spectrum antimicrobial agent is declining due to its ability to sensitize workers, its known toxicity and its potential carcinogenicity.

Alkalis

Many microbial pathogens are susceptible to high pH values. Sodium hydroxide and potassium hydroxide are used extensively for cleaning surfaces, especially when grease and tissue debris are present. At high concentrations, these caustic alkalis have marked micro-biocidal properties. Caustic alkali solutions are effective against many viruses including foot-and-mouth disease virus, adenoviruses and swine vesicular disease virus. Although sodium carbonate at a 4% concentration is used primarily as a cleaning agent, it is particularly effective against the virus of foot-and-mouth disease.

Both sodium hydroxide and potassium hydroxide are corrosive for metals especially aluminium. Eye protection,

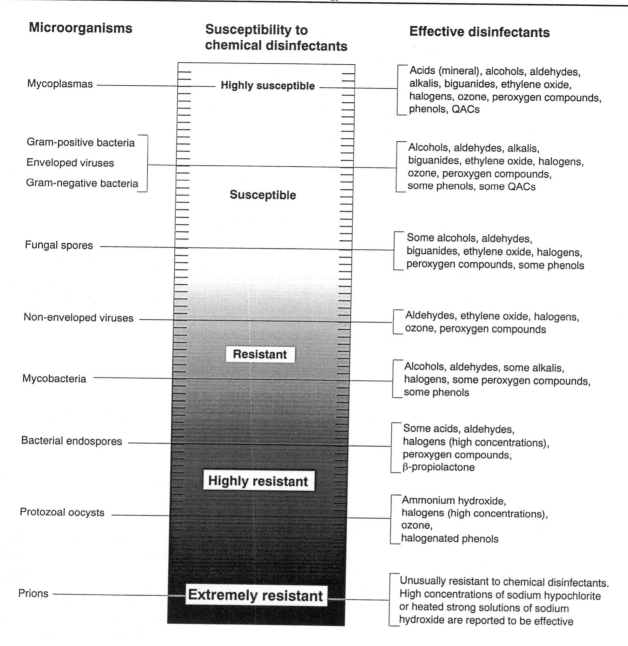

Figure 83.4 Microorganisms ranked according to their relative susceptibility to chemical disinfectants. The composition and concentration of the disinfectant together with the presence of organic matter, the ambient temperature and the contact time influence the effectiveness of the disinfection procedure. QACs, quaternary ammonium compounds.

rubber gloves and protective clothing should be worn by workers using caustic alkalis. At appropriate concentrations, sodium hydroxide has a wide antimicrobial spectrum including endospores. The reported susceptibility of prions to treatment with 1M NaOH at a temperature of 100°C is of importance because these unconventional agents resist most standard chemical decontamination procedures (Taylor, 2001). Ammonium hydroxide, a weak base, has marked activity against coccidial oocysts which resist inactivation by the majority of standard disinfectants.

At concentrations as low as 1% this compound has potent antibacterial activity.

Biguanides

The most important member of this group of cationic compounds is chlorhexidine which is widely used for handwashing and preoperative skin preparation. Although available as a dihydrochloride and diacetate, chlorhexidine gluconate is frequently used as it is the most water-soluble preparation. Its activity is reduced by the presence of

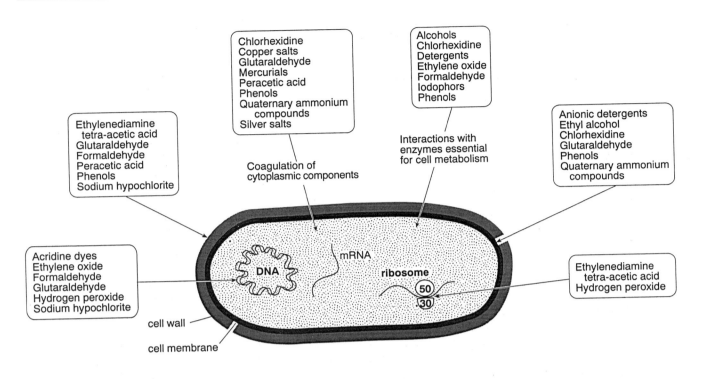

Figure 83.5 Sites of interaction or changes induced in cytoplasmic components of a bacterial cell by chemicals with antibacterial activity.

organic matter and it is incompatible with anionic detergents and inorganic anionic compounds. It is more active at alkaline than acid pH values.

Chlorhexidine is more active against Gram-positive bacteria than Gram-negative bacteria. Some Gram-negative bacteria, particularly *Pseudomonas* species and *Proteus* species, may be resistant to low concentrations of chlorhexidine gluconate. It has limited fungicidal activity. This biguanide is neither mycobactericidal nor sporicidal. Although it may be active against some enveloped viruses, the antiviral activity of chlorhexidine is variable and it cannot be considered as a reliable virucide.

Alcoholic chlorhexidine solutions are superior to aqueous solutions. Toxicity arising from absorption through the skin has not been demonstrated for this compound. Because it has longer residual activity on teat skin than many other disinfectants, chlorhexidine is used extensively in teat dips for mastitis control programmes in dairy cattle.

Halogen compounds

Compounds of chlorine and iodine are widely used as disinfectants and antiseptics. In addition to their long-established place in water treatment, chlorine and chlorine-releasing compounds are used extensively in food processing industries. Iodine-based compounds are also used in food processing and as teat dips in the dairy industry.

Chlorine compounds

Sodium hypochlorite, chlorine dioxide, chloramine T and dichloroisocyanurate are the chlorine compounds most widely used as disinfectants. In aqueous solutions, most chlorine compounds with disinfectant activity release hypochlorous acid which is considered to be the active principle. These disinfectants are most effective at pH values below 7 and the optimum pH for hypochlorites is close to pH 5.

Hypochlorites, which are extensively used in veterinary medicine, are potent virucides and are also mycobactericidal and sporicidal. When used at high concentrations, they are reported to inactivate prions gradually. Chlorination, a standard water treatment for preventing the spread of infectious disease, is generally considered to be safe, although concern has been expressed recently about the safety of water chlorination because trihalomethanes have been detected in treated water. Trihalomethanes are reported to be carcinogenic in laboratory animals.

Sodium hypochlorite is fast-acting, non-staining and inexpensive. Its general use, however, is limited by its corrosive effects and its relative instability. The two most important factors limiting the biocidal activity of hypochlorites are the presence of organic matter and the neutralization of hypochlorous acid by alkaline substances. Low levels of chlorine compounds are ineffective as disinfectants when used in dirty environments. The stability of free available chlorine in solution depends on chlorine concentration, pH, presence of organic matter and exposure to light. Because of their instability, hypochlorites can lose up to 50% of their concentration within one month if stored in open containers.

Environmental risks arising from the use of chlorine-based products appear to be limited. Advantages of these disinfectants over other compounds include low toxicity at effective concentrations, ease of use and relatively low cost.

Iodine compounds

Although they are less chemically reactive than chlorine compounds, iodine compounds are more active in the presence of organic matter. Iodine compounds are available as aqueous solutions, tinctures and iodophors. Despite its low solubility, iodine was formerly used as an aqueous solution. When dissolved in ethyl alcohol (tincture of iodine) high levels of free iodine were obtained. Disadvantages of using iodine solutions include instability, staining of skin and fabrics, toxicity and skin irritation. Inorganic iodine has been largely replaced by iodophors in which iodine is complexed with surface-active compounds or polymers that allow both increased solubility and sustained release of free iodine. When complexed, free iodine levels are limited and the disadvantages of using aqueous and alcoholic solutions are avoided. In many iodophor preparations, the carrier is a non-ionic surfactant and the iodine is present as micellar aggregates. An iodophor in which iodine is complexed with polvinylpyrrolidone, referred to as povidone-iodine, is commonly used. Because the amount of free iodine in an iodophor solution depends on the concentration used, more concentrated solutions have less antimicrobial activity than diluted solutions. The increased antimicrobial activity of dilute solutions reflects the level of free iodine present. For maximum antimicrobial effect, iodophor solutions should be diluted in accordance with manufacturers' instructions.

Iodophors have a broad range of antimicrobial activity when used at appropriate dilutions and at pH values below 5. They are bactericidal, fungicidal and virucidal. Some non-enveloped viruses are less sensitive than enveloped viruses to iodophors. Reports of prolonged survival of *Pseudomonas aeruginosa* and *Burkholderia cepacia* in povidone-iodine solution have been attributed to the presence of organic matter, inorganic material or biofilm formation on items being treated.

Iodophors retain much of their antimicrobial activity in the presence of organic matter and are effective at both low and high temperatures. In many countries iodophors are the most common teat dips used. Acidic iodophor solutions are widely used as sanitizers in the dairy industry and in the food industry.

Peroxygen compounds

Hydrogen peroxide, peracetic acid and ozone are powerful oxidizing agents with broad antimicrobial spectra. The characteristics of each compound determine their usefulness as disinfectants in veterinary medicine.

Hydrogen peroxide is a non-polluting compound which decomposes to oxygen and water. Because hydrogen peroxide solutions are unstable, benzoic acid or other suitable substances are usually added as stabilizers. This oxidizing agent is bactericidal, fungicidal, virucidal and, at high concentrations, sporicidal. However, its activity against mycobacteria is questionable. Greater activity is evident against Gram-positive bacteria than Gram-negative bacteria. The presence of catalase or other peroxidases in some bacteria can increase their tolerance to low levels of hydrogen peroxide. Formation of hydroxyl radicals, which react with cell components including lipids, protein and nucleic acid, account for the antimicrobial activity of this compound. In addition to its use as a disinfectant and antiseptic, hydrogen peroxide is used in the food industry for aseptic packaging.

Peracetic acid, a strong oxidizing agent which is more potent than hydrogen peroxide, retains its activity in the presence of organic matter. It is lethal for bacteria, including mycobacteria, fungi, algae, endospores and viruses but it may be hazardous to handle. It can corrode steel, copper and other metals; natural and synthetic rubber are also affected. Concern has been expressed about the safety of peracetic acid as it may have carcinogenic properties.

Ozone (O_3) an allotropic form of oxygen, has strong oxidizing properties. It is bactericidal, virucidal and sporicidal. Ozone is sometimes used for disinfection of water because it can react with protein and nucleic acids.

Phenolic compounds

Phenols are widely used as disinfectants and sometimes as preservatives. These general purpose disinfectants have marked antibacterial activity but are not sporicidal. Activity is dependent on the particular formulation used. Phenol, the original standard against which many disinfectants were compared, is rarely used today for its antibacterial properties. Formerly, most of the phenolic compounds used for the manufacture of disinfectants were obtained by distillation of coal. Today, many phenolic compounds are synthesized. Simple and substituted phenols constitute a complex group of chemicals. Because of differences in formulation, generalizations concerning the antimicrobial activity of phenolic compounds are inappropriate. The antimicrobial activity of phenolic disinfectants depends on the exact formulation and concentration of each active constituent.

At recommended concentrations (usually above 2%), many phenolic compounds are considered to be bactericidal, tuberculocidal and fungicidal. They are not sporicidal and their activity against viruses is unpredictable; some enveloped viruses may be susceptible, whereas non-enveloped viruses may be resistant. *Ortho*-phenylphenol, an effective phenolic compound with less toxic and corrosive activity than many other phenols, is active against mycobacteria and many animal viruses.

Phenolic compounds are usually inexpensive and not seriously affected by the presence of organic matter. Contact with the skin should be avoided because of the irritation and depigmentation produced by some compounds. Pigs and cats are particularly susceptible to the toxic effects of phenolic disinfectants. Because they impart a tarry odour and leave a residual film on surfaces that can cause tainting of food and agricultural products, phenolic compounds should not be used in meat plants and dairies or for disinfecting surfaces or containers which come into direct contact with food for human consumption.

Quaternary ammonium compounds

These cationic compounds have surface-active properties but they are incompatible with soaps and other anionic compounds. Because they are non-staining, odourless, non-toxic and usually non-corrosive they are used extensively as disinfectants in food processing industries. Quaternary ammonium compounds (QACs) are most effective at neutral or slightly alkaline pH values. Their antimicrobial activity appears to result from the disruption of the cell membrane, inactivation of enzymes and denaturation of proteins (Fig. 83.5). They should be applied to clean surfaces as their activity is reduced by organic matter such as faeces, blood and milk.

This group of compounds have a limited antimicrobial spectrum and are moderately expensive. They exhibit greater activity against Gram-positive than Gram-negative bacteria. Some Gram-negative bacteria such as *Pseudomonas* species and *Serratia marcescens* can survive and grow in solutions of QAC. One of the most commonly used members of this group is benzalkonium chloride which is bactericidal and fungicidal. Quaternary ammonium compounds are neither sporicidal nor mycobactericidal. Although some of these compounds have activity against enveloped viruses, non-enveloped viruses are resistant and, as a group, they are considered unreliable as virucides.

Ethyl alcohol potentiates the action of QACs. Dilute solutions of these compounds are used as antiseptics for preoperative preparation of the skin and mucous membranes. High concentrations can cause skin irritation. Apart from organic matter and soaps, material such as gauze pads and cotton can reduce the microbiocidal activity of QACs.

Microbial resistance to disinfection

Resistance of bacteria and fungi to disinfectants may be intrinsic or acquired. In many instances, intrinsic resistance relates to the impermeability of microbial structures to individual disinfectants. Components of the cell wall of Gram-negative bacteria, particularly the outer membrane may prevent uptake of quaternary ammonium compounds. Bacterial endospores exhibit a high degree of resistance to many chemical compounds. This intrinsic resistance is attributed to the spore coats and other structures which prevent entry of many commonly used disinfectants. Some bacterial pathogens appear to have the inherent ability to breakdown chlorhexidine and this form of resistance is reported to be chromosomally mediated. The basis of the extreme resistance of prions to the majority of chemical disinfectants is poorly understood. The agents of bovine spongiform encephalopathy and scrapie are considered to be composed of abnormally-folded proteins which exhibit marked thermal stability and, in addition, they are minimally affected by the majority of standard disinfectants at concentrations effective against bacteria, viruses and fungi. They are reported to be inactivated by high concentrations of sodium hypochlorite and by hot 1M NaOH. Acquired bacterial resistance to antiseptics and disinfectants resembles that which occurs with antimicrobial therapeutic drugs. Mutations, plasmids or transposons are the usual methods whereby some bacteria acquire resistance to disinfectants. Plasmid-encoded resistance may relate to decreased uptake of disinfectants, their inactivation, or their elimination by efflux mechanisms. Gram-negative bacteria from environments where disinfectants are in constant use, tend to be less sensitive to these compounds than bacteria isolated from other locations. Selection and mutation may account for some of the observed resistance in these instances. Fungal resistance to disinfectants may be intrinsic or acquired but little is known about the underlying mechanisms.

Disinfection procedures

The correct choice of disinfectant is fundamental to the success of a disinfection programme. For optimal activity, disinfectants should be used at the correct concentration and allowed sufficient contact time with the surfaces or equipment. Thorough cleaning of all surfaces before application of disinfectant is essential for the inactivation of infectious agents as the antimicrobial activity of many chemical compounds is seriously impaired by residual organic matter such as faeces, blood, exudates, food and bedding. Moderate amounts of organic matter interferes with the activity of halogen disinfectants, particularly sodium hypochlorite, whereas phenolic disinfectants retain much of their activity under similar conditions.

A high pressure washer set at low pressure can be used

Chapter 84

Infection and immunity

Protection against infectious agents is a fundamental requirement for survival. Without such protection, animals would be overwhelmed rapidly by a variety of opportunistic infections of environmental origin. Pathogenic microbial agents pose an even greater threat to the survival of susceptible animals. To counter these infectious threats, animals, both avian and mammalian, have evolved elaborate defence mechanisms which offer some immediate protection against invasion by micro-organisms.

The first barrier to infection which offers a rapid, non-discriminating response is termed innate or non-specific immunity. After the animal encounters an infectious agent, lymphocytes which interact with the invading pathogen undergo functional changes. They proliferate and secrete soluble factors which promote the involvement of other cells of the immune system in an attempt to contain the infection. This response is referred to as a specific immune response. Moreover, following an encounter with a microbial pathogen, the body's immune system learns from the experience by responding in a specific manner to the pathogen and by 'remembering' the interaction. Immunological memory resides in lymphocytes which are produced in the course of a response to an infectious agent and these cells react quickly to subsequent invasion by the same agent. The immune system, which is composed of specific and non-specific components, is a remarkable array of structures, cells and secretions which is at its most advanced form in higher vertebrates (Fig. 84.1). It provides effective protection against a vast array of actual or potential pathogens present in the immediate environment of animals. Immune responses are not confined to infectious agents, and by responding to innocuous substances such as pollens, foreign proteins and some therapeutic drugs, potentially destructive hypersensitivity reactions can develop. Although the primary activity of the immune system is usually considered to be associated with protection against infectious agents, it has a distinct role to play in immune surveillance, whereby neoplastic tissue changes can be detected and, in some instances, eliminated by immune mechanisms. Soon after birth, the external surfaces of the body, extensive portions of the alimentary tract and regions of the respiratory tract become colonized by bacteria. The host and colonizing bacteria live in a relatively peaceful state of coexistence, with micro-organisms restricted to parts of the body where they can be tolerated and microbial invasion of tissues prevented by natural antibacterial defence mechanisms. Bacteria which colonize many parts of the body without producing disease

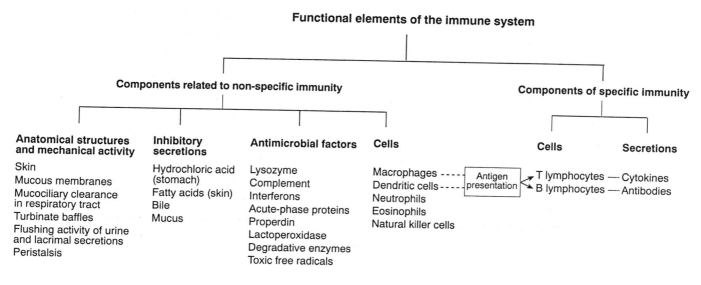

Figure 84.1 Anatomical structures, cells and secretions which form the functional elements of the immune system.

constitute part of the normal flora. This harmonious relationship between animals and their environment can be reinforced by good management systems, optimal nutrition, adequate floor space and effective disease control programmes (Fig. 84.2). Negative factors which can tilt the balance in favour of potential or actual pathogens include overcrowding, uncontrolled environmental temperature, nutritional imbalances and absence of a disease control programme. Even if bacteria, fungi or viruses succeed in entering the tissues and causing infection, disease is not an inevitable outcome. Characteristics of the infectious agent, environmental influences and the susceptibility of the infected animal usually determine the outcome of infection. If infection is not quickly eliminated, clinical disease or subclinical infection is the likely result (Fig. 84.3).

Normal flora

Soon after birth, neonatal animals are exposed through contact, ingestion or inhalation to microorganisms present on the dam. Bacteria, yeasts and perhaps other microorganisms from the animal's immediate environment may colonize particular sites on the skin and regions of the alimentary, respiratory or urogenital tracts. Microorganisms that compete successfully for particular

sites gradually form a stable normal flora. Different regions of the body may have a distinctive resident flora suggesting that regional colonization may reflect a selective advantage on the part of successful microorganisms. The ability to survive acidic conditions in the alimentary tract or tolerance for some naturally-occurring antimicrobial factors confers particular survival capabilities on some resident flora. Adherence to host cells or elaboration of metabolic substances antagonistic to competitors may enhance colonization of the skin, mucous membranes or parts of the alimentary tract by some bacteria and by yeasts. There is evidence that the normal flora can compete with and sometimes prevent establishment of pathogenic microorganisms. This may be achieved by competition for nutrients, formation of inhibitory substances or by attachment to receptors on cell surfaces, thereby preventing colonization by invading pathogens. Although the normal flora is not directly associated with non-specific immunity, their competitive role can be considered beneficial for the host. In addition, normal flora may gently challenge the naive immune system of young animals at an early age thereby preparing them for subsequent encounters with virulent pathogens. As the animal matures, the normal flora may play a vital part in digestion, especially in ruminants. In some species, the normal flora may contribute to synthesis of B vitamins

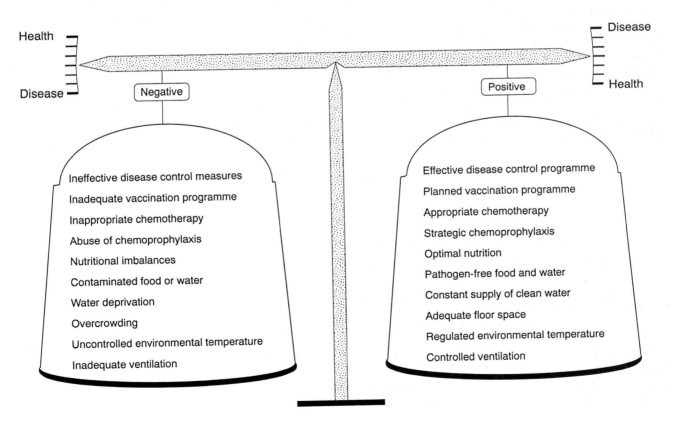

Figure 84.2 The dynamic equilibrium between positive and negative factors which influence the health status of animal populations.

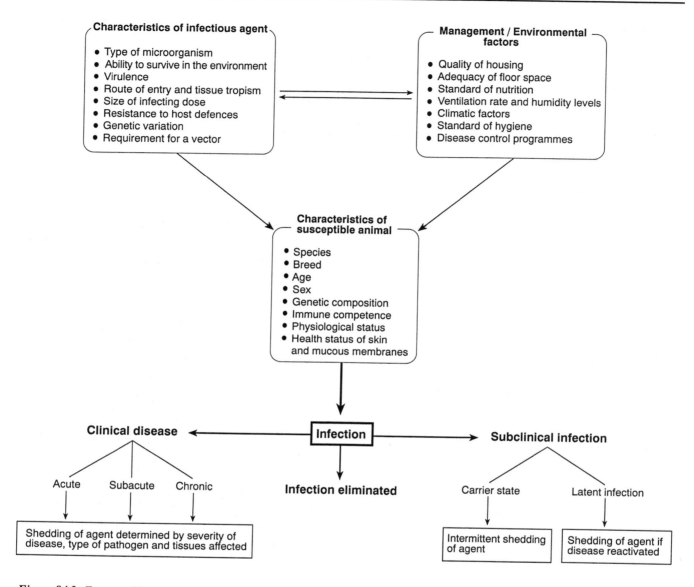

Figure 84.3 Factors which influence host-pathogen interactions and the possible outcome of a primary infection in a surviving animal.

and vitamin K. Prolonged therapy with antimicrobial drugs may interfere with normal intestinal microorganisms, permitting the survival and proliferation of organisms resistant to the drugs used. This can lead to the emergence of resistant strains of bacteria which may replace the normal flora and lead to digestive upsets and disease. In the absence of resident microorganisms in the alimentary tract, overgrowth by the pathogenic yeast, *Candida albicans* can occur leading to tissue invasion.

Comparative aspects of non-specific and specific immunity

During embryological development, myeloid and lymphoid cells arise from a pluripotent stem cell in the bone marrow (Fig. 84.4). Myeloid cells, along with

natural killer cells, are part of non-specific immune defences. From the bloodstream, monocytes migrate to tissues where they become either fixed or free macrophages. Among the polymorphonuclear leukocytes, neutrophils play the most prominent role in combating pyogenic bacterial infections. Polymorphonuclear leukocytes move into tissues from the bloodstream in response to release of soluble factors from damaged host cells. In addition, soluble factors in the blood or in body fluids attract inflammatory cells to developing lesions. Two types of lymphocytes referred to as T lymphocytes and B lymphocytes arise from a lymphoid stem cell in the bone marrow. Following maturation in appropriate tissues, these specialized cells, through their secretions or direct involvement, constitute specific immunity.

Non-specific immunity and specific immunity are

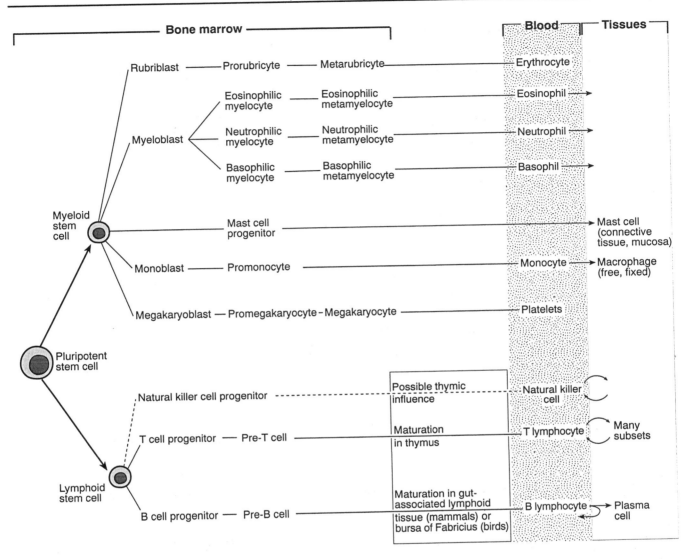

Figure 84.4 Stages in the development of myeloid and lymphoid cells from a pluripotent stem cell in the bone marrow.

compared in Table 84.1. Non-specific resistance to infection which is innate, is demonstrable in both vertebrates and invertebrates. Physical barriers, mechanical action, physiological factors, soluble antimicrobial substances and phagocytic cells contribute to this natural resistance to infection characterized by a rapid response but without a 'memory' for the pathogens encountered. Other factors which can alter susceptibility to microbial pathogens are presented in Box 84.1. Specific immunity, a response to infection which is confined to vertebrates, requires induction either through infection or vaccination. The T and B lymphocytes which participate in this specific response release soluble factors called cytokines. These low molecular weight regulatory proteins or glycoproteins which serve as chemical messengers between cells, are

produced by many cell types especially by subsets of T lymphocytes. Antibodies, which have a high specificity for the infectious agents which induced their formation, are produced by plasma cells which arise from B lymphocytes (Fig. 84.5).

Non-specific immune responses could be considered as the first line of defence against opportunistic pathogens whereas specific immunity, although relatively slow in developing, ultimately produces an effective response to a wide range of virulent microorganisms. Because of the production of memory cells, secondary responses involving B and T lymphocytes are more rapid than primary responses. A comparison of T lymphocytes and B lymphocytes and their roles in specific immune responses is presented in Table 84.2.

Table 84.1 Comparison of non-specific immunity with specific immunity.

Feature	Non-specific immunity	Specific immunity
Occurrence	Vertebrates and invertebrates	Vertebrates only
Induction	Innate	Induced by exposure to pathogens or by vaccination
Physical barriers	Skin, mucous membranes, muco-ciliary clearance, turbinate baffles	—
Mechanical action	Flushing activity of tears and urine, peristalsis	—
Physiological influences	Low pH values on skin, gastric acidity, bile	—
Participating cells	Macrophages, monocytes, poly-morphonuclear leukocytes, natural killer cells, mast cells	T and B lymphocytes (antigen-presenting cells required to initiate some responses)
Principal soluble factors	Complement, lysozymes, interferons, degradative enzymes	Cytokines, antibodies
Rate of response to infection	Moderately fast, minutes to hours	Relatively slow, days to weeks
Immunological memory	Absent	Present
Contribution to body defenses	First line of defence against opportunistic pathogens; offers limited protection against virulent microorganisms	Produces an effective response to a wide range of virulent microorganisms, effectiveness of the response improves with time

Complement

The plasma of animals contains a group of approximately 30 proteins, collectively referred to as the complement system, which play an important role in non-specific immunity and, in addition, amplify specific immune reactions. Complement components participate in many immune reactions ranging from degranulation of mast cells to solubilization of immune complexes. More than 90% of plasma complement components are produced in the liver; some components are synthesized in a number of cell types including monocytes, macrophages, endothelial cells, lymphocytes, glial cells, renal epithelium and intestinal epithelium (Prodinger *et al.*, 1999). With onset of inflammation, plasma levels of complement may increase by a factor of three.

For historical reasons, complement components are numbered from C1 to C9. The biochemical reaction sequence is C1-C4-C2-C3-C5-C6-C7-C8-C9. The nomenclature of complement components is complicated by the number of different proteins involved and by fragments produced in the course of activation of individual components. Additional proteins involved in complement activation are identified by letters, such as B and D. Fragments are designated, according to the component from which they derived, by a lower case letter such as C3b. By convention, smaller fragments are denoted by the letter "a" and larger fragments by the letter "b". When cleavage products form an active complex, such a complex is indicated by a bar over the components. The complex $\overline{C4b, 2a}$ illustrates an important example referred to as C3 convertase.

Activation of the complement system involves a sequential enzyme cascade in which the proenzyme product of one step becomes an enzyme catalyst for the next step. Several molecules of each sequential component are activated causing marked amplification of the response. Following activation, complement components have short half lives. Consequences of complement activation include release of factors which promote inflammatory reactions and lysis of target cells such as mammalian red blood cells, nucleated cells and bacteria.

Two distinct pathways of complement activation are recognized, the classical pathway and the alternative pathway (Fig. 84.6). The classical pathway is activated by an immune complex such as one molecule of IgM or two molecules of IgG bound to a target cell. In plasma, C1 exists as a macromolecular complex composed of C1q, C1r and C1s stabilized by calcium ions. Following formation of the immune complex, C1q binds to the Fc portion of the bound antibody. Binding of C1q activates C1r which, in turn activates C1s. When activated, these three subcomponents form $\overline{C1}$ which then cleaves C4. From the point after which C3 becomes activated, the classical pathway and the alternative pathway merge (Fig. 84.7).

Box 84.1 Factors which can limit colonization by pathogenic bacteria or alter susceptibility to microbial pathogens.

- Competition occurs between normal flora and bacterial or fungal pathogens for nutrients and attachment sites on host cells
- Normal body temperature can render some species resistant to particular pathogens
- Some species of animals are innately resistant to specific microbial pathogens

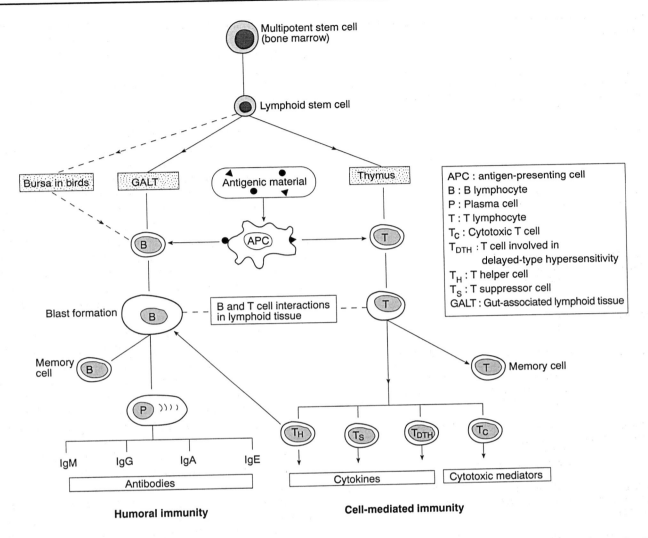

Figure 84.5 Differentiation and maturation of cells of the immune system which participate in cell-mediated and humoral immunity. In birds, lymphoid stem cells which migrate to the bursa of Fabricius differentiate into B cells.

The alternative pathway is activated directly by bacterial cell surfaces, components of infectious agents such as lipopolysaccharide, yeast cell walls and some viruses and virus-infected cells. This method of activating complement is of major importance in non-specific immune responses.

Classical pathway

Details of the classical pathway are illustrated in Fig. 84.7. Following sequential activation of C1q, r, s to generate $C\overline{1}$ (recognition unit), C4 is cleaved by the activated first complement component into $C\overline{4}b$ and C4a. The $C\overline{4}b$ fragment attaches to the target surface in the vicinity of C1. The third subcomponent of C1, C1s, splits C2 into two fragments, $C\overline{2}a$ and C2b. When $C\overline{2}a$ binds to C4b, the union ($C\overline{4}b,\overline{2}a$) is referred to as classical pathway C3 convertase. Two fragments are formed from C3 cleavage, $C\overline{3}b$ and C3a. When $C\overline{3}b$ binds close to the existing

complex on the cell membrane, the union, $C\overline{4}b,\overline{2}a,\overline{3}b$, generates the last enzyme of the classical pathway which is referred to as classical pathway C5 convertase. Subsequently, C5 is split into C5a and $C\overline{5}b$. The bound $C\overline{5}b$ initiates formation of the membrane attack complex, the terminal stage of the classical pathway, which involves the sequential activation of C6, C7, C8 and C9. The membrane attack complex displaces membrane phospholipids, forming a large transmembrane channel in the membrane that allows loss of potassium ions and entry of sodium ions and water leading to hypotonic lysis of the target cell.

Alternative pathway

In this non-antibody dependent pathway for complement activation, the early acting complement components C1, C2 and C4 are not required. Thus, this pathway can be activated before the establishment of an immune response

Table 84. 2 Comparison of T lymphocytes and B lymphocytes and their roles in specific immune responses.

Feature	T lymphocyte	B lymphocyte
Origin	Bone marrow	Bone marrow
Site of maturation	Thymus	Bursa of Fabricius in birds; bone marrow and gut-associated lymphoid tissue in mammals
Antigen receptors	T cell receptors	Membrane-bound immunoglobulins. Following interaction with antigen, B cells differentiate into plasma cells which produce antibody
Soluble factors produced	Cytokines	Antibodies
Protective role	Subsets of T lymphocytes participate in a wide range of cell-mediated immune responses	Antibodies, which have a protective role against many infectious agents, are the effector molecules of humoral immunity
Participation in hypersensitivity reactions	Participate in type IV reaction	Participate in types I, II and III reactions
Contribution to the development of immunological memory	Memory T cells produced	Memory B cells produced

to infectious agents.

Availability of C3b is essential for the activation of the alternative pathway. Because C3 contains an unstable thioester bond, it is subject to spontaneous hydrolysis to yield C3a and $\overline{\text{C3b}}$. Free $\overline{\text{C3b}}$ can bind to foreign surfaces or infectious agents such as bacteria, yeasts and viruses. The membranes of most mammalian cells have high levels of sialic acid which causes rapid inactivation of bound $\overline{\text{C3b}}$ molecules on host cells. The cell walls of many infectious agents such as bacteria and yeasts have low levels of sialic acid and, accordingly, $\overline{\text{C3b}}$ bound to these surfaces remains active for some time. Bound $\overline{\text{C3b}}$ can attach to another protein called factor B (Fig. 84.7). This binding of C3b exposes a site on factor B that serves as a substrate for the circulating enzyme factor D which cleaves factor B into Ba and $\overline{\text{Bb}}$. The fragment Ba diffuses away leaving the $\overline{\text{C3b}}$, $\overline{\text{Bb}}$ complex which has C3 convertase activity analogous to $\overline{\text{C4b}}$, $\overline{\text{2a}}$ in the classical pathway. The $\overline{\text{C3b}}$, $\overline{\text{Bb}}$ complex, which is stabilized by properdin, can cleave C3, producing more $\overline{\text{C3b}}$ and C3a generating $\overline{\text{C3b}}$, $\overline{\text{Bb}}$, $\overline{\text{C3b}}$. The formation of $\overline{\text{C3b}}$,$\overline{\text{Bb}}$,$\overline{\text{C3b}}$ can cleave C5 to C5a

and $\overline{\text{C5b}}$ thereby acting as alternative pathway C5 convertase. The sequence of reactions which follow initiate the formation of the membrane attack complex.

In addition to the classical and alternative pathways of complement activation, another pathway, the mannose-binding lectin pathway can lead to activation of complement. Mannose-binding lectin is activated by binding to repetitive sugar residues, and associated serine proteases which are homologues of C1r and C1s, are recruited. Activation of C4 and C2 lead to the formation of the classical pathway C3 convertase.

Regulation of the complement system

Because of its ability to damage not only pathogenic microorganisms but also host cells, complement activation is highly regulated. Several regulatory proteins prevent uncontrolled complement activation. These include C1 inhibitor, a protein that blocks the enzymatic function of activated C1 thereby preventing further activation of C4 and C2 in the classical pathway of activation. Factor I is a serine protease that splits C3b while factor H, a glyco-protein, binds to C3b and facilitates dissociation of the alternative complement pathway component $\overline{\text{C3b}}\overline{\text{Bb}}$ into $\overline{\text{C3b}}$ and $\overline{\text{Bb}}$. Decay accelerating factor, a membrane bound glycoprotein present on many cells, accelerates decay of C3 convertase. A circulating serum protein called S protein can bind to $\overline{\text{C5b,6,7}}$ complex thereby preventing its insertion into the membrane of cells. This regulatory protein also prevents C9 from binding to the $\overline{\text{C5b,6,7,8}}$ complex and, as a consequence, formation of the membrane attack complex does not occur.

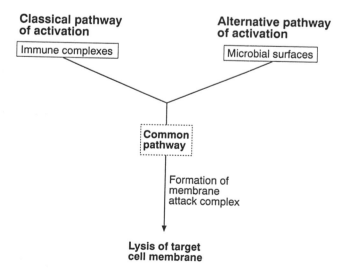

Figure 84.6 Activation of complement through the classical or alternative pathways. The formation of immune complexes (antigen bound to antibody) initiates the classical pathway whereas microbial surfaces such as yeast cell walls or lipopolysaccharide can activate the alternative pathway without the requirement of antibody.

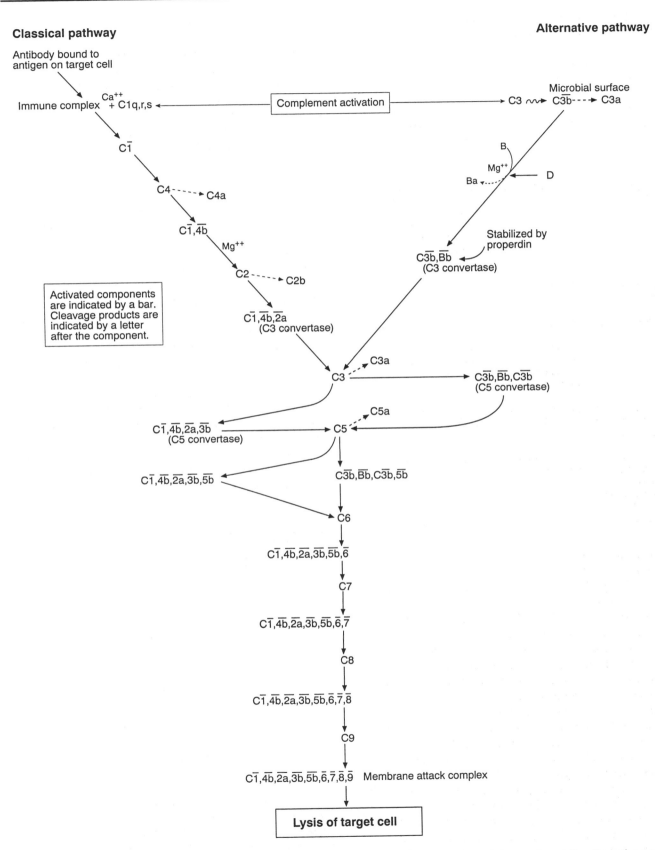

Figure 84.7 Complement activation pathways. The classical pathway is activated by immune complexes whereas the alternative pathway can be activated by surface components of microbial agents.

Complement-binding receptors

Many of the biological activities of complement depend on receptors on various cells for complement fragments. These receptors (CR1, CR2, CR3, CR4) bind breakdown products of C3 and, in addition, some have a role in the regulation of the classical pathway, binding C4b and immune complexes to cells. The CR1 receptor binds C3b and C4b. It is present on many cell types including neutrophils, monocytes, macrophages, B cells, T cells, eosinophils, follicular dendritic cells and primate red blood cells. The CR2 receptor, present on B cells, can bind breakdown products of C3 and may be involved in B cell activation. The CR3 receptor, present on monocytes, macrophages, neutrophils and natural killer cells, binds C3 degradation products. This receptor also binds cell adhesion molecules and immune complexes. The CR4 receptor, present in neutrophils, some T cells, macrophages and natural killer cells, binds breakdown fragments of C3.

Receptors for C3a, C4a and C5a fragments, which are referred to as anaphylatoxins because of their ability to induce degranulation of mast cells and basophils and release vasoactive amines, are present on many cell types. There is a common receptor on mast cells for C3a and C4a and these fragments can also bind to receptors on basophils and granulocytes. Receptors for C5a are widely distributed on mast cells, basophils, granulocytes, monocytes, platelets and endothelial cells.

Biological activity of complement

The central role of complement in inflammatory reactions relates to the diversity of immune reactions in which complement components and fragments participate (Box 84.2). The formation of the membrane attack complex on target cells is effective in lysing many Gram-negative bacteria. The majority of Gram-positive bacteria are resistant to the lytic effects of complement, probably as a consequence of their thick peptidoglycan layer preventing access of C5b-9 to the inner membrane. Because of their rigid, relatively impermeable cell walls, most fungi can resist the lytic action of the membrane attack complex. Some strains of Gram-negative bacteria appear to be resistant to the lytic action of complement by confining complement activation to a subset of lipopolysaccharide molecules with longer than normal 'O'-polysaccharide side chains, thereby preventing the C5b-9 complexes from reaching the complement-sensitive sites on the outer membrane (Law and Reid, 1995).

Complement levels in domestic animals and complement deficiencies

On the basis of haemolytic activity, complement levels in domestic animals show wide variation. Canine serum has low haemolytic activity while guinea-pig serum has an exceptionally high level of activity. Ruminants have an intermediate level of complement activity and horses have

---

> **Box 84.2** Biological activities of complement.
>
> - Modification of inflammatory responses and destruction of pathogens
>   — opsonization of infectious agents through binding of C3b
>   — lysis of microorganisms, erythrocytes and nucleated cells by formation of the membrane attack complex on target cells
>   — promotion of phagocytosis through receptors on phagocytic cells for complement fragments
>   — chemotaxis of neutrophils and macrophages mediated by C5a, C3a and C5b,6,7
> - Removal of immune complexes through binding of C3b
> - Degranulation of mast cells and basophils by C3a, C4a, C5a leading to release of vasoactive amines and increased vascular permeability
> - Virus neutralization through the activation of the classical or alternative pathways; lysis of enveloped viruses producing envelope fragmentation

moderately low levels.

Complement deficiencies are reported in humans and animals. Brittany spaniels with a congenital deficiency of C3 have been reported and rabbits with a C6 deficiency have been described. Other deficiencies of complement components have been described in humans and in laboratory animals. Such deficiencies invariably lead to recurring bacterial infections and sometimes to glomerular lesions if immune complexes are not cleared from the circulation.

The role of phagocytic cells in non-specific immune responses

From a pluripotent stem cell in the bone marrow two important groups of cells arise: those that belong to the myeloid series and those that belong to the lymphoid series. Neutrophils, eosinophils and basophils, described as polymorphonuclear cells, arise from myeloblasts, whereas cells of the monocyte-macrophage series arise from monoblasts (Fig. 84.4). Although many cell types are capable of engulfing particles, two cell types, macrophages and neutrophils, are the phagocytic cells of greatest importance in non-specific immunity.

Neutrophils are formed in the bone marrow, move to the bloodstream and later into the tissues. During their life span of only a few days, they are capable of rapid response to invading microorganisms, especially bacteria. Monocytes and macrophages respond slowly to bacterial invasion but they are better equipped to engulf and destroy invading pathogens, especially those microorganisms which can multiply intracellularly.

Neutrophils

When the tissues are invaded by pyogenic bacteria, neutrophils are the first cells to arrive at the site of inflammation. Damaged endothelial cells at the site express adhesive proteins which bind neutrophils. Rolling and arrest of neutrophils on the endothelium is mediated by successive interactions with selectins and β-integrins that can overcome hydrodynamic force (Mollinedo *et al.*, 1999). When intercellular adhesion molecule 1 is highly expressed on activated endothelial cells, neutrophil adhesion proceeds through direct β_2-integrin-intercellular adhesion molecule 1 interaction. Adhesion is followed by diapedesis when the neutrophils pass through the endothelial cell junctions and, stimulated by chemotactic factors such as C5a, migrate to the site of tissue invasion. Chemotaxis is followed by adherence to the pathogens and then phagocytosis. In the absence of opsonins, phagocytosis of many bacteria is ineffective.

The neutrophil extends pseudopodia around the pathogen to engulf it in a vacuole termed a phagosome. The phagosome fuses with neutrophil granules which release their digestive enzymes and other toxic factors thereby destroying the engulfed pathogen. Neutrophils contain lytic enzymes and bactericidal substances within primary and secondary granules. The larger primary granules contain cationic antimicrobial proteins, bactericidal permeability-inducing protein, a variety of hydrolytic enzymes, peroxidase and lysozyme. The smaller secondary granules contain collagenase, lactoferrin and lysozyme. Both oxygen-dependent and oxygen-independent pathways are used by neutrophils to generate antimicrobial substances. Two oxygen-dependent mechanisms, the respiratory burst and the hydrogen peroxide-myeloperoxidase-halide system are employed. Toxic metabolites produced during the respiratory burst include superoxide anion, hydrogen peroxide, singlet oxygen and hydroxyl radicals. In the hydrogen peroxide-myeloperoxidase-halide system, hydrogen peroxide produced by the respiratory burst, myeloperoxidase from the primary granules and a halide such as a chloride combine to yield chlorine and hydroxyl ions both of which are toxic for the engulfed bacteria. The oxygen-independent mechanisms of neutrophil killing involve lysozyme, cathepsins, elastase and lactoferrin.

Mononuclear phagocytes

Although they share a common progenitor cell with neutrophils, monocytes and macrophages are different in many respects. Circulating monocytes move to tissues and become resident tissue macrophages (Fig. 84.4). Tissue macrophages occur throughout the body and have different names and functions depending on the tissue: alveolar marophages in the lungs, Kupffer cells in the liver, microglial cells in the brain. Unlike neutrophils, macrophages are long-lived cells that are better equipped to deal with virulent microorganisms. Macrophages have many important functions which include phagocytosis, antigen presentation to T cells to initiate specific immune responses and secretion of cytokines to activate lymphocytes and promote inflammatory responses.

In common with neutrophils, macrophages are actively phagocytic. The steps involved in engulfment of bacteria by both phagocytic cells have much in common. However, the macrophage membrane has receptors for the Fc portion of IgG and for C3b. Thus, when an antigen is coated (opsonized) with appropriate antibody or complement component, the antigen binds more readily to the macrophage membrane and phagocytosis is enhanced. Among the antimicrobial factors produced by these phagocytic cells lysozyme, proteases, collagenases and elastases feature prominently. Nitric oxide produced by macrophages in some species of animals has marked bactericidal activity.

Unlike neutrophils, macrophages continue to differentiate after they leave the bone marrow and they can become activated if stimulated in an appropriate manner. When acted on by interferon gamma, a lymphokine produced by T cells, macrophages can become activated. Such activated cells exhibit enhanced phagocytosis and intracellular killing of bacteria. In addition to their antibacterial role in defence, macrophages secrete an array of cytokines including interleukin-1, interleukin-6, interleukin-12, tumour necrosis factor and interferon alpha. These factors stimulate immune and inflammatory responses. Other secreted products of macrophages include complement components, coagulation factors, fibronectin and prostaglandins.

Specific immunity

At a particular stage in its development, the foetus acquires the ability to recognize foreign antigenic material and respond to infectious agents encountered *in utero*. Newborn animals, transferred from a sterile intrauterine environment to a world abounding in microorganisms, have an innate ability to resist invasion by many environmental organisms. Without colostral protection, however, neonatal animals are susceptible to many enteric and respiratory pathogens. As an animal matures, its immune system develops in tandem with other anatomical and physiological alterations. Within weeks of birth, most young animals are immunologically competent and, if challenged by infectious agents can respond in an appropriate manner to prevent or limit tissue invasion.

The immune system can distinguish foreign material such as cells or soluble substances introduced into the body from 'self' components. This recognition of 'self' and tolerance to its own tissue antigens occurs during embryological development. In exceptional circumstances, some individual animals produce an immune response against their own tissues and this condition is termed autoimmunity.

Lymphocytes can interact with foreign material through surface receptors. On B cells, the receptors are membrane-bound immunoglobulins. In contrast, T cell receptors are not immunoglobulins and can only react with antigen in association with other molecules. Lymphocyte receptors can recognize a diverse range of foreign molecules including the components or products of bacteria, viruses, fungi, protozoa and helminth parasites. These foreign substances are collectively referred to as antigens. An antigen can be defined as any substance capable of binding specifically to components of the immune system such as specific antibodies or T cell receptors. An immunogen is any agent or substance capable of inducing an immune response. This differentiation of antigens and immunogens is necessary because some low-molecular weight compounds, referred to as haptens, which include breakdown products of some antibiotics, cannot induce immune responses unless coupled with large molecules such as proteins. Haptens, however, can bind to components of the immune system specifically produced against them. For a substance to be immunogenic, it must have certain characteristics. These include foreignness, high molecular weight, chemical complexity and biodegradability. In general, compounds that have molecular weights less than 1,000 Da are not immunogenic, whereas those with molecular weights between 1,000 and 6,000 Da may be immunogenic in some instances. Compounds with molecular weights greater than 6,000 Da are usually immunogenic. Proteins are highly immunogenic, carbohydrates moderately immunogenic, while lipids and nucleic acids are usually poor immunogens.

Infectious agents are composed of structures containing molecules of great complexity. Accordingly, an individual bacterium can have a vast array of complex surface antigens which a lymphocyte receptor can recognize. The lymphocyte receptor can recognize only a small portion of a complex molecule and this small part of the molecule is referred to as an antigenic determinant or epitope. Complex antigens consist of a mosaic of individual epitopes and, when similar determinants are present on different infectious agents, cross-reactions may occur in serological test procedures involving these infectious agents.

Specific recognition of antigen is possible because lymphocytes possess two structurally similar types of receptors, membrane-bound immunoglobulins on B cells and T cell receptors on T cells. These cellular receptors serve two functions: they bind to antigenic material and they trigger responses in the cells on which the receptors are expressed. Naive B lymphocytes express two classes of membrane-bound antibodies, IgM and IgD. Activation of B lymphocytes is followed by proliferation of antigen-specific cells, a process referred to as clonal expansion. Differentiation of these proliferating cells results in the production of antibody-secreting plasma cells and memory cells. The secreted antibodies have the same specificity as the naive B cell membrane receptors that combined with antigen and initiated the response.

The antigen receptors on B cells and T cells recognize chemically different structures. While B lymphocytes are able to recognize native macromolecules such as proteins, lipids, carbohydrates and nucleic acids, T cells can recognize peptides only if they are presented on antigen-presenting cells in association with membrane proteins encoded in the major histocompatibility complex (MHC) genetic locus. The MHC molecules can be considered as a third set of recognition molecules for antigen in addition to antigen-specific T cell receptors and B cell receptors. Although most nucleated cells in the body express class 1 MHC molecules, class II molecules are expressed mainly on B lymphocytes and antigen-presenting cells such as macrophages and dentritic cells. The peptide-binding clefts of MHC molecules bind peptides derived from protein antigens and display them for recognition by T cells. Although each MHC molecule can present only one peptide at a time, it is capable of presenting many different peptides. The function of class 1 MHC molecules is to present peptides derived from protein antigens to the subset of T cells known as $CD8^+$ cells (cytotoxic T cells). When cytotoxic T cells recognize class 1 MHC-associated peptides on host cells such as cells infected with a virus, they attack and destroy such cells. This destruction of an infected host cell by a cytotoxic T lymphocyte is an example of cell-mediated immunity. The function of class II MHC molecules is to present peptides to lymphocytes known as $CD4^+$ T cells. These $CD4^+$ T cells, referred to as T helper cells, promote the engulfment and intracellular destruction of pathogens by macrophages and they enhance B cell responses leading to plasma cell formation and antibody production.

Immune responses are initiated when an animal encounters foreign antigenic material, often an infectious agent. Within days, the infected animal responds by producing antibody molecules specific for the antigenic determinants of the infectious agent and by expansion and differentiation of antigen-specific regulatory and effector T lymphocytes. As a consequence of the encounter, lymphocytes with an immunological memory are produced. If challenged later by the same infectious agent, a more rapid and sustained antibody response occurs (Fig. 84.8). A similar enhanced and more effective T cell response usually occurs in secondary immune responses. This is the basis of vaccination which ensures a rapid and usually protective immune response to antigenic material, injected or otherwise administered to susceptible animals. Following vaccination, animals do not all respond in an identical manner; the antibody responses of vaccinated animals follow a normal distribution (Fig. 84.9). An outline of the principal elements of specific immunity and its induction is presented in Fig. 84.10.

Antibodies produced against infectious agents have the ability to neutralize bacterial toxins and viruses. They can

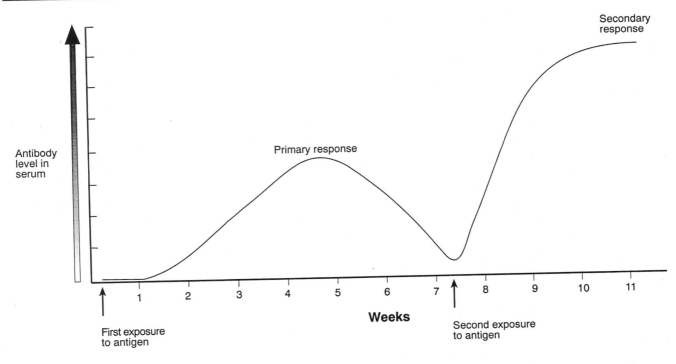

Figure 84.8 Primary and secondary antibody responses following natural exposure to an infectious agent or after vaccination. The primary response occurs after an interval of almost ten days and the predominant immunoglobulin is IgM. The secondary immune response reaches higher levels and lasts longer, and the antibodies produced are mainly IgG.

opsonize microbial pathogens for phagocytosis by macrophages and neutrophils. Some antibodies such as IgA, produced locally in the gastrointestinal and respiratory tracts, prevent attachment of pathogens to host cells, thereby hindering colonization and minimizing the likelihood of disease production. This form of local immunity, referred to as mucosal immunity, is of particular importance in young animals. By activating the classical complement pathway, antibodies can initiate responses which lead to lysis of microbial pathogens and opsonization through fixation of C3b on the target membrane to which they have attached. They can also

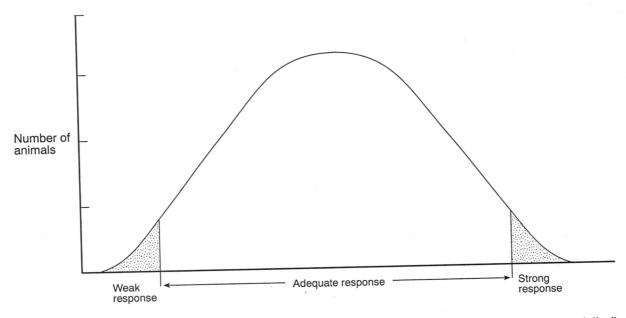

Figure 84.9 The antibody responses of a randomly selected population of vaccinated healthy animals follows a normal distribution.

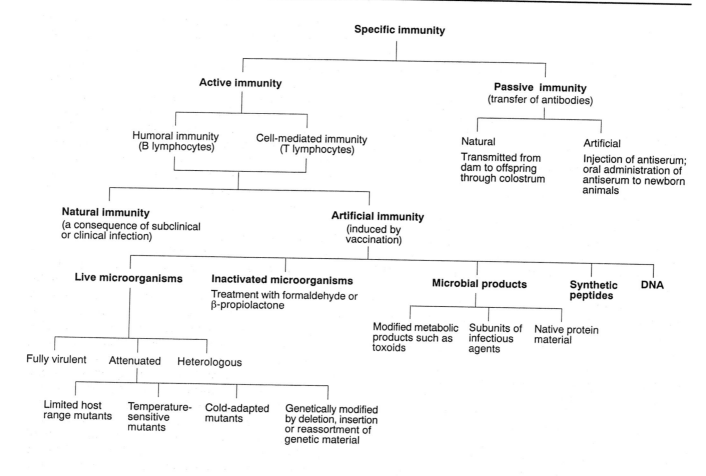

Figure 84.10 An outline of the principal elements of specific immunity. The methods used to confer passive immunity and to induce active immunity are shown.

promote inflammatory responses through the generation of cleavage components once the complement system is activated. Antibodies produced by the dam and secreted in colostrum passively protect newborn animals against a wide range of respiratory and enteric pathogens.

Passive immunity refers to the transfer of antibodies from an actively immune animal to a susceptible animal. This form of immunity occurs naturally when neonatal animals ingest colostrum. Antiserum specific for a particular pathogen or toxin can be administered by injection to give immediate short-term protection against infectious agents. Newborn animals can be given antiserum orally to protect them against infection with certain enteropathogens. Mouse monoclonal antibodies to the K99 pilus antigen of *E. coli* are used to protect calves against enteric disease caused by this organism. Following administration of antiserum the duration of passive immunity is shorter in a heterologous species than in a homologous species (Fig. 84.11).

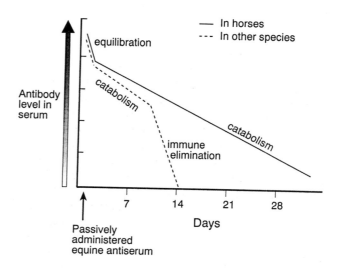

Figure 84.11 The duration of passive immunity following administration of equine antiserum to horses and to other species of animals. The dose of antiserum administered influences the duration of protection in the homologous species which may be up to three weeks when the recommended amount of antiserum is administered.

Vaccination

Active immunization, which generally refers to the administration of a vaccine that can induce a protective immune response, can produce long-lasting protection against infectious agents. The duration of protection is influenced by many host factors including age, immune competence and the presence of maternal antibodies in the animal's circulation. Many attributes of the vaccine itself affect the type of immune response and its duration. The duration of protection achieved with inactivated vaccines is usually shorter than that induced by modified live vaccines.

When feasible, effective and safe, vaccination is one of the most cost-effective measures for controlling infectious disease not only in companion animals but also in food-producing animals. Some infectious diseases with wildlife reservoirs, such as rabies, can also be controlled in particular animal species through vaccination. The benefits of vaccination, therefore, are not confined to reduced morbidity and decreased mortality in vaccinated animals as transmission of zoonotic diseases such as rabies in the human population can be substantially reduced by dog and cat vaccination. Although many of the vaccines currently licensed for use in animals are produced by conventional methods, the advent of biotechnology has provided an opportunity for developing vaccines with improved efficacy and greater safety. Inactivated vaccines often contain many irrelevant antigenic substances, some with undesirable biological activity. Live attenuated vaccines can produce adverse reactions including immuno-suppression. Despite these limitations, conventional vaccines will continue to be used until superseded by safer more effective subunit or genetically engineered live vaccines.

Inactivated vaccines

Infectious agents can be killed without substantially altering the immunogenicity of their protective antigens. Although most inactivating chemicals do alter the immunogenicity of infectious agents, some such as formaldehyde, cause limited antigenic change. When preparing inactivated vaccines, care has to be taken to ensure complete inactivation of the infectious agents as the chemicals used can cause aggregation of particles thereby allowing survival of some microorganisms in the centre of aggregated material. Chemicals used for the preparation of inactivated bacterial and viral vaccines include formaldehyde, β-propiolactone and etylenimine. Many bacterial vaccines used in animals are prepared by inactivating bacterial cultures (bacterins) or rendering their toxins inactive (toxoids) by chemical treatment.

A major limitation of inactivated vaccines is that some protective antigens are not produced readily *in vitro*. In addition, some components of killed vaccines can interfere with host immune responses. Inactivated viral or bacterial preparations can be partially purified and combined with adjuvants to enhance their immunogenicity. Because they are processed as exogenous antigens in the body, many inactivated vaccines can induce high levels of circulating antibody but are less effective at stimulating cell-mediated and mucosal immunity. As inactivated vaccines do not contain agents which can replicate, a greater antigenic mass and more frequent administration of vaccine (booster injections) are required to achieve results comparable to those obtained with live attenuated vaccines. Advantages of inactivated vaccines include stability at ambient temperatures, safety for recipients due to their inability to revert to a virulent state, and a long shelf life.

Live attenuated vaccines

Apart from the orf vaccine which is used in sheep, few virulent living organisms are used as vaccines in animals. The virulence of living organisms is reduced by attenuation, a process which involves adapting them to grow under conditions whereby they lose their affinity for their usual host and do not produce disease in susceptible animals. Bacteria such as the bacillus of Calmette-Guérin, a strain of *Mycobacterium bovis*, was attenuated by culture in a bile-supplemented medium over many years. Bacteria can also be rendered avirulent using genetic manipulation.

Viruses can be attenuated by growing them in monolayers prepared from species to which they are not naturally adapted. Chick embryo attenuation has been employed successfully for rabies virus. Prolonged culture of canine distemper virus in canine kidney cells produced strains of reduced virulence suitable for immunization of dogs.

Even without attenuation, antigenically-related viruses can be used to induce active immunity in certain species which they do not normally infect. Measles virus has been used to vaccinate dogs against distemper and, although these viruses cross-react, maternal antibodies to distemper virus in pups do not neutralize the live measles vaccine virus. The use of turkey herpesvirus to control Marek's disease in chickens is another example of protection induced by an antigenically-related virus.

Live attenuated vaccines have many potential advantages over inactivated vaccines. They can be administered by a number of routes and present all the relevant antigens required for the induction of protective immunity since they multiply in the recipient. They usually induce a satisfactory level of cell-mediated and humoral immunity at sites where protection is required such as mucosal surfaces. Because they replicate in the body, adjuvants are not required. Booster doses, if required, can be given at widely-spaced intervals as these vaccines induce a good immunological memory.

Disadvantages of these modified live vaccines include their possible immunosuppressive effects, especially in young animals or where an immunodeficient state exists. While live attenuated vaccines have been used for decades, the exact nature of the genetic change responsible for attenuation is usually unknown. As attenuating mutations are often produced at random, it is not possible to predict accurately the circumstances in which reversion to virulence might occur. Live attenuated viral vaccines can be contaminated by extraneous agents which can induce disease in recipients. In young animals, maternal antibodies can neutralize live attenuated viral vaccines. Accordingly, vaccination of young animals should be deferred until maternal antibodies have declined to low levels in recipients.

The presence, in a vaccine, of tissue culture fluid and cells in which the virus was grown can produce adverse reactions in some animals. The limited shelf-life and the requirement for refrigeration to ensure viability are additional disadvantages of live attenuated vaccines.

Vaccines produced by recombinant technology

Recombinant vaccines are classified into three categories by the U.S. Department of Agriculture (Mackowiak *et al.*, 1999). Type I vaccines are composed of antigens produced by genetic engineering. Type II vaccines consist of genetically attenuated microorganisms while Type III vaccines are composed of modified live viruses or bacteria into which DNA encoding a protective antigen is introduced.

Type I vaccines are composed of subunit proteins produced by recombinant bacteria or other microorganisms. The DNA coding for the required antigen is isolated and introduced into a suitable bacterium or yeast in which the recombinant antigen is expressed. These vaccines usually contain adjuvants which are required to enhance the immunogenicity of the purified antigen derived from the recombinant organism. Type I vaccines have been developed for a number of bacterial and viral diseases. They have been used against the virus of foot-and-mouth disease, feline leukaemia virus and against *Borrelia burgdorferi*, the cause of Lyme disease.

Type II recombinant vaccines consist of virulent microorganisms which are rendered less virulent by gene deletion or site directed mutagenesis. The genome of large DNA viruses, such as herpesviruses, contain many genes not required for *in vitro* replication. Using recombinant DNA technology, a pseudorabies vaccine lacking the gene for thymidine kinase has been produced. As thymidine kinase is required by this herpesvirus to replicate in non-dividing cells such as neurons, viruses from which the gene encoding for this enzyme has been deleted are able to infect neurons but unable to replicate in these cells. Such deletion mutants induce a protective immune response in pigs. Deletion of the gene encoding for the glycoprotein gI on the pseudorabies virus permits differentiation of infected pigs, which produce antibodies against gI, from vaccinated pigs which lack such antibodies. Thus, vaccination programmes can proceed in countries where the disease is being eradicated without interfering with serological recognition and removal of infected pigs.

The failure of some vaccines used in veterinary medicine to induce a protective immune response can result from problems related to delivery. Development of delivery systems, therefore, that are effective, safe and convenient for administration and suit producers' needs is a challenge for those engaged in vaccine production. The use of live viruses for the delivery of veterinary vaccines is a possible solution to current difficulties. Type III vaccines are composed of modified live organisms called vectors into which a gene is inserted and this organism also serves as a delivery system in the recipient. In order to produce safe viral vaccine vectors it is necessary to ensure that the vector itself does not pose any threat to vaccinated animals or to humans. This is usually achieved by attenuating the viral vector or by generating live attenuated viruses with precise genetic changes that ensure their suitability as vectors.

Recombinant DNA technology offers a greater understanding of the genetic organization of many viruses, permitting selection of suitable regions for insertion of foreign genetic material. Numerous types of potentially useful viral vectors from a variety of viruses including pox viruses, adenoviruses, herpesviruses and retroviruses have been developed (Sheppard, 1999). Potential advantages of viral vectors for vaccine delivery include possible administration to large groups of animals by aerosols or in water rather than by injection of individual animals. Such mass administration procedures would be particularly relevant to poultry and pig producers. If properly designed, the vector would only express those antigens from the pathogen that are required to induce a protective immune response thereby reducing or eliminating the chance of disease in animals exposed to the infectious agent in a modified live form. A distinct advantage of vectored vaccines is that they induce both humoral and cell-mediated immune responses, including strong cytotoxic T cell immunity. In addition, some vectored vaccines may be capable of inducing local immune responses on mucosal surfaces.

To ensure vector stability and the appropriate expression of the foreign genetic material, only a limited amount of that genetic material can be incorporated into the vector genome. Consequently, each vectored vaccine can only deliver one or a relatively small number of foreign antigens to the host animal for the induction of a protective immune response. A possible complication of vectored vaccines is that they may express altered tissue tropism as a result of the acquisition of foreign genetic material. Prior exposure of animal populations to the virus used to construct the vector would substantially limit the effectiveness of a vectored vaccine.

Currently a small number of viral vectored vaccines have been approved for use in animals. A vaccinia virus vector carrying the rabies G glycoprotein gene has been used successfully as an oral vaccine administered to wild carnivores in bait. The G glycoprotein induces virus-neutralizing antibodies in vaccinated animals which protect against rabies.

Synthetic peptide vaccines

If the structure of epitopes which can induce a protective immune response is known, it is possible to synthesize peptides corresponding to these antigenic determinants. Only a small portion of antigenic molecules interact with specific receptors on B cells and T cells. For B cells, an antibody interacts with three to five amino acids in its antigen-combining site. Epitopes for T cell receptors can be composed of 12 to 15 amino acids.

The general approach with synthetic peptide vaccines is to identify potential epitopes in the protein antigen and to synthesize a series of peptides corresponding to that amino acid sequence. The immunological activity of these molecules is then evaluated *in vivo*. This approach is appropriate only for epitopes consisting of contiguous amino acids referred to as linear epitopes. The majority of natural epitopes are non-linear and are, therefore, dependent on the conserved three-dimensional structure of the molecule. Antibodies induced by peptide vaccines may not react with the native molecule and, in addition, peptides are usually poor immunogens due to their small size. Immunogenicity can be enhanced with appropriate carrier molecules or adjuvants. Limited progress has been made with synthetic peptides for the induction of protective immune response against infectious agents.

DNA vaccines

One of the most significant developments in vaccine production in recent years involves the use of DNA, encoding microbial antigens in a bacterial plasmid, for immunization. The procedure involves injection of a plasmid encoding the DNA sequence for a protective antigen linked to a strong mammalian promoter sequence. Injection of plasmids encoding for protective antigens into the skin or muscle of animals may result in protein expression and immunity against an infectious agent carrying that protein. This leads to the expression in host cells of the encoded genes with the development of a significant immunological response to the gene product in the recipient. Unlike viral vectors, the plasmid cannot replicate in mammalian cells but transfected host cells express the vaccine antigen. Methods of delivery include direct intramuscular injection and the use of liposomes or coated gold particles fired by a 'gene gun'. Although transfection rates appear to be low, antigen production has been detected in animals vaccinated with DNA intramuscularly six months after injection. Because DNA vaccination induces intracellular processing of antigen, it seems to mimic a natural infection and is, therefore, an effective method of inducing T cell responses. Even small amounts of DNA can stimulate strong cell-mediated responses. Humoral responses, however, may not be as high as those obtained by injection of a purified antigen.

A strategy in which priming with DNA vaccines is followed by boosting with attenuated viral vectors such as fowlpoxvirus or modified vaccinia virus has produced exceptionally strong immune responses (Ramshaw and Ramsay, 2000). The success of consecutive use of DNA vaccines and attenuated viral vectors was attributed to the ability of the DNA vaccines to generate T cells of high affinity which were further stimulated by boosting with non-replicating viral vectors. Although immune responses may be delayed following DNA vaccination, a persistent response may occur. In contrast to modified live viral vaccines, maternal antibody does not appear to affect the immune response in young animals. An advantage of immunizing with purified DNA is the possibility of antigen presentation in its native form as it would occur during replication of an infectious agent in the body. By this method of vaccination, it is also possible to select genes for the antigen of interest without the need for a complex viral or bacterial vector.

The safety of DNA vaccines is still unresolved. The possibility that the DNA in a vaccine might integrate into chromosomes and induce neoplastic changes or other cellular alterations has been suggested. It has also been suggested that DNA introduced into the body by this method of vaccination might induce anti-DNA antibodies to the recipient's DNA.

Vaccines for clinical coliform mastitis

Despite many years of research, vaccination has proved to be of limited value for preventing mastitis in dairy cattle. The large number of bacterial pathogens involved and the vulnerability of the mammary gland to opportunistic infection militate against the development of a single effective vaccine. The introduction of core antigen vaccines for clinical coliform mastitis marks an important advance in attempts to induce a protective immune response against opportunistic pathogens infecting the mammary gland.

Mutant strains of *Escherichia coli* and *Salmonella* Typhimurium have been used to develop these vaccines. Because these bacteria are unable to produce complete lipopolysaccharide molecules, they are referred to as rough mutants. The ability of the lipopolysaccharide core antigen of *E. coli* to induce protection against a wide range of Gram-negative bacteria is attributed to the production of antibody which cross-reacts with these organisms, especially when they are growing rapidly. The rough mutant, *E. coli* J5, has been extensively evaluated in field trials with encouraging but sometimes inconsistent results (Yancey, 1999).

Vaccination with core antigen should be confined to the dry period as there may be a short-term reduction in milk production if lactating cows are vaccinated. Although vaccination with core antigens did not consistently reduce the incidence of new coliform intramammary infections at calving, the percentage of quarters which developed clinical coliform mastitis when intramammary infection occurred was significantly lower in vaccinated cows.

In ovo vaccination

Formerly, vaccination against Marek's disease was carried out manually. Newly hatched chickens were vaccinated subcutaneously with a bivalent herpesvirus of turkeys. Following the demonstration in the early 1980s that embryonated eggs responded to vaccination at 18 days of incubation, *in ovo* vaccination against Marek's disease became an established procedure in the early 1990s and an automated egg injection system was developed (Ricks *et al.*, 1999).

Using the automated egg injection system, vaccination is carried out between 17.5 and 18.5 days of incubation at a time when transfer from incubators to hatcheries normally takes place.

It is reported that more than 80% of the broiler industry in the U.S. employs *in ovo* vaccination for the control of Marek's disease. This procedure, which is considered to be a safe and effective method for vaccination of poultry, may be employed for the control of endemic viral diseases such as infectious bronchitis and infectious bursal disease. It may be used in the future for administration of bacterial and parasitic vaccines when safe and effective antigenic preparations become available.

Although many aspects of vaccine production are closely monitored and vaccination schedules are carefully devised, vaccination failure can still occur. Both animal-related factors and vaccine-related factors can contribute to vaccination failure (Fig. 84.12). In addition to vaccination failure, adverse consequences of vaccination can emerge. These include granuloma and fibrosarcoma development at the vaccination site, the development of hypersensitivity reactions, toxic effects or even clinical disease in immunologically competent animals (Box 84.3). The use of live viral vaccines in pregnant animals is usually contraindicated as it can result in congenital infections.

Adjuvants

Substances that have the ability to enhance humoral and cell-mediated immune responses to inactivated microorganisms or their products are termed adjuvants. Purified antigens and low molecular weight antigenic material are often weakly immunogenic unless combined with an effective adjuvant. A large number of substances can enhance the immune response as adjuvants, as carriers for antigenic material, or as vehicles in which vaccines can be administered (Fig. 84.13).

Adjuvants differ in their chemistry and in their modes of action. Aluminium salts were among the first substances used to enhance the immune response to soluble toxoid by creating microparticulate antigen and thereby enhancing immunogenicity. In recent years many substances with adjuvant activity have been evaluated (Edelman, 1997). The modes of action of substances which enhance immune responses include prolongation of antigen release, recruitment of antigen-presenting cells, activation of macrophages and stimulation of T and B lymphocytes (Box 84.4).

Aluminium compounds

Aluminium salts are used to precipitate toxoids in many veterinary vaccines and to establish an antigen depot at the site of injection. They stimulate an earlier, higher and longer-lasting antibody response after primary immunization than occurs with soluble vaccines. Their stimulatory effect relates only to the primary immune responses as secondary immune responses are not affected. These adjuvants promote antibody production through stimulation of T_H2 cell responses. Cell-mediated

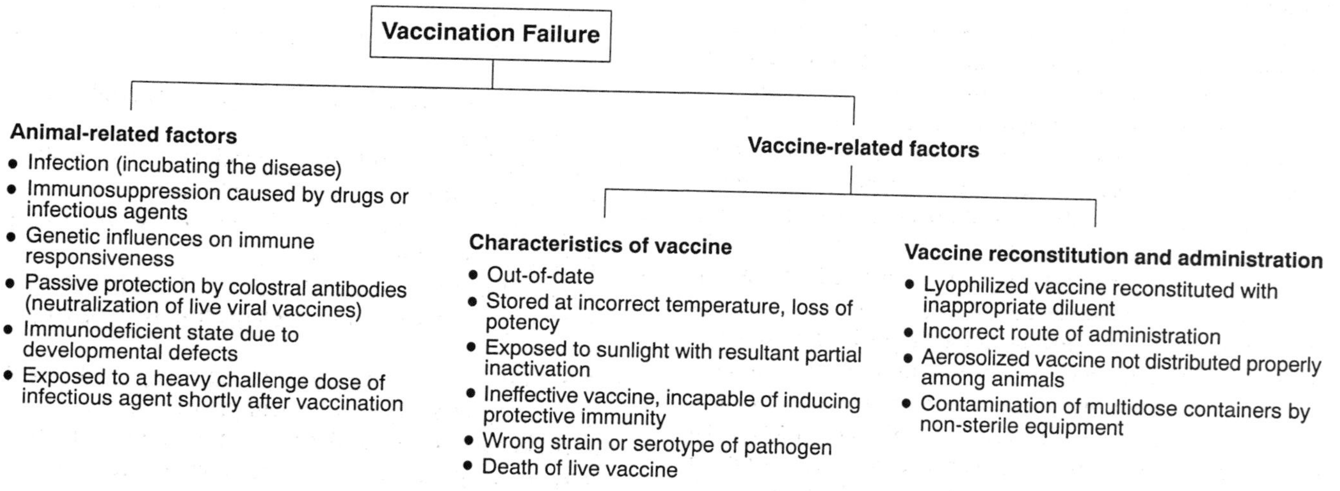

Vaccination Failure

Animal-related factors
- Infection (incubating the disease)
- Immunosuppression caused by drugs or infectious agents
- Genetic influences on immune responsiveness
- Passive protection by colostral antibodies (neutralization of live viral vaccines)
- Immunodeficient state due to developmental defects
- Exposed to a heavy challenge dose of infectious agent shortly after vaccination

Vaccine-related factors

Characteristics of vaccine
- Out-of-date
- Stored at incorrect temperature, loss of potency
- Exposed to sunlight with resultant partial inactivation
- Ineffective vaccine, incapable of inducing protective immunity
- Wrong strain or serotype of pathogen
- Death of live vaccine

Vaccine reconstitution and administration
- Lyophilized vaccine reconstituted with inappropriate diluent
- Incorrect route of administration
- Aerosolized vaccine not distributed properly among animals
- Contamination of multidose containers by non-sterile equipment

Figure 84.12 Factors which may contribute to vaccination failure.

Box 84.3 Potential adverse reactions following vaccination.

- Local or systemic infection caused by contamination of live vaccine with extraneous agents
- Disease produced by the survival of infectious agents in a supposedly killed vaccine
- Disease produced by resistant infectious agents such as prions surviving in inactivated vaccines
- Disease production by live vaccine in immuno-suppressed animals
- Vaccine-induced immunosuppression
- Development of hypersensitivity reactions to vaccine components (immediate or delayed responses)
- Induction of neoplastic changes due to the presence of oncogenic infectious agents or from the action of adjuvants
- Disease produced by the presence of infectious agents in live vaccines undectable by current conventional methods

responses are stimulated minimally, a serious limitation of aluminium-based adjuvants for vaccines aimed at intra-cellular pathogens. Aluminium salts tend to induce a granulomatous reaction at the injection site and they can be detected where they are deposited for up to one year after administration.

Oil emulsion-based adjuvants

Water-in-oil emulsions, consisting of droplets containing soluble antigen, have been used to form depots in the tissues. Freund's incomplete adjuvant consists of light mineral oil and an emulsifying agent in which the antigenic material is dispersed. Freund's complete adjuvant contains heat-killed mycobacteria in mineral oil to enhance further the immune response to antigenic material. Because mycobacteria contain immuno-stimulating substances such as muramyl dipeptide, Freund's complete adjuvant is a potent stimulator of macrophages, T cells and B cells. It induces strong cell-mediated responses and stimulates antibody production.

Oil-based adjuvants have a number of undesirable attributes. They may induce local and systemic inflamma-tory reactions. Granuloma and abscess formation may occur at the inoculation site. The use of Freund's complete adjuvant is not permitted in food-producing animals as oil remains at the injection site and the killed mycobacteria in the adjuvant induce a positive reaction in the tuberculin test. Injection of mineral oils into tissues is a questionable procedure as some may have carcinogenic activity. Alternatives to Freund's adjuvants have been proposed and evaluated. These include vegetable oil emulsions composed of peanut oil, olive oil or sesame oil with emulsifying agents.

Bacterial products

Muramyl dipeptide, a mycobacterial cell wall component, is a potent macrophage stimulator which induces secretion of interferon-gamma, tumour necrosis factor-alpha and interleukin-1, and also promotes T helper cell activity.

Lipopolysaccharides, which are B cell mitogens, enhance antibody production and some of their derivatives also augment cell-mediated immunity. Much of the toxicity and adjuvanticity of lipopolysaccharide is associated with the lipid A portion of the molecule. Using mild hydrolysis, the lipopolysaccharide of *Salmonella* Minnesota has been detoxified without destroying its adjuvant activity and the resultant monophosphoryl lipid A has been used in many adjuvant preparations. Monophosphoryl lipid A induces cytokine production, including interleukin-1, interleukin-2, interleukin-12 and interferon-gamma. It exerts an adjuvant effect on both humoral and cell-mediated responses and can be combined with other adjuvant preparations.

Saponins and immunostimulating complexes

Triterpene glycosides isolated from the bark of the South American tree *Quillaja saponaria Molina*, referred to as saponins, have both toxic activity and the ability to stimulate non-specifically immune responses. A partially purified saponin, Quil A, has been widely used as an adjuvant in veterinary vaccines. Immunostimulating complexes (ISCOMs), formed by mixing antigen with cholesterol, phospholipids and Quil A, are stable, cage-like structures with a diameter of 30 to 40 nm. An important characteristic of ISCOMs is their ability to stimulate not only high titres of long-lasting antibodies but also potent cytotoxic T cell responses. In experimental animals, ISCOMs induced mucosal immunity after intranasal, intravaginal or parenteral administration. An ISCOM-based equine influenza vaccine has been licensed for use.

Box 84.4 Modes of action of adjuvants.

- Retention and slow release of antigenic material from the site of injection
- Increased immunogenicity of small or antigenically weak synthetic or recombinant peptides
- Improved speed of response and persistence of response to effective antigens
- Increased immune response to vaccines in immuno-logically immature, immunosuppressed or ageing animals
- Stimulation of macrophage activity and the processing of antigen by antigen-presenting cells
- Modulation of humoral or cell-mediated immune responses by the subset of T lymphocyte activated
- Stimulation of T and B lymphocytes

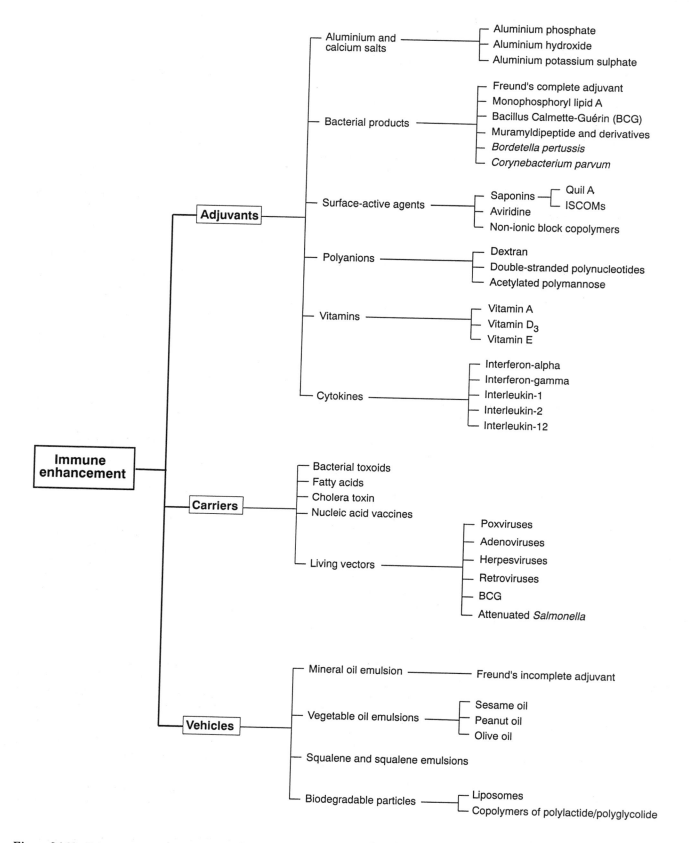

Figure 84.13 Substances which can be used to enhance immune responsiveness to vaccines either on their own or in combination with other compatible compounds.

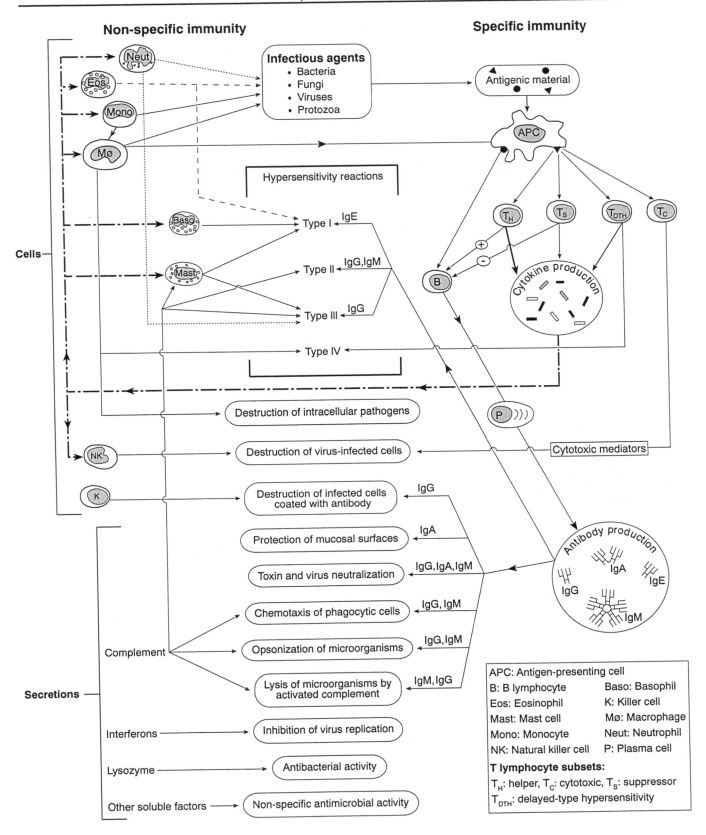

Figure 84.14 A diagrammatic illustration of the principal cells and secretions which collectively constitute non-specific immunity and specific immunity. The cooperation between elements of non-specific immunity and specific immunity enhances body defences against infectious agents, but may occasionally generate deleterious responses such as hypersensitivity reactions.

Biodegradable particles

Liposomes are membranous vesicles of naturally-occurring phospholipids which can be degraded by macrophages, especially in the liver and spleen. Various types of biologically-active substances, including antigens, can be incorporated into liposomes by encapsulation, surface absorption or covalent linkage. Both humoral and cell-mediated responses can be induced by antigen incorporated into liposomes.

Biodegradable polymer particles can be designed to serve as a method for controlled release of vaccines by trapping antigen in solution in the cavity formed by the polymeric membrane or by dispersing antigen throughout the polymeric matrix. A compound composed of copolymers of polylactide/polyglycolide, which has been used for many years as a biodegradable suture material, has been used for antigen delivery. This compound, which is non-reactive in tissues, is degraded by hydrolysis. Biodegradable microparticles can induce effective cell-mediated immunity in addition to antibody formation.

Cytokines

Many cytokines can act as effective vaccine adjuvants, especially if administered repeatedly. The cytokines with the greatest potential are those given as a single dose, close to the time of vaccine administration. They include interferon-alpha, interferon-gamma, interleukin-1, interleukin-2 and interleukin-12.

Concluding comments

An integrated outline of the principal cells and secretions which collectively constitute non-specific immunity and specific immunity is illustrated in Fig. 84.14. The two branches of immunity are mutually complementary and provide an effective defence against many pathogenic microorganisms. The immune system has the capacity to respond to a vast array of antigenic determinants present on infectious agents and on non-infectious material such as foreign protein, pollens and cells from other animals. This ability to produce antibodies or cell-mediated responses to foreign antigenic material does not necessarily correlate with the development of protective immunity. Many antigenic substances encountered by animals are non-infectious and some responses, such as those produced in response to the secretions of biting insects may lead to the development of allergic reactions. In addition, many of the antigenic determinants on infectious agents are not directly involved in disease production and, accordingly, do not induce protective immune responses.

An animal's genome influences and may sometimes determine susceptibility to infectious agents. Because of the complexity of host-pathogen interactions, however, it is often difficult to assess accurately the contribution that genetic factors make to resistance against many infectious agents. Observed variation in innate resistance to particular pathogens may be related to the virulence of the pathogens, route of entry into the host, size of the infecting dose and resistance of the agents to host defences.

At extremes of age, inadequate body defences may be unable to halt tissue invasion by pathogenic microorganisms. In domestic animals, maternally-derived passive immunity offers temporary protection to the offspring against opportunistic invasion by environmental pathogens to which the dam has been exposed. Without colostral protection, neonatal animals are at particular risk of acquiring enteric and respiratory infections. As animals approach the end of their normal life span, their tissues again become vulnerable to invasion by opportunistic pathogens reflecting the decline in immunological competence which results from thymic atrophy and reduced lymphoid activity.

References

Edelman, R. (1997). Adjuvants for the future. In *New Generation Vaccines*, Second Edition. Eds. M.M. Levine, G.C. Woodrow, J.B. Kaper and G.S. Cobon. Marcel Dekker Inc., New York. pp. 173–192.

Law, S.K.A. and Reid, K.B. (1995). *Complement*. IRL Press, Oxford.

Mackowiak, M., Maki, J., Motes-Kreimeyer, L., Harbin, T. and Van Kampen, K. (1999). Vaccination of wildlife against rabies: successful use of a vectored vaccine obtained by recombinant technology. In *Advances in Veterinary Medicine*, **41**. *Veterinary Vaccines and Diagnostics*. Ed. R.D. Schultz. Academic Press, San Diego. pp. 571–583.

Mollinedo, F., Borregaard, N. and Laurence, A.B. (1999). Novel trends in neutrophil structure. *Immunology Today*, **20**, 535–537.

Prodinger, W.M., Würzner, R., Erdei, A. and Dierich, M.P. (1999). Complement. In *Fundamental Immunology*. Fourth Edition. Ed. W.E. Paul. Lippincott-Raven, Philadelphia. pp. 967–995.

Ramshaw, I.A. and Ramsay, A.J. (2000). The prime-boost strategy: exciting prospects for improved vaccination. *Immunology Today*, **21**, 163–165.

Ricks, C.A., Avakian, A., Bryan, T. *et al.* (1999). *In ovo* vaccination technology. In *Advances in Veterinary Medicine*, **41**. *Veterinary Vaccines and Diagnostics*. Ed. R.D. Schultz. Academic Press, San Diego. pp. 495–515.

Sheppard, M. (1999). Viral vectors for veterinary vaccines. In *Advances in Veterinary Medicine*, **41**. *Veterinary Vaccines and Diagnostics*. Ed. R.D. Schultz. Academic Press, San Diego. pp. 145–161.

Yancey, R.J. (1999). Vaccines and diagnostic methods for bovine mastitis: fact and fiction. In *Advances in Veterinary Medicine*, **41**. *Veterinary Vaccines and Diagnostics*. Ed. R.D. Schultz. Academic Press, San Diego. pp. 257–273.

Further reading

Benjamini, E., Coico, R. and Sunshine, G. (2000). *Immunology A Short Course*. Fourth Edition. Wiley-Liss, New York.

Pastoret, P.-P., Blancou, J., Vannier, P. and Verschueren, C. (1997). *Veterinary Vaccinology*. Elsevier, Amsterdam.

Schaechter, M., Engleberg, N.C., Eisenstein, B.I. and Medoff, G. (1998). *Mechanisms of Microbial Disease*. Williams and Wilkins, Baltimore.

Tighe, H., Corr, M., Roman, M. and Raz, E. (1998). Gene vaccination: plasmid DNA is more than just a blueprint. *Immunology Today*, **19**, 89–97.

Tizard, I.R. (2000). *Veterinary Immunology*. Sixth Edition. W.B. Saunders Company, Philadelphia.

Index

All numbers refer to page numbers. Those in **bold** refer to major entries.